FUNDAMENTALS
OF UROLOGY

JACK LAPIDES, M.D.

Professor of Surgery and Head
Section of Urology
University of Michigan Medical Center

1976   W. B. SAUNDERS COMPANY
Philadelphia, London, Toronto

W. B. Saunders Company: West Washington Square
Philadelphia, PA 19105

1 St. Anne's Road
Eastbourne, East Sussex BN21 3UN, England

833 Oxford Street
Toronto, Ontario M8Z 5T9, Canada

Library of Congress Cataloging in Publication Data

Main entry under title:

Fundamentals of urology.

Based on the 4th rev. ed. of Fundamentals of urology by
R. M. Nesbit, J. Lapides, and W. C. Baum.

1. Urology.   I. Lapides, Jack, 1914–   II. Nesbit, Reed
Miller, 1898–   Fundamentals of urology. [DNLM:
1. Urologic diseases. WJ100 L313f]

RC871.F83   616.6   75–12490

ISBN 0–7216–5629–3

Fundamentals of Urology   ISBN 0-7216-5629-3

Last digit is the print number: 9   8   7   6   5   4   3   2   1

DEDICATION

Dedicated to Reed M. Nesbit, a distinguished
teacher, ardent investigator, superb surgeon,
and great human being.

CONTRIBUTORS

ROBERT E. ANDERSON, M.D.

Male Infertility
Clinical Instructor, Department of Internal Medicine and Department of Surgery, Section of Urology, University of Michigan Medical School, Ann Arbor, Michigan.

WILLIAM C. BAUM, M.D., M.S.

Physiology of the Male Genital System
Former Associate Professor, Department of Surgery, Section of Urology, University of Michigan Medical School, Ann Arbor; Practicing Urologist, St. Mary's Hospital, Grand Rapids, Holland City Hospital, Holland, North Ottawa Community Hospital, Grand Haven, and Zeeland Community Hospital, Zeeland, Michigan.

WILLIAM J. BUTLER, M.D., M.S.

Obstructive Uropathy—Ureterohydronephrosis
Clinical Associate Professor, Department of Surgery, Section of Urology, University of Michigan Medical School, Ann Arbor; Attending Urologist, University Hospital, Ann Arbor, and Borgess Hospital, Kalamazoo, Michigan.

C. E. CARLTON, JR., M.D.

Traumatic Lesions of the Urogenital Tract
Professor and Head of Urology, Baylor College of Medicine, Houston, Texas.

CHENG-YANG CHANG, M.D.

Genitourinary Tuberculous Infection
Former Assistant Professor, Department of Surgery, Section of Urology, University of Michigan Medical School, Ann Arbor; Attending Urologist, McLaren General Hospital, Hurley Medical Center, and Genesee Memorial Hospital, Flint, Michigan.

ANANIAS C. DIOKNO, M.D.

Urine Transport, Storage, and Micturition
Assistant Professor, Department of Surgery, Section of Urology, University of Michigan Medical School; Staff Urologist, University

v

Hospital, Ann Arbor, and Wayne County General Hospital, Eloise, Michigan.

PAUL W. GIKAS, M.D.

Uropathology
Professor, Department of Pathology, University of Michigan Medical School; Staff Pathologist, University Hospital and Veterans Administration Hospital, Ann Arbor, Michigan.

KARL R. HERWIG, M.D.

Gonorrhea, Adrenal Gland
Associate Professor, Department of Surgery, Section of Urology, University of Michigan Medical School; Staff Urologist, University Hospital and Veterans Administration Hospital, Ann Arbor, Michigan.

WILLIAM HYNDMAN, M.D., FRCS[C]

Congenital Anomalies of the Genitourinary Tract
Assistant Professor, Division of Surgery and Pediatrics, University of Calgary; Staff Urologist, Holy Cross Hospital, Foothills General Hospital, and Alberta Children's Hospital, Calgary, Alberta, Canada.

ROBERT D. JOHNSON, M.D.

Calculus Disease
Professor, Department of Internal Medicine, Division of Endocrinology and Metabolism, University of Michigan Medical School, Ann Arbor, Michigan.

LESTER KARAFIN, M.D.

Obstructive Uropathy—Prostatism
Professor of Urology and Head, Section of Urology, Medical College of Pennsylvania; Clinical Professor of Urology, Temple University School of Medicine, Philadelphia, Pennsylvania.

A. RICHARD KENDALL, M.D.

Obstructive Uropathy—Prostatism
Professor and Chairman, Department of Urology, Temple University School of Medicine; Professor of Urology, Medical College of Pennsylvania; Consulting Urologist, St. Christopher's Hospital for Children, Philadelphia, Pennsylvania.

JOHN W. KONNAK, M.D.

Normal and Abnormal Renal Function, Renal Transplantation
Associate Professor, Department of Surgery, Section of Urology, University of Michigan Medical School; Staff Urologist, University Hospital, Veterans Administration Hospital, Ann Arbor, and Wayne County General Hospital, Eloise, Michigan.

JACK LAPIDES, M.D., M.A.

Normal and Abnormal Renal Function; Urine Transport, Storage, and Micturition; Urinary Infection
Professor, Department of Surgery, and Head, Section of Urology, University of Michigan Medical School and University Hospital, Ann Arbor, Michigan.

HAROLD E. MARDEN, JR., M.D.

Neoplasms of the Genitourinary System
Associate Professor of Surgery, Division of Urology, Albany Medical College; Urologist-in-Chief, Child's Hospital; Urologist, Albany Medical Center Hospital; Consulting Urologist, Veterans Administration Hospital, Albany, New York.

WILLIAM S. OBERHEIM, M.D.

Neoplasms of the Genitourinary System
Assistant Professor of Surgery, Division of Urology, Albany Medical College; Urologist, Albany Medical Center Hospital and St. Peter's Hospital; Consulting Urologist, Veterans Administration Hospital, Albany, New York.

RUSSELL SCOTT, JR., M.D.

Traumatic Lesions of the Urogenital Tract
Professor of Urology, Baylor College of Medicine, Houston, Texas.

RALPH A. STRAFFON, M.D.

Renovascular Hypertension
Head, Department of Urology, Cleveland Clinic Foundation, Cleveland, Ohio.

JOHN R. THORNBURY, M.D.

Uroradiology
Professor, Department of Radiology, University of Michigan Medical School; Uroradiologist, University Hospital, Ann Arbor, Michigan.

JEREMIAH G. TURCOTTE, M.D.

Renal Transplantation
Professor and Chairman, Department of Surgery, University of Michigan Medical School; Surgeon, University Hospital, Veterans Administration Hospital, Ann Arbor; Surgeon, Wayne County General Hospital, Eloise, Michigan.

RUSSELL T. WOODBURNE, Ph.D.

Anatomy of the Excretory Tract
Professor Emeritus of Anatomy, University of Michigan Medical School, Ann Arbor, Michigan.

MARVIN W. WOODRUFF, M.D.

Neoplasms of the Genitourinary System
Professor of Surgery and Director, Division of Urology, Albany Medical College; Associate Director, New York State Kidney Disease Institute, Albany; Urologist-in-Chief, Albany Medical Center Hospital; Consulting Urologist, Veterans Administration Hospital, Memorial Hospital, and Child's Hospital, Albany, New York.

ANDREW J. ZWEIFLER, M.D.

Medical Management of the Hypertensive Patient
Professor, Department of Internal Medicine, University of Michigan Medical School; Chief, Hypertension Clinic of the Hypertension Service, University Hospital, Ann Arbor, Michigan.

PREFACE

In 1942 Dr. Reed M. Nesbit published the first edition of a text entitled *Fundamentals of Urology,* written entirely by him with the express purpose of providing the third year students at the University of Michigan Medical School with a comprehensive survey of the principles of urology. His effort was eminently successful as measured by the acceptance of the paperback book not only at Michigan but at many teaching centers throughout the nation, and by residents and men in practice in addition to medical students. In fact, so much of the material was timeless that, to this very day, 23 years after the fourth and final edition, requests are still being received for copies of his outstanding work.

Because the volume has been so durable, some of Dr. Nesbit's "boys and grandboys" decided to dust off the work, make a few changes, add the important advances made in urology during the past score of years, and publish it. An effort has been made to retain the flavor of the original writing in all of its aspects. Unfortunately, knowledge has expanded to such a degree through the years that some of the facets of the original work, e.g., brevity and the number of contributors, required alteration.

The present contributing authors are dedicated teachers who continue to impart knowledge in a fashion common to all good mentors. We have had the extreme good fortune of being able to call upon colleagues in the basic and clinical sciences who have special interests in genitourinary matter to write the sections on anatomy, pathology, radiology, calculus disease, and fertility.

As in the original text, basic principles are emphasized and delineated in a manner to aid the student in solving clinical problems. A considerable amount of discussion has been devoted to lower urinary tract physiology and pathology since it is believed that most upper urinary tract disease is secondary to structural and functional abnormalities of the bladder, urethra, and prostate.

The present text represents a considerable amount of time and effort given ungrudgingly and cheerfully by the authors, the Saunders' editor Brian Decker, and my secretary Anita Lavin; I am deeply grateful to them.

JACK LAPIDES, M.D.

CONTENTS

Chapter Sixteen

ADRENAL GLAND 445

Karl R. Herwig

Chapter Seventeen

RENOVASCULAR HYPERTENSION 466

Ralph A. Straffon

Chapter Eighteen

MEDICAL MANAGEMENT OF THE HYPERTENSIVE PATIENT............ 491

Andrew J. Zweifler

Chapter Nineteen

RENAL TRANSPLANTATION 503

John W. Konnak and Jeremiah G. Turcotte

Chapter Twenty

MALE INFERTILITY 521

Robert Anderson

Chapter One

ANATOMY
OF THE
EXCRETORY TRACT

Russell T. Woodburne

KIDNEYS

The kidneys lie paravertebrally at lower thoracic and upper lumbar levels. The right kidney may be slightly lower than the left. Their posterior relationships are to the diaphragm over the upper one-third of their surfaces and to the psoas major muscle medially, then to the quadratus lumborum, and, most laterally, to the transversus abdominis muscle over the lower two-thirds of their surfaces. Their anterior relationships differ on the two sides and are to the upper abdominal viscera generally. Both kidneys are capped superomedially by the suprarenal glands. The kidneys measure from 10 to 12 cm in length and from 5 to 6 cm in width and are about 3 cm thick. (See Figs. 1–1, 1–2, 1–3, 1–21.)

The retroperitoneal kidneys are embedded in a thick mass of adipose and fibrous connective tissue derived from the layer of extraperitoneal connective tissue and fat. Thus, fat lies over and around the kidney, as a fatty capsule (perirenal fat) and external to the renal fascia, as pararenal fat. The *renal fascia*, formed from the connective tissue component of extraperitoneal connective tissue, surrounds both the kidney and the suprarenal gland, but a thin extension runs between the glands to form separate renal and suprarenal compartments. The renal fascia provides anterior and posterior laminae, which unite laterally and medially, except where they are in relation to the renal artery and vein. Here the laminae continue across the vertebral column anterior and posterior to the aorta and inferior vena cava, but adhere so closely to the adventitia of the vessels that no communication exists from one kidney compartment to the other. Inferomedially a delicate extension of the renal fascia is prolonged along the ureter as periureteric fascia.

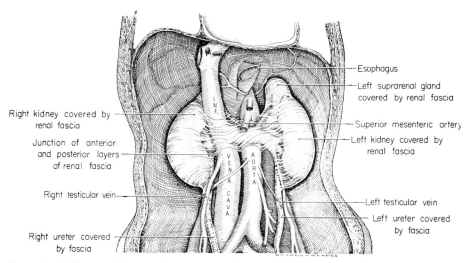

Figure 1–1   The renal fascia and its extensions. (From Hayes, M. A.: Abdominopelvic fasciae. Am. J. Anat., 87:119–161, 1950. Copyright by The Wistar Press. Reprinted by permission.)

The *renal arteries* arise at the level of the upper border of the second lumbar vertebra and about 1 cm below the superior mesenteric artery. Passing directly laterally to the hilum of the kidney, the right renal artery passes behind the inferior vena cava, the head of the pancreas, and the second part of the duodenum. The left renal artery, usually a little higher than the right, lies behind the left renal vein, the pancreas, and the splenic vein. At the hilum of the kidney, renal arteries and veins break up into branches which enter the sinus of the kidney both anterior and posterior to the renal pelvis. (Interlobar arteries derived from the anterior branches are somewhat larger, and their distribution therefore goes somewhat past the midcoronal plane of the kidney.) Each renal artery provides an inferior suprarenal artery and a ureteric branch. Accessory renal arteries are frequent (23 per cent of cases) and tend to pass directly from the aorta to the surface of the kidney and frequently to its inferior pole. These lower pole accessory vessels cross the ureter and may cause back pressure in the ureter leading to hydronephrosis.

It has been found that branches of the anterior and posterior renal arteries demarcate constant *vascular renal segments*. (See Fig. 1–2.) The anterior artery (or arteries) branches separately to an apical, an upper anterior, a middle anterior, and a lower segment of the kidney, while the posterior artery distributes to a posterior segment that represents parenchyma opposite the upper and middle anterior segments. Apical and lower segments are through and through portions. There are no intrarenal anastomoses between these vascular segments. It is to be noted that accessory renal arteries are always found to be normal segmental arteries with usually a more proximal (renal artery or aorta) origin.

In section (Fig. 1–2) the kidney exhibits *cortical and medullary*

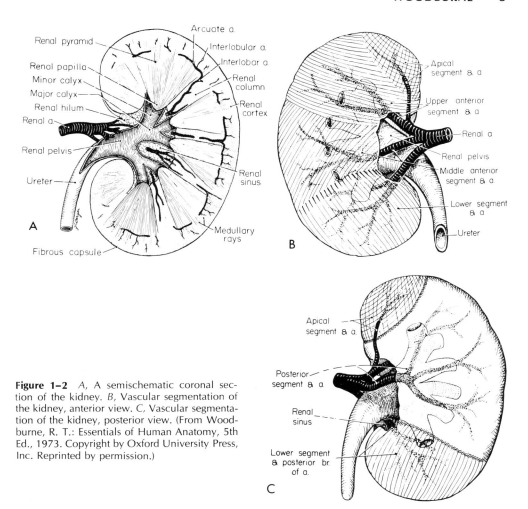

Figure 1–2 *A,* A semischematic coronal section of the kidney. *B,* Vascular segmentation of the kidney, anterior view. *C,* Vascular segmentation of the kidney, posterior view. (From Woodburne, R. T.: Essentials of Human Anatomy, 5th Ed., 1973. Copyright by Oxford University Press, Inc. Reprinted by permission.)

portions related respectively to relative concentrations of renal glomeruli and more vertically oriented tubular and collecting duct portions. However, both zones contain the various parts of the nephron in a mixture. Thus, the *pars radiata* of the cortex is due to radiating tubules, and the *renal columns* are glomerular concentrations extending deeply toward the renal sinus between the *medullary pyramids* of the medulla. Traversing each renal column is an interlobar artery; its name is a reflection of the lobar character of a single medullary pyramid and the cortical tissue on all sides of it.

The unit of renal structure is the tubular nephron, of which there are over a million in each human kidney. The *nephron* begins in a double-walled cup, the glomerular capsule, which encloses a capillary tuft, the glomerulus. The glomerular capsule leads into a proximal convoluted tubule. After several turns, this tubule runs toward the medulla of the kidney; it has a total length of about 14 mm. It tapers abruptly into the thin-walled straight tubule, or descending limb of Henle's loop. The straight tubule may be 20 mm long or quite short. It in turn passes into the ascending limb and then into the distal convoluted tubule. The distal tubule ends in a collecting duct which, joining many other collecting tributaries, is directed toward the hilum of the kidney where it ends on the surface of a pyramidal eminence, the *renal papilla.* Just before its entry into the glomerular capsule, the afferent arteriole of the glomerulus exhibits a differentiated region, the juxtaglomerular apparatus. The cells of the media here exhibit granules instead of myofibrils, and the nuclei of these cells are rounded, not elongated. Adjacent to the juxtaglomerular complex a knuckle of the distal convoluted tubule inserts itself between the afferent and efferent arterioles and is modified as the *macula densa.* Its wall is thickened and heavily nucleated and lies against the glomerular root. This very brief enumeration of the principal components of the nephron is merely introductory to the finer detail which must be considered in relation to the histophysiology of the kidney (pp. 166–189).

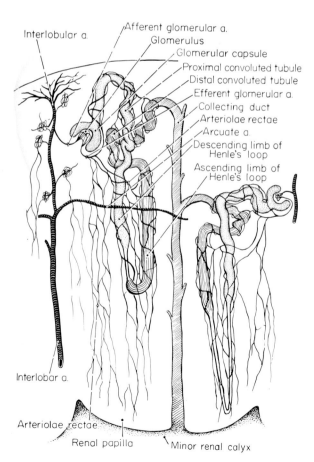

Figure 1–3 The kidney tubule — its parts and vascular relations. (From Woodburne, R. T.: Essentials of Human Anatomy, 5th Ed., 1973. Copyright by Oxford University Press, Inc. Reprinted by permission.)

The *renal papillae*, on which open the collecting ducts of the kidney, are usually received into eight cup-shaped *minor calyces*, several papillae into one calyx at times. Recognized as the first element in the duct system of the kidney, the minor calyces empty into two or three larger *major calyces*, draining the superior, middle, and inferior portions of the kidney. Still within the renal sinus, the major calyces converge to a common chamber, the *renal pelvis*, which in turn narrows extrarenally to become the *ureter*. The epithelium of the large collecting ducts is continuous with that of the calyces, and the connective tissue capsule of the kidney turns in to line the renal sinus and become continuous with the connective tissue outer wall of the calyces. A muscular wall characterizes the calyces, pelvis, and ureter, providing for peristaltic action in the duct system.

Doubling of the ureter is an occasional developmental anomaly (3 per cent). Embryologically, it appears to be due to a very early division of the primary renal pelvis with a subsequent extension of this division inferiorly. The division may stop somewhere short of the bladder, producing a Y-shaped ureter, or it may be complete. When two complete ureters occur on one side, the one arising from the superior renal pelvis terminates in the bladder in an orifice which is lower than that in which the ureter arising from the inferior pelvis terminates.

PELVIC KIDNEY; HORSESHOE KIDNEY

The kidneys develop in the pelvis with subsequent apparent migration to the upper lumbar levels. Occasionally the migrational change is aborted or abbreviated, and the kidney may then be found in the pelvis, at the sacral promontory, or at some level below the normal. Such kidneys are apt to be misshapen and to receive their blood supply from the iliac vessels or lower aorta. Horseshoe kidneys are characterized by a fusion across the midline of the lower poles of the primordia of the two sides. The two organs are unrotated, their hila are directed forward, and their ureters lie anteriorly across their lower portions. Their arteries are derived from iliac vessels or the lower aorta, and the inferior mesenteric artery frequently descends across their interconnecting band as though the upward migration of the organ had been prevented by the obstructing presence of that vessel.

URETER

The ureter is a thick-walled muscular tube with a much folded mucosal lining of transitional epithelium. It continues from the renal pelvis to the ureterovesical junction and has a length of about 25 cm. The ureter lies in the extraperitoneal connective tissue of the abdomen, within a sheath of periureteric fascia prolonged downward along it from the renal fascia. Closely adherent to the overlying peritoneum, the ureter is crossed by the testicular or ovarian vessels, on the left by the left colic vessels, and on the right by the right colic and ileocolic vessels. (See Figs. 1–1, 1–4, 1–5, and 1–17.)

The ureters descend on the psoas muscles, until, crossing the bifurcation of the common iliac arteries or the commencement of the external iliac arteries, they enter the pelvis. The pelvic one half of the ureter descends retroperitoneally on the side of the pelvic wall, curving forward and medialward. Medially crossing the obturator nerve and vessels and the umbilical artery, the ureter inclines toward the posterolateral aspect of the bladder in front of the upper end of the seminal vesicle. Here the ductus deferens passes downward over the fundus of the bladder, crossing the termination of the ureter. The end of the ureter is surrounded by the vesical plexus of veins. At the ureterovesical junction, the ureter runs obliquely through the wall of the bladder over a distance of about 1.5 cm.

Two laminae of smooth muscle generally characterize the ureteric wall. These have been designated internal longitudinal and external circular, but in truth, the fascicles run obliquely and blend into one another, giving a meshlike character to the total thickness. Terminally the musculature of the ureter becomes primarily longitudinal, is finely fasciculated, and is intermingled with connective tissue. It is in this state that it penetrates the wall of the bladder.

A somewhat confusing muscular relationship exists as the ureter meets the bladder. Here coarse detrusor fascicles from the bladder wall reflect onto the terminal ureter, mounting as much as 3 cm up that tube. These coarse fascicles, connected by scanty connective tissue, hold the ureter to the bladder but are not ureteric muscle. They are designated in the urologic literature as Waldeyer's sheath.

The ureter is arterialized by means of one or several vessels which run longitudinally on the tube. Since this long tube runs through several territories, however, vessels feed into these longitudinal vessels at several sites. The number of such vessels varies from three to nine, with an average of five. There is usually a renal artery contribution at the level of the renal pelvis followed sometimes by a branch from the testicular or ovarian artery. The aorta (bifurcation level) and common iliac arteries frequently provide ureteric branches. The pelvic portion of the ureter frequently receives a branch from the internal iliac artery, and lower down there may be ureteric branches of the superior and inferior vesical arteries, the umbilical artery, and, in the female, the uterine artery. Branches of the longitudinal ureteric arteries form anastomosing offsets which encircle and penetrate the ureteric wall along its length.

The ureter propels jets of urine in a manner similar to peristalsis. The lumen is almost totally closed between intervals of passage, and at such times the mucous membrane is infolded on itself, frequently forming the cross-sectional appearance of a five-pointed star. As the lumen opens, spaces develop between the sides of the star, and the opening proceeds to a squarish lumen and then to a circular one at full distention. In a typical experiment the collapsed lumen had a cross-sectional area of 0.12 mm^2 and it enlarged to 2 mm^2 in diuresis. This 17-fold en-

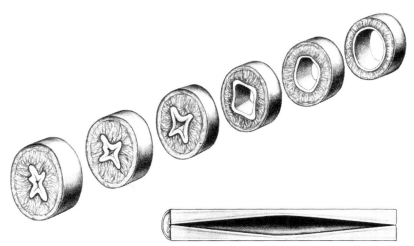

Figure 1–4 Successive blocks of tissue to illustrate luminal change in the ureter. (From Woodburne, R. T., and Lapides, J.: The ureteral lumen during peristalsis. Am. J. Anat. *133*:255–258, 1972. Copyright by The Wistar Press. Reprinted by permission.)

largement of the lumen occurred over a 3 cm length of the peristaltic wave. There was relatively little gross enlargement of the segment, increase of luminal size being largely accommodated by thinning of the muscle coats and attenuation of the mucous membrane.

URINARY BLADDER

The urinary bladder is the reservoir for the urinary system. It occupies the anterior half of the pelvis, bounded in front and at the sides by the symphysis pubis and the diverging walls of the pelvis and behind by the rectovesical septum. Flattened superiorly when empty, it becomes globular as urine fills it, and it has a capacity of about 500 ml of urine. The superior surface and the uppermost one or two centimeters of the posterior aspect of the bladder are covered by peritoneum, which sweeps off the bladder into the rectovesical (or vesicouterine) pouch. Inferiorly, the bladder rests on and is firmly attached to the base of the prostate in the male; in the female it lies on the pelvic diaphragm. The bladder is enveloped in endopelvic fascia. Sweeping from the neck of the bladder and the base of the prostate, a sheet of this fascia attaches to the parietal fascia on the back of the pubis and to the superior fascia of the pelvic diaphragm. This is the puboprostatic ligament or lateral true ligament of the bladder. It is the pubovesical (pubourethral) ligament in the female. Lying posteriorly and inferiorly, the seminal vesicles and the ampulla of the ductus deferens are embedded in endopelvic fascia against the fundus of the bladder. In the female the fundus is loosely attached to the anterior wall of the vagina. (See Figs. 1–5 to 1–12; 1–17, and 1–22.)

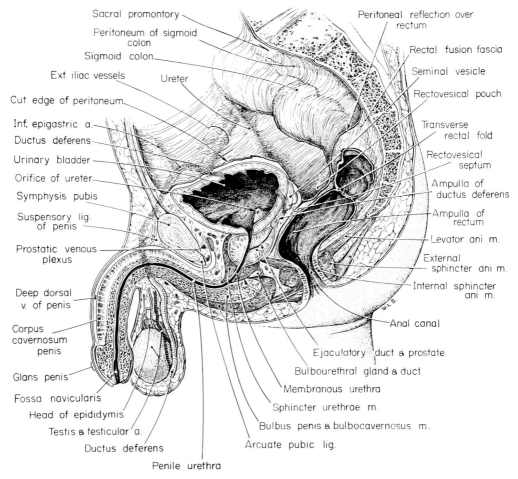

Sacral promontory

Peritoneum of sigmoid colon

Sigmoid colon

Ext. iliac vessels

Ureter

Cut edge of peritoneum

Inf. epigastric a.

Ductus deferens

Urinary bladder

Orifice of ureter

Symphysis pubis

Suspensory lig. of penis

Prostatic venous plexus

Deep dorsal v. of penis

Corpus cavernosum penis

Glans penis

Fossa navicularis

Head of epididymis

Testis & testicular a.

Ductus deferens

Penile urethra

Peritoneal reflection over rectum

Rectal fusion fascia

Seminal vesicle

Rectovesical pouch

Transverse rectal fold

Rectovesical septum

Ampulla of ductus deferens

Ampulla of rectum

Levator ani m.

External sphincter ani m.

Internal sphincter ani m.

Anal canal

Ejaculatory duct & prostate

Bulbourethral gland & duct

Membranous urethra

Sphincter urethrae m.

Bulbus penis & bulbocavernosus m.

Arcuate pubic lig.

Figure 1–5 A median section of the male pelvis. (From Woodburne, R. T.: Essentials of Human Anatomy, 5th Ed., 1973. Copyright by Oxford University Press, Inc. Reprinted by permission.)

Traditionally the bladder wall has been described as consisting of three muscular layers: outer longitudinal, middle circular, and inner longitudinal. All close analyses of the muscular arrangements have denied such a rigid schema, for the coarse detrusor fascicles do not run in continuous planes, but crisscross and decussate and change direction and level so that there is a meshwork character to the muscular wall. Nevertheless, the inner layer of musculature shows a tendency to longitudinal convergence on the urethral aperture and much of it is continuous with the internal longitudinal musculature of the urethral wall. Observation of the external aspect of the bladder shows much longitudinal and oblique musculature but with areas of interposed transverse fascicles and with the turning in of many bundles of muscle fibers to become continuous with bundles of differing orientation. A rather

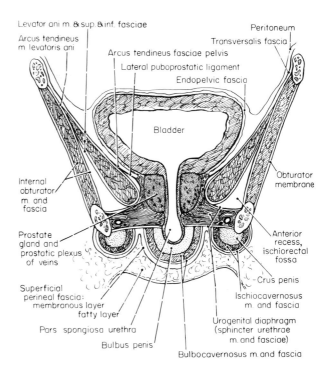

Figure 1–6 A semischematic frontal section of the pelvis and perineum through the bladder and prostate gland. (From Woodburne, R. T.: Essentials of Human Anatomy, 5th Ed., 1973. Copyright by Oxford University Press, Inc. Reprinted by permission.)

prominent longitudinal band on the posterior wall of the bladder thickens toward the prostate and divides, diverging around the neck of the bladder and the base of the prostate, and its fibers appear to end in the stroma of the prostate laterally and anteriorly.

Though an internal sphincter has been credited to the bladder neck, no annular sphincter has ever been described. Instead, certain

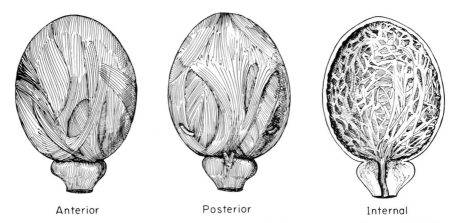

Anterior   Posterior   Internal

Figure 1–7 The muscular fasciculation of the human bladder. (From Woodburne, R. T.: The sphincter mechanism of the urinary bladder and the urethra. Anat. Rec., *141*:11–20, 1961. Copyright by the Wistar Press. Reprinted by permission.)

arching bundles have been considered to form opposing loops of detrusor muscle capable of constricting the urethral aperture between them. The divergence of the posterior detrusor bundles described above has been ascribed such a looping function. Another observable bundle lies transversely across the anterior vesical neck region, and curving backward, sprays out posterolateral to the aperture. This bundle (of Heiss) is archiform in character.

The pubovesical muscle is another derivative of the external muscular coat, this time of the anteroinferior surface of the neck of the bladder. Such bundles peel off the superficial sheet mainly to form bilaterally symmetric slips that descend external to the prostate and sphincter urethrae muscle in the male or to the sphincter urethrae muscle in the female. The muscle fibers terminate in the retropubic connective tissue and thereby gain traction on the pubis. The descending character and inferior attachments of both the pubovesical muscles and the posterior detrusor bundles suggest downward traction on the bladder as bladder contraction takes place. The bundle of Heiss, likewise, may be thought of as drawing the bladder fundus downward and forward.

The *ureterovesical junction* and the *trigone region* are special and related areas of the urinary bladder. The ureters penetrate the bladder wall just lateral to the posterior strip of longitudinal detrusor muscle. In this penetration the superficial fascicles of the detrusor medial to the ureter are elevated, and fascicles both medial and lateral to it are forced aside. Medially the ureter penetrates under the deeper layers of muscle and so traverses the wall of the bladder, lying intramurally for about 5 mm. Internal detrusor bundles arch over the ureter as it bulges internally. It then runs submucosally about 1 cm to its aperture.

As the ureters approach the bladder wall, detrusor fascicles reflect onto them over their terminal 2 to 3 cm, such fibers gaining attachment into the adventitia of the ureteric wall. Contrary to certain statements in

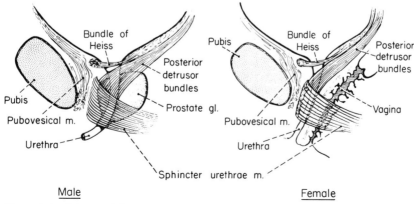

Figure 1–8 Scheme of the principal muscular relations of the bladder neck and urethra. (From Woodburne, R. T.: Anatomy of the bladder and bladder outlet. J. Urol., *100*:474–487, 1968. Copyright by Williams and Wilkins Co. Reprinted by permission.)

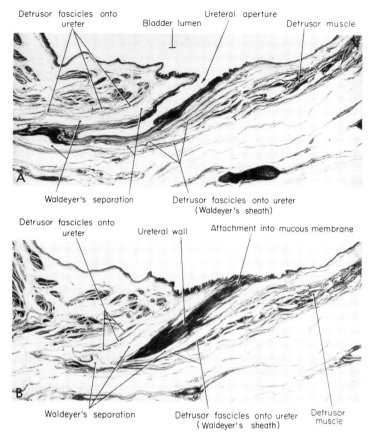

Detrusor fascicles onto ureter — Ureteral aperture — Bladder lumen — Detrusor muscle

A

Waldeyer's separation — Detrusor fascicles onto ureter (Waldeyer's sheath)

Detrusor fascicles onto ureter — Ureteral wall — Attachment into mucous membrane

B

Waldeyer's separation — Detrusor fascicles onto ureter (Waldeyer's sheath) — Detrusor muscle

Figure 1–9   *A*, Section longitudinal to the intramural ureter. *B*, Section through long axis of terminal ureter. Human. (From Woodburne, R. T.: Anatomy of the ureterovesical junction. J. Urol., 92:431–435, 1964. Copyright by Williams and Wilkins Co. Reprinted by permission.)

the literature, they do not represent ureteric musculature but are clearly detrusor in nature. They are not closely applied, a small separation (Waldeyer) existing between the detrusor fascicles and the ureteric wall short of their termination. Coupled by these fascicles, the ureter penetrates loosely through the wall of the bladder; there is no close fibrous or muscular investment of the terminal ureter.

The ureteric aperture is slitlike and makes an extremity of the ureteric triangle within the bladder. It has been noted that the ureter is represented terminally by finely fasciculated, closely connected muscular fibers. In their transit through the bladder wall, muscle fibers of the ureter progressively roll aside to become located lateral and deep to the lumen, allowing the lumen to migrate to the surface. A few fine fibers of the ureter decussate just proximal and also distal to the ureteric aperture, and the wall of the ureter becomes progressively thinner over the lumen until the lumen debouches onto the surface.

The *vesical trigone* represents the termination of the ureter. The

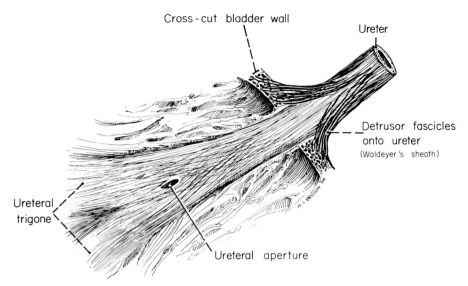

Cross-cut bladder wall

Ureter

Detrusor fascicles
onto ureter
(Waldeyer's sheath)

Ureteral
trigone

Ureteral aperture

Figure 1–10 Detail of dissection of extramural and intramural ureter. (From Woodburne, R. T.: Anatomy of the ureterovesical junction. J. Urol., 92:431–435, 1964. Copyright by Williams and Wilkins Co. Reprinted by permission.)

trigone form is produced by the blending of the continuing muscle of the ureters across the midline to form the interureteric fold plus a fanning downward toward the urethral aperture. This trigone area represents the termination of the ureter. It is quite clear in microscopic sections that the ureteric musculature attaches firmly into the mucous membrane of the trigone area, forming a thin layer of muscle internal to the true detrusor muscle of the bladder. This is the termination and attachment of the ureter. The ureter is loose as it passes through the bladder wall, but it is firmly attached in the trigone area. Contrary to statements in the early literature, its fibers do not reach the urethral aperture.

The *vesical neck* constitutes a region of some accumulation of muscle bundles of the bladder. It is the site of any bladder sphincter, if such exists. However, it is noted that no annular sphincter has ever been confirmed in the region, although components of certain looping or arching bundles exist. Maceration studies of the dog confirm that there are no annular bundles. In fact, these studies confirm arching bundles, but they appear to arch away more than they arch around the urethral aperture. The vesical neck region is also an area of great elaboration of elastic tissue. In the bladder wall generally small amounts of elastic tissue are found in the submucosa and between the muscular layers. However, as the vesical neck region is approached, the submucosal area accommodates a thick collection of elastic tissue which is also interspersed among the muscle bundles, particularly the more centrally lying longitudinally oriented muscle fascicles. This elaboration of elastic tissue continues into the urethral wall below.

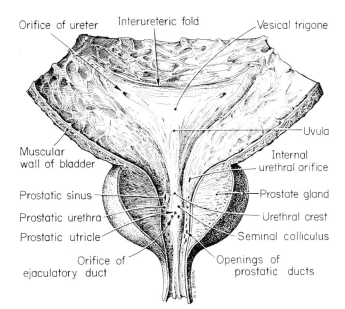

Orifice of ureter Interureteric fold Vesical trigone

Muscular wall of bladder

Uvula

Internal urethral orifice

Prostatic sinus Prostate gland

Prostatic urethra Urethral crest

Prostatic utricle Seminal colliculus

Orifice of ejaculatory duct Openings of prostatic ducts

Figure 1–11 A frontal section of the bladder and prostate gland to show the vesical trigone and prostatic urethra. (From Woodburne, R. T.: Essentials of Human Anatomy, 5th Ed., 1973. Copyright by Oxford University Press, Inc. Reprinted by permission.)

URETHRA

The posterior urethra of the male and the proximal three-fourths of the urethra of the female have certain characteristics and functions in common. As urinary passages, their epithelium is transitional, and the subepithelial mucosa is a loose tissue well supplied with thin-walled

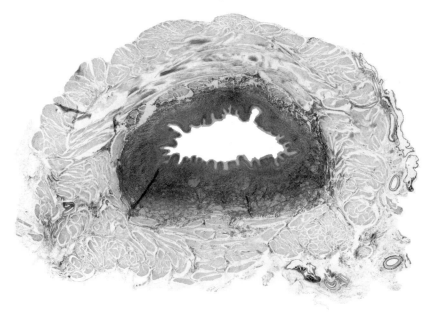

Figure 1–12 A cross section of the canine bladder neck. Elastic tissue block. Weigert stain. (From Woodburne, R. T.: Anatomy of the bladder and bladder outlet. J. Urol., *100*:474–487, 1968. Copyright by Williams and Wilkins Co. Reprinted by permission.)

mucosal veins. The principal constituent of the urethral wall is a mass of longitudinally oriented smooth muscle, a layer which is prolonged downward from the internal longitudinal layer of the bladder. Circular bundles are minimally represented in the female but form a complete layer in the male. The muscular bundles are heavily infiltrated with elastic tissue in both sexes. (See Figs. 1–5, 1–6, 1–8, 1–11, 1–13, 1–14, and 1–18.)

In the male, prostatic tissue and the sphincter urethrae muscle surround the urethra; in the female, only the sphincter urethrae muscle is present. This voluntary striated muscle, external to the prostate in the male, extends up to the neck of the bladder and down beyond the apex of the prostate. In the female its vertical extent is similar. It arches across the front of the prostate (urethra in the female) and forms a true sphincter for the male beyond the apex of the prostate. It has a shape somewhat like a chariot in the female, more open behind, with only minor sphincteric accumulations around the urethra and behind the vagina. Its general form is arching posterior and lateralward where its fibers end in the connective tissue around the internal pudendal vessels and the pudendal nerve. The muscle rests on and is limited below by the perineal membrane (inferior fascia of the urogenital diaphragm). It is capable of abrupt voluntary termination of micturition. The general relations of the male urethra and the features of its parts will be described according to region.

The female urethra is about 4 cm long and has a slightly curved

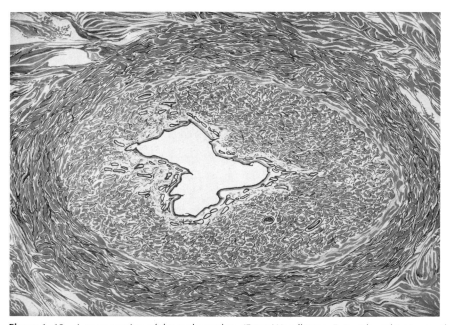

Figure 1–13   A cross section of the male urethra. (From Woodburne, R. T.: The sphincter mechanism of the urinary bladder and the urethra. Anat. Rec., *141*:11–20, 1961. Copyright by the Wistar Press. Reprinted by permission.)

course, the concavity of which is forward. Its external orifice lies about 2.5 cm behind the glans clitoridis and immediately anterior to the vaginal opening. The urethra is so intimately related to the anterior vaginal wall in its lower portion as to appear to be embedded in it. It is less closely held in its upper portion. Fixation of the urethra anteriorly is principally by the pubourethral (pubovesical) ligaments, two strong collagenous bundles that sweep off the back of the pubis and the superior fascia of the pelvic diaphragm. Investigators have also described an anterior pubourethral ligament arising as deeper fibers of the suspensory ligament of the clitoris and an intermediate sheet or ligament that extends from the posterior pubourethral ligament under the symphysis pubis to the anterior pubourethral ligament. Among the urethral glands in the female, one group opens by the *paraurethral ducts* in the vestibule at the sides of the external urethral orifice.

PENIS

Fundamentally the penis consists of three cavernous bodies surrounded by a firm fascia penis (deep fascia of penis), subcutaneous connective tissue, and skin. The skin of the penis is thin, hairless, and dark; it is only loosely connected to the deeper structures. On the ventral or urethral surface of the penis, the skin shows a median raphe continuous with the raphe of the scrotum. Along the base of the glans penis the skin forms a free fold, the prepuce (foreskin), which overlaps the glans to a variable extent. The skin of the inner surface of the prepuce is continuous with that covering the glans and resembles mucous membrane. The skin over the glans is firmly attached to the underlying erectile tissue. The frenulum of the prepuce passes as a small median fold from the deep surface of the prepuce to a point immediately below the external urethral orifice. Numerous sebaceous glands are present in the skin, especially on the urethral surface of the penis. Circumcision, or the amputation of the prepuce, a traditional rite of certain religions, is also common as a simple hygienic measure. (See Figs. 1–5 and 1–14.)

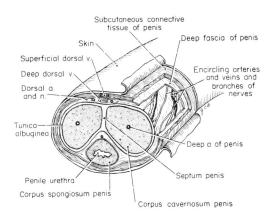

Figure 1–14 The structures of the penis as seen in a cross section of its body. (From Woodburne, R. T.: Essentials of Human Anatomy, 5th Ed., 1973. Copyright by Oxford University Press, Inc. Reprinted by permission.)

Subcutaneous connective tissue of penis

Skin

Deep fascia of penis

Superficial dorsal v.

Deep dorsal v.

Dorsal a. and n.

Encircling arteries and veins and branches of nerves

Tunica albuginea

Deep a. of penis

Penile urethra

Corpus spongiosum penis

Septum penis

Corpus cavernosum penis

The subcutaneous connective tissue of the penis is loose areolar tissue without fat but characterized by smooth muscle fibers prolonged from the tunica dartos scroti. In the dorsal midline of the penis the superficial dorsal vein passes toward the root of the penis where it communicates with the superficial external pudendal veins of the upper thigh. The superficial external pudendal veins are tributary to the greater saphenous vein of each side.

A deep fascia (fascia penis) encloses the cavernous bodies and the main vessels and nerves of the penis. It is attached distally in the groove between the shaft of the penis and the corona of the glans and extends backward over the roots of the cavernous bodies and their muscles in the superficial perineal space.

Two of the cavernous bodies of the penis, the *corpora cavernosa penis*, lie side by side on the dorsum of the penis, whereas the third, the *corpus spongiosum penis*, lies ventrally in the median plane. Distally, the penis has a conical extremity, the glans penis. The glans is formed by an expansion of the corpus spongiosum penis which fits over the blunt terminations of the corpora cavernosa penis. The corona of the glans projects backward beyond the ends of the corpora cavernosa penis. The urethra traverses the corpus spongiosum penis and opens near the summit of the glans in a slitlike opening, the external urethral orifice.

Erectile tissue is composed of a meshwork of interlacing and intercommunicating spaces lined by an endothelium directly continuous with that of the veins which drain the meshwork. Each *corpus cavernosum penis* is enclosed in a dense, white fibrous coat (tunica albuginea) that fuses with the coat of the other side at their contact to form the median septum of the penis. This septum is incomplete, so that the spaces of the two cavernous bodies communicate. The structure of the corpus spongiosum penis is generally like that of a corpus cavernosum, but the fibrous tunica albuginea is thinner and more elastic and the cavernous meshwork is finer. The glans penis is also composed of erectile tissue but does not have a strong tunica albuginea. The urethra is expanded vertically within the glans as the fossa navicularis.

At the root of the penis, the two corpora cavernosa penis diverge as the crura of the penis. Slightly swollen at first, these taper posteriorly and end just in front of the ischial tuberosity. Each crus is firmly attached to the periosteum of the medial side of the ischiopubic ramus, and each is covered by an ischiocavernosus muscle. Continuing backward in the median line, the corpus spongiosum penis becomes enlarged posteriorly to form the bulb of the penis. The bulb is firmly attached to the inferior fascia of the urogenital diaphragm (perineal membrane) through which the urethra passes to enter the bulb and traverse the corpus spongiosum. The bulb of the penis is invested by the bulbocavernosus muscle.

The root of the penis is firmly held to the underside of the pubic arch by the *suspensory ligament* of the penis. This median, triangular band of strong fibrous tissue extends from the symphysis pubis and the arcuate pubic ligament to the deep fascia of the penis. A more superficial *fundiform ligament* also serves to support the penis at its dorsal flexure.

The *bulbocavernosus and ischiocavernosus muscles* are associated with the corpus spongiosum and its bulb and with the crura of the corpora cavernosa, respectively. The muscle fibers are directly applied to these cavernous bodies, and their fiber fascicles run generally oblique to the bodies and end in their dorsal aspects and in the perineal membrane dorsal to them. They are capable of compressing the cavernous tissue.

The *deep fascia of the penis* loosely surrounds the three cavernous bodies of the penis, distally attaching at the junction of the body and the glans of the penis. The fascia encloses the dorsal artery and nerve of the penis and the deep dorsal vein. The deep fascia continues backward into the perineum, becoming the investing fascia of the bulbocavernosus and ischiocavernosus muscles and terminating with the posterior extent of these muscles. Extravasation of fluid within the chamber defined by the attachments of the deep fascia produces a fusiform swelling of the penis that extends backward into the perineum. There is no natural egress from this space.

PENILE URETHRA

The penile or cavernous portion of the urethra is its longest portion. Extending from the sphincter urethrae muscle and the perineal membrane to the external urethral orifice, it is about 15 cm long. It is of fairly uniform caliber (6 mm) but is dilated proximally in the bulb and again anteriorly in the fossa navicularis of the glans penis. A transverse slit through most of its extent, it ends in a vertical slit at the external urethral orifice. This is also its narrowest and least distensible point. (See Figs. 1–5 and 1–14.)

The lining membrane presents the orifices of numerous mucous urethral glands. Besides these there are a number of small pitlike recesses, or lacunae. Their orifices are directed distally so they may intercept the point of a catheter in its passage along the canal. An especially large lacuna, lacuna magna, is situated on the upper surface of the fossa navicularis. The *bulbourethral glands* open into the penile urethra about 2.5 cm distal to the perineal membrane.

SCROTUM

The scrotum is a cutaneous pouch, formed of bilateral contributions, which contains the testes and parts of the spermatic cords. (See Fig. 1–5.) It is developed from the skin of the abdominal wall in the region of the genital swellings. Its bilateral derivation is evident in a midline scrotal raphe which continues forward to the under surface of the penis and backward along the median line of the perineum to the anus. Internal to the raphe, the scrotal sac is divided into two chambers by the scrotal septum.

The layers of the scrotum are the skin and the tunica dartos. The skin of the scrotum in the adult exhibits scattered coarse hairs and has well developed sebaceous glands. The underlying subcutaneous connective tissue is the *tunica dartos scroti.* There is no fat in the tunica dartos, but it contains smooth muscle intermingled with its areolar tissue. This muscle is the cause of the wrinkling of the skin of the scrotum. The tunica dartos scroti has continuities with the more generalized subcutaneous areas adjacent to it. At the posterior border of the scrotum it goes over into the subcutaneous tissues of the perineum. These are characterized by a fatty external layer and a deeper membranous layer (Colles' fascia). The membranous layer has bony and membranous attachments which enclose and define the superficial space of the perineum: the inferior pubic and the ischial rami laterally and the posterior border of the perineal membrane posteriorly. A similar lamination exists in the lower portion of the abdominal wall; here the membranous layer attaches to the fascia lata of the thigh just inferior to the inguinal ligament, to the pubic tubercle, and to the pubic symphysis. It is not attached between these pubic landmarks (over the pubic crest), and this deficiency is known as the abdominoscrotal opening.

The various attachments and continuities alluded to are important for understanding the containment and spread of extravasations under Colles' fascia. Such extravasations may spread through the superficial perineal space but do not descend into the thighs; they will extend forward to fill the scrotal sac deep to tunica dartos scroti and the penis deep to tunica dartos penis. Fluid can ascend through the abdominoscrotal opening into the lower abdominal wall and will tend to accumulate in the flanks, again prevented from entering the thighs by the attachments of the membranous layer of superficial fascia.

TESTIS

The testes are paired, oval bodies which elaborate the spermatozoa. Each testis is from 4 to 5 cm in length, 3 cm in width, and about 2 cm thick and has its long axis directed upward and slightly forward and lateralward. The lateral and medial surfaces of the testis are flattened; its rounded anterior border is free, whereas its posterior border provides an attachment for the epididymis. (See Figs. 1–5, 1–15, and 1–16.)

The thick external covering of the testis is the tunica albuginea, composed of dense, white fibrous connective tissue. At the posterior border of the gland the tunica albuginea indents the substance of the testis and is broken up into the more open meshlike mediastinum testis. The latter is traversed by the major ducts of the testis and by its arteries, veins, and lymphatics. From the internal aspect of the mediastinum, numerous connective tissue septa radiate to the surface of the organ, where they blend with the tunica albuginea. The tunica vasculosa, a delicate network of vessels, is formed on the septa and on the deep surface of the tunica albuginea. In the compartments between the septa lie a large number of fine threadlike convoluted seminiferous tubules. There are estimated to be 800 or more such tubules in the testis. The convoluted tubules unite to form a smaller number of straight seminiferous tubules which enter the mediastinum testis. These anastomose in a network of epithelial-lined channels in the fibrous stroma which constitute the rete testis. At the upper end of the mediastinum the channels of the rete testis coalesce to form from 12 to 15 efferent ducts. These perforate the tunica albuginea and form convoluted masses, the lobuli epididymidis, which together constitute the head of the epididymis. The efferent ducts, each from 15 to 20 cm in length if uncoiled, open opposite the bases of the cones into a single duct which constitutes the duct of the epididymis.

The *epididymis* is a comma-shaped structure which invests the back and upper end of the testis and bulges onto its lateral surface posteriorly. The duct of the epididymis is essentially an irregularly twisted tube that has a total uncoiled length of from 15 to 20 feet and a diameter of about 1 mm. The head of the comma is represented by the head of the epididymis. The mass of coils is somewhat reduced at the back of the testis, where it is called the body of the epididymis. This portion is separated from the posterior part of the lateral surface of the testis by a recess of the visceral layer of the tunica vaginalis testis, which constitutes the sinus of the epididymis. The tail of the epididymis is the

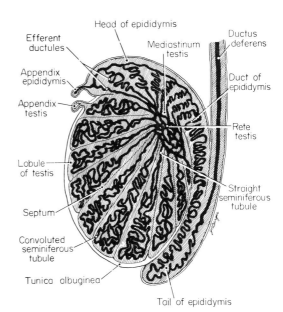

Figure 1–15 A schematic vertical section of the testis and epididymis. (From Woodburne, R. T.: Essentials of Human Anatomy, 5th Ed., 1973. Copyright by Oxford University Press, Inc. Reprinted by permission.)

smaller inferior end. It is attached to the inferior pole of the testis by loose areolar connective tissue and by the tunica vaginalis testis. In the tail portion the duct of the epididymis increases in thickness and diameter to become continuous with the ductus deferens.

On the upper extremity of the testis, usually emerging from under the head of the epididymis, is a minute oval remnant of the upper end of the paramesonephric duct; this is the appendix of the testis. On the head of the epididymis is a second small appendage, the stalked appendix of the epididymis, usually regarded as a detached efferent duct.

The *tunica vaginalis testis* is an invaginated serous sac covering most of the testis, the epididymis, and the lower end of the spermatic cord. It represents the lowermost pinched-off portion of the processus vaginalis of the peritoneum. Its visceral layer dips between the posterolateral surface of the testis and the body of the epididymis as the sinus of the epididymis. The tunica vaginalis reflects on itself to leave the posterior border of the testis uncovered; here the blood vessels and nerves of the testis enter from the spermatic cord.

DESCENT OF THE TESTIS

The testis develops in the extraperitoneal connective tissue of the upper lumbar region and remains in the abdominal cavity until nearly the end of intrauterine life. The testes form in close association with the mesonephros. As their bulk increases, the peritoneum covering them is pushed out until, at seven weeks of development, each testis is intraperitoneal and is suspended by a mesorchium. At either end the peritoneum is thrown into folds, the inferior one extending caudalward in the celomic cavity. At the same time, a peritoneal fold progresses backward from the anterolateral abdominal wall. Fibrous connective tissue of the inferior fold from the testis and the mesonephros, known as the genitoinguinal ligament, coalesces with the connective tissue of the fold from the abdominal wall to form the gubernaculum testis. The gubernaculum thus becomes a connection between the developing testis in the lumbar region and the abdominal wall at the site of the future deep inguinal ring. The fold of peritoneum superior to the testis is its vascular fold and contains its blood vessels. (See Fig. 1–16.)

Meanwhile, a celomic evagination begins in the inguinal region at the site of attachment of the gubernaculum. This peritoneal protrusion is the processus vaginalis; it pushes into the scrotal swelling, and the muscular and fascial layers of the abdominal wall are evaginated between the external skin and the internal peritoneum. As the processus vaginalis is deepened, its mouth becomes constricted. It would be incorrect to say that the gubernaculum draws the testis downward, for inequality in development and growth rates is probably fundamental to the apparent migrations of embryonic organs, but the net effect is much the same.

At the third month of fetal life the testis lies in the iliac fossa, and by the fifth month it is close to the inguinal ring. The testis begins to

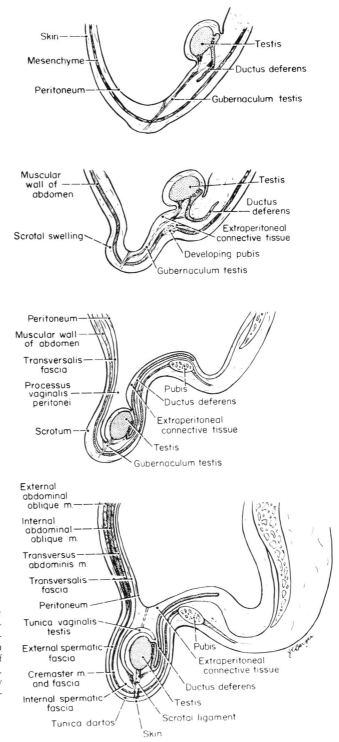

Figure 1–16 The descent of the testis and the formation of its coverings and of the scrotum, diagramed in four stages. (From Woodburne, R. T.: Essentials of Human Anatomy, 5th Ed., 1973. Copyright by Oxford University Press, Inc. Reprinted by permission.)

pass through the ring during the seventh month of gestation and ordinarily lies in the scrotum by the eighth month. The passage of the processus vaginalis into the scrotal pouch thins out and carries down the inguinal portion of each of the abdominal wall layers and accounts for the presence in the adult scrotum of their derivatives, the internal and external spermatic fasciae and the cremaster muscle and its fascial layer. The gubernaculum testis becomes much reduced in the adult, its remnant constituting the scrotal ligament, which extends from the inferior pole of the testis and the tail of the epididymis to the skin of the bottom of the scrotum.

As development nears completion, the processus vaginalis forms a thin tubular connection between the peritoneum of the abdominal cavity and that over the testis in the scrotal sac. Normally, both the abdominal and scrotal ends of this tube pinch off, and the intervening part becomes atrophied, an indistinct connective tissue remnant being all that remains. The peritoneum covering the anterior and lateral aspects of the testis then forms a closed serous sac, the tunica vaginalis testis, and only a dimple in the abdominal peritoneum remains to indicate the site of the evagination. However, the processus vaginalis is said to be open in 50 per cent of infants until a month after birth, and irregularities in its obliteration are implicated in certain forms of inguinal hernia and hydrocele. Occasionally the testis fails to descend or fails to make a complete descent. This condition is known as cryptorchidism. Abnormal descent may occur, as into the thigh or the perineum. Such testes are ectopic in position.

COVERINGS OF CORD AND TESTIS

The genital swellings of the inguinal region of the abdominal wall accommodate to the descent of the testis and form the scrotum. The muscular and fascial layers carried down by the testis are (1) the external spermatic fascia from the fascia of the external abdominal oblique muscle, (2) the cremaster muscle and fascial layer from the internal abdominal oblique muscle layer, and (3) the internal spermatic fascia from the transversalis fascia of the abdomen. (See Fig. 1–5.) Abdominal extraperitoneal connective tissue invests the ductus deferens and the arteries, veins, nerves, and lymphatics associated with the testis, and peritoneum is represented by the now pinched-off and isolated tunica vaginalis testis.

The spermatic cord itself consists of the ductus deferens, the deferential artery and vein, the testicular artery, the pampiniform plexus of veins, lymphatics, and autonomic nerves. Subsidiary to the coverings and skin are the cremasteric artery, the genital branch of the genitofemoral nerve, and the anterior scrotal branch of the ilioinguinal nerve.

DUCTUS DEFERENS

The ductus deferens begins in the tail of the epididymis as the continuation of the duct of the epididymis. (See Figs. 1–5 and 1–17.) About 45 cm in length, it ascends in the spermatic cord, traverses the inguinal canal and then, running backward and medialward, descends on the fundus of the bladder. Tortuous like the epididymis at its beginning, it straightens out behind the testis and ascends on the medial aspect of the epididymis. The ductus deferens lies in the center of the other constituents of the spermatic cord and can be identified by its hard and cordlike character when rolled between the fingers, owing to its small lumen and very thick muscular coat. It is this thick muscular layer which, by its peristaltic action, provides for delivery of the semen to the prostatic urethra. Emerging from the deep inguinal ring, the ductus deferens passes lateral to the inferior epigastric artery and ascends obliquely across the external iliac arteries. Reaching the pelvic brim, it descends between the peritoneum and the lateral wall of the pelvis medial to the obliterated umbilical artery and the obturator nerve and vessels. It then curves onto the back of the bladder, crossing to the medial side of the ureter. The ductus deferens descends on the fundus of the bladder medial to the ureter and the seminal vesicle, where it becomes dilated and tortuous in its ampullary portion. This enlarged portion narrows markedly just above the base of the prostate gland and, joined there by the duct of the seminal vesicle, forms the ejaculatory duct.

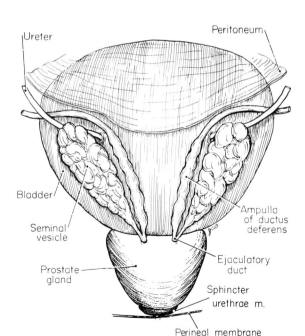

Figure 1–17 A posterior view of the urinary bladder, prostate gland, and seminal vesicle. (From Woodburne, R. T.: Essentials of Human Anatomy, 5th Ed., 1973. Copyright by Oxford University Press, Inc. Reprinted by permission.)

SEMINAL VESICLES

The seminal vesicles, each roughly the size and shape of a small finger, are lobulated "blind" pouches which secrete an alkaline constituent of the seminal fluid. (See Fig. 1–17.) They lie against the fundus of the bladder, diverging like the limbs of a V. They are enclosed by endopelvic fascia, and the ductus deferentes descend along their medial surfaces. The upper ends of the vesicles are rounded and they taper toward their lower ends. Above the base of the prostate, each vesicle is constricted to form a short duct which joins the lateral side of the narrowed ductus deferens at an acute angle. The common duct formed by this union is the ejaculatory duct. The seminal vesicles are related through the rectovesical septum to the rectum behind them. They are more intimately connected to the bladder by the rectovesical portion of the endopelvic fascia. The seminal vesicle and the ampulla of the ductus deferens are similar in structure. They are thin-walled and their mucous membranes present a honeycomb appearance.

EJACULATORY DUCTS

The ejaculatory ducts (Figs. 1–17 and 1–18) are formed just above the base of the prostate by the union of the ducts of the seminal vesicles with the narrowed ends of the ductus deferentes. About 2 cm in length, each ejaculatory duct lies almost completely within the prostate. Each duct passes downward and forward through the prostate, converging on its fellow of the opposite side. The ducts open by slitlike apertures into the prostatic urethra on the colliculus seminalis at either side of the opening of the prostatic utricle. The walls of the ejaculatory ducts are extremely thin.

PROSTATE

The prostate is an accessory gland in the seminal tract. It underlies the male bladder, resting by its apex on the pelvic diaphragm and the sphincter urethrae muscle. The ampulla of the rectum abuts it from behind with the rectovesical septum intervening. The greatest breadth of the prostate is superior in relation to the bladder; it is narrow inferiorly and thus has the shape of a blunted cone. The prostate measures about 4 cm transversely across its base; it is about 3 cm in its vertical diameter and about 2 cm in its anteroposterior diameter. Most of the base of the prostate is structurally continuous with the bladder wall. The lateral surfaces of the prostate are convex and are related to the superior fascia of the pelvic diaphragm. (See Figs. 1–8, 1–11, 1–17, and 1–18).

The urethra enters the prostate near the middle of the base of the gland and leaves it on its anterior surface immediately above the apex of the gland. The ejaculatory ducts enter at the posterior border of the base and run obliquely downward and forward to open at either side of the prostatic utricle. The gland is formed by the enlargement of the urethral glands and is developmentally divisible into two lateral lobes which surround the urethra and fuse anteriorly in an isthmus that is largely muscular. However, the wedge of prostate above the course of the ejaculatory ducts is frequently designated as its middle lobe; clinical usage also designates the portion of the prostate below the ejaculatory ducts as the posterior lobe.

A sheath for the prostate is supplied by a condensation of endopelvic fascia. The sheath is continuous with the puboprostatic ligaments, two fibrous sheets which unite the anterior and lateral surfaces of the gland with the back of the pubis and the superior fascia of the pelvic diaphragm along the arcus tendineus fasciae pelvis.

The prostate consists of a fibromuscular stroma and enclosed glandular elements. A condensation of the stroma forms the capsule of the gland from which septa pass into it, dividing it into about 50 lobules. The glandular tissue is composed of minute, slightly branched tubules which lead into from 20 to 30 prostatic ducts. Most of these empty into the prostatic sinuses at either side of the urethral crest of the posterior urethral wall. The prostate is formed from enlarged urethral glands, and its fibromuscular stroma is thus derived from the urethral wall. Its involuntary musculature is also continuous from the neck of the bladder. Peripherally the fibromuscular prostate is not sharply separable from the surrounding striated muscle fibers of the sphincter urethrae muscle.

The *prostatic portion of the urethra* is from 3 to 4 cm long and traverses the prostate in a gentle curve, the concavity of which is forward. The lumen is somewhat spindle-shaped, wider in its middle than above or below. A narrow, longitudinal ridge in the posterior wall, the urethral crest, indents the lumen, so that it is crescentic in cross section. The grooves on either side of the crest are the prostatic

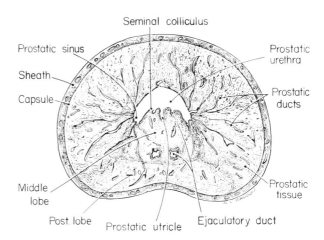

Figure 1–18 A semischematic cross section of the prostate gland. (From Woodburne, R. T.: Essentials of Human Anatomy, 5th Ed., 1973. Copyright by Oxford University Press, Inc. Reprinted by permission.)

sinuses, and it is here that most of the ducts of the prostate gland open. A minority open along the sides of the urethral crest. Beyond the midlength of the crest there is a rounded eminence, the seminal colliculus. In the median plane of the colliculus, a small slit leads into a "blind" pouch less than a centimeter in length which is directed backward and upward into the prostate; this is the prostatic utricle. It is formed from the fused ends of the paramesonephric ducts and is the male homologue of the uterus and the vagina. On each side of the mouth of the prostatic utricle there is the more minute opening of the ejaculatory duct. The urethral crest diminishes in height both above and below the seminal colliculus but may have continuity with the uvula of the bladder above. Inferiorly, it frequently divides into two inconspicuous elevations in the membranous portion of the urethra.

The *membranous portion of the urethra* merely traverses the sphincter urethrae muscle and the perineal membrane. As the shortest part of the urethra, its length is about 1 cm and it enters the sphincter urethrae muscle about 2.5 cm behind the pubic symphysis. The wall of the membranous portion is thin.

BULBOURETHRAL GLANDS

These pea-size glands are embedded in the fibers of the sphincter urethrae muscle posterolateral to the membranous urethra. Their ducts perforate the perineal membrane into the bulb of the urethra and, after a course of about 2.5 cm, open into the lumen of the bulbous urethra by minute apertures. (See Fig. 1–15.)

ARTERIES AND VEINS IN THE URINARY SYSTEM

The renal arteries and the contributions to the blood supply of the ureters have been considered. Other major vessels to the urinary system are the testicular and internal iliac arteries. (See Figs. 1–19 and 1–20.)

The long, slender *testicular arteries* arise from the anterior aspect of the abdominal aorta just below the renal arteries. They descend retroperitoneally across the psoas muscles to the deep inguinal ring, crossing the ureters in course and being crossed by various colic and sigmoid vessels. In the inguinal canal, the testicular artery is accompanied by the ductus deferens and is enmeshed by the pampiniform plexus of veins. The principal branches of the artery pierce the posterior part of the tunica albuginea of the testis and supply the gland; others supply the epididymis and ductus deferens.

The internal iliac artery is the principal artery of the pelvis and perineum. The *umbilical artery,* one of its earliest branches, provides the *superior vesical artery,* from which several branches reach the superior and lateral aspects of the bladder, and the tiny *artery of the ductus deferens* to the ductus. The *inferior vesical artery* may arise separately or in

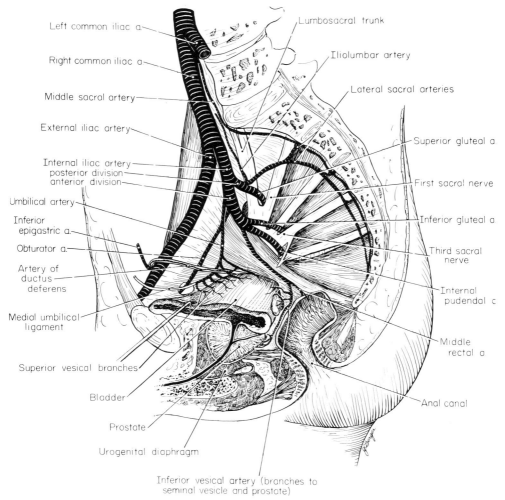

Left common iliac a.

Right common iliac a.

Middle sacral artery

External iliac artery

Internal iliac artery
posterior division
anterior division

Umbilical artery

Inferior
epigastric a.

Obturator a.

Artery of
ductus
deferens

Medial umbilical
ligament

Superior vesical branches

Bladder

Prostate

Urogenital diaphragm

Inferior vesical artery (branches to
seminal vesicle and prostate)

Lumbosacral trunk

Iliolumbar artery

Lateral sacral arteries

Superior gluteal a.

First sacral nerve

Inferior gluteal a.

Third sacral
nerve

Internal
pudendal c

Middle
rectal a

Anal canal

Figure 1–19 The common pattern of branching of the internal iliac artery. (From Woodburne, R. T.: Essentials of Human Anatomy, 5th Ed., 1973. Copyright by Oxford University Press, Inc. Reprinted by permission.)

common with the middle rectal artery. It reaches the underside of the bladder, giving branches to the fundus, the prostate, and the seminal vesicles. Its prostatic branch anastomoses within the prostatic sheath with the artery of the opposite side.

The *middle rectal artery* may be the source of the inferior vesical artery; it also has branches to the prostate and seminal vesicle.

The *internal pudendal artery*, one of the terminal branches of the internal iliac artery, is the principal artery of the perineum. Its *perineal* branch supplies the bulbocavernosus and ischiocavernosus muscles. There is also an *artery of the bulb of the penis*, a *urethral artery*, and finally the *deep artery* and the *dorsal artery of the penis*.

Veins generally accompany and are related to the same structures as the arteries. However, there is both a superficial and a deep dorsal vein of the penis. The superficial vein ends in the superficial external pudendal vein while the deep dorsal vein penetrates between the arcuate pubic ligament and the transverse ligament of the perineum to enter the prostatic plexus of veins clustered around that organ. Within the basin of the pelvis numerous intercommunicating thin-walled veins give rise to the visceral tributaries of the internal iliac vein. These include the middle rectal plexus, the vesical plexus, and the prostatic venous plexus.

LYMPHATIC DRAINAGE

Due to embryonic derivation, there is some diversity in the lymphatic drainage of the various parts of the excretory system. Within the perineum, the scrotum, penis, and other perineal structures drain their lymph to superficial inguinal lymphatic nodes. On the other hand, lymphatic flow from the testis and epididymis and the distal ductus deferens is along the route of the testicular vessels, reaching the lumbar chain of nodes at the renal level. Lymphatic drainage from the pelvic part of the ductus deferens, seminal vesicle, prostate gland, urinary bladder, and prostatic and membranous urethra is by way of internal iliac nodes, the posteromedial nodes of the external iliac group, and the sacral nodes. Lymphatic drainage of the kidneys follows the renal veins to the lumbar lymph nodes. Drainage of the ureter is regional: to the

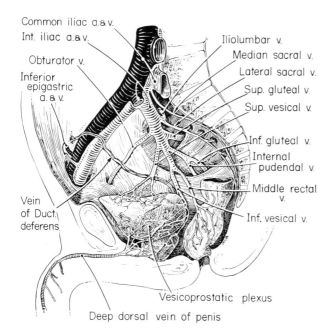

Common iliac a. & v.
Int. iliac a. & v.
Obturator v.
Inferior epigastric a. & v.
Vein of Duct. deferens

Iliolumbar v.
Median sacral v.
Lateral sacral v.
Sup. gluteal v.
Sup. vesical v.
Inf. gluteal v.
Internal pudendal v.
Middle rectal v.
Inf. vesical v.

Vesicoprostatic plexus
Deep dorsal vein of penis

Figure 1–20 The internal iliac vein and its tributaries. (From Woodburne, R. T.: Essentials of Human Anatomy, 5th Ed., 1973. Copyright by Oxford University Press, Inc. Reprinted by permission.)

lumbar nodes from the upper abdominal ureter, to the lower lumbar and common iliac nodes from the lower abdominal ureter, and to the internal iliac nodes from the pelvic ureter.

NERVE SUPPLY

NERVES OF THE KIDNEY

An autonomic and afferent innervation is provided for the kidney by the nerves of the renal plexus. (See Figs. 1–21 and 1–22.) Its nerves are derived from the celiac plexus, the lesser thoracic splanchnic and least thoracic splanchnic nerves, and the aorticorenal ganglion.

The renal plexuses consist of an open meshwork of nerves along the renal arteries, supplemented by nerves which run both superior and inferior to the arteries. The plexuses receive from four to eight branches from the celiac and aorticorenal ganglia. These convey both sympathetic and parasympathetic (vagal) fibers, branches from the first (sometimes second) lumbar splanchnic nerve, renal branches from the intermesenteric nerves, and contributions from the superior hypogastric plexus. The contributions from the superior hypogastric plexus are

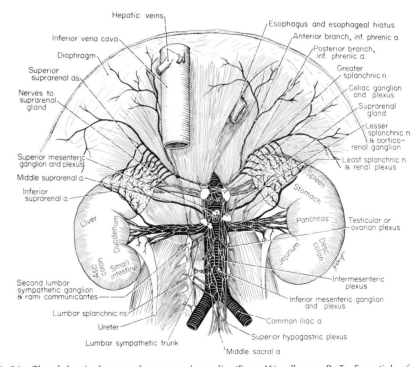

Figure 1–21 The abdominal nerve plexuses and ganglia. (From Woodburne, R. T.: Essentials of Human Anatomy, 5th Ed., 1973. Copyright by Oxford University Press, Inc. Reprinted by permission.)

thought to be the pathways for the parasympathetic innervation of the renal pelvis and the upper end of the ureter. In addition, the lesser splanchnic nerve ends in the aorticorenal ganglion and the least splanchnic nerve in the renal plexus; contributions from these nerves join the renal plexus on either side. Renal ganglia are usually found along the posterosuperior aspect of the renal artery but, occasionally, are anterior to it. There are communications between the renal and suprarenal plexuses and also with the ureteric plexus below. The renal plexus sends offshoots to the testicular plexus and the inferior vena cava on the right side.

The principal efferent innervation of the kidney is vasomotor, autonomic nerves being supplied to the muscular coats of the afferent and efferent arterioles. Nerves appear to influence urine formation only by changing the blood supply to the kidney; it is doubtful if there are any true secretory nerves to the organ. Afferent fibers probably reach the spinal cord through the tenth, eleventh, and twelfth thoracic nerves.

NERVES TO THE URETER AND TESTIS

The ureteric plexuses are composed of nerves which interlace along the ureters; the plexuses are both abdominal and pelvic in location. Nerves to the upper portions of the ureters are derived from the renal plexuses, the intermesenteric plexus, and the superior hypogastric plexuses. The latter contributions probably provide parasympathetic nerves from the pelvic splanchnic nerves. Tiny nerve filaments to the midportions of the ureters arise from the superior hypogastric plexuses and from the hypogastric nerves. The nerve supply of the lower portions of the ureters comes from the hypogastric nerves and the inferior hypogastric plexuses and is associated with the innervation of the ductus deferens, the seminal vesicle, and the urinary bladder.

The testicular plexuses are closely related to the ureteric plexuses and receive branches from the same sources regionally. These plexuses lie on and follow the testicular arteries. The testicular plexus supplies the spermatic cord, the epididymis, and the testis. It may be predicated, on embryologic and reflex grounds, that the parasympathetic fibers of the testicular plexuses are vagal in origin.

HYPOGASTRIC PLEXUSES AND NERVES

The *superior hypogastric plexus* of the abdomen continues into the pelvis as the hypogastric nerves and the inferior hypogastric plexuses. The superior hypogastric plexus is continuous with the intermesenteric plexus; it lies against the lower part of the abdominal aorta, its bifurcation, and the median sacral vessels. Its extent is from the lower border of the third lumbar vertebra to the middle of the first sacral segment. The superior hypogastric plexus consists of a broad, flattened band of intercommunicating nerve bundles that descend over the aortic bifurcation. In addition to its continuity with the intermesenteric

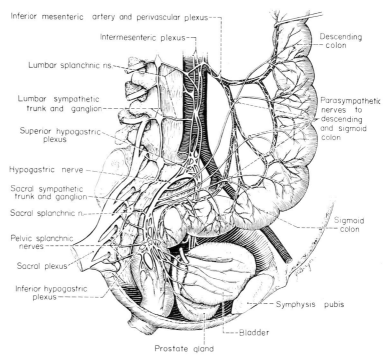

Inferior mesenteric artery and perivascular plexus

Intermesenteric plexus

Lumbar splanchnic ns.

Lumbar sympathetic trunk and ganglion

Superior hypogastric plexus

Hypogastric nerve

Sacral sympathetic trunk and ganglion

Sacral splanchnic n.

Pelvic splanchnic nerves

Sacral plexus

Inferior hypogastric plexus

Descending colon

Parasympathetic nerves to descending and sigmoid colon

Sigmoid colon

Symphysis pubis

Bladder

Prostate gland

Figure 1–22 The autonomic nerves of the pelvis. (From Woodburne, R. T.: Essentials of Human Anatomy, 5th Ed., 1973. Copyright by Oxford University Press, Inc. Reprinted by permission.)

plexus, it receives the lower two lumbar splanchnic nerves. Broadening below, the plexus divides opposite the first sacral segment into the right and left hypogastric nerves. There are few, if any, parasympathetic neurons in the superior hypogastric plexus, but the afferent (pain) fibers it contains are sometimes clinically more important than its efferent bundles. (See Fig. 1–22.)

The right and left *hypogastric nerves* are formed from the bifurcation of the superior hypogastric plexus. The relatively solid nerve trunks diverge on either side of the rectum and curve outward, downward, and backward into the pelvis. They are from 7.5 to 10 cm in length and contain no ganglia. They interconnect the superior hypogastric and inferior hypogastric plexuses and are the principal sympathetic roots of the latter. The hypogastric nerves lie in the extraperitoneal connective tissue lateral to the rectum and medial to the internal iliac vessels; they are in the base of the rectouterine fold in the female (or the rectovesical fold in the male). Near their upper extremities, the hypogastric nerves provide branches to the sigmoid colon and the descending colon. A prominent vascular branch of each hypogastric nerve joins the internal iliac or the external iliac artery, and there may also be branches to the testis and the ureter.

The *inferior hypogastric plexuses* are fanlike expansions of the hypogastric nerves located, in the male, on either side of the rectum, the prostate, and the seminal vesicles, and against the inferolateral surface of the bladder. In the female the relationships are similar, the cervix of the uterus and the lateral vaginal fornices taking the place of the seminal vesicles and the prostate. The intercommunicating nerves and ganglia that constitute the plexus form a thin meshwork, the dimensions of which are about 6 cm in the anteroposterior direction and about 4 cm from above downward. The plexus lies medial to the internal iliac vessels and their radicles and is separated from the viscera by endopelvic fascia. The ureter crosses the superior border of the plexus from without inward, and the terminal ureter is related to the inner surface of the anterior part of the plexus. The hypogastric nerves which join the inferior plexuses at their superolateral angles are their principal sympathetic roots, but the sacral splanchnic branches also convey sympathetic filaments to each plexus. The pelvic splanchnic nerves contribute the parasympathetic supply for the pelvic viscera. The inferior hypogastric plexuses may be divided into rectal and vesical parts in the male, and rectal, uterovaginal, and vesical parts in the female.

The *pelvic splanchnic nerves* represent the sacral portion of the craniosacral (parasympathetic) portion of the autonomic nervous system. With cells of origin in the second, third, and fourth sacral spinal cord segments, these preganglionic nerves supply the parasympathetic innervation of all the pelvic and perineal viscera and of the abdominal viscera supplied by the inferior mesenteric artery. The pelvic splanchnic nerves spring from the ventral rami of the second, third, and fourth sacral nerves shortly after their emergence from the pelvic sacral foramina, the contribution from the third sacral nerve usually being the largest. From three to ten strands of nerves pass forward to and become incorporated in the inferior hypogastric plexus, where they become indistinguishable from other components in the plexus as they distribute through its branches. These nerve strands synapse in the ganglia of the inferior hypogastric plexus and in minute ganglia in the muscular walls of the pelvic viscera.

The subsidiary plexuses of the inferior hypogastric plexus are the middle rectal, the vesical, the deferential, and the prostatic.

NERVES OF THE BLADDER AND ADNEXA

The vesical plexus is a continuation of the anterior portion of the inferior hypogastric plexus and contains postganglionic sympathetic and preganglionic parasympathetic fibers. The vesical plexus of each side invests the terminal portion of the ureter and lies against the posterolateral aspect of the bladder (Fig. 1–22). It supplies the bladder, the lower portion of the ureter, the seminal vesicle, and the ductus deferens as far as the epididymis. The parasympathetic innervation of the bladder serves the emptying reflex, causing contraction of the musculature of the wall of the bladder (detrusor muscle). The sympathetic supply of the bladder reaches the trigonal muscle and the blood vessels. Its stimulation results in closure of the ureteral orifices and movement of the fundus of the bladder toward its base. Afferent impulses are conducted along both the sympathetic and parasympathetic sets of nerves, impulses of pain due to an overstretched bladder traveling with the sympathetic fibers. Initiated by normal stretching of the muscle layers as the viscus fills, the more important proprioceptive impulses from the muscular wall travel over the parasympathetic fibers. Their stimulation results in reflex emptying of the bladder.

Recently developed histochemical methods for differentiating parasympathetic and sympathetic nerve fibers have led to the revival of the concept of postganglionic synapses in the bladder wall. In 1936, Mosely reported that in cats approximately 40 per cent of the intramural ganglia in the bladder received preganglionic fibers exclusively from the hypogastric nerves, 40 per cent exclusively from the pelvic nerves, and about 20 per cent from both sets of nerves. It is now thought that neurons in either the sympathetic or the parasympathetic pathway may effect synapses with ganglion cells of the other modality and thus provide a modulating interaction between the two systems in the control of bladder activity.

The deferential plexus consists of several nerves which accompany and supply the ductus deferens as far as the epididymis. They are offshoots of the inferior portion of the vesical plexus.

The prostatic plexus is derived from the larger nerves of the anterior inferior part of the inferior hypogastric plexus. It lies along the side of the prostate gland, and its nerves communicate with twigs to the neck of the bladder and to the seminal vesicle. It supplies the prostate gland, the prostatic urethra, and the ejaculatory ducts. Terminals communicate with the pudendal nerve, and branches of both sets innervate the penile vessels, the corpora cavernosa, the corpus spongiosum, the membranous and penile portions of the urethra, and the bulbourethral glands. This distribution is occasionally by way of definite greater and lesser cavernous nerves. The former accompanies the dorsal nerve of the penis and supplies the corpora cavernosa; the latter supplies the corpus spongiosum and the urethra. Both the sympathetic and parasympathetic nerve mechanisms are necessary to sexual activity. Erection depends on stimuli transmitted through the parasympathetic nerves that lead to engorgement of the corpora cavernosa by dilatation of their arteries or, possibly, by relaxation of their vascular tone. Contraction of the bulbocavernosus and ischiocavernosus muscles helps maintain erection by interference with the venous return of blood from the cavernous tissues. Stimulation of sympathetic nerves leads to constriction of the arteries and subsidence of erection. Ejaculation consists of two phases: emission and ejaculation proper. Emission, or the delivery of semen to the membranous urethra, follows reflex peristalsis in the ductus deferentes and seminal vesicles and contraction of the smooth muscle of the prostate gland. This is a sympathetic response. Ejaculation, or expulsion of the seminal fluid, follows parasympathetic stimulation and is accompanied by clonic spasm of the bulbocavernosus and ischiocavernosus muscles. (In the female the comparable parasympathetic stimulation leads to increased vaginal secretion, erection of the clitoris, and engorgement of the erectile tissue of the vestibule.) Afferent fibers from the viscera accompany both sympathetic and parasympathetic fibers.

SELECTED REFERENCES

Edvardsen, P.: Nervous control of urinary bladder in cats. Acta Physiol. Scand., 72:151–171 (Part I, The collecting phase); 172–182 (Part II, The expulsion phase); 183–193 (Part III, Effects of autonomic blocking agents in the intact animal); 234–247 (Part IV, Effects of autonomic blocking agents on response to peripheral nerve stimulation), 1968.

Elbadawi, A., and Schenk, E. A.: A new theory of the innervation of bladder musculature (Part III). Postganglionic synapses in uretero-vesico-urethral autonomic pathways. J. Urol., *105*:372, 1971.
The two references above are representative of the current revision of opinion on the control of micturition.

Hodson, J.: The lobar structure of the kidney. Brit. J. Urol., *44*:246, 1972.
Emphasizes the fundamental lobation of the human kidney in relation to arterial distribution.

Mitchell, G.A.G.: Anatomy of the Autonomic Nervous System. Baltimore, Williams and Wilkins Co., 1953.
Probably the best reference concerning innervation.

Woodburne, R. T.: Anatomy of the bladder and bladder outlet. J. Urol., *100*:474, 1968.
A source of additional detail on excretory tract anatomy.

Woodburne, R. T.: Essentials of Human Anatomy, 5th Ed. New York, Oxford University Press, 1973.
A general reference.

Chapter Two

CONGENITAL ANOMALIES OF THE GENITOURINARY TRACT

C. William Hyndman

A thorough knowledge of anatomy and embryology must be achieved before congenital anomalies of the genitourinary tract can be fully understood. The dynamic development of the entire tract must be approached by specifically considering each organ. However, it must be remembered that the organs are developing simultaneously, and an aberration during the development of one will affect others further along in the process. This effect is apparent in the genitourinary tract, where the presence of multiple anomalies is common. It is estimated that between 10 and 15 per cent of individuals have at least one genitourinary anomaly.

KIDNEY

Normal Development

The kidney develops in three stages from the intermediate mesoderm of the embryo. The pronephros appears first in the cervical and upper thoracic mesoderm at three weeks following conception and does not function as an excretory organ. The mesonephros begins to develop in the lumbar region during the fourth week while the pronephros is degenerating. It is caudal to the pronephros and has some limited excretory function. The metanephros is composed of two systems—the ureteric bud which forms at the junction of the cloaca and mesonephric duct (Wolffian duct) and the metanephrogenic tissue from the caudal intermediate mesoderm. The ureteric bud extends dorsocranially, enlarging at the distal end to form the pelvis. Division of the pelvis results in the formation of major and minor calyces, and finally the collecting ducts of the kidney. Aggregates of tissue from the

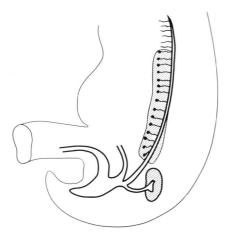

Figure 2–1   Normal development of the kidney.

nephrogenic tissue invest the tips of the branching ducts, forming caps which are on the ampullae or terminal portion of the ducts. These go on to form the nephron. Urine formation occurs at approximately three months following conception.

During the seventh and eighth week the kidney ascends from the pelvis by a combination of differential growth and a straightening of the fetal curvature. With ascent, the anteriorly located renal pelvis rotates medially to complete kidney development.

Abnormal Development

ANOMALIES OF NUMBER

Renal Agenesis. Renal agenesis results from a failure of the nephrogenic ridge or the metanephros to develop. It is bilateral in approximately 1 in 2700 births, and unilateral in 1 in 500 to 1200 births. Bilateral renal agenesis is incompatible with life, whereas in unilateral disease life is dependent upon the status of the solitary kidney.

Absence of urine formation by the fetus causes oligohydramnios and associated compression of the fetal chest, resulting in pulmonary hypoplasia. Cardiac and orthopedic anomalies are also common with this aberration.

In unilateral renal agenesis the functional kidney has a much higher incidence of anomalies. The diagnosis is made when the agenetic kidney cannot be visualized by intravenous pyelography and the absence of the trigone on the affected side is observed at cystoscopy.

Occasionally a blind ended ureter may be present in aplasia. Consequently, the presence of two ureteric orifices at cystoscopy does not rule out aplasia.

Supernumerary Kidneys. Supernumerary kidneys are formed as a result of a splitting of the metanephric blastema or a development of two separate metanephric blastemas. This condition is the rarest of all kidney anomalies, and it is asymptomatic unless associated with other anomalies. The ureter from a supernumerary kidney usually joins the ipsilateral ureter, but it may enter the bladder separately. The diagnosis is made when three kidneys are apparent on an intravenous pyelogram.

ANOMALIES OF POSITION

Ectopic Kidney. Ectopia may be due to persistent fetal blood vessels preventing the kidney's normal ascent to its definitive position. Unilateral ectopic kidney occurs in approximately 1 in 800 births and is bilateral in 1 in 2200 births. Most ectopic kidneys are found in the pelvis but rarely may be found in the thorax.

A pelvic kidney may be confused with a pelvic tumor, and its presence may complicate the management of labor. Occasionally the kidney may cause pain by pressing on nerves and other surrounding structures. Using intravenous pyelography, the diagnosis is made when one kidney is seen in the pelvic area. Visualization of the kidney may be difficult because the contrast material is masked by the bony pelvic structures.

There is a higher incidence of ureteric anomalies associated with pelvic kidneys.

Crossed Renal Ectopia. In crossed renal ectopia one kidney crosses the midline to lie on the same side as its mate. Usually the dystrophic or abnormal kidney crosses over to fuse with the normal one. The incidence of those having crossed renal ectopia is uncertain, but it

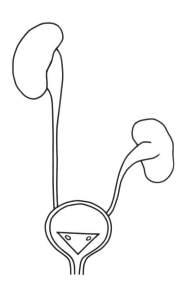

Figure 2–2 Pelvic kidney.

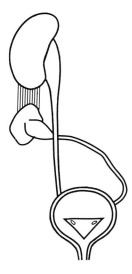

Figure 2–3 Crossed renal ectopia.

is estimated to be approximately 1 in 2000 births. The blood supply to the ectopic kidney arises from the lower aorta or iliac vessels. Clinically, the ectopic kidney is silent unless an obstruction or infection supervenes. The diagnosis is made by intravenous pyelography when two kidneys are visualized on one side of the midline. The ureters usually enter the bladder in the normal position. However, on rare occasions only one ureter may conduct urine from both poles.

ABNORMAL FORM OR SIZE

Renal Dysplasia. Renal dysplasia results from a failure of the metanephros to develop normally. Primitive glomeruli, cysts, fibrous tissue, and fatty tissue may be present. This is a rare lesion. As with agenesis, it is discovered by intravenous pyelography.

Renal Hypoplasia. Renal hypoplasia is thought to be caused by a failure of development of the normal blood supply to the kidney. This anomaly is found in approximately 1 in 500 autopsies. Clinically, renal hypoplasia may be totally asymptomatic, but there is evidence to indicate that it may be a cause of hypertension. Distinguishing hypoplastic kidneys from pyelonephritic kidneys is a challenge. On an intravenous pyelogram, a small kidney and renal pelvis suggest hypoplasia. Pyelonephritic kidneys frequently have distorted calyces. Some blunting of the calyces indicates infection, but this is not an invariable finding. The prognosis depends on the condition of the remaining kidney. Nephrectomy is indicated in cases of hypertension only after other causes of the hypertension have been ruled out and the response to medical management is unsatisfactory.

Horseshoe Kidney. Horseshoe kidney usually results from the fusion of the lower poles of the metanephros blastema in front of the inferior vena cava and aorta. The kidney is located in the lower lumbar region where an isthmus joins the lower poles of the definitive kidneys. Since each kidney fails to rotate to its normal position, its pelvis is anterior. The incidence of horseshoe kidney varies between 1 in 600 and 1 in 1800 births. Clinically, a horseshoe kidney may be asymptomatic but there is a higher incidence of renal calculi, infection, and obstruction. One third of newborns with this anomaly have associated chromosomal aberrations (Turner's syndrome) and cardiovascular, gastrointestinal, and central nervous system lesions. Diagnosis is made by intravenous pyelography which reveals the anterior displaced pelves and a reversal of the normal renal axes. Uncomplicated horseshoe kidney requires no surgery.

ABNORMAL STRUCTURE

Simple Cysts. Simple cysts are thought to be the result of urinary obstruction and impaired circulation during development. The cysts are very rare in children but common in adults. Clinically, such cysts are important in the differential diagnosis of tumors of the kidney.

Infantile Polycystic Kidneys (Potter Type 1). Infantile polycystic kidneys are thought to be due to hyperplasia of the interstitial portion of the collecting tubules during development. The cystic changes are bilateral and symmetric and are not associated with other lower urinary tract anomalies. The glomeruli are normal. The liver is also affected by proliferation and dilatation of the bile ducts and periportal hyperplasia. This disease is inherited as an autosomal recessive trait. Clinically, it presents with bilateral abdominal masses, uremia, or signs of portal hypertension. The diagnosis is made by intravenous pyelography when large, poorly functioning kidneys are found. Renal and liver biopsies confirm the diagnosis. The prognosis for infantile polycystic kidneys is poor, but renal transplantation is a suitable treatment for older children.

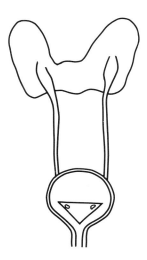

Figure 2–4   Horseshoe kidney.

Multicystic Kidney (Potter Type 2). Multicystic kidneys are thought to be due to an inhibition of the ampullary portion of the kidney and are the most common cause of a nonfunctioning kidney in the newborn. The disorder is not hereditary and although usually unilateral, a bilateral condition may exist. When both kidneys are affected, the infant dies shortly after birth. The affected kidney does not function, is not always larger than normal, and is associated with an atretic ureter. The opposite kidney has a greater than normal incidence of anomalies such as atretic ureteral segments and reflux. The diagnosis is made usually by palpation of an abdominal mass in a newborn infant, and transillumination of the flank may help to establish the presence of cysts. On an intravenous pyelogram only one kidney is visualized. Surgical exploration, however, may be necessary to confirm the diagnosis. If the disease is unilateral and the opposite kidney is normal, then the prognosis is excellent. The liver is not involved in this disease.

Adult Polycystic Kidney (Potter Type 3). Adult polycystic kidneys are caused by a combination of abnormal development in the interstitial and ampullary portions of each kidney. Usually this disease is bilateral, but it may be unilateral. It is inherited as an autosomal dominant trait, and one third of those patients with adult polycystic kidney have liver involvement. Clinically, patients present with large bilateral abdominal masses, and an intravenous pyelogram reveals large cystic kidneys. In early childhood, an intravenous pyelogram may show the kidneys to be normal in size and shape. The prognosis depends on the age when symptoms appear. Transplantation is an effective treatment when renal function is poor.

Medullary Sponge Kidney. Medullary sponge kidney is a congenital dilatation of the collecting tubules. Occasionally it is familial. Clinically, it is asymptomatic unless complicated by calculus or infection. The diagnosis is made by intravenous pyelography when a blush phase is seen near the calyces, indicating dilatation of the collecting tubules. The prognosis is excellent unless infection and stone formation supervene. There is also an association with hemihypertrophy.

Pyelogenic Cysts. These cysts are spaces communicating with calyces. Most of them are asymptomatic, but they are associated occasionally with stone formation and infection. Usually no treatment is necessary, but some require heminephrectomy and the removal of the infected portion of the kidney.

Microcystic Disease. Microcystic disease is a cystic dilatation of the proximal tubule of the kidney, resulting in a congenital nephrotic syndrome. Patients with this condition do not have large kidneys as in other forms of cystic disease.

ABNORMAL BLOOD SUPPLY

The fetal kidney takes its blood supply from the mesonephric artery which in turn arises from the aorta. Around the pelvis of the kidney there is a plexus of arteries which enters the kidney and divides. Usually, one of these branches persists as the solitary renal artery, but anomalies such as aneurysms, arteriovenous malformations, and aberrant vessels can occur. Approximately 1 per cent of people have a renal artery anomaly. Aberrant arteries are important when surgery on the kidney is contemplated since they are end arteries, and damage to the vessel or ligation results in an infarct of the kidney. Congenital arteriovenous malformations are very rare, but large malformations can result in congestive heart failure and aneurysmal dilatation of the renal arteries. Arteriography is useful in delineating these abnormal vessels. The treatment of such arterial anomalies will depend on the clinical problem.

ANOMALIES OF THE PELVIS

Ureteral Pelvic Junction Obstruction. The pelvis develops from the distal end of the ureteric bud, which originates at the junction of the mesonephric duct and the cloaca. Obstruction may be caused by fibrous bands, blood vessels, or an intrinsic defect at the junction. Hydronephrosis or dilatation proximal to this obstruction is one of the commonest causes of abdominal masses in children who present with pain and urinary tract infection. Intravenous pyelography reveals a dilated pelvis, and retrograde pyelography at the time of cystoscopy confirms a normal ureter below the obstructed ureteric pelvic junction. Treatment consists of pyeloplasty or remodeling of the ureteric pelvic junction so that a normal funnel is present.

Duplication of the Pelvis and Ureter. Duplication varies from a complete duplication of the ureters and pelvis to a bifid pelvis. This is the most common anomaly of the upper collecting system. Complete duplication is caused by the development of two separate ureteric buds from the mesonephric duct. During development of the bladder, the

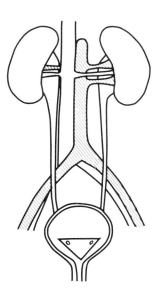

Figure 2–5 Abnormal blood supply.

terminal portion of the mesonephric duct is absorbed into the bladder. The first ureteric bud (to the lower portion of the kidney) is the first to be incorporated into the bladder and, by a peculiar pattern of growth of the bladder, shifts cephalad and laterally. The second ureteric bud (draining the upper kidney) terminates caudal to the first. Thus, the upper pole of the kidney drains to the lowest portion of the bladder. Unilateral duplication can occur in approximately 1 in 200 births, while bilateral duplication occurs in approximately 1 in 1200 births.

The duplication may be complete, resulting in two orifices in the bladder, or the ureters may join one another before entering the bladder. The position of each orifice determines the clinical manifestations. The upper pole ureter empties lower than the lower pole ureter, and it also tends to be ectopic. If so, it may join the urethra, vagina, uterus, or seminal vesicle. Obstruction may be present and may cause infection. In the female, an ectopic ureter entering the vagina or lower urethra may cause dribbling and incontinence. The lower pole ureter has a tendency to vesicoureteral reflux because of its rather perpendicular course through the bladder musculature. Ectopic ureter will be discussed further under *Ureter*.

The diagnosis is made by intravenous pyelography when two ureters are seen. If the obstruction is severe, then both ureters may not be visualized, but the upper pole of the kidney may be pushed laterally because of the hydronephrosis. Cystoscopy, retrograde pyelography and occasionally antegrade pyelography may be useful in delineating the abnormality further. Simple duplicating requires no treatment. If the ureter is ectopic, then its reimplantation into the bladder is necessary. When the kidney is severely damaged by obstruction, heminephrectomy and uretectomy must be considered.

URETER

Normal Development

The ureter develops from the ureteric bud at the junction of the mesonephric duct and the cloaca as described previously. The ureter then fuses with the metanephrogenic mesoderm, forming the kidney and upper collecting system.

Abnormal Development

DUPLICATION ANOMALY

See *Kidney*.

URETEROCELE

Ureteroceles are thought to be caused by persistence of the epithelium at the junction of the ureteric bud and the mesonephric duct

(Chwalla's membrane). The result is a narrowing at the ureteric orifice as it enters the bladder and a ballooning proximal to the point of obstruction. The ureterocele then consists of bladder mucosa, fibrous tissue and muscle, and the lining of the ureter as it bulges into the bladder itself. Ureteroceles may be unilateral, bilateral, ectopic, or in the normal position.

In 1 to 2 per cent of cystoscopy reports, varying degrees of ureteroceles are described; 15 per cent are bilateral. A large ureterocele may obstruct the opposite ureteric orifice, causing hydronephrosis or prolapse through the urethra in the female. The presenting sign is a perineal mass with protrusion of the ureterocele through the urethra, or there may be a history of urinary tract infection and hematuria. Radiologically a ureterocele is seen as a filling defect in the bladder, giving a "cobra head deformity."

The diagnosis is made by intravenous pyelography and also by cystoscopy. Treatment is surgical. If an ectopic ureter with a nonfunctioning portion of kidney is present, then heminephrectomy is necessary. If the kidney is functional, then a transurethral resection of the stenotic ureteric orifice or reimplantation of the ureter into the bladder is necessary.

ECTOPIC URETER

Ectopic ureter has been described briefly under duplication anomalies and development of the ureter, and its incorporation into the bladder has also been discussed. Ectopic ureter is more common in the female than in the male and is more often associated with duplication in the female than in the male. The position of the ectopic ureter determines the clinical manifestations: If near the bladder neck, no symp-

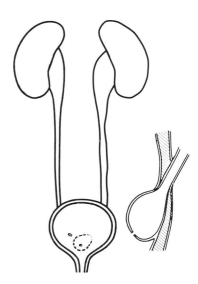

Figure 2-6 Ureterocele.

toms are present; if in the urethra, obstruction may occur resulting in infection; if in the vagina or lower urethra, then dribbling incontinence associated with normal periodic voiding may be the typical history. Incontinence does not occur in the male because the ureter always enters above the membranous urethra where the external sphincter is located.

The diagnosis may be difficult to make if dribbling is not present, but cystoscopy, urethroscopy, vaginoscopy, and voiding cystourography may delineate the lesion. Treatment varies from the removal of a nonfunctioning kidney to a ureteric reimplantation if the kidney is functioning.

RETROCAVAL URETER

Normally the inferior vena cava is formed by a persistence of the right subcardinal vein. If the posterior cardinal vein persists, then the right ureter lies posterior to the inferior vena cava. This causes partial obstruction of the midureter. On a radiograph, the ureter is found to be more medially placed than normal, and it also may have a characteristic S curve as it travels from the kidney to the bladder. Treatment depends on the degree of obstruction; and if severe, division of the ureter and reanastomosis of the ureter in its normal position may be necessary. The transection is usually done in the dilated part of the ureter to take advantage of the large uniform lumen.

BLADDER

Normal Development

The urinary bladder develops from the cloaca or expanded end of the hindgut. The cloaca is connected to the allantois (cephalad) and

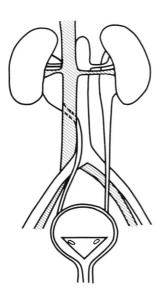

Figure 2–7 Retrocaval ureter.

the mesonephric ducts. Caudally the ectoderm comes in very close approximation to the cloaca and is called the cloacal membrane. At approximately the fourth week a septum (urorectal septum) divides the cloaca into the rectum posteriorly and the urogenital sinus anteriorly. The urogenital sinus differentiates further into the vesicourethral canal which forms the bladder and upper urethra, and the definitive urogenital sinus from which the main portion of the urethra is formed. The mesonephric duct is incorporated along with the ureters during bladder development.

Abnormal Development

CONGENITAL BLADDER NECK OBSTRUCTION

At one time bladder neck obstruction was thought to be a common cause of recurrent urinary tract infections and reflux in children. At the present time, however, most urologists feel that vesical neck contracture is a very rare anomaly and that the previously diagnosed obstruction was in fact a normal bladder neck which had a varying appearance on voiding cystourethrograms and at the time of cystoscopy and urethroscopy.

EXSTROPHY OF THE BLADDER

Exstrophy of the bladder results from a failure of the mesoderm to cover the lower anterior abdominal wall and causes exposure of the posterior bladder in the lower abdomen. This occurs in approximately 1 in 40,000 births. Clinically the child presents with an obvious congenital anomaly where the posterior bladder fuses with the lateral abdominal wall. Diastasis of the pubic symphysis pubis is also present. Club feet, cleft palate, rectovaginal fistula, and imperforate anus are associated anomalies. Children with exstrophy of the bladder are totally incontinent of urine. They also have a higher incidence of pyelonephritis, umbilical hernias, inguinal hernias, and chronic inflammation of the exposed bladder surface. Squamous metaplasia is present, and malignancy (adenocarcinoma) may occur in later life. Intravenous pyelography is useful in delineating other associated anomalies of the upper tract, such as ureteric duplication.

At present, controversy surrounds the selection of treatment for exstrophy of the bladder. Closing the bladder with reconstruction of the urethra in order to attain a normal functioning bladder with continence is successful in approximately 10 per cent of cases. Some urologists feel that diversion of the urinary stream by ureterosigmoidostomies or ileal loop diversion is preferable in early childhood.

URACHAL CYSTS AND PATENT URACHUS

A patent urachus is present when the urachal canal fails to close. A discharge of fluid from the umbilicus, which at the time of voiding

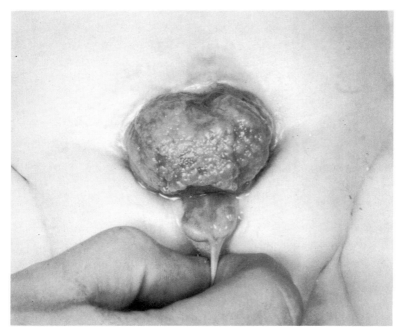

Figure 2–8   Bladder exstrophy.

increases in volume, is the usual presenting sign. Urethral obstruction is frequently present and must be relieved before the patent urachus is closed. Cystograms and cystoscopies are useful when delineating this lesion.

Urachal cysts result when only the central portion of the canal remains patent. Children with urachal cysts present with abdominal masses. An infected cyst may simulate an intra-abdominal abscess. The diagnosis may be difficult and is usually made at the time of surgery. Treatment consists of removal of the cyst if it is uninfected, and drainage and marsupialization if an abscess is present.

DUPLICATED BLADDER

Duplicated bladder is a very rare anomaly in which the bladder may be totally or partially duplicated. The septum usually lies in the sagittal plane. Rarely an hourglass bladder occurs. Duplication of the urethra is also associated with this anomaly.

URETHRA AND PENIS

Normal Development

The male urethra develops from the vesical anlage above the verumontanum and the urogenital sinus. The female urethra is derived from the vesical anlage only. External genitalia in the male and female begin with the same embryonic structures. The genital tubercle forms between the tail and umbilical cord. The urogenital membranes become a longitudinal groove surrounded by the urogenital folds. By 90 days after conception, the genital tubercle is elongated to become the phallus in the male and the clitoris in the female. The urethral folds come together, forming the urethra in the male, and remain as the labia minora in the female. The genital swellings become the scrotum in the male and the labia majora in the female. The determining factor in this development is the formation of the gonads which occurs during this period of time. In individuals with the Y chromosome, testicles develop, resulting in androgen production (and male development). The absence of the Y chromosome results in female development.

Abnormal Development

4% = reflux (¾ abate)

POSTERIOR URETHRAL VALVES

Posterior urethral valves are the most common cause of obstruction in the male infant. Their origin is uncertain. They may stem from the persistence of the urogenital membrane. There are three types of valves described according to their relationship to the verumontanum. Type 1 originates at the verumontanum and balloons into the distal prostatic urethra, and it is by far the most common form. Type 2 extends from the verumontanum to the vesical neck and is very uncommon. Type 3 is a diaphragm at the level of the verumontanum. Urine formation begins during the third month, and consequently, the fetus develops dilatation of the urinary tract behind the valves prior to birth. The degree of obstruction determines the amount of renal function available at birth. Symptoms of obstruction vary from renal failure to a decrease in the flow of urine or the development of urinary tract infections in later life. The diagnosis is made with a voiding cystourethrogram and substantiated by urethroscopy. Treatment consists of transurethral resection of the valves. The dilatation and decompensation of the urinary tract above the obstruction may be so severe that removal of

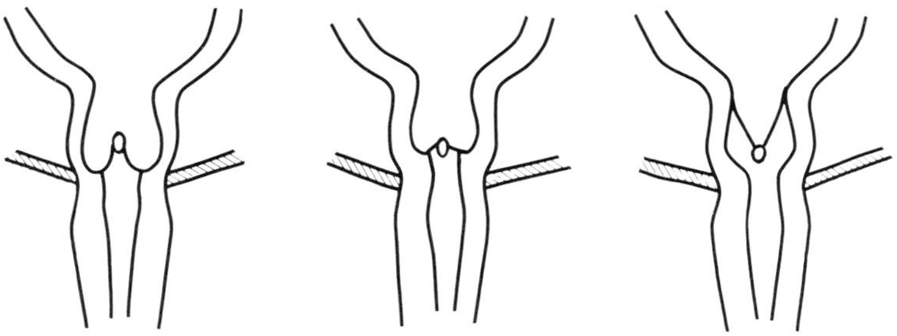

c̄ Rx :
38% = stress incont.
⅓ = total "
— better by puberty

Figure 2–9　Posterior urethral valves.

I　　　　　II　　　　　II

the valves may not allow necessary drainage of the upper tract, and loop ureterostomies or nephrostomies may be necessary as a temporary measure.

ANTERIOR URETHRAL VALVES

This is a rare lesion occurring in the anterior urethra or the urethra distal to the membranous urethra. A voiding cystourethrogram may visualize these valves, and treatment consists of either a resection of the valve transurethrally or an open excision.

MEATAL STENOSIS AND URETHRAL STRICTURE

Meatal stenosis is a common cause of obstruction in the infant. Damage to the urinary system depends on the degree of stenosis, which is treated by simple meatotomy.

Congenital urethral strictures can occur at other portions of the urethra, but they are very rare.

URETHRORECTAL FISTULA

Congenital communication between the urethra and colon is most commonly seen in association with imperforate anus.

HYPOSPADIAS

Hypospadias is a very common anomaly in which the urethral meatus does not attain its normal position at the end of the penis. Hypospadias occurs in the female but is far more common in the male. It is thought to be caused by a failure of androgen production by the fetal testicle, resulting in incomplete fusion of the urethral folds. The folds close from proximal to distal, and types of hypospadias are classified as glandular, penile, penile scrotal, and perineal, depending on where the opening is situated. A familial incidence of this anomaly has been reported, but the mode of inheritance is uncertain. In the extreme form of perineal hypospadias with bifid scrotum and cryptorchidism, intersex problems must be considered. Chordee or ventral curvature of the penis is present in almost all types of hypospadias. This is due to the fibrous nature of the undeveloped corpus spongiosum distal to the meatal opening. Other genitourinary anomalies are commonly associated with hypospadias. It is imperative that circumcisions not be performed on boys with this condition because the foreskin may be used in surgical repair of the anomaly at a later age. Treatment depends upon the degree of involvement. The penis must be straightened to allow normal intercourse, and the meatus must be brought out to the end of the phallus to allow the boy to void like his peers. Many operations have been devised which consist of one stage or multiple stage proce-

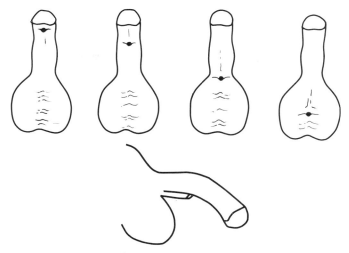

Figure 2–10   Hypospadias.

dures. Most physicians feel that surgical treatment should be performed before school age.

EPISPADIAS

Epispadias is a rare congenital anomaly in which the urethra is incompletely fused on the dorsum of the penis. Epispadias may be considered a mild form of exstrophy of the bladder, since their embryogenesis is similar. Treatment consists of the formation of a tube extending to the end of the penis.

TESTES

Normal Development

The gonads develop along the medial aspect of the mesonephros. The germinal cells migrate from the yolk sac. The gonad is divided into

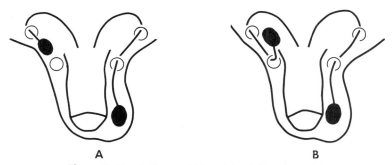

A   B

Figure 2–11   *A,* Cryptorchid testicle. *B,* Ectopic testicle.

a cortical area and a medullary area. The cortex forms the ovary, and the medullary portion forms the testicle depending on the chromosomal makeup of the fetus. A ligament between the caudal portion of the gonad and the inguinal canal, the gubernaculum, along with hormonal influences may be involved in the descent of the testicle. Descent occurs gradually in the retroperitoneum until the scrotum is reached in the eighth or ninth month in utero. A pinched-off portion of peritoneum forms a tunica vaginalis for the testicle in the scrotum. Development of the testicles stimulates the formation of the external male genital system. Absence of the gonad or the presence of an ovary results in female development. This is important when considering the embryogenesis of intersex problems.

Abnormal Development

CRYPTORCHIDISM

There are two types of undescended testicles: (1) A failure to descend along the normal path, and (2) the ectopic or malpositioned testicle.

The cryptorchid or undescended testicle may be found intra-abdominally in the inguinal canal or at the external ring. Ectopic testicles may be found superficial to the external oblique after having passed through the external ring) at the base of the penis, or in the opposite groin or perineal area.

An infant's testicles are very mobile, and manipulation of the genitalia or simply the removal of a diaper may cause them to retract into the inguinal canals. They can be drawn down into the scrotum easily and must not be confused with cryptorchid testicles. If a testicle has not descended spontaneously by age 1, it is unlikely to descend on its own. Human chorionic gonadotropin therapy can be given in cases of bilateral involvement. This form of therapy is effective in approximately 30 per cent of those males with cryptorchid testicles. In unilateral instances, descent occurs in less than 15 per cent of those patients having hormonal therapy. Orchidopexy is the procedure necessary to bring the testicle down into its normal position. Several operations have been devised which effectively place the undescended testicle in the scrotum.

The incidence of tumors in cryptorchid testicles, even after being placed in the scrotum, is approximately 40 times the normal incidence of testicular neoplasms. A sudden descent of a previously undescended testicle in a young adult suggests the possibility of tumor development in the testicle.

SELECTED REFERENCES

Arey, L. B.: Developmental Anatomy. A Textbook and Laboratory Manual of Embryology. 7th ed. rev. Philadelphia, W. B. Saunders Company, 1965.
  A complete text on embryology.

Campbell, M. F., and Harrison, J. H. (eds.): Urology. vol. 2. 3rd ed. Philadelphia, W. B. Saunders Company, 1970, pp. 1379–1712.
The standard text on urology.

Emmett, J. L., and Witten, D.: Clinical Urography. vol. 3. 3rd ed. Philadelphia, W. B. Saunders Company, 1971.
A radiologic approach to urology.

Netter, F. H.: Kidney, Ureter, Bladder. vol. 6. *In* Shapter, R. K. (ed.): Ciba Collection of Medical Illustrations. Summit, N. J., Ciba Pharmaceutical Co., 1973.
Excellent drawings by Netter of genitourinary anomalies.

Williams, D. I. et al.: Urology in Childhood. New York, Springer-Verlag New York, Inc., 1973.
A text reviewing pediatric anomalies by a noted pediatric urologist.

REFERENCES

Bernstein, J.: Developmental abnormalities of renal parenchyma: Renohypoplasia and dysplasia. Pathol. Annu., 3:213, 1968.

Blyth, H., and Ockenden, B. G.: Polycystic disease of kidney and liver presenting in childhood. J. Med. Genet., 8:257, 1971.

Campbell, M.: Ureterocele: Study of 94 instances in 80 infants and children. Surg. Gynecol. Obstet., 93:705, 1951.

Cherry, J. W.: Patent urachus: Review and report of case. J. Urol., 63:693, 1950.

DeWeerd, J. H., and Simon, H. B.: Simple renal cysts in children: Review of literature and report of five cases. J. Urol., 75:912, 1956.

Hawthorne, A. B.: Embryologic and clinical aspect of double ureter. J.A.M.A. 106:189, 1936.

Hendren, W. H.: Posterior urethral valves in boys. A broad clinical spectrum. J. Urol., 106:298, 1971.

Hesse, V. E.: Retrocaval ureter. S. Afr. Med. J., 43:561, 1969.

Honke, E. M.: Ectopic ureter. J. Urol., 55:460, 1946.

Kelalis, P. P., Culp, O. S., Stickler, G. B. et al.: Ureteropelvic obstruction in children: Experiences with 109 cases. J. Urol., 106:418, 1971.

Malek, R. S., Kelalis, P. P., Burke, E. C. et al.: Observations on ureteral ectopy in children. J. Urol., 107:308, 1972.

Muecke, E. C.: The role of the cloacal membrane in exstrophy: The first successful experimental case. J. Urol., 92:659, 1964.

Osathanordh, V., and Potter, E. L.: Pathogenesis of polycystic kidneys. Type 1 due to hyperplasia of interstitial portions of collecting tubules. Arch. Path., 77:466, 1964.

Patten, B. M., and Barry, A.: Genesis of exstrophy of bladder and epispadias. Am. J. Anat., 90:35, 1952.

Stephens, F. D.: Intramural ureter and ureterocele. Postgrad. Med. J., 40:179, 1964.

Tanagho, E. A.: Anatomy and management of ureteroceles. J. Urol. 107:729, 1972.

Uhlir, K.: Rare malformations of the bladder. J. Urol., 99:53, 1968.

Williams, D. I., and Royle, M.: Ectopic ureter in the male child. Br. J. Urol., 41:421, 1969.

Williams, D. I., and Savage, J.: Reconstruction of the exstrophied bladder. Br. J. Surg., 53:168, 1966.

Young, N. H., Frantz, W. A., and Baldwin, J. C.: Congenital obstruction of the posterior urethra. J. Urol., 3:289, 1919.

Chapter Three

URORADIOLOGY

John R. Thornbury

This chapter presents the basic precepts of uroradiologic examination, which can provide information for making decisions about diagnosis and management of patients' health problems. For the medical student, this initial exposure to the complexities of the diagnostic process is often a confusing experience. His confusion is further compounded by the plethora of other information with which he is confronted in a relatively short period of time. To aid the beleaguered student, this chapter is designed to provide a framework on which he can build a useful store of diagnostic knowledge while gaining experience in patient care. For the house officer, this chapter should be a reacquaintance with many of the uroradiologic precepts that were introduced to him as a student.

The major emphasis of the chapter is on the most commonly used uroradiologic examination, *excretory urography* (see Table 3–1). *Retrograde pyelography* is discussed from the standpoint of its use when excretory urography has failed to provide useful information. *Cystography* and *urethrography* receive less emphasis since the specific clinical problems for which they are best suited are less frequently encountered than the problems requiring excretory urography. This reduced emphasis does not mean that cystogram or urethrogram information is less useful than that obtained from the excretory urogram. On the contrary, for *certain clinical problems* (e.g., vesicoureteric reflux or urethral stricture) these procedures provide more specific information about abnormalities that involve the bladder or urethra than does the urogram.

Brief mention is also made of the uroradiologic examinations that require manipulative expertise by the radiologist. These are *selective renal arteriography, percutaneous renal needle aspiration,* and *percutaneous antegrade pyelography.* These examinations are minor surgical procedures that require special training of the radiologist. They also involve more risk, more radiation, and more expense to the patient than does urography, cystography, or urethrography. However, for the specific clinical problems for which their use is recommended, the information they provide is critical for optimum decision-making by the physician.

TABLE 3–1   Type of Uroradiologic Examinations

TYPE	NUMBER PERFORMED°
Excretory urography	3835
Retrograde pyelography	92
Cystography	53
Urethrography	241
Selective renal arteriography	218
Renal needle aspiration	30
Antegrade pyelography	2

°At the University of Michigan Hospital, July 1973 through June 1974.

Diagnostic Strategy

The proper selection of radiologic procedures that will solve clinical diagnostic or management problems is best understood if considered from a decision theory standpoint. Diagnostic decisions are made on the basis of information gathered by the physician from the patient and his record (i.e., history and physical examination) and from testing procedures (e.g., laboratory studies and radiologic examinations). These decisions are made within the context of the physician's general medical knowledge and prior clinical experience.

Two principles that pertain to the acquisition of information must be appreciated. First, the value of information is in its changing probabilities. In medical diagnosis, this means that *useful* information changes a physician's diagnostic certainty. Second, there is always a "cost" involved in obtaining information. This cost is divided into five categories: (1) *radiation exposure* to the patient, (2) *risk* to the patient from injection of radiopaque contrast materials, (3) *dollar cost* of the examination, (4) *time* away from the patient's income-producing work, and (5) *discomfort* experienced by the patient.

When the physician selects a uroradiologic examination to gain diagnostic information, he must balance the expected return of useful information against the overall cost (radiation, risk, dollars, time, and discomfort) to the patient. The medical student learns about guidelines for the "useful information expectation" aspect by reading about "indications" for examinations that are listed in texts and by observing how experienced clinicians make the choices of what to do and when to do it. However, the student seldom learns the "cost" aspect of the choice unless he asks the physician.

The disquieting thing about asking the attending physician to estimate the overall cost is that often the physician does not know the answer. Often a better source for answering this cost question is the radiologist. Students and house officers should make it a point to ask *both* attending physicians and radiologists these questions in regard to their patients so that they will know the cost aspect and learn to make more informed choices of examinations.

A physician should not request a radiologic examination simply because it is a means of extending the physical examination to areas he cannot see, palpate, or auscultate. There should be a sound reason why a particular examination is ordered for a specific patient and that reason should be based on an expected useful diagnostic information return. If a urogram is requested and performed merely to satisfy the idle curiosity of the physician and that patient happens to be the 1 of 40,000 patients having a urogram who dies unexpectedly from a severe contrast material reaction, then the physician has been judgmentally and ethically wrong in requesting the urogram.

To avoid this difficulty, the physician should be certain that he first forms a problem statement from the clinical information at hand. Based on this statement, he then formulates a diagnostic hypothesis to explain the cause of the problem that he has identified. Only then does he consider the array of examinations available and select the one which is most likely to give him further useful information in solving the problem. After obtaining the radiologic information, he then revises his diagnostic hypothesis in light of that information. If this information fully supports his diagnosis, he can then make treatment decisions. If not, he has to use other tests to verify his diagnosis to the extent that he is willing to make such treatment decisions.

Tailored vs. Routine Uroradiology

It is the author's conviction that the optimum information from a uroradiologic examination results from a knowledgeable radiologist monitoring and modifying (i.e., "tailoring") the examination to each patient with the aim to providing radiologic answers to those clinical questions raised in that particular patient's case. This technique runs counter to the procedure of doing a "routine" fixed sequence of radiographs on every patient regardless of the problem involved. In other words, a directed information search is employed in individual cases rather than a routine general screening approach to all problems.

This approach means that the radiologist has to know the pertinent clinical information available at the time of the examination and the diagnoses being considered. The best procedure to follow in radiologic consultation has the physician personally telling the radiologist this information. However, such personal contact is not usually feasible or possible except in very complex cases. A compromise is to have the patient's record in hand for review before doing the examination and to use the attending physician's problem statement or his diagnosis from the x-ray requisition. Occasionally the radiologist will have to call the physician for additional information before doing the examination. On rare occasions the radiologist will have to confer in depth with the physician since, from the radiologic viewpoint, the examination is not indicated, or a different examination would provide more useful information.

URORADIOLOGIC EXAMINATIONS

Excretory Urography

Most common of the uroradiologic examinations, excretory uro-graphy also may be called intravenous pyelography (IVP) or intra-venous urography. The student should understand that the basic exami-nation concept is the same, regardless of the name. Excretory urography requires the intravenous injection of a radiopaque contrast material in order to make the urinary tract more visible on radiographs of the abdomen. The contrast material is opaque to x-rays because it contains three atoms of iodine per molecule. Iodine has a relatively high atomic number (53) and absorbs a greater proportion of the x-ray beam striking it than do the lower atomic number components of ab-dominal soft tissue structures and body fluids such as blood and urine.

The intravenous contrast material reaches the heart as a bolus, traverses the pulmonary circuit, is ejected from the left ventricle, and is dispersed to the arterial circulation quite rapidly. Normally, the first contrast material reaches the kidney within 15 seconds after the start of the injection. Upon reaching the kidneys (via the aorta and renal arte-ries), the contrast material is excreted by the individual nephrons and follows the route of urine production and flow. The mechanism of con-trast material excretion is by glomerular filtration. As the nephron lumen is traversed, the contrast material is concentrated within the urine that flows through the proximal and distal convoluted tubule. The mechanism of concentration is by water reabsorption through the tubular wall cells.

Upon leaving the nephron, the contrast laden urine travels to the tip of the renal papilla via collecting ducts and flows into the adjacent draining minor calyx. Radiopaque urine is then transported to the exter-nal environment via the collecting system (minor and major calyces and renal pelvis), ureter, bladder, and urethra. Contrast material first reaches the bladder four to five minutes after the start of injection.

Excretory urography is made possible by this serial opacification of the urine in the kidney, ureter, and bladder. By taking radiographs at proper intervals, the gross anatomy of these portions of the urinary tract can be demonstrated. Since 50 per cent of the injected contrast material normally is filtered from the plasma by the glomeruli within 30 to 60 minutes, and the peak of the urine flow is induced by the hyperosmolar contrast material in 10 to 12 minutes after injection, the filming sequence is planned accordingly. (See Fig. 3–1.)

EXCRETORY UROGRAM FILMING IN NORMAL ADULTS

Prior to the Injection. A preliminary radiograph of the abdomen, known as a scout film, preliminary film, or KUB, is taken to see the ini-tial aspects of the patient's anatomy prior to opacification by the con-

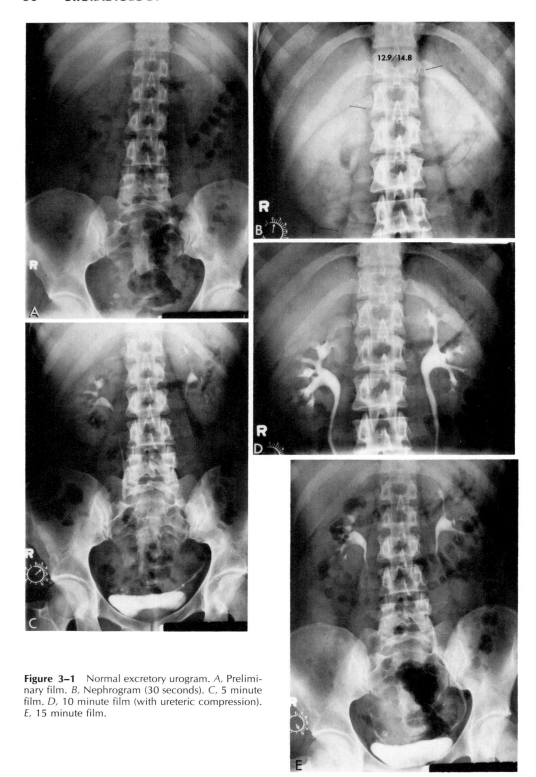

Figure 3–1 Normal excretory urogram. *A,* Preliminary film. *B,* Nephrogram (30 seconds). *C,* 5 minute film. *D,* 10 minute film (with ureteric compression). *E,* 15 minute film.

trast material. In particular, one should look for urinary calculi and calcifications that might be subsequently obscured by opacified urine.

At the End of the Injection.   A small radiograph of the kidneys, known as a nephrogram film or 30 second film, is taken to capture the transient general opacification of the renal parenchyma when contrast material first reaches the kidneys and is in the nephrons and collecting ducts. Defects in the parenchyma that are due to scarring, cysts, or tumors are often highlighted in this view.

Five Minutes After Injection.   A radiograph of the abdomen is taken that includes the kidney and bladder regions. By this time early filling of the collecting systems, ureters, and bladder has occurred, and the nephrogram effect in the kidneys has faded. The symmetry of bilateral fill of the collecting systems and ureters plus a degree of concentration of the opacified urine provides early clues as to the presence of obstruction or renal parenchymal abnormality.

Ten Minutes After Injection.   A small radiograph of the kidneys is obtained during ureteric compression (a compression device that wraps around the patient has been in place since the five minute film was obtained). Collecting system distension is greatest at this point, and fine detail of calyceal anatomy is best shown. A film at this stage is particularly useful for detecting signs of pyelonephritis or destruction that is due to a tumor. Oblique views may be obtained for a better assessment of the anterior and posterior aspects of the kidneys.

Fifteen Minutes After Injection.   A large abdominal radiograph is taken for an overall survey of the kidneys, ureters, and bladder with the compression device having been removed as soon as the ten minute film was obtained. By now the collecting systems are less full, different portions of the ureters are visible than were seen on the five minute film, a result that is due to intermittent peristalsis, and the bladder is more completely filled and opacified.

GROUND RULES FOR LOOKING AT UROGRAMS

The useful diagnostic information is seldom restricted to one radiograph out of the sequence. The series of films must be regarded as a whole. However, the viewer has to look at each film in detail, understand its relationship to the normal sequence of contrast excretion, and then integrate each film's information into a total diagnostic information package.

In order to make optimum use of the urogram in decision-making, the radiologic findings must be correlated with clinical information about the problem at hand. The prime risk in this correlation is that the clinician may unconsciously restrict his visual search of the urogram films to that of looking for clues that are specific for the problem hypothesis he has previously framed from the patient's history, physical examination, and laboratory test results. To avoid this tendency, the clinician must make a second and third effort after his initial search of the films to look specifically for (1) calculi or calcifications in the urinary tract and (2) abnormal anatomy in other regions included on the urograms, such as the liver, spleen, skeleton, retroperitoneal soft tissue, or intestines. This search is most commonly useful in turning up evidence of destruction that is due to malignancy or for multiorgan disease, such as hematologic disorders.

One should always keep in mind that the density, or "whiteness," of the contrast opacified urine on the radiograph does *not* quantitatively relate to the number of functioning nephrons or to the efficiency with which they either filter the contrast material at the glomerular level or concentrate the contrast material laden urine at the tubular level. Kidneys with considerable parenchymal loss can still excrete and concentrate contrast material to a normal degree. In addition, anatomically normal kidneys may *not* excrete or concentrate contrast material to normal density on the film in the face of high urine flow from diuresis or low renal blood flow, as in hypotension due to shock. To measure renal function, one must do specific renal function tests.

OVERALL COST OF UROGRAPHY

Radiation exposure to the patient is inherent in all x-ray examinations. The aim of the radiologist is to take as few radiographs as are necessary to provide the most useful information for the individual patient's specific problem. The exposure dosage is diminished by limiting the x-ray beam to the margins of the film size for each exposure.

The gonads are the most sensitive organs to the radiation that occurs during urography. Testes receive a higher dose than do ovaries from the same exposure. The ovaries are protected by a relatively large amount of intervening abdominal soft tissue that absorbs a large portion of the x-ray beam and results in about one tenth the dose received by the testes. In some circumstances, lead gonad shields can be used to diminish gonad irradiation.

Gonad irradiation is of concern because it has been shown that in experimental animals chromosome abnormalities and resultant genetic problems can be caused. The *minimum* dosages required to produce these effects in humans are not known when x-ray beam quality and dosage ranges on the order of those used in diagnostic radiology are considered. This radiation danger is primarily of concern in adults in the child bearing age (to age 35 years or so) and in children.

A related radiation risk is in pregnancy, particularly during the first eight to twelve weeks when the fetus is most sensitive to radiation. Urography should be avoided during pregnancy to prevent an increased incidence of congenital malformations. The estimated risk using modern equipment and filming techniques is very low but still is one to consider. If urography is required during pregnancy because of life threatening reasons, the examination should be restricted to the most essential films.

Risk of reaction to contrast material injection falls into two categories: *minor reactions* and *major reactions*. Major reactions are those that rapidly lead to death and feature either precipitous respiratory arrest or cardiovascular collapse. The frequency of death has been documented to be about 1 in 40,000 urogram injections. The mechanism of major reaction is unknown and thus cannot be prevented. Likewise, preinjection testing to detect fatal reactors is not possible. Therefore, though of low incidence, the potential major reaction risk must be balanced by the clinician against the expected useful information return when he is deciding whether to request urography.

Minor reactions most commonly consist of nausea or vomiting, generalized flushing, or a peculiar taste or sensation in the tongue or throat. These reactions occur individually or in combination in about 5 to 10 per cent of patients. Less common are hives, edema about the eyes or mouth, or an asthmaticlike breathing difficulty. The mechanism of minor reactions also is unknown, and they cannot be prevented by prophylactic medication. Most disappear within 15 minutes after injection. Some may require antihistamine or steroid medication for alleviation. The most important thing to know about minor reactions is that they do *not* make it more likely for an individual to have a subsequent major, fatal reaction.

The *dollar cost* of excretory urography varies slightly from institution to institution.* Compared with the cost of other radiologic contrast examinations, this is not high, but someone has to pay the bill, whether it be the patient, the insurance carrier, or the federal government. The latter two primarily collect from the public.

Time required away from work is often a full day, even though the individual's status as an outpatient may be terminated by the end of the morning. Many people having urography may still be upset through the afternoon following the examination from the effects of dehydration and the laxative. For patients in the hospital about half a day is required for urography, which includes waiting without breakfast until the examination is performed and the transportation time to and from the radiology department.

Discomfort to the patient includes the minor reaction sensations discussed previously, venipuncture, the necessity of lying on an x-ray table (padded or otherwise) for a minimum of 20 to 30 minutes clad in a skimpy hospital gown, and the worry about the risk of reaction and the results of the examination.

Contrast Material

Urographic contrast materials in current use are triiodinated, benzene ring based, organic molecular compounds. A physiologically normal kidney excretes and concentrates the contrast material quite efficiently, utilizing the route of urine formation. The mechanisms of

---

*The late 1974 cost at University Hospital, Ann Arbor, Michigan was $41.50.

excretion and concentration involve glomerular filtration and tubular water reabsorption, respectively.

The usual intravenous dosage for normal adults is 50 ml. This should be increased to 100 ml if

1. The serum creatinine is 1.5 to 2.0 mg/100 ml or greater.

2. There is prior information that severe renal damage or urinary obstruction is present, or clinical evidence now indicates this to be very likely.

3. The patient is quite large or obese (despite having a normal creatinine).

4. The patient is being examined in an unprepared state.

The contrast material dose is usually injected as a *bolus*, that is, the total volume is rapidly injected (50 ml within 15 to 20 seconds, 100 ml within 30 to 45 seconds). Rarely, a dilute form of the contrast material is injected slowly as an *infusion* when fragile veins or precarious venipuncture precludes rapid injection. About 200 to 300 ml of half strength contrast material is infused in five to eight minutes. Experimental work indicates that using the larger volume of dilute contrast material does not improve the diagnostic quality of the urogram. The use of a larger volume only increases the cost and the time it takes to do the urogram.

Radiologists or clinicians responsible for injecting urographic contrast material should understand that they must be prepared to handle effectively the rare unexpected cardiac or respiratory arrest. They must be able to resuscitate patients, treat cardiac arrest or fibrillation, interpret EKG's, and have proper equipment available. If they cannot do this procedure personally, then they must have rapid access to a formal cardiac arrest team's expertise.

PATIENT PREPARATION

Under usual circumstances, the patient should have oral food and fluid intake withheld for 6 to 15 hours before urography. This lack of intake makes it less likely that the patient will be in a diuretic high urine flow state, and such fasting enhances the tubular reabsorption of water. The added reabsorption results in greater contrast material density (whiteness) on the radiograph. In addition, at a reasonable length of time before the examination, the patient should receive a laxative to cleanse the colon of feces. Colonic contents commonly obscure details of radiographic anatomy, particularly of the kidneys.

Exceptions to the above general rules are

1. Patients who are off oral intake and are receiving intravenous fluid therapy. The rate of infusion should be slowed for several hours, if possible, prior to the urogram.

2. Patients who have acute abdominal emergency problems.

3. Patients who have established, or strongly suspected, severe diabetes mellitus, multiple myeloma, or uric acid nephropathy. *In a dehydrated state* these patients' kidneys are more sensitive to contrast material and have a tendency to develop renal failure. Therefore, they

should have urography performed when their kidneys are in a normal state of hydration, using the 100 ml dosage of contrast material.

URETERIC COMPRESSION

As mentioned in the section entitled "Excretory Urogram Filming in Normal Adults," the technique of ureteric compression enhances distension of the collecting system and upper ureter. This is accomplished by applying a compression band around the patient at the level of the lower anterior abdomen. The band does not secure the patient to the table since it simply fits tightly around the lower part of the torso. Thus, the patient can be turned into oblique positions for filming with the compression band still in place.

Placed between the underside of the compression band and the skin are two small inflatable balloons positioned so that they overlie the sacral wing bilaterally. They are inflated after the five minute film and remain inflated until the ten minute films are obtained. The aim is to compress the ureters as they cross over the sacral wings. This compression consequently creates a low grade temporary obstruction of the ureteric urine flow so that the collecting systems can be mildly distended for optimum visualization.

Ureteric compression is used on all adults except those who have symptoms of ureteric colic, recent abdominal surgery, acute abdominal pain, abdominal aortic aneurysm, or colostomy or ileostomy stomas. It is effective in distending the collecting systems in about 75 per cent of patients with the failures the result of obesity or improper positioning of the compression balloons. Patient discomfort is mild and transient.

MODIFICATION OF THE BASIC UROGRAM: "TAILORING" *

The procedural variables that can be managed to better obtain answers to urologic clinical questions are listed below.

Contrast Material Dosage. See page 60 for the discussion on contrast material.

Timing of the Filming Sequence. When obstruction is present, the appearance of opacified urine in that part of the urinary tract will be delayed. The more severe the obstruction, the longer the delay. Therefore, *delayed films* of the abdomen may be necessary to delineate a collecting system or ureter even up to 24 or 48 hours after injection.

Early filming between the nephrogram and five minute films is of value when looking for clues to unilateral renal artery stenosis. Films are obtained at two and three minutes after injection so that one may

---

*The author is indebted to Dr. Anthony F. Lalli of the Cleveland Clinic for coining the term *tailored urography.*

look for any asymmetry between the initial appearance of contrast in the calyces, comparing one kidney to the other.

Changing Position of the Patient. When clinical interest is focused on the mid or distal ureter, the patient is turned into the *prone position* to obtain optimum filling of the ureter. One is usually looking for an extrinsic retroperitoneal mass that is leaning on the ureter, or one is trying to encourage (by gravity) the ureter to accept contrast when a partial ureteric obstruction is present.

Emptying the Bladder. Having the patient void accumulated bladder contrast will make the most distal ureter more visible. Most commonly this film is used to look for the precise site of an obstruction due to a small calculus or stricture.

A postvoiding film also indicates to what extent the bladder has emptied at that voiding. If the bladder contrast is emptied normally, it can be assumed that the patient does not carry a large residual urine. If contrast is still retained in the bladder after voiding, *no* assumptions can be made about the presence of residual urine. Some people cannot void on command, and some people are bashful about voiding in strange places. On the other hand, the patient may not be able to empty the bladder for reasons of disease. Which is the true state cannot be determined from this type of postvoiding film result.

Use of Laminagraphy. *Laminagraphy,* also known as tomography or body section radiography, is a special filming technique used to highlight local areas within a section of the kidney (coronal plane). The x-ray tube and film are moved, but in *opposite directions,* during the exposure. The pivot point about which they move defines a plane in which structures at that level are in focus. Structures not in that plane are blurred. Laminagraphy is used primarily to define renal margins or to look for nephrogram defects that differentiate renal cyst from malignant tumor of the kidney. The technique also improves visualization of the kidney when overlying feces obscure detail.

Some radiologists recommend that laminagraphy be done on all urogram cases for the most complete assessment of the kidney possible. It is the author's opinion that if a normal dense nephrogram is obtained, the collecting system detail is well seen, and all the renal margins are clearly defined, then laminagraphy is not necessary in those cases. Short of these criteria, laminagraphy should be carried out.

UROGRAPHY IN CHILDREN

Children provide a different urographic challenge than adults. Contrast material dosage is less than for adults, varying as to age and weight. On the whole, once calyceal filling begins, children have a more rapid serial opacification of the upper urinary tract than do adults. Children normally distend their collecting systems better than adults, and ureteric compression is not required, except in adolescents on occasion.

Preparation by dehydration and laxative administration is seldom necessary and in fact is contraindicated in infants and small children. Particular attention should be paid to limiting the number of films to those necessary for obtaining the optimum information required by the clinical problem. It is not unusual to end up with a three film urogram on children who indicate no obstruction or tumor problems (a preliminary, five minute, and ten minute film).

Besides having the examination tailored by a radiologist, two other factors are essential for obtaining optimum films in urography on children. An interested, sympathetic, and knowledgeable technologist is very important for the successful urography of any patient, but the presence of such an individual is particularly important when handling children. Of equal importance is expertly done venipuncture for contrast material injection.

RECOGNITION AND DIAGNOSIS OF ABNORMAL STATES

Pathologic states that affect the excretion and concentration of contrast material fall into three basic categories:

1. *Parenchymal damage* to the kidney (e.g., chronic pyelonephritis), which results in a diminished nephron population and decreased renal function.

2. *Obstruction* of the flow of urine (e.g., due to a calculus impacted in the ureter), which can occur at any level in the urinary tract from the renal tubules to the tip of the urethral meatus. Obstruction affects the handling of contrast material by the kidney by causing higher fluid pressures within the nephrons, thus creating a backpressure phenomenon.

3. *Abnormal blood supply* to, or within, the kidney. This category includes *functional* causes (e.g., hypotension in shock states) and *anatomic* causes (e.g., renal artery stenosis from atherosclerosis) of abnormal blood flow.

The above three basic states may afflict the kidney independently or in combination, depending on the particular pathologic entity involved. To complicate matters, pathologic entities commonly exist together and not in isolation. For example, in an older man an enlarged prostate may prevent normal bladder emptying and cause obstruction of the ureters. This obstruction results in increased urinary pressure, which affects glomerular and tubular function. These nephrons are often already handicapped by considerable atherosclerotic changes in the renal arteries of this older man.

Thus, the clinician and the radiologist are confronted daily with multivariable, coexistent problems of varying complexity rather than with those of a simple nature. Effectively dealing with the ambiguous information that results from these many differently weighted variables is what diagnosis is all about.

It is very important for students and house officers to develop their own categorical frameworks from reading and lecture material upon which they can base problem solving. It is just as important that they accumulate as much experience as they can in order to learn about the exceptions to the rules. However, it is critical that they regularly look at their experience in retrospect so that errors in judgment or testing are revealed. This constant reevaluation is the only way basic rules and their exceptions can be updated, thus assuring that the student and house officer *learn*. This process should not end when the student enters into practice but should expand as further experience accumulates and new methods of diagnosis and treatment are developed.

Perplexing as these concepts may be, the student and house officer should be comforted by the fact that pathologic states which affect contrast material handling and alter anatomy are often indicated by rather simplistic signs on the urogram. Anatomy is either normal or it is not. Normal serial opacification of the urinary tract follows injection, or it does not. Contrast density (whiteness) is either normal, diminished, or greater than normally expected.

Consequently, the primary goal for the student should be to learn normal radiographic anatomy and contrast handling. Secondarily, the student should absorb the much more interesting and exciting findings of abnormal states. However, he must learn early on to recognize the normal state so that he subsequently can identify the presence of any early abnormality. He should familiarize himself with as many normal urogram images as possible during his clinical training in order to learn normal variations of anatomy and function. Following the same approach, the house officer should, in addition, strive to increase his knowledge of the exceptions to the rules and store the images of a wider spectrum of abnormalities in his visual memory bank.

The best opportunity a young physician has to learn from his mistakes and the mistakes of others is during his student and house officer days. Most people have to sink a few times before they learn how to swim.

Retrograde Pyelography

This is a radiographic examination that requires a urologic procedure for its performance. Through a cystoscope placed in the bladder via the urethra, the ureteric orifices are cannulated by the urologist under direct vision using the telescopic viewing system of the cystoscope. A small caliber plastic ureteric catheter is passed up the ureter to about the level of the renal pelvis. A preliminary film is obtained, and then a small amount (6 to 10 ml) of contrast material is injected into the collecting system via the catheter, thus delineating the collecting system and ureter (Fig. 3–2).

Retrograde pyelography is reserved for cases in which excretory urography has failed to provide satisfactory diagnostic information. Usually this occurs when the kidney has become affected by a disease process and has been unable to either excrete enough opacified urine

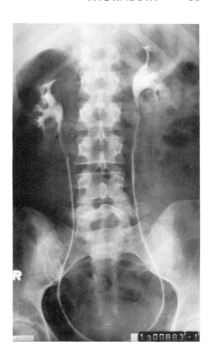

Figure 3–2 Normal retrograde pyelogram with ureteric catheters in place.

or concentrate it sufficiently to permit the delineation of the collecting system or ureter. Pathologic states commonly causing such conditions are obstruction (e.g., ureteric obstruction by tumor) or severe renal damage (e.g., from extensive renal tumor). (See Figure 3–3.)

The disadvantages of retrograde pyelography are (1) the requirement of an additional procedure (cystoscopy), and (2) the risk of causing urinary infection or of stirring up pre-existing infection through the manipulation of the urinary tract. This examination involves more dollar cost, discomfort, and time off from work for the patient than does excretory urography. Radiation exposure is usually less than with excretory urography because fewer films are obtained.

From the standpoint of overall information about the urinary tract, retrograde pyelography provides only direct information about the collecting system and ureters. It does not provide information about the status of blood flow to the kidney, the capabilities of the nephrons to excrete and opacify urine, or the efficiency of the collecting system and ureter in the undisturbed state to transport opacified urine to the bladder. However, when the use of retrograde pyelography is indicated, the information it does provide is often crucial for optimum patient management.

Cystography and Urethrography

These examinations may be done separately or in combination. Their use is reserved for clinical problems which focus attention

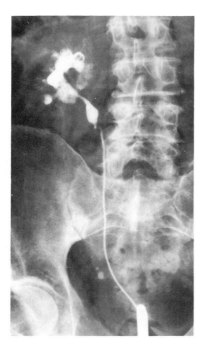

Figure 3–3 Right retrograde pyelogram with grossly deformed collecting system due to transitional cell carcinoma.

primarily on the bladder or urethra rather than on the upper urinary tract. *Cystography* (Fig. 3–4) is accomplished by placing a Foley catheter into the bladder through the urethra. Contrast material is then injected, using gravity filling, until the bladder is distended to the point that the patient has the urge to void. Radiographs are obtained in frontal and occasionally oblique projections. The contrast material delin-

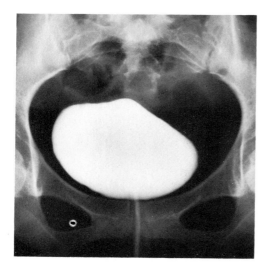

Figure 3–4 Normal cystogram.

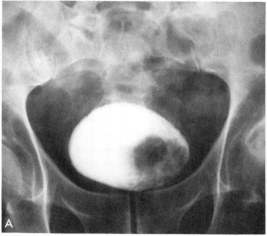

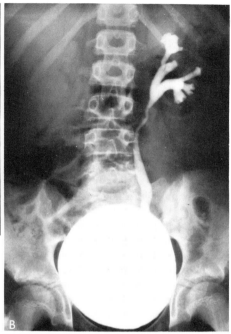

Figure 3–5 Abnormal cystograms. *A*, Large bladder tumor intruding on bladder lumen. *B*, Left vesicoureteric reflux in recurrent cystitis.

eates the inside surface of the bladder and vesicoureteric reflux of opacified urine if it is present (Fig. 3–5).

At this point two options are available to obtain further information. The catheter may be removed, the patient asked to void, and radiographs of the urethra obtained during voiding. This provides a voiding urethrogram study. When combined with the original cystogram films and a subsequent postvoiding film, the entire sequence is known as *voiding cystourethrography* (Fig. 3–6).

The second option is to simply empty the bladder via the catheter

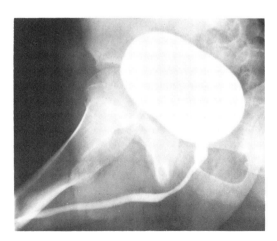

Figure 3–6 Normal voiding cystourethrogram.

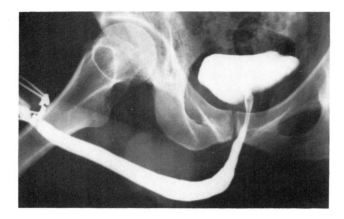

Figure 3–7 Normal   retrograde urethrogram.

and obtain a postdrainage film. The examination combining the cystogram and the drainage film is still called simply *cystography.* It does not provide information about the urethra or the functional emptying capability of the bladder. However, it does demonstrate the bladder and its contents, frequently to better advantage than seen on excretory urography.

Another method to demonstrate the male urethra which does not involve catheterizing the bladder is *retrograde urethrography* (Fig. 3–7). Using a widemouthed syringe, very thick, jellylike contrast material is injected into the external urethral meatus. A radiograph taken at the end of an injection of about 20 to 25 ml shows the anterior urethral lumen and occasionally a glimpse of the urethra proximal to the urogenital diaphragm. This is a simple examination primarily intended only to provide gross information about strictures and extravasation involving the anterior urethra (Fig. 3–8). The female urethra cannot be adequately examined by this technique, and voiding cystourethrography is used instead.

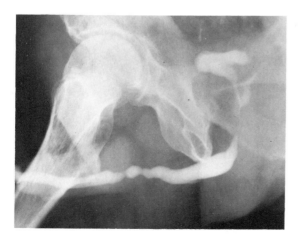

Figure 3–8 Anterior urethral stricture on retrograde urethrogram.

The overall cost of these examinations of the lower urinary tract varies from that of excretory urography. *Radiation exposure* to the gonads is usually more in cystography and urethrography since the gonads are more directly in the x-ray beam. How much more depends on the number of films taken. *Risk of reaction* to contrast material, either major or minor, is practically nonexistent. However, an additional new risk of stirring up existing infection or introducing new infection (inherent in catheterization) has been added. The frequency of this complication is low but must be considered particularly in those with previous urinary infection.

The *dollar cost* is generally less than that for excretory urography.* *Time* required off work varies with the incidence of complicating infection; in its absence, one-half day would be the usual requirement. *Discomfort* occurs primarily from the catheter being passed through the urethra into the bladder or by the distension of the male urethra by retrograde injection. Neither sensation is pleasant, but both are transient.

URORADIOLOGIC SPECIAL EXAMINATIONS

The examinations in this category are (1) *selective renal arteriography*, (2) *needle aspiration* (i.e., cyst puncture), and (3) *antegrade pyelography*. These examinations are reserved for use in specific clinical problems when the information they provide is critical for diagnosis or patient management decisions. The more specific information that they provide is purchased at greater overall cost as compared to the more general information-gathering type of examination such as excretory urography.

The proper performance of these examinations requires that the radiologist possess minor surgical skills and the training necessary to execute and interpret them. In addition, he must be performing these examinations in sufficient numbers to maintain his expertise since they are not simple procedures that can be performed in a casual fashion by partially trained people. With the advance of technology, the number of these special procedures has increased, creating a subspecialty procedural area within diagnostic radiology.

Selective Renal Arteriography

Sophisticated x-ray equipment and facilities are required for arteriography. These examinations are generally performed in an angiography suite within the radiology department. The basic equipment components include (1) an image intensified fluoroscopy with televi-

---

*At University Hospital in Ann Arbor, Michigan, the cost of cystography in late 1974 was $30.00; voiding cystourethrography, $48.00; and retrograde urethrography, $18.00.

sion monitoring, (2) rapid filming devices, and (3) pressure injection devices for the rapid injection of contrast material.

The examination sequence generally involves the following. After skin antisepsis and local anesthesia of the femoral triangle has been administered, the radiologist pierces the femoral artery through the skin using a special needle. He then passes a flexible guide wire into the lumen of the artery via the channel provided by the special needle. The needle is withdrawn, leaving several inches of the guide wire in the arterial lumen. A radiopaque plastic vascular catheter, larger in caliber than the guide wire, is passed over the guide wire, through the skin, and into the artery. This method of percutaneous vascular catheterization is known as the Seldinger Technique and has the advantage of not requiring surgical exposure of the artery for catheter introduction.

The radiologist now can advance the catheter containing the guide wire up the femoral and iliac arteries and into the aorta. Once he has reached the level of the renal arteries, the radiologist can manipulate the catheter into the proximal renal artery using the television fluoroscope to chart his course. Once the catheter is hooked into the renal artery, a small volume of contrast material is injected within one to two seconds, and the renal arterial supply is opacified for a brief time. Stages of filling and emptying of the renal arterial tree are captured on serial films exposed at a rate of two to three films per second for three to four seconds. Several slightly delayed films will normally demonstrate the main draining renal veins (Fig. 3–9). Additional injection in the oblique position can be done, or the catheter can be inserted in the opposite renal artery and injection performed to see the contralateral

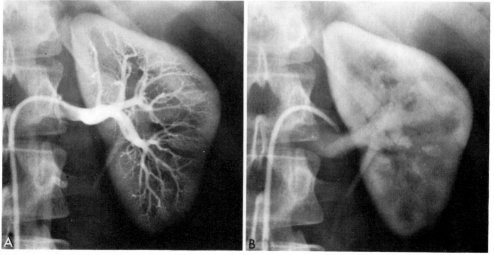

Figure 3–9 Normal selective renal arteriogram. *A,* Early in arterial filling phase (at 1.5 seconds). *B,* Main renal vein well opacified late in filming sequence (at 8 seconds). Corticomedullary junction is well delineated.

kidney and its vasculature. If the aorta is of interest, an injection can be made using the same catheter, but with its tip in the aortic lumen, and serial filming done.

Information from arteriography can be used to

1. Evaluate blood flow dynamics (e.g., when looking for renal artery stenosis in hypertensive patients).

2. Document abnormal vasculature (e.g., characteristic patterns of vessels supplying malignant tumors).

3. Determine the cause of scarring of the renal parenchyma (e.g., differentiation of chronic pyelonephritis from arteriolonephrosclerosis).

4. Determine the cause of renal space-occupying lesions discovered on urography (e.g., differentiation of tumor from cyst or cortical nodule).

The overall cost of arteriography is as follows. The *dollar cost* is considerably more than that for urography.* *Radiation risk* varies greatly from patient to patient depending upon how complicated the problem is under study. The total minimum fluoroscopic and filming radiation dosage is about 10 to 15 times that experienced with excretory urography. However, the gonads are not in the direct x-ray beam, and only scattered radiation reaches them. Thus the total gonad exposure is only three to four times that of urography. Needless to say, arteriography should be avoided during pregnancy it at all possible.

Risk of a fatal reaction to the contrast material is less of a possibility than that from urography. However, vascular complications add another risk factor. Delayed bleeding from the puncture site occurs in about 1 of 500 patients. Thrombosis at the puncture site occurs in about 1 of 800 patients and results in the loss of the lower extremity in about 1 of 10,000 patients. One other complication is contrast induced renal failure, which occurs in about 1 of 700 patients.

These potential complications require that the patient be in the hospital for observation following arteriography. Thus a minimum of two patient days is usually necessary from the patient's *working time.* *Patient discomfort* is greater than that experienced in urography and includes pain and swelling at the puncture site, vague abdominal pain, and prominent hot flush sensations during injection. Complete bed rest is required for 8 to 12 hours after injection.

Needle Aspiration (Cyst Puncture)

This examination is reserved for the evaluation of patients in whom urography has provided evidence of a cystic lesion in the kidney. Information from a previous ultrasound examination of the kidney may further increase the certainty that the lesion is fluid filled. The question to be answered is whether the "cystic lump" in the kidney is a benign

---

*The 1974 dollar cost at University Hospital, Ann Arbor, Michigan was $273 for a study of both kidneys.

simple renal cyst or a necrotic, cystic renal adenocarcinoma (hypernephroma).

Needle aspiration is performed in the following manner. Contrast material is given as in excretory urography to opacify the kidney and its collecting system. The patient is placed in the prone position five minutes after injection, and the renal area of interest is observed on the television fluoroscope. Following skin antisepsis and local anesthesia down to the renal capsule, the radiologist passes a 20 gauge, eight inch needle percutaneously into the renal lesion. He watches the television image of the course of the needle as he advances it into the lesion to assure that his aim is true.

The fluid contents of the lesion are partially aspirated for visual and cytologic inspection. Contrast material is injected into the lumen of the cyst to determine characteristics of its wall and inner surface. This is documented on frontal and oblique single radiographs (Fig. 3–10). Then the total lesion contents are aspirated.

If no free fluid is obtained because the seemingly cystic lesion is actually an avascular tumor or a dysplastic anomaly of the kidney, a small cytologic specimen is aspirated. Then a small contrast injection is made into the lesion, and the contrast distribution pattern of the solid lesion is documented on a radiograph.

The information from needle aspiration falls into three categories:

1. Appearance of the aspirate.
2. Cytologic diagnosis from the aspirate.
3. X-ray appearance of the lesion.

The interpretation of this information is discussed in the section entitled "The Renal Cyst/Tumor/Cortical Nodule Problem."

The overall cost of needle aspiration includes the following. The

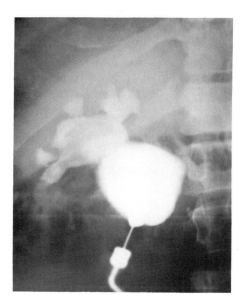

Figure 3–10 Cyst puncture. Medially situated smooth benign cyst lumen is shown by injected contrast material. Collecting system is opacified lateral to the cyst from previous intravenous injection.

1974 *dollar cost* was $89.00.* *Contrast reaction* risk is similar to that expected in excretory urography, both as to major and minor reactions. *Radiation risk* is probably slightly greater than with urography. Fewer films that include the gonad area are taken than in urography, but secondary radiation scatter from the fluoroscopic beam restricted to the kidney section elevates the total gonad dosage over that of urography. Fluoroscopic radiation dosage, however, is less than that from renal arteriography.

Experience indicates that *complications* from placing a needle into the renal lesion are low in frequency and minor in consequence. Transient abdominal pain (20 minutes or so in duration) can occur from the leaking of hyperosmolar contrast material from the puncture site in the lesion. This happens in 8 of 100 patients and disappears spontaneously. About 5 of 100 patients will have transient hematuria for several hours after needle placement. The author has not encountered renal or perirenal hemorrhage in cases of benign simple cysts or malignant tumors.

The potential risk of spreading malignant cells along the needle tract or disseminating cells intravascularly from puncturing a tumor has been raised in the past as a reason not to do renal needle aspiration. It has been documented in the Karolinska experience that this is not a real risk, and the experience in other large case groups supports these findings.

The potential minor complications do not require hospitalization for observation, and aspiration can be done on an outpatient basis. Therefore, *patient time off work* varies from one-half to one day, depending upon scheduling circumstances. *Patient discomfort* ranges from minor subjective responses to contrast injection (as in urography) to the uncommon occurrence of transient abdominal pain following puncture. Brief pain during placement of local anesthesia to the level of the renal capsule occurs prior to needle placement.

Antegrade Pyelography

This examination is seldom used, but for the isolated specific instances when it is indicated, the information it provides is uniquely valuable. The usual reason for employing antegrade pyelography is to determine the site and cause of obstruction of the ureter or renal pelvis when the obstruction is so severe that the kidney cannot excrete urographic contrast material (Fig. 3–11). Commonly, retrograde pyelography is performed as an alternative to excretory urography in this circumstance. However, occasionally it is not technically possible to catheterize the ureteric orifice, or the urologist does not want to introduce instruments into the bladder when obvious urinary infection is present.

_____

*At University Hospital.

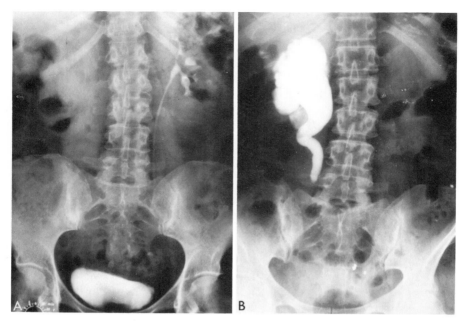

Figure 3–11 Antegrade pyelogram. A, Prior urogram shows nonopacification of the right collecting system or ureter in a patient with carcinoma of the cervix. B, Antegrade pyelogram delineates dilated collecting system and ureter to level of obstruction by metastatic neoplasm.

The basic procedure is identical to that used in needle aspiration with two exceptions. The target for puncture is a very dilated (hydronephrotic) collecting system instead of a "cystic lump." In addition, the dilated collecting system may be only faintly opacified by the urographic contrast material or only a slightly more dense nephrogram of very thin renal parenchyma will be visible. When even these faint images are absent in very severe obstruction, the radiologist has to imagine the location of the kidney on the television monitor, basing his judgment on previous laminagrams done during urography, in order to locate the renal margins.

The types of information gained from antegrade pyelography include the

1. Appearance of the aspirate.

2. Cytologic diagnosis from the aspirate.

3. Degree of dilatation of the collecting system or ureter and features of the obstructing lesion and its location.

The overall cost factors are the same as with needle aspiration with one exception. The risk of aggravating infection in the upper urinary tract is added to the complications of needle aspiration. When severe obstruction of the upper tract is present, chronic infection is also often present to some degree. Therefore, when infection is strongly suspected, prophylactic antibiotic therapy is given for 24 hours prior to and 48 hours after needle aspiration to avoid an acute flare of chronic pyelonephritis.

NORMAL RADIOGRAPHIC ANATOMY AND LANDMARKS

Kidneys

A right and left kidney characterized by fairly similar gross anatomic features are present in most humans. However, the right and left kidneys are rarely a mirror image of each other (Fig. 3–12). This asymmetry applies within a single kidney as well. Very seldom does the upper half of the internal renal architecture match even closely the lower half. Normal asymmetry is understandable in view of the embryologic pattern of renal development. The ureteric bud ascends from the pelvis toward the future retroperitoneum and begins its rapid serial dichotomous branching that stimulates the nephrogenic blastema to form nephrons and other renal elements. The possibilities for variation in rate and speed of this process are many. Actually, it is surprising that asymmetry is not more pronounced.

The left kidney lies slightly more cephalad than the right and commonly is slightly longer than the right. Renal length is measured as the longest dimension from the tip of the upper pole to lower pole. Usually this dimension parallels the margin of the psoas muscle. Most normal adult kidneys fall within the 11 to 15 cm range for renal length. Usually the difference in length between the right and left kidney is no more than 1.5 cm. During urography, as diuresis is caused by the hyperosmolar contrast material, the length of each kidney increases by 0.5 cm or so if one measures the renal length on all the urogram films. This variation is limited in older individuals by changes in the renal interstitium caused by aging and by the development of arterionephrosclerosis.

The outline of the kidney is best delineated on the nephrogram just after injection, and it gives the visual impression of the normal reniform shape in a fashion similar to a silhouette. The shape of normal

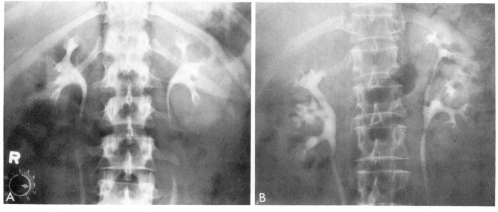

Figure 3–12 Normal renal collecting system asymmetry. A, Fairly symmetrical. B, Quite asymmetrical. Right upper calyx in A and both upper calyces in B show examples of normal compound calyx variation.

kidneys can range from short and wide to long and thin but commonly will resemble the familiar "kidney bean." Frequently, the renal outline will be smooth, but occasionally it will have normal but irregularly shaped indentations known as fetal lobulations (see Fig. 3–14). The nephrogram film also provides an indication of the uniformity of distribution of nephrons and collecting ducts within the renal parenchyma. Normally this uniformity should appear as a homogenous "lighting up" of the renal substance within the confines of the renal outlines.

The density, or whiteness, of the nephrogram depends upon the rapidity of contrast material injection and the amount of contrast material used. It also depends upon the number of normally functioning nephrons present and a normal renal blood supply. If 50 ml of one of the currently used urographic contrast agents is injected intravenously within 10 to 15 seconds, the nephrogram will be quite distinct and bright in normal individuals. The normal nephrogram whiteness usually fades almost completely within three to five minutes after injection.

As the patient's age increases beyond 40 to 45 years, nephrosclerosis and aging processes begin to diminish the number of nephrons, and the usual nephrogram will be less "white" than in younger patients. Another cause of diminished nephrogram density is decreased renal blood flow. Two pathologic states, severe renal artery stenosis and severe shock, are examples in which the nephrogram density is very low or even nonexistent.

The configuration of the collecting system (minor and major calyces and renal pelvis) *and* its relation to the size and shape of the kidney are major factors that lead an observer to decide whether a kidney is normal or abnormal on a urogram. Usually there are 8 to 14 minor calyces per kidney. Often they are clustered in upper, mid, and lower groups. Occasionally they will cluster only in an upper and a lower group. Urine in each cluster of minor calyces drains through a major calyx, or infundibulum, to the renal pelvis.

The term *calyx* means cup in Latin, and a minor calyx resembles a cup when seen in profile. Its shape is due to the insertion of the renal papilla into the minor calyx. The brim of the cup, or fornix portion of the calyx, is normally sharply marginated. When a single papilla inserts into a minor calyx, the calyx will be small and delicate. When several papillae fuse and insert into a calyx as a larger more irregularly surfaced structure, a much different calyceal appearance results. This peculiar looking, but still normal, minor calyx is commonly called a "compound calyx" (see Fig. 3–12).

The major calyces, or infundibula, vary from long and thin to short and wide. Sometimes they are practically nonexistent, with the minor calyces looking as if they drain directly into the renal pelvis. The variation in normal major calyx configuration is great even within a single kidney.

The renal pelvis also exists in all sizes and shapes. Basically there

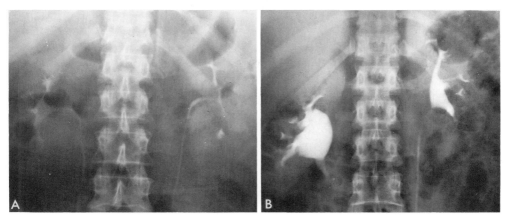

Figure 3–13   Normal renal pelvis variations. *A,* Intrarenal. *B,* Extrarenal.

are two types, intrarenal and extrarenal (Fig. 3–13). The *intrarenal* pelvis is relatively small in volume and narrow in caliber. It lies deep within the renal substance in the renal hilum and is firmly clutched by the surrounding renal parenchyma. The *extrarenal* pelvis is located for the most part outside the grasp of the kidney and is larger in volume and caliber than the intrarenal variety. It distends to a much greater degree under the influence of diuresis than does the more tightly constrained intrarenal pelvis.

Under the influence of a changing rate of urine flow and intermittent peristalsis, the collecting system volume and size changes somewhat from film to film during urography. The student and resident must learn the normal range of this change in shape by putting together the images from all of the films of the urogram.

Appreciating the collecting system anatomy is important, but it is critical that the observer relates it to the overall size and shape of the renal parenchyma. Normally on a urogram, an imaginary line joining the tips of the minor calyces follows the same course as the accompanying renal margin (Fig. 3–14). This assessment is important to make in order to perceive renal parenchymal scarring.

Occasionally this guideline for normal parenchymal thickness does not hold when more cortical than medullary tissue is present in one part of a kidney. Then the minor calyx appears farther away than usual from the renal margin, and the nephrogram often is more dense in this area. This variation of normal anatomy is known as a benign cortical nodule, or prominent column of Bertin, and must not be confused with a renal tumor (see Fig. 3–34).

Ureters

Normally, the ureter gently curves downward and medially from its origin at the ureteropelvic junction. It goes over the anterolateral aspect

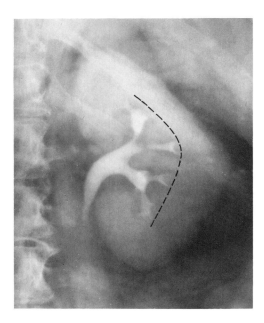

Figure 3–14 Normal relationship of minor calyceal tips to the renal margin. Dromedary kidney shape and fetal lobulation variations (lower lateral margin) are also present.

of the psoas muscle, and on the urogram it is seen to cross the tips of the lower lumbar transverse processes. Then it passes over the lateral extent of the sacrum and dips into the confines of the bony pelvis. The distal third of the ureter then more or less follows the curve of the pelvic wall and finally heads medially and downward to enter the bladder at the trigone.

How much of the entire length of the normal ureter is seen on the serial films of a urographic study depends on the amount of contrast material injected and the instant in time the film is exposed in relation to the peristaltic activity of the ureter at that instant. If 100 ml of contrast medium is injected, greater diuresis will ensue and more urine per unit time will have to be transported down the ureter. The ureter will thus tend to be more full and distended than if 50 ml of contrast medium had been injected. On the urogram films the portion of the ureter not contracted by peristalsis will be well delineated, while the intervening contracted portions will not. Often, different portions of a ureter will be seen on the five minute, fifteen minute, and postvoiding films.

There are three normal points of apparent narrowing of the ureter. These are located at the ureteropelvic junction, the point where the ureter crosses over the iliac artery and vein, and at the ureterovesical junction. These points are clinically important, for they mark the common sites of impacted ureteric calculi.

The ureter commonly is kinked proximally and narrowed transiently owing to buckling from the movement of the kidney with respiration. The distal ureter varies a great deal in position from patient to patient. It may be tightly applied to the pelvic wall or it may even take a straight line from pelvic brim to the bladder.

Bladder

The bladder is a very distensible organ since it normally can accommodate up to about 425 ml of urine in adults. Its shape when fully distended is ellipsoidal, and its lining is smooth. When partly distended it assumes a variety of shapes. When empty the crinkled pattern of the normal mucosa folded upon itself often is outlined by the normal small amount (less than 15 ml) of opacified urine that remains after emptying (Fig. 3–15). When the bladder is only partly distended, the outline of the interureteric ridge may be seen, particularly in men.

Two variations from the usual ellipsoidal shape are commonly encountered. In women the uterus causes a smooth curving indentation on the superior surface of the partly distended bladder. Anterior prolongation of the bladder produces a second density overlying the usual oval density of opacified urine in the bladder. This second density is superimposed on the upper anterior aspect of the bladder and should not be mistaken for a diverticulum.

Normal Renal Variants and Minor Anomalies

About the time the student has an image fixed in his mind that corresponds to a "normal kidney," there appears a kidney which seems "normal" but looks peculiar because of its shape, position, size, or collecting system configuration. Once he has seen one of these normal variants or renal anomalies, the student will usually recognize it the next time he sees it. Recognition is more easily accomplished and retained if the basic anatomic deviation that accounts for the peculiar image is understood.

DROMEDARY KIDNEY

This normal variation almost always involves the left kidney. It appears as though the lateral margin of the kidney has a "humplike" pro-

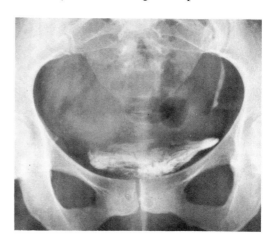

Figure 3–15 Normal bladder mucosal pattern on postvoiding film.

trusion that often gives the left kidney an overall triangular shape. The protrusion deformity most commonly affects the midportion of the lateral margin but may be skewed superiorly or inferiorly. The thickness of the renal cortex is equal to that of the rest of the kidney. Commonly a mid or lower minor calyx extends laterally more than its neighbors and points right at the "hump" (see Fig. 3–14).

ABNORMAL ROTATION

This minor anomaly often gives one the impression that the kidney has been rotated about its longitudinal axis more than usual. Actually what has happened embryologically is that the kidney has not rotated medially as much as usual. The result is that the calyces point more posteriorly, the renal pelvis is more anteriorly placed, and the proximal ureter courses more laterally than usual to join the most inferior portion of the renal pelvis (Fig. 3–16). Occasionally, there is less lower pole parenchyma than usual, giving the impression that the kidney is somewhat "top-heavy."

This anomaly should not be confused with a kidney that has been rotated laterally by an enlarging retroperitoneal mass medial to the kidney. In the latter case, the kidney usually is farther away from the psoas margin, and the ureter appears "stretched" in its course to join the renal pelvis. Another, less common variation on the rotation theme is the abnormal rotation of the kidney about its horizontal axis. This rotation causes a foreshortened appearance of the kidney on the frontal view.

DUPLICATION

Duplication of the kidney and ureter is a common anomaly, particularly in females. In duplication the ureteric bud either begins abnor-

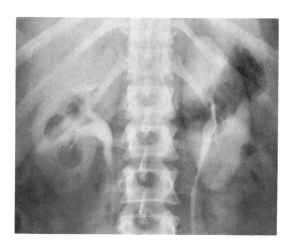

Figure 3–16 Incomplete rotation of the left kidney about its vertical axis.

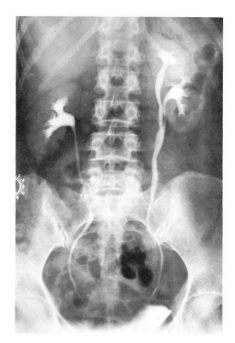

Figure 3–17 Duplication of the left kidney with partial duplication of the proximal left ureter. Normal right upper urinary tract.

mally or branches prematurely before stimulating the nephrogenic blastema. The result is two separate collecting systems draining into their respective ureters. Thus the kidney is functionally two separate units, but there is no discrete anatomic separation. The ureters may unite before reaching the bladder or remain separate, each having its own orifice in the bladder (Fig. 3–17). The orifice of the ureter from the upper renal segment always is located more medial and distal than the orifice of the lower renal segment ureter. Duplication anomaly may be unilateral or bilateral. The duplicated kidney is always longer than its nonduplicated mate unless atrophy has ensued from infection or obstruction.

COMPENSATORY HYPERTROPHY

The most common cause of unilateral renal enlargement is compensatory hypertrophy. This usually follows the surgical removal of the opposite kidney, the development of contralateral severe parenchymal atrophy, or results from agenesis or severely retarded development of the opposite kidney. The kidney enlarges because of hypertrophic changes in the interstitium and proximal convoluted tubules. No new nephrons are developed in this process. On the urogram the renal size and shape will simply be larger (the long axis is usually more than 15 cm in length) with a continuing normal relationship of the size and shape of the collecting system to the renal outline (Fig. 3–18).

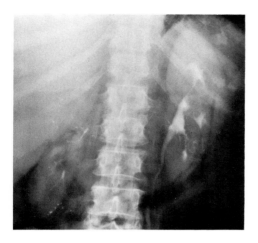

Figure 3–18 Large left kidney (17 cm) due to compensatory hypertrophy secondary to right renal pyelonephritic atrophy (10.5 cm).

A greater potential for renal hypertrophy exists in children and young adults than in older patients. Hypertrophy can occur after the age of 50 years but will usually be in the 0.5 to 1.0 cm range of increase in length rather than the 1.0 to 2.0 cm increase seen in normal younger kidneys. Focal hypertrophy within one kidney can occur when severe focal atrophy, such as in chronic pyelonephritis, affects only a portion of a kidney.

ABNORMAL STATES

An example of the range of diagnoses that resulted from a study of uroradiologic examinations appears in Table 3–2, which lists the general categories of all the diagnoses coded in that study.*

The vast majority of the diagnoses were the result of the most frequently done examination, excretory urography (3762 urograms). In the remainder of this chapter, the most common diagnostic problems in the general categories listed in Table 3–2 are presented with primary emphasis on excretory urography findings. The discussion concentrates on the basic principles of diagnosis rather than attempting to illustrate all of the pathologic variations in detail.

The diagnostic problems to be covered include the following:
1. Acute and chronic pyelonephritis.
2. Renal insufficiency and failure.
3. Obstruction affecting the kidney.
4. Urinary calculi, calcifications, and colic.
5. Renal cyst versus tumor versus normal cortical nodule.
6. Renal artery stenosis and hypertension.

---

*The examinations were conducted by the author and his associates from Sept. 1, 1970, through Aug. 31, 1971.

TABLE 3–2 Range of Diagnoses Resulting from Uroradiologic Examinations

Diagnostic Category	Number	Per Cent of Total
Normal (including anomalies)	3480	53
Inflammation	330	5
Neoplasm (including prostatic hyperplasia and benign renal cyst)	787	12
Trauma (including postoperative state)	583	9
Calculi, obstruction, and circulatory disease	1405	21
	6585	100

Pyelonephritis

In daily practice this diagnostic problem usually is identified by the clinician in one of two general contexts or clinical settings. The patient presents a sign and symptom cluster that indicates involvement by an infectious process of either the kidney *or* the bladder. In either context the clinician requests an excretory urogram in order to look for radiologic signs of acute or chronic pyelonephritis.

When the bladder site predominates clinically, the urogram is obtained to detect infectious involvement of the kidney secondary to cystitis. Experts still are not in agreement as to whether the pyelonephritis is caused by the ureteric reflux of infected urine due to recurrent cystitis or is hematogenously spread from the chronically infected bladder wall. The usual clinical clues for pyelonephritis often are subtle, absent, or obscured by the patient's attention to the urgent bladder symptoms.

The type of infection most commonly encountered in either primary or secondary pyelonephritis is pyogenic in nature with Escherichia coli the predominant organism. Rarely will tuberculosis or a fungus be the infectious agent. With the possible exception of tuberculosis, the specific organism cannot be predicted with certainty from the radiologic findings.

RADIOLOGIC FINDINGS IN ACUTE PYELONEPHRITIS

Clinical experience* indicates that slightly over one fourth (28 per cent) of these patients will have abnormal urographic findings caused by acute pyelonephritis. The rest will have normal urograms. In most of the abnormal urograms, the findings will be multiple and obvious. In some, however, the abnormal findings will be few and subtle (Fig. 3–19).

---

*At the University of Michigan.

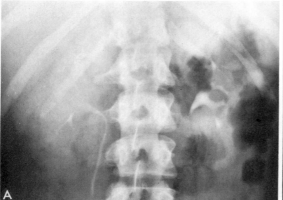

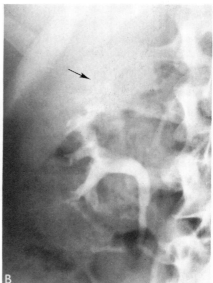

Figure 3–19 Acute pyelonephritis, excretory urography. *A,* Mild right renal enlargement, decreased contrast concentration, and attenuated collecting system. *B,* Upper pole corticomedullary contrast streaking as the only abnormality in a different patient.

Obvious multiple findings include the following:
1. Gross renal enlargement.
2. Decreased concentration of contrast material.
3. Delayed calyceal contrast appearance time.
4. Collecting system dilatation.

These obvious findings usually exist together and may be focal or generalized in a kidney, depending on whether the infection involves all or a portion of the kidney. The abnormalities will be unilateral or bilateral, depending on the involvement of one or both kidneys.

Subtle, rare findings include
1. Minimal renal enlargement.
2. Blurred streaklike collections of contrast material that extend from the renal papilla into the cortex.

Varying aspects of the inflammatory process account for the radiologic abnormalities. Renal enlargement is due to edema. Decreased contrast material density in the collecting system is due to the inhibited concentrating capability of nephrons plus the dilution of contrast material in unopacified urine that is retained longer in the collecting system as a result of diminished peristalsis. Collecting system dilatation is also an effect of the peristaltic defect. The infrequent streaklike parenchymal contrast material collections are due to the stasis of opacified urine in collecting ducts where pus has accumulated in the urine.

RADIOLOGIC FINDINGS IN CLASSIC CHRONIC ATROPHIC PYELONEPHRITIS

The variety and combination of findings in this disease are many but fall into two main categories:

1. Abnormalities in the size and shape of the renal outline.

2. Abnormalities in the collecting system, particularly the minor calyces.

The pathologic hallmark of chronic atrophic pyelonephritis is focal renal parenchymal scarring. The extent and degree of scarring depend on the frequency, length, and severity of the recurrent episodes. Additional factors are the patient's immune response and the effectiveness of antibiotic therapy.

Hodson's excellent radiologic-pathologic correlation studies of chronic pyelonephritis highlight the focal, through-and-through parenchymal involvement typical of the disease. In *advanced* scarring, the radiologic findings include

1. Blunting of the minor calyces from retractive scarring of adjacent papillae.

2. Prominent focal indippings of the renal margin.

3. Narrowed parenchymal thickness between the sites of margin intrusion and calyceal blunting.

4. Decreased overall length and width of the kidney. The end result is a small, irregularly contracted renal outline and grossly deformed minor calyces (Fig. 3–20).

It must be appreciated that in chronic atrophic pyelonephritis the degree of concentration, or whiteness, of the contrast material in the collecting system will frequently be the same as that seen on normal urograms. It is only very late in the course of the disease when a large enough portion of the nephron population has been destroyed that the concentrating capability of the kidney is sufficiently impaired to result in faint opacification of collecting system urine. The density of the contrast material in the urine is *not* a quantitative indication of the state of renal function.

Early in the scarring process, the radiologic abnormalities are subtle. The earliest change is usually a minimal decrease in parenchymal thickness. This decrease frequently is discernible before calyceal

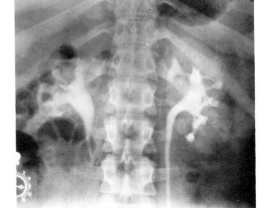

Figure 3–20 Severe bilateral chronic atrophic pyelonephritis with grossly deformed minor calyces and severe parenchymal scarring.

blunting begins, particularly in children. Prominent incursion of the renal margin also is not developed yet. Previous urograms for comparison are especially helpful in detecting early parenchymal loss.

UNUSUAL TYPES OF PYELONEPHRITIS

Another type of chronic pyelonephritis that occurs but does *not* produce the image of an irregularly contracted kidney with blunted calyces is *interstitial pyelonephritis.* This uncommon variety features uniform involvement of the renal parenchyma, rather than focal involvement. The scarring process involves the entire kidney, and the margin of the kidney remains smooth despite the fact that destruction is progressing. Additionally, the calyces seldom show blunting.

Thus, as the kidney gradually becomes smaller while still maintaining normal contrast material concentration, the disease process becomes perceptible relatively late in its course. Commonly, this process is bilateral, and the kidney does not reach as small a size as found in typical focal chronic atrophic pyelonephritis. When interstitial pyelonephritis involves both kidneys equally, the resultant urographic image of smooth surfaced, moderately contracted kidneys with intact minor calyces is indistinguishable from that due to chronic glomerulonephritis and arteriolonephrosclerosis.

Tuberculous pyelonephritis is rare in clinical practice today. However, when the disease is *well established* in the kidney, its urographic image has specific features that enable the observer to make the diagnosis with great certainty. These features are

1. Ragged irregularity of the minor calyces with narrowing of the adjacent draining major calyces.

2. Parenchymal abscess formation.

3. Calcification in areas of necrotic parenchyma undergoing healing.

When the disease is just beginning to involve the kidney, these obvious findings will *not* be present. Similarly, when the disease has been present a long time and has destroyed the major portion of the parenchyma, the midstage of the disease featuring the above specific findings has been long passed.

The urographic findings can be related to the pathogenesis of renal involvement. Renal tuberculosis results from the hematogenous spread of acid fast organisms that originate in an extrarenal primary site of infection, most commonly the pulmonary region. As the bacilli become established in the medullary portion of the parenchyma, they produce caseation necrosis of the renal papillae. As the papillae necrose, this causes the earliest but still nonspecific urographic sign of tuberculosis: *irregularity* of the margins of the adjacent *minor calyces.* As the necrotic infection progresses within the kidney, *narrowing* of the draining *major calyx* and the development of a *parenchymal abscess* becomes predominant. As healing begins as a result of the patient's immune response or antibiotic therapy, gradual *calcification* commonly develops in the scarring area of necrosis.

It is important to understand that the normal healing response to tuberculous infection is characterized by extensive progressive scarring. Thus, even though the infection is controlled and eradicated by therapy, *cicatricial scarring* at previously infected sites involving the major calyces, renal pelvis, or ureter can occur without symptoms and in the face of repeated negative urine cultures and smears for acid fast organisms. Severe obstruction of the urinary tract due to scarring at any of these sites causes destruction of the kidney, or a portion thereof, from obstructive atrophy. Therefore, it is mandatory that excretory urography be performed in these "cured" patients at about four to six month intervals for one to two years to detect this asymptomatic complication.

Renal Insufficiency and Failure

These two terms indicate functional derangement of the kidneys and indicate different degrees of loss of normal nephron population. Renal *insufficiency* is an intermediate state characterized by a moderate elevation of serum creatinine and BUN levels and some loss of urine concentrating capability. Renal *failure* is much more severe, and oliguria or anuria is added to the progressing features of insufficiency previously noted. Neither term indicates the cause of the nephron population destruction. The discussion of the use of excretory urography in the evaluation of the clinical problem is limited to the examination of adult patients.

The radiologist is faced with a considerable task in tailoring the urogram to gain useful information. The nephron deficit, particularly regarding urine concentration, results in faint opacification of collecting systems and ureters. In addition, most of these patients have copious intestinal contents that obscure the upper urinary tract. Added to these handicaps is the problem that results from these patients not being examined in a dehydrated state. In fact, overnight dehydration is contraindicated because the kidney in moderate to severe insufficiency is prone to go into failure when assaulted with hyperosmolar contrast material if the patient is in a dehydrated state.

To offset the nephron deficit, a larger amount of contrast material is used (100 ml instead of the usual 50 ml dosage). To get a better view of the obscured, faintly opacified structures, laminagraphy is mandatory (Fig. 3–21). In the face of parenchymal disease it is critical that the laminagrams be obtained within 25 minutes after injection since what little density is achieved becomes progressively more dilute after that time. This situation is the opposite to that when obstruction is present. Contrast density increases and accumulates slowly over several hours or even a day or so in an obstructed urinary tract.

In considering the many possible causes of renal insufficiency, the

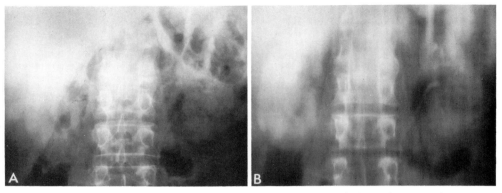

Figure 3–21 Bilateral nephrosclerosis. *A,* 15 minute urogram film (high dose) showing only faint renal outlines. *B,* Laminagram at 20 minutes delineating some normal calyces and normal renal pelvis on left and faint normal right pelvis.

clinician can expect to gain useful information from urography that answers two basic questions:

1. Is there evidence of chronic renal parenchymal disease, and if so, what kind of parenchymal disease?

2. Is urinary obstruction present?

If the kidneys are smaller than normal, show an irregular, asymmetrical outline, and have blunted calyces, a diagnosis of chronic atrophic pyelonephritis can be made with great certainty. If the kidneys are small, smooth surfaced, and have no calyceal blunting, then any one of the next four most common diagnoses could be equally likely: chronic glomerulonephritis, interstitial pyelonephritis, arteriolonephrosclerosis, or collagen disease. Patient history, physical, and laboratory findings may help sort out these possibilities, but renal biopsy is often necessary for a definitive diagnosis. Thus, high dose urography is specific only for a diagnosis of chronic atrophic pyelonephritis.

Infrequently, chronic bilateral ureteric obstruction is present that has itself caused either severe renal atrophy or made worse already existent chronic parenchymal disease. The most common clinical setting in this latter category is the elderly male with bilateral ureteric obstruction from prostatic enlargement who also has arteriolonephrosclerosis.

When excretory urography has failed to indicate whether obstruction is present, retrograde pyelography offers an alternative diagnostic method. However, its attendant risks of instrumentation and infection in a patient already in a precarious physiologic state pose a real dilemma to the clinician. He must be prepared to accept the patient as an operative candidate if he finds evidence of a surgically correctable obstruction. In addition, he must also accept the increased risk of the retrograde pyelogram.

When the clinical problem is frank renal failure, the need for urography can be easily discarded *if* all clinical evidence indicates acute tubular necrosis. If such is not the case, then the diagnostic considerations and type of useful information from high dose urography with laminagraphy are the same as discussed under the condition of insufficiency.

Two major differences, however, are that the likelihood of sufficiently opacifying the urinary tract for diagnosis is much less, and that the risk of renal contrast toxicity is greater. To make matters even more difficult, the risks of retrograde pyelography are also greater. Most of the time, if the patient's life expectancy is otherwise reasonable for his circumstances, the urogram should be done in a *nondehydrated* patient. If the serum creatinine is 12 mg/100 ml or over, the expectation of diagnostic useful information return is 10 per cent or less, but the overall risk is less than doing a retrograde pyelogram in these very fragile patients.

Obstruction Affecting the Kidney

Obstruction to the flow of urine at any level in the urinary tract potentially can affect the kidney. Obstruction may affect one or both kidneys, depending upon the site of obstruction. The ultimate results of such obstruction are dilatation of the collecting system and the inhibition of urine formation by the nephrons that is due to increasing urinary back pressure. The serious renal pathologic consequence of obstruction is irreversible atrophy of the renal parenchyma and the loss of renal function. The factors that determine whether renal atrophy develops are basically the severity and length of time the obstruction has existed. A secondary, but important, factor is whether or not infection develops subsequent to the onset of obstruction. Urinary infection commonly accompanies obstruction.

An understanding of how obstruction affects urine formation is critical to explaining the variations of contrast material excretion by nephrons that produce the radiologic signs of obstruction seen on excretory urograms. Recall that urographic contrast agents are excreted by glomerular filtration with subsequent concentration in the tubules by a process of water reabsorption.

Glomerular filtration is controlled by a balance of forces. Glomerular arteriolar pressure is opposed by the sum of the hydrostatic pressure in Bowman's space and the plasma oncotic pressure in the glomerular capillary. Normally, the arteriolar pressure force predominates, and the flow of filtrate from the glomerular tuft into Bowman's space ensues. This causes a positive pressure that is the driving force for the urinary filtrate, which moves along the tubules and collecting ducts, eventually reaching the collecting system. As the filtrate passes through the proximal and distal convoluted tubules, it is concentrated by water reabsorption through the tubular epithelium.

In obstruction, the hydrostatic pressure increases and is transmitted back to the level of the nephrons. If the pressure rise is small, filtrate continues to be formed by the glomeruli, but it flows very slowly along the tubules. Therefore, the degree of water reabsorption relatively increases, and the filtrate is *hyperconcentrated.* On the other hand, if the pressure rise is great, glomerular arteriolar pressure is overcome and *no filtrate* is formed. If intrarenal pressure remains elevated sufficiently high and long enough, blood flow to the kidney diminishes and parenchymal atrophy develops progressively.

In obstruction involving a modest increase in hydrostatic pressure, the urographic signs related to the kidney are as follows:

1. Collecting system
   a. Dilatation.
   b. Delay in contrast appearance time.
2. Nephrogram
   a. Slowly and progressively increasing nephrogram density (whiteness).

When hydrostatic pressure is greatly increased such that glomerular arteriolar pressure is overcome, little if any filtrate is formed. Thus, the urographic signs range from

1. Collecting system
   a. Dilatation (if opacified).
   b. Faint and delayed to nonopacification.
2. Nephrogram
   a. Diminished to absent.

When signs of obstruction are detected on the early films of a urogram, the radiologist's strategy is to obtain delayed films while waiting for the contrast material to seep downward from the kidney in the dilated urinary tract in order to detect the level at which the obstruction is located (Fig. 3–22). In some instances this procedure will take an hour or so, and occasionally even up to a day or more may be required. When obstruction results in very faint opacification, only a little contrast is diluted in a large volume of stasis urine. Laminagrams are commonly obtained to detect the faintly opacified collecting system(s) and ureter(s).

A larger than normal amount of urographic contrast often is used when moderate to severe obstruction is suspected from the clinical setting. This is influenced somewhat by the serum creatinine and BUN (blood urea nitrogen) level results. If the creatinine and BUN levels are normal and the suspected obstruction is most likely unilateral, there is nothing to be gained from using more than the usual 50 ml intravenous dosage of contrast material. On the other hand, if the creatinine and BUN levels are elevated, the same 100 ml dosage that is used for renal insufficiency would be employed.

The causes of obstruction are often apparent on the urogram. The most common causes are

1. Urinary calculi (particularly ureteric).
2. Idiopathic stenosis of the ureteropelvic junction.
3. Pelvic and retroperitoneal malignancy.
4. Neurogenic bladder dysfunction.
5. Prostatic enlargement.

Infrequently, even high dose urography (including laminagraphy)

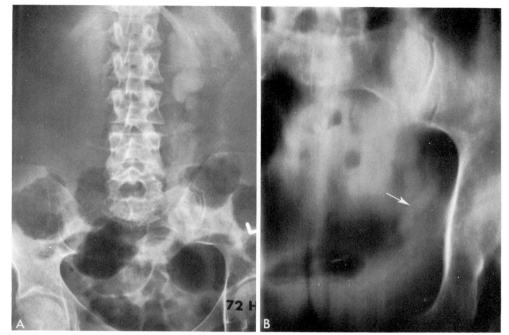

Figure 3–22 Delayed urogram filming in ureteric obstruction from carcinoma of the cervix. A, At 72 hours contrast material persists in the dilated left collecting system and ureter. B, Laminagram at 72 hours shows the point of distal obstruction to better advantage.

does not demonstrate the obstructed portion of the upper urinary tract. Two other radiologic examinations are available to solve the problem. The more frequently used is *retrograde pyelography*, in which a ureteric catheter is placed into the ureter by the urologist during cystoscopy. If the obstruction is complete, injection of contrast material demonstrates the ureter distal to the obstruction (Fig. 3–23). If the obstruction is partial, the portion of ureter at the obstructed site is seen, and some contrast material streams past the site proximally into the dilated portion of the urinary tract.

The other examination for evaluating severe obstruction, particularly the ureteric or ureteropelvic junction type, is *antegrade pyelography*. Here the radiologist inserts a needle (under fluoroscopic control) into the dilated renal collecting system and injects contrast material to opacify the upper tract down to the level of the obstructing lesion. This method delineates the anatomic features of the obstructing lesion and occasionally permits a specific diagnosis to be made (see Fig. 3–11).

Two points about renal size in obstruction should be appreciated. Early in severe obstruction, before renal atrophy develops, the kidney is larger than its preobstructive size. As atrophy develops, the kidney gradually shrinks to a somewhat smaller size than normal.

If the obstruction is relieved, e.g., by the removal of a calculus or

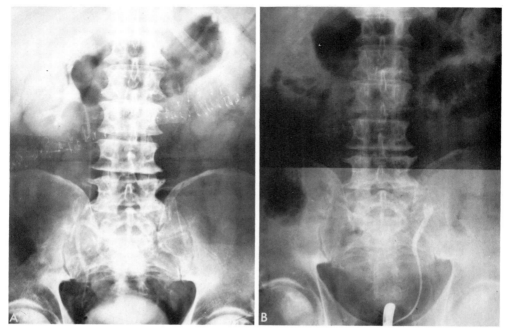

Figure 3–23 Severe obstruction of the left mid ureter from primary ureteric carcinoma. *A,* Urogram showing nonopacification of the left upper urinary tract. *B,* Left retrograde ureterogram showing complete obstruction to contrast flow by a round surfaced intraluminal tumor.

the response of a malignancy to chemotherapy or radiation therapy, and atrophy has begun, the kidney, even though no longer obstructed, gradually continues to shrink over the next three to six months. Eventually it appears normal although slightly reduced in size with sharp, normal minor calyces. The parenchymal thickness is uniform and slightly less than normal. This process is best appreciated if a previous urogram is available for comparison.

Urinary Calculi, Calcifications, and Colic

Urinary calculi, or "stones," are commonly encountered urologic abnormalities. Their radiologic appearance is specific and distinctive when they contain enough calcium to be radiopaque (white) on x-ray films. Fortunately, most calculi (90 per cent) that involve the *kidney* and *ureter* are radiopaque and readily demonstrated even on a plain film. The remainder are nonopaque and require contrast material in the urine to be ascertained. This proportion is not true in the bladder, where only about 50 per cent are radiopaque, and the rest are chalklike, fibrinous, and nonopaque in nature.

This discussion is restricted to the more common upper urinary tract calculi and calcifications and does not discuss bladder calculi further. Almost all ureteric calculi originate in the kidney.

There are two general categories of renal calcifications:

1. *Nephrolithiasis* (common): calculi that reside in, or are immediately adjacent to, the minor calyces or are in the renal pelvis.
2. *Nephrocalcinosis* (rare): calcifications that generally occur within the renal parenchyma, most commonly in the medullary portion.

NEPHROLITHIASIS

Most renal calculi are composed of calcium carbonate, oxalate, or phosphate and are quite radiopaque. Stones composed of other substances such as cystine or urate salts are usually of low density or even nonopaque. Calculi may be single or multiple, unilateral or bilateral.

The appearance of the calculus is determined primarily by the site in which it is located (Fig. 3-24). A calculus in the tip of the renal papilla or in the fornix of the minor calyx is usually quite small and either punctate or plaquelike. As such stones migrate into the lumen of the calyx, they begin to float about the collecting system.

A stone free in the renal pelvis will usually be oval or spherical since its entire surface is exposed to calcium deposition from the surrounding urine. When it becomes large enough to fill the cavity in which it lies (calyx or pelvis), it will assume the shape of that cavity.

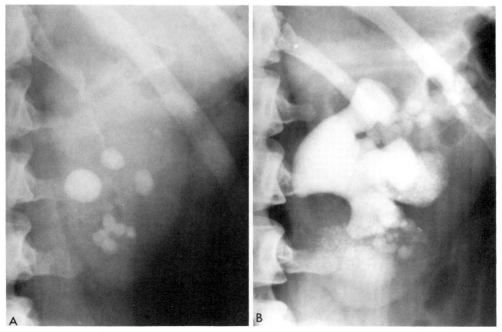

Figure 3-24 Opaque renal calculi (plain films). *A,* Multiple varying sized calculi in pelvis and calyces. *B,* Large staghorn calculus with multiple small peripheral calculi.

Thus, it may form a cast of a calyx or of the entire collecting system (a "staghorn" calculus).

Extrarenal calcifications may simulate renal calculi on the supine abdominal film. These include gallstones, vascular calcifications, and calcified costal cartilages. The radiologist utilizes oblique views of the kidney to help sort out these densities. To be in the kidney, the density must remain within the outline of the renal margin on both the supine and oblique films. These must be obtained before contrast injection, or the contrast material may obscure the density and prevent localization.

To determine the precise location of the opaque calculus in the kidney, excretory urography must be done. Besides relating the calculus to the internal renal anatomy, the urogram delineates the obstructive nature of the calculus. Nonopaque calculi are visualized as a negative defect within the collecting system contrast material (Fig. 3–25).

NEPHROCALCINOSIS

There are two subtypes of this calcification that occur in the renal parenchyma: metastatic and dystrophic. Metastatic calcification is due to calcium deposited in otherwise normal tissue because of metabolic disease. Dystrophic calcification, on the other hand, occurs in tissue previously damaged by a disease process or injury.

Disease entities characterized by metastatic calcification include: hyperparathyroidism, renal tubular acidosis, sarcoidosis, and idiopathic hypercalciuria. Diseases which occasionally result in dystrophic renal calcification include: chronic pyelonephritis, recurrent nephrolithiasis, medullary sponge kidney, and tuberculosis.

The pattern of calcification is not specific for any of these entities with the exception of medullary sponge kidney (Fig. 3–26) and renal

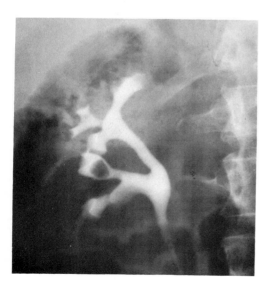

Figure 3–25 Nonopaque calculus in the middle calyx (excretory urogram).

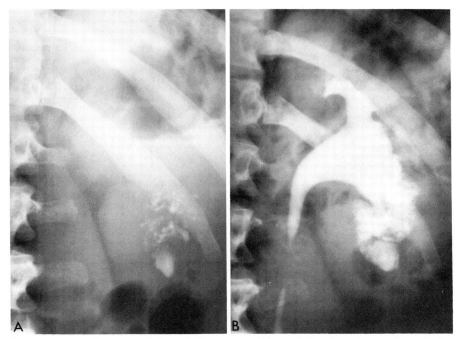

Figure 3–26 Nephrocalcinosis in medullary sponge kidney. *A,* One large lower calyx calculus and multiple punctate medullary calculi in the lower pole. *B,* 15 minute urogram film showing partial obscuration of the individual calculi by excreted contrast material.

tubular acidosis (Fig. 3–27). In both of these diseases the calcification is restricted to the tips of the renal papillae. In medullary sponge kidney, the calcifications are quite small and usually short and rodlike, clustering in the papillae and radiating out from the minor calcyes. The stones develop and are located within collecting ducts that are abnormally

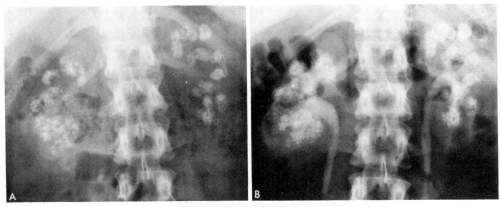

Figure 3–27 Nephrocalcinosis in renal tubular acidosis. *A,* Plain film delineation of bilateral multiple clusters of punctate stones distributed in the medullary region. *B,* 15 minute urogram film showing decreased contrast concentration and persistence of discrete calculous densities.

dilated, usually in a fusiform manner. Thus, as contrast material is excreted, surrounding the intraductal calculi, they seem to be increased in size owing to the accumulation of surrounding opacified urine. These calcifications may be unilateral or bilateral and may involve all or a portion of the papillae of a kidney.

Renal tubular acidosis also often causes papillary calcifications that cluster about the minor calyces in a radiating fashion. However, they are usually larger, of more uniform size, and more generally involve all the papillae than in medullary sponge kidney. In addition, the calculi do not appear to enlarge during contrast material excretion since they do not lie within dilated collecting ducts but instead are in the interstitium of the papillae as well as in *nondilated* collecting ducts.

COLIC

Colic is a specific type of abdominal pain characterized by paroxysms of severe pain with intermittent periods of relief. When the pain distribution suggests a urinary origin, i.e., flank pain radiating to the groin, the cause is almost always sudden obstruction of the ureter. Most commonly this is due to impaction of a calculus in the ureter. Rarely is

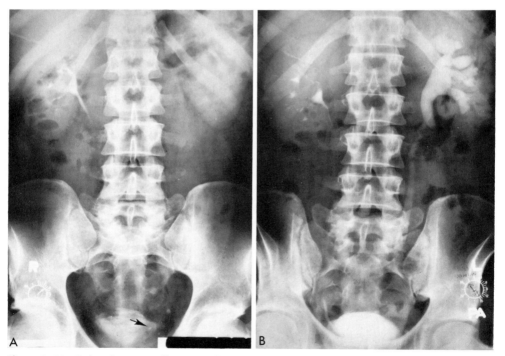

Figure 3–28 Delayed urogram filming in obstruction from a distal left ureteric calculus. *A,* 5 minute urogram film showing dense nephrogram and no collecting system filling. Opaque calculus barely discernible at arrow. *B,* 30 minute urogram film delineating left upper tract dilatation down to the level of the calculus.

the obstructing lesion a blood clot, soft tissue debris, or a ureteric tumor.

In this clinical setting, the clinician can confirm the urinary origin and document the site and severity of the ureteric obstruction by requesting an excretory urogram (Fig. 3–28). A specific diagnosis can usually be made since most ureteric calculi are opaque and detectable even on the preliminary film. If the obstructing lesion is not opaque and a radiolucent defect is seen within the ureteric lumen at the point of obstruction, the true diagnosis may be a nonopaque calculus, blood clot, tumor, or debris.

Upon discovering an opaque density in the vicinity of the ureter on a supine plain film of the abdomen, one must not *automatically* assume that the density is a urinary calculus. Instead, the possibility of commonly encountered densities that mimic ureteric calculi must be considered and ruled out. These include phleboliths, tips of transverse processes, film artifacts, and intestinal contents. Oblique views usually help to sort these out, except in the case of small pelvic phleboliths. Using urography to define the course of a ureter in relation to the density often is the only way to distinguish a phlebolith from a distal ureteric calculus (Fig. 3–29).

Most opaque ureteric calculi are small (1 to 3 mm) and only temporarily obstruct the ureter because they have an irregular shape and surface when viewed upon recovery after passage. They are not like a cork with a smooth surface totally plugging a pipe but are more like sticking a cockleburr into a collapsible muscular-walled tube. As peristalsis struggles to move the calculus on down the ureter, the muscular wall goes into spasm about the calculus, and the normal transport of urine is inhibited.

As urine distends the ureter above the level of spasm at the site of the calculus, ureteric peristalsis becomes more pronounced and pain

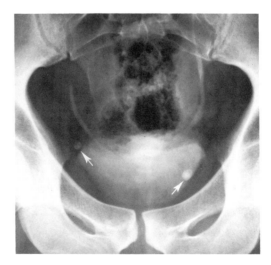

Figure 3–29 Normal relation of two phleboliths (arrows) to the distal ureters and bladder (excretory urogram).

becomes intense. Finally the ureteric wall becomes fatigued and relaxes, with a temporary easing of the pain. The calculus then may move further down the ureter pushed on by the increased urinary pressure behind it. Repetition of this sequence accounts for the typical intermittent nature of ureteric colic.

The urogram in ureteric colic that is due to a calculus reflects the signs of obstruction described in the preceding section. Depending on how severe a degree of partial ureteric obstruction results, findings will range *from a*

1. Moderately increased and transiently prolonged nephrogram density,

2. Slight delay of appearance time of contrast material in the calyces,

3. Mild to moderate dilatation of the collecting system and ureter down to the calculus,

to a

1. Progressively more dense and persistent intense nephrogram.

2. Prolonged delay of calyceal appearance time of contrast material.

3. Severe dilatation of the collecting system and ureter to the level of the calculus.

Since these patients are often examined in the acute state and are not prepared with dehydration and bowel catharsis, a large (e.g., 100 ml) dosage of contrast material is often used. This results in hyperosmolar diuresis modified by the degree of urinary back pressure caused by the obstruction. Occasionally this extra physiologic "shove" can cause immediate passage of the calculus. In this event, the urogram initially shows the obstructive phase as above. Then the opaque calculus is no longer seen, and the intense nephrogram and upper tract dilatation rapidly resolve within minutes.

If the calculus has stimulated mucosal edema at the site it impacted, the return to normal may be slower since the edema still causes partial obstruction. This seems more often the case with distal ureteric calculi than with those more proximal in position.

If the calculus persists in obstructing the ureter during urography (even if it moves a short distance), delayed films must be obtained, even up to 24 hours later (see Fig. 3–28). This procedure permits the excreted contrast material to filter slowly down through the distended collecting system and ureter to the level of the opaque calculus. The subsequent films should confirm the calculus as the cause of the obstruction, and a less likely, but still possible, associated abnormality (such as ureteric stricture or anomaly) can be ruled out.

If the cause of acute ureteric colic is not due to an opaque calculus, the urogram still documents the presence and level of the obstructive ureteric lesion.

A nonopaque intraluminal obstructing lesion often produces the appearance of a convex defect in the end of the contrast medium column at the level of obstruction. The differential diagnosis then is nonopaque calculus, polypoid ureteric tumor, or blood clot (see Fig. 3–23). The urographic appearance is often nonspecific and *retrograde pyelography* is commonly used to sort out these three possibilities. Cytology of the urine sampled from the site of the lesion often provides helpful information about tumors.

All ureteric calculi are not passed spontaneously. If the calculus remains impacted for a period of days, or even several weeks, and is associated with constant pain or hydroureteronephrosis, surgical removal (ureterolithotomy) usually is considered. A repeat urogram at this point provides important information about the state of the obstruction and its effects on the kidney.

Several times a year a patient is encountered who has a persistent opaque calculus impacted in the ureter, but who has no pain or urographic evidence of obstruction. In this circumstance, the calculus has so many protruding surface irregularities that it actually occludes less than half the ureteric lumen even though it may be quite large. Additionally, it may have been eccentrically incorporated into the ureteric wall by inflammation response, thus losing its obstructing potential.

The Renal Cyst/Tumor/Cortical Nodule Problem

When a space-occupying lesion, or "lump," that creates a bulge or exists within an adult kidney is suggested by urogram evidence, one of three diagnoses is the cause in about 93 per cent of such cases. These diagnostic possibilities are benign simple cyst, malignant primary renal tumor, and a normal renal anatomic variant known as a benign cortical nodule, or prominent column of Bertin.

In the author's urographic experience the frequency of these three diagnoses is

Cyst	59%
Tumor	19%
Cortical nodule	15%
Other	7%
	100%

"Other" here includes rarely encountered lesions such as segmental renal dysplasia, renal abscess, and localized fat accumulation in the renal sinus. This discussion is restricted to the three most common diagnoses.

The urographic criteria for differentiating the three possibilities are related to their anatomic and pathologic characteristics.

BENIGN SIMPLE CYST

A *benign simple cyst* is a slowly developing spherical or ellipsoidal "lump" which compresses and gently pushes aside adjacent renal parenchyma and collecting system. If it begins near the surface of the kidney, it bulges out from the surface. However, it may arise from deep within the kidney, and no bulge will be apparent. When centrally and medially located it is called a parapelvic cyst and primarily affects the renal pelvis and infundibula.

A cyst has *no* blood vessels within its confines and is considered *avascular*. For radiologic diagnosis, this is an important distinction since tumor and cortical nodule are vascular lesions. A benign simple cyst rarely contains calcium in its wall, but when it does the calcification may be curvilinear, punctate, or amorphous in appearance.

The usual uncomplicated benign simple cyst is thin-walled, contains watery, clear yellow fluid, and has a smooth inner lining surface. Cytologic examination of the fluid may show a few benign epithelial cells but nothing resembling malignant cells. Rarely, a cyst will bleed, and hemorrhagic contents will accumulate within the cyst lumen. The fluid then is no longer clear yellow, but instead is a dirty, turbid yellow or, more commonly, a reddish or chocolate brown; the fluid is also more viscous. Cytologic examination of such fluid shows cellular debris and peculiar crystalloid elements but no neoplasticlike cells.

Urographic criteria (Fig. 3–30) that indicate typical cyst are

1. A spherical or ellipsoidal shaped lesion.

2. A lesion that is radiolucent and sharply demarcated from the normal surrounding radiodense renal parenchyma.

3. Adjacent calyces that are smoothly stretched and not obliterated. These criteria are *all* optimally fulfilled on about 85 of 100 urograms taken of patients who actually have a benign simple cyst. The urogra-

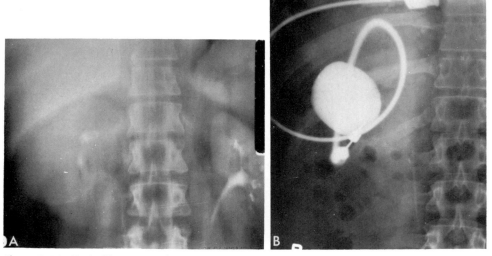

Figure 3–30 Typical benign simple renal cyst. *A*, Laminagram from excretory urography showing a large (8 cm) round radiolucent right renal cystic lesion. *B*, Cyst puncture delineating the cyst's smooth ovoid lumen. Fluid was clear yellow and evidence of cellular abnormality was negative.

phic diagnosis in this circumstance is quite certain. In the remaining 15 of 100 cysts, the criteria are only partly fulfilled, and the urographic diagnosis much less certain.

MALIGNANT PRIMARY RENAL TUMOR

The most common primary malignant renal tumor encountered is renal adenocarcinoma, or "hypernephroma." It is a more rapidly growing lesion than simple cyst and tends to destroy, rather than push aside, adjacent structures. Unfortunately, this tendency is characteristic of *later* stages of growth. Early on the tumor does push aside, rather than destroy, such things as calyces. Hypernephromas are much more likely to contain calcification than cysts. About 15 per cent of hypernephromas contain calcium with a pattern ranging from curvilinear to punctate to amorphous in nature.

Hypernephroma is a highly vascular tumor and contains bizarre tumor blood vessels within its confines. Ninety-five of every 100 hypernephromas will be solid tumors. The other 5 of 100 will have extensive, severe central necrosis and fewer central tumor vessels than usual.

One of these five will have almost its entire contents so necrotic that liquefaction will have occurred. This results in a thin-walled shell of tumor tissue surrounding dark, turbid fluid contents. Cytologic examination of such fluid may permit a diagnosis of adenocarcinoma if a few intact cells remain in the necrotic fluid contents. This rare form of hypernephroma, known as "cystic" hypernephroma, mimics very closely on gross pathologic examination a benign simple cyst that has been bled into.

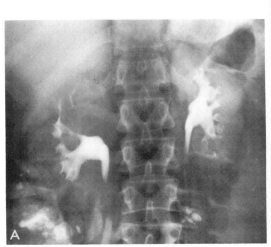
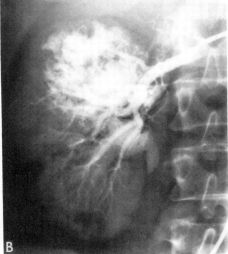

Figure 3–31 Typical hypernephroma. *A*, 10 minute excretory urogram film showing a 4 cm bulging lesion in the medial aspect of the right upper pole. *B*, Selective arteriogram delineating malignant tumor vasculature at the site of the urogram lesion.

Urographic criteria (Fig. 3–31) for typical large solid hyper-nephroma are

1. An irregularly shaped lesion.

2. A lesion that is of about the same or slightly greater density than the surrounding normal renal parenchyma but is *not* sharply demarcated from it.

3. Adjacent calyces which are destroyed.

These criteria are completely fulfilled on about 75 of 100 urograms taken of patients having a hypernephroma, and diagnostic certainty is high. If calcification is also present, certainty is even greater (Fig. 3–32). In the remaining 25 of 100 tumors, the criteria is only partially met, and diagnosis is much less certain. One of these 25 will be the rare "cystic hypernephroma," which can confuse the urographic diagnosis of benign simple cyst (Fig. 3–33).

CORTICAL NODULE

This normal renal anatomic variation simply means that in one portion of the renal parenchyma there is cortical tissue which dips prominently into the medulla between the renal pyramids. When this intrusion is extensive enough, it slightly displaces adjacent calyces, thus simulating a space-occupying lesion.

Cortical nodules are supplied by normal renal blood vessels which in no way resemble tumor vessels. Since there is more cortical thickness (and more normal vessels) than usual in the area of the cortical nodule, this area appears more radiodense than the surrounding parenchyma on the nephrogram phase immediately after injection.

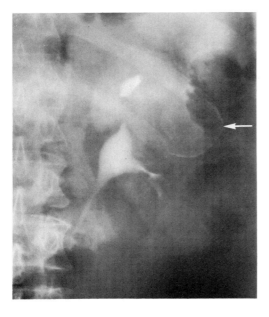

Figure 3–32 Spherical, shell-like calcification of a hypernephroma in the midlateral region of the kidney.

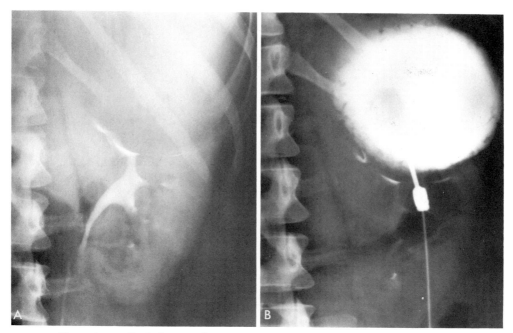

Figure 3–33 Cystic hypernephroma. *A,* Large left upper pole cystic-appearing lesion on 15 minute urogram film. *B,* Cyst puncture film delineating irregular lumen margins and an intraluminal tumor defect. Fluid was dark brown, and cytologic report indicated adenocarcinoma.

Urographic criteria (Fig. 3–34) for cortical nodule are

1. A hemispherically shaped lesion with its base adjoining the cortical portion of the renal parenchyma.

2. A lesion of the same or slightly greater density than neighboring parenchyma which appears on the nephrogram; it is *not* sharply demarcated from normal parenchyma.

3. A mild degree of smooth stretching of adjacent calyces.

Complete fulfillment of these criteria is found in about 50 of 100 cases when the true diagnosis is normal cortical nodule, and certainty of the diagnosis is high. In the remaining 50 of 100 cases, the criteria are only partly met, and diagnosis of cortical nodule is quite uncertain. Cyst and tumor are mistakenly diagnosed with equal frequency in this group when cortical nodule actually is the true diagnosis.

DEFINITIVE RADIOLOGIC DIAGNOSIS

The urogram provides evidence for the (1) presence of a lesion and (2) the type of lesion. However, the resulting urographic diagnosis is not certain enough to decide the issue of whether a benign or malignant process is present, but it does provide reasonable information to select one of the two radiologic procedures that provide a very certain (greater than 99.5 per cent) diagnostic solution to the cyst/tumor/cor-

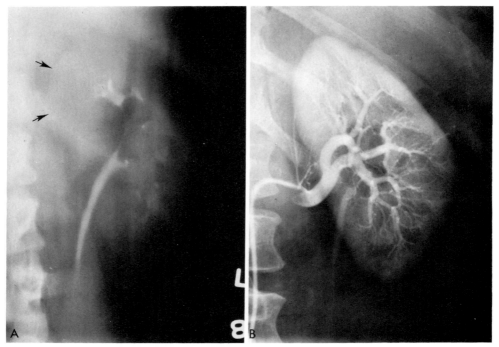

Figure 3–34   Benign cortical nodule. A, Laminagram from excretory urography showing bulging deformity of the medial aspect of left upper pole. B, Selective arteriogram showing normal arterial supply and more than usual (but still normal) cortical thickness at the site of the urogram deformity.

tical nodule problem. These competing procedures are renal cyst needle *aspiration* and selective renal *arteriography*.

The optimum decision concerning the use of aspiration versus arteriography is as follows. If the lesion is a benign simple cyst, needle aspiration is the procedure of choice (see Fig. 3–30). If the lesion is a tumor or cortical nodule, arteriography is the proper choice (see Figs. 3–31 and 3–34). The consequences of this decision are very important. If cyst is proven by aspiration, no further treatment is necessary. If tumor is proven by arteriography, its extent is then known, and decisions about surgery or chemotherapy can be made. If cortical nodule is proven, no further treatment is necessary.

Using the most likely diagnosis from the urogram evidence as the basis for the choice, the appropriate procedure is chosen in about 90 per cent of cases. In the remaining 10 per cent of cases, most are cysts that were incorrectly evaluated by arteriography, and needle aspiration is done to sort out the common benign cyst from the rare cystic hypernephroma. A smaller proportion are tumors incorrectly examined by needle aspiration, and arteriography is then done in order to arrive at the proper preoperative evaluation of the extent of tumor involvement. Rarely, a cortical nodule is needled, and an arteriogram is then required for final diagnosis.

Some clinicians use ultrasound as an intermediate sorting test after urography to distinguish cystic (for aspiration) from noncystic (for arteriography) lesions. Experience at the University of Michigan indicates that ultrasound has its own inherent false diagnosis results and does not really diminish the difficulty of correctly choosing between arteriography and aspiration based on the urogram alone. Using *tailored* urography, the usual practice at the University of Michigan is to recommend needle aspiration or renal arteriography on the basis of the urogram evidence alone.

The basic information provided by arteriography as opposed to needle aspiration is important to understand. Arteriography makes possible the diagnosis of hypernephroma by delineating the bizarre tumor vessels characteristic of this tumor. Additionally, it provides evidence of the extent of tumor involvement. It also clearly defines the normal vascular nature of a cortical nodule normal variant. Thus, arteriography is appropriate for a diagnosis of vascular lesions, specifically malignant tumor and cortical nodule.

Renal needle aspiration is designed for the diagnosis of cystic lesions, specifically benign simple cyst and the rare cystic hypernephroma. The diagnostic information aspiration provides can be grouped into three categories:

1. Appearance of aspirated fluid.
2. Cytologic examination of the aspirated fluid.
3. Configuration and smoothness of the lining of the cystic lumen.

If the aspirated fluid is clear and yellow, the cytologic examination is negative for tumor, and the lumen shown on the injection radiograph indicates a smooth lining. The diagnosis of benign simple cyst is then so certain that *no* further treatment, including surgery, is required. On the other hand, if any of these three criteria are not precisely met, then further diagnostic investigation is required. Usually this means arteriography and occasionally surgical exploration.

Renal Artery Stenosis and Hypertension

Hypertension is a common vascular disorder in adults. The vast majority of cases are due to primary, or "essential," hypertension, but a small portion (about 5 per cent) are due to renal artery stenosis. In the past 20 years a great deal of interest has been focused on the detection of patients with potentially surgically curable renal artery stenosis. Two radiologic examinations, rapid sequence excretory urography and renal arteriography, have been widely used in this diagnostic problem. Now that long term clinical experience has been accumulated, valid measurements of the usefulness of these two examinations have begun to emerge from a welter of controversial claims.

Rapid sequence, or "hypertensive," excretory urography is a slight modification of the usual program in that films of the kidneys at two and three minutes after injection are added to the usual filming sequence previously described in the section on uroradiologic examinations. The purpose of these early films is to detect slight changes in the appearance time of contrast material in the minor calyces of one kidney compared to the other. In the absence of obstruction of the kidney or ureter, a unilateral delay in the appearance of contrast material in the calyces most commonly indicates slowed blood flow to the kidney.

Renal artery stenosis means that there is a narrowing of the renal artery which obstructs renal blood flow. Depending on the severity, location, and duration of the stenosis, this causes renal parenchymal ischemia (and, ultimately, renal atrophy) which, for a still unknown reason, causes an increase in renin and aldosterone secretion. This secretion in turn results in hypertension.

The excretory urogram is used to detect the changes in renal anatomy and urine formation that are due to unilateral renal ischemia. These urographic signs (Fig. 3–35) are

1. A unilateral delay of at least one minute in calyceal appearance time of contrast material (normally, appearance time should be equal and within two to three minutes after the *start* of injection).

2. A difference of 1.5 cm or more in renal length of the smaller (ischemic) kidney compared to the contralateral normal kidney.

3. Hyperconcentration (increased whiteness) of contrast material in the collecting system of the ischemic kidney.

4. Ureteric "notching" defects that are due to increased size and tortuosity of the ureteric artery when it acts as a collateral channel to bypass the renal artery stenosis.

Of these four signs, only the first, delayed appearance time, is a *fairly* reliable predictor of the presence of a *severe* renal artery stenosis. Even this sign has about a 10 per cent probability of falsely predicting renal artery stenosis in patients who actually have "essential" hypertension and not renal artery stenosis.

In predicting the surgical curability of patients who prove to have

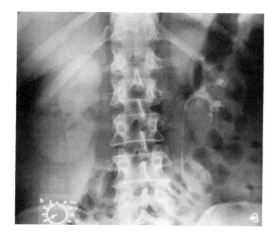

Figure 3–35 Hypertensive excretory urogram showing delayed calyceal appearance time on the right (3 minutes).

renal artery stenosis, the urogram provides an even less discriminating power. The "hypertensive" urogram provides *normal* results in many patients who ultimately have surgical cure of their hypertension by aortorenal bypass graft. This false normal prediction rate is from about 30 to 50 per cent, depending on the type and location of the renal artery stenosis. Therefore, the hypertensive urogram is not a reliable separator of the essential from the renovascular type of hypertension and is a *poor* predictor of surgical cure in those patients who have severe renal artery stenosis.

Renal arteriography is used to document the presence, location, and type of stenosis as well as to assess its "significance," i.e., to predict whether surgical cure is likely. Two main types of renal artery stenosis are most common: (1) those due to changes of fibrodysplasia in the arterial lining or wall and (2) those due to atherosclerotic lesions in the arterial lining.

Fibrodysplasia exists in several forms, but the most common arteriographic appearance is that of a "string of pearls." This condition is caused by serial small aneurysmal dilatations of the arterial lumen separated by concentric constricting lesions (Fig. 3–36). Lesions of fibrodysplasia are located more distally in the main renal artery and its segmental branches. On the other hand, lesions of atherosclerosis occur more commonly in the main renal artery close to its aortic origin and are localized concentric or eccentric constricting lesions (Fig. 3–37).

Arteriographic criteria for the prediction of surgical cure are based

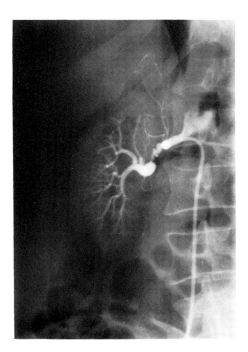

Figure 3–36 Selective arteriogram in the same patient as Figure 3–35 showing typical "string of pearls" deformity of the main renal artery due to fibromuscular dysplasia.

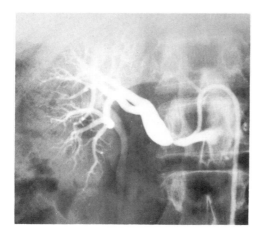

Figure 3–37 Selective arteriogram in a hypertensive patient with a main renal artery atherosclerotic lesion. Hypertension was later cured surgically.

primarily on the demonstration of collateral arterial channels bypassing a severe stenosis or the effects of collaterals on blood flow dynamics. These findings coupled with renin assays from renal veins or split renal function studies provide a reliable prediction of surgical cure or significant improvement in about 85 to 90 per cent of patients afflicted with severe renal artery stenosis.

To sum up, hypertensive urography is not a reliable screening examination to separate hypertensive patients who have renal artery stenosis from those who do not. Therefore, the choice of which hypertensive patients should have aortography cannot reasonably be based on urogram findings. Features of the clinical setting such as age and sex of the patient, response of the hypertension to drug therapy, duration of the hypertension, evidence of extrarenal vascular disease, and the patient's ability to withstand surgery are much more important arteriographic decision criteria. On the other hand, renal arteriography is an important part of the clinical assessment of a patient who has a high risk of having renal artery stenosis based on the preceding clinical criteria.

SELECTED REFERENCES

Emmett, J. L., and Witten, D. M.: Clinical Urography. 3rd ed. Philadelphia, W. B. Saunders Company, 1971.
In general this three volume reference work is beyond the level of medical students in the first two years. After learning the concepts of this chapter, medical students in clinical clerkships can cope with the wide and complete range of diagnostic topics that are covered in encyclopedic fashion by this work.

Lalli, A. F.: The Tailored Urogram. Chicago, Year Book Medical Publishers, 1973.
This monograph, devoted primarily to the "bread and butter" urographic techniques and diagnosis, is intermediate in complexity for the medical student and is highly recommended for basic information and concepts.

Thornbury, J. R., and Culp, D. A.: The Urinary Tract: Roentgen Diagnosis. Chicago, Year Book Medical Publishers, 1967.
This 430 page handbook is particularly designed to acquaint medical students and house officers with basic concepts and to illustrate in topical fashion the gamut of radiologic diagnoses in all types of uroradiologic examinations.

REFERENCES

Ansell, G.: Adverse reactions to contrast agents; Scope of problem. Invest. Radiol., 5:374, 1970.

Batson, P. G., and Keats, T. E.: The roentgenographic determination of normal adult kidney sizes related to vertebral height. Am. J. Roentgenol. Radium Ther. Nucl. Med., 116:737, 1972.

Bookstein, J. J., and Walter, J. F.: The role of abdominal radiography in hypertension secondary to renal or adrenal disease. Med. Clin. North Am., 59:169, 1975.

Bozniak, M. A., and Schweizer, R. D.: Urographic findings in patients with renal failure. Radiol. Clin. North Am., 10:433, 1972.

Cooperman, L. R., and Lowman, R. M.: Fetal lobulation of the kidneys. Am. J. Roentgenol., 92:273, 1964.

Craven, J. D., and Lecky, J. W.: The natural history of postobstructive renal atrophy shown by sequential urograms. Radiology, 101:555, 1971.

Foster, J. H. et al: Ten years experience with the surgical management of renovascular hypertension. Ann. Surg., 177:755, 1973.

Frimann-Dahl, J.: Normal variations of the left kidney. Acta Radiol., 55:207, 1961.

Green, W. M. et al: "Column of Bertin": Diagnosis by nephrotomography. Am. J. Roentgenol. Radium Ther. Nucl. Med., 116:714, 1972.

Hodson, C. J. et al: The radiological contribution toward the diagnosis of chronic pyelonephritis. Radiology, 88:857, 1967.

Hodson, J.: The lobar structure of the kidney. Br. J. Urol., 44:246, 1972.

Lalli, A. F.: Roentgen aspects of renal calculus disease. Urol. Clin. North Am., 1:213, 1974.

Little, P. J. et al: The appearance of the intravenous pyelogram during and after acute pyelonephritis. Lancet, 1:1186, 1965.

Moell, H.: Size of normal kidneys. Acta Radiol., 46:640, 1956.

Olsson, O.: Diagnostic Radiology, vol. 1. In Alken, C. E. et al: Encyclopedia of Urology. Berlin, Springer-Verlag, 1962.

von Schreeb, T. et al: Renal adenocarcinoma: Is there a risk of spreading tumor cells in diagnostic puncture? Scand. J. Urol. Nephrol., 1:270, 1967.

Stanley, J. C., and Fry, W. J.: Renovascular hypertension secondary to arterial fibrodysplasia in adults: criteria for operation and results of surgical therapy. Arch. Surg., 111:922, 1975.

Talner, L. B.: Urographic contrast media in uremia; Physiology and pharmacology. Radiol. Clin. North Am., 10:421, 1972.

Thornbury, J. R.: Needle aspiration of avascular renal lesions. Radiology, 105:299, 1972.

Watson, R. C. et al: Arteriography in the diagnosis of renal carcinoma; review of 100 cases. Radiology, 91:888, 1968.

Chapter Four

UROPATHOLOGY

Paul W. Gikas

KIDNEY

This discussion on the pathology of the kidney focuses on the inflammatory, vascular, and neoplastic disorders. The important congenital anomalies are the subject of a previous chapter.

Although urologists are concerned primarily with the so-called surgical diseases, they must consider several of the medical disorders of the kidney because of the overlap of signs and symptoms between the two basic categories. Hematuria, pyuria, and flank pain can herald afflictions in either group, and it behooves the student of urology to achieve at least a rudimentary knowledge of the common nonsurgical renal entities.

Inflammation

The renal inflammatory lesions can be broadly grouped into two categories: those that result from a reaction in the glomerulus to immunologic injury and those inflammations that are due to direct action in the kidney by pathogenic organisms which lodge there or toxic substances such as certain medications which pass through the organ. The generic term *glomerulonephritis* encompasses the first category, and *interstitial nephritis* is the term which characterizes the second group. With the exception of some cases of infectious interstitial nephritis, the inflammatory conditions to be described are bilateral when both kidneys are present.

Glomerulonephritis

Glomerulonephritis is a renal disease in which there is an inflammatory reaction in the glomeruli. Secondary changes may be seen in vessels, tubules, and interstitia.

Greater than eight out of ten cases of glomerulonephritis are initiated by an immunologic glomerular injury. Considering the fact that the primary function of the glomerulus is to filter blood, it is not surprising to learn that the trapping by the glomerulus of immune complexes consisting of antigen and antibody accounts for about 80 per cent of the cases of glomerulonephritis. Another 5 per cent are triggered by circulating antibodies to the glomerular basement membranes, which for some unknown reason serve as an antigen (anti-GBM nephritis).

Pathogenesis. Immunofluorescence studies utilizing antisera to the immunoglobulins IgG, IgM, and IgA have confirmed the presence of antibodies in glomerular capillary walls. The immune complex type of glomerulonephritis is characterized by a granular pattern of fluorescence. The ultrastructural counterpart exhibited by the use of the electron microscope is the presence of aggregates of electron dense deposits believed to be immune complex in a subepithelial, intramembranous, or subendothelial position in glomerular capillary walls (Fig. 4–1). The antigenic component of the immune complex may be of endogenous or exogenous origin. Bacterial products are examples of exogenous antigen while nuclear material such as DNA may serve as an endogenous antigen. Several antigens in both groups have been defined in the production of human glomerular disease. The glomeruli from patients with circulating antibodies to glomerular basement membranes display a linear pattern of fluorescence in the capillary walls when reacted with antisera to immunoglobulins, particularly IgG. In such cases no electron dense deposits are seen with electron microscopy.

Prototypical examples of immune complex glomerulonephritis are poststreptococcal glomerulonephritis and lupus nephritis. Goodpasture's disease and some forms of so-called rapidly progressive glomerulonephritis belong to the less common group of anti–basement membrane disorders. In Goodpasture's disease, the circulating antibodies apparently react to both glomerular basement membrane and pulmonary capillary basement membrane, thus accounting for the renal disease as well as for the often fatal hemoptysis seen in these patients.

The pathogenesis of the glomerular damage in both the immune complex disease and anti-GBM disease is similar and related to the activation of complement by the antigen-antibody reaction. This results in chemotaxis of polymorphonuclear leukocytes and their subsequent release of lysozymes that attack various components of the glomerulus, particularly the basement membrane. Coagulation within the glomerulus and the action of kinins and vasoactive amines probably also play a role in stimulating glomerular reaction that is revealed by alterations in the capillary basement membrane, or proliferation of the intrinsic glomerular cells (mesangial, endothelial, and epithelial). This may result in proteinuria, hematuria, and a decrease in renal function, which accompanies the glomerulonephritides.

In the acute phases of glomerulonephritis, the kidney may be of

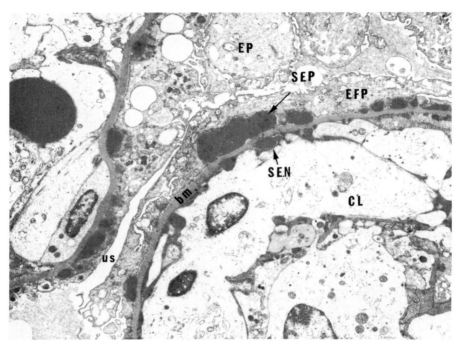

Figure 4–1 Electron micrograph of two glomerular capillary walls showing prominent sub-epithelial (SEP) and subendothelial (SEN) electron dense deposit from a patient with acute post streptococcal glomerulonephritis. (Original magnification 3700×.) Epithelial cytoplasm (EP); Basement membrane (bm); Urinary space (us); Capillary lumen (CL); Epithelial foot process (EFP).

normal size or enlarged. Petechial hemorrhages sometimes dot the subcapsular surface in severe cases. Using the light microscope, one sees glomerular hypercellularity as a result of endothelial, mesangial, and sometimes epithelial cell proliferation (Fig. 4–2). Neutrophilic leukocytes may also contribute to the increased cellularity. When the majority of glomeruli exhibit proliferation of the parietal epithelium of Bowman's capsule with the formation of crescents, the disease is classified as rapidly progressive glomerulonephritis, which generally carries a grave prognosis with progression to terminal renal failure in a matter of weeks or months. During the acute attack of glomerulonephritis, the tubules often contain erythrocytes, and the interstitium may be edematous. Vascular changes are minimal unless the glomerulonephritis accompanies a systemic vasculitis.

Chronic long-standing glomerulonephritis decreases the size of the kidney, and the organ exhibits a uniformly granular cortical surface as a result of foci of subcapsular tubular and glomerular atrophy between normal or dilated hypertrophic tubules (Fig. 4–3). The glomeruli show varying degrees of hypercellularity and are partially to completely sclerotic. There is considerable tubular atrophy, chronic interstitial inflammation, and arteriolosclerosis. The severity of these alterations

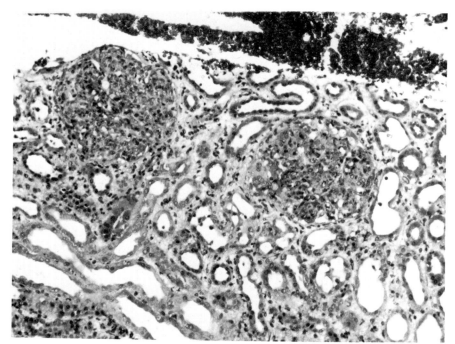

Figure 4–2   Two glomeruli from the same case as Fig. 4–1, exhibiting marked diffuse hyper-cellularity due to proliferation of intrinsic glomerular cells. Marked interstitial edema is also present. (Original magnification 163×.)

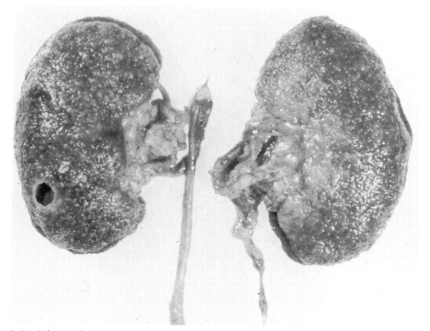

Figure 4–3   Subcapsular granularity in kidneys with long-standing chronic glomerulonephritis. Hypertension of long duration with arteriolonephrosclerosis also produces this change.

increases as the disease progresses, ultimately resulting in the so-called end-stage kidney. Proteinuria, hematuria, and casts may be present in any stage of the disease; however, hematuria is usually more prominent in the acute phases.

When the term glomerulonephritis is used without modification, it usually refers to a generalized process involving all or most glomeruli. If only scattered or occasional glomeruli are involved by the disease process, the glomerulonephritis is designated as focal. It is virtually impossible to prognosticate on the basis of focal versus generalized involvement. Diseases in either category may resolve with no significant loss of renal function, or they may progress at varying velocities to terminal renal disease. The urologist should be particularly aware of focal glomerulonephritis as one of the causes of so-called benign essential hematuria.

The pathogenic scheme depicted involving immune complex activation of complement with the resulting attraction of neutrophils and lysosomal enzyme release and the subsequent glomerular damage and cellular reaction is generally accepted; however, such a scheme does not adequately account for all of the histologic patterns seen with immune complex glomerulonephritis. One notable exception is membranous glomerulonephritis, better designated as epimembranous nephropathy, in which one sees abundant immune complexes manifested as electron dense deposits in an epimembranous location in glomerular capillary walls; yet typically in this disease, there is no significant glomerular hypercellularity. Patients with this disorder often present with the nephrotic syndrome. This glomerular lesion may be etiologically related to gold therapy, penicillamine therapy, syphilis, lupus erythematosus, or occur on an idiopathic basis. There are no distinguishing gross features; however, microscopically, there is a diffuse thickening of the glomerular capillary walls with minimal or no hypercellularity. The diagnosis is confirmed by the ultrastructural findings described above (Fig. 4–4).

Interstitial Nephritis

The glomerulus is initially spared in this form of nephritis, and the abnormality appears to manifest itself in the interstitium. Interstitial nephritis is subclassified into noninfectious and infectious types.

Noninfectious. The noninfectious form may be associated with nephrotoxic agents including certain common medications. Most notable in this regard is analgesic nephropathy seen in patients who consume large quantities of aspirin and phenacetin-containing compounds. Certain antibiotics may be nephrotoxic and result in a predominantly interstitial nephritis. Penicillin, methicillin, and ampicillin, to mention a few, have been incriminated in the production of interstitial nephritis.

The pathogenetic mechanisms in analgesic nephropathy are not

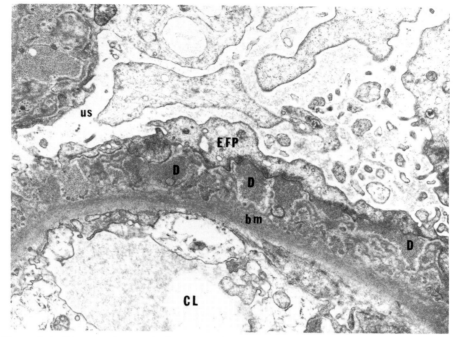

Figure 4–4 Electron micrograph showing a glomerular capillary wall with abundant electron dense deposit (D) in an epimembranous location with overlying fused epithelial foot processes. Idiopathic epimembranous nephropathy. (Original magnification 10,900×.) Capillary lumen (CL); Basement membrane (bm); Epithelial foot processes (EFP); Urinary space (us).

clearly understood. There is some evidence to incriminate immunologic injury at a tubular site as the inciting factor in some antibiotic induced nephropathy. The presence of immune complexes, presumably with methicillin as an antigen in tubular epithelium, which is the site of 90 per cent of the antibiotic excretion, is suggested by electron microscopic and immunofluorescence studies.

There are no characteristic gross changes in the kidney. In analgesic nephropathy, there is tubular atrophy, periglomerular fibrosis, chronic inflammatory cell infiltrate, and increased collagen in the interstitium. There is some evidence to suggest the lesion begins in the medulla and progresses to the cortex. The tubular damage is reflected in the earliest functional abnormality, which is impaired ability to concentrate the urine. Renal failure may result if analgesic abuse continues.

The interstitial nephritis associated with antibiotics such as methicillin is characterized by foci of inflammatory cell infiltrates, chiefly lymphocytes, plasma cells, and eosinophils, predominantly in the cortical region. Interstitial edema and focal tubular necrosis are also evident. Clinically, these patients present with hematuria, proteinuria, and azotemia. Resolution appears to be the rule; however, an occasional patient may exhibit residual morphologic and functional damage.

Infectious. This form of interstitial nephritis is also known as pyelonephritis, and it implies an inflammatory reaction in a kidney as a direct result of the presence of pathogenic organisms in the renal parenchyma. The microorganisms may arrive in the kidney via the hematogenous route or ascend from the lower urinary tract. Obstruction to outflow of urine in the lower tract renders the kidney more susceptible to infection via either route. The coliform, proteus, klebsiella, pseudomonas, enterococcal, aerobacter, and staphylococcal organisms are the most frequent offenders, but theoretically, any bacterium or fungus can be involved. Instrumentation of the urinary tract may introduce organisms and incite infection. For some unknown reason, females possess a higher incidence of bacteriuria than males of all ages. Pregnancy also places the female at a greater risk for the development of renal infection as a result of urinary retention and the dilatation and decrease in tone of the ureters, related to the enlarged uterus or in response to the altered hormonal environment of pregnancy. As males grow older and reach the age when prostatic hyperplasia and neoplasm are more frequent, their incidence of urinary infection rises.

The acute form of pyelonephritis is clearly the result of infection with microorganisms; however, the relationship of infection to the origin of chronic pyelonephritis is less lucid. In those cases associated with the retention of urine, bacteria can often be identified as the cause of the continuing inflammatory process; however, in patients with chronic pyelonephritis who do not show evidence of urinary tract obstruction or stasis, there is a notorious inability to identify organisms in the urine or renal tissue.

One possible explanation for the perpetuation of the chronic inflammatory process in such cases would be the presence of bacterial products acting as antigens. The evidence for this supposition is fragmentary and inconclusive. It is possible that some forms of chronic pyelonephritis have no connection with infection as an initiating or perpetuating event.

The acute disease is characterized by purulent and often suppurative inflammation. Grossly, one may see small 1 to 5 mm yellow-white abscesses in the cortex. Histologically, there is interstitial edema, hyperemia, and infiltrates of neutrophilic leukocytes in between tubules (Fig. 4–5). Purulent casts are seen within tubules, and foci of suppurative necrosis may be seen. Coalescence of suppurative foci may lead to an extensive abscess or renal carbuncle. When the suppurative process violates the renal capsule, a perinephric abscess may form. The inflammatory process may be diffuse, involving the parenchyma of the entire organ, or it may have a patchy distribution, sparing large areas. When the disease is present in a hydronephrotic kidney with obstruction to outflow, the purulent exudate collects in the renal pelvis and produces pyonephrosis.

The gross appearance of chronic pyelonephritis varies markedly depending on the extent and distribution of the destructive inflammatory process. Local involvement results in delineated depressed sub-

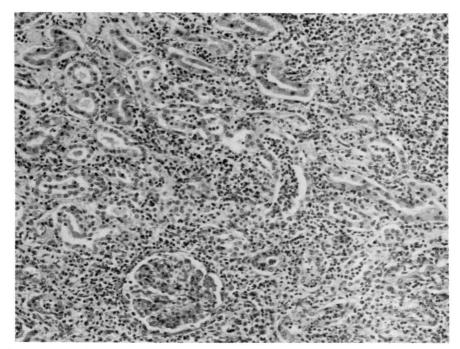

Figure 4–5 Purulent casts in tubules and acute interstitial inflammation in a kidney with acute pyelonephritis. (Original magnification 100×.)

capsular scars which may be indistinguishable from old infarcts that are the result of vascular occlusion. As it progresses, the more diffuse disease produces a shrunken kidney with many coarsely irregular sub-capsular scars. When these changes are combined with those of hydro-nephrotic atrophy, as frequently is the case, the renal parenchyma is reduced to a thin scarred rim around the ectatic calyces and pelvis.

Chronic pyelonephritis is the most difficult disease to diagnose with certainty from renal biopsy because of the oftentimes focal nature and the fact that no single histologic alteration is specific (Fig. 4–6). The following changes, all nonspecific when they occur individually, should be present for a diagnosis of chronic pyelonephritis:
1. Periglomerular fibrosis
2. Atrophy of tubules and dilatation of tubules with colloidlike casts
3. Interstitial infiltrate of chronic inflammatory cells
4. Inflammatory cell infiltrate in pelvic mucosa
5. Vascular sclerosis

LIPOGRANULOMATOUS PYELONEPHRITIS

A unique variety of interstitial nephritis bearing the appellation lipogranulomatous pyelonephritis is seen in occasional patients. There is a high association with infection by proteus organisms.

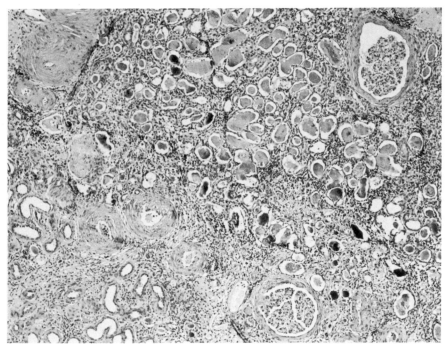

Figure 4–6 Chronic pyelonephritis exhibiting periglomerular fibrosis, dilated atrophic tubules with colloid-like casts, vascular sclerosis, and chronic interstitial inflammation. (Original magnification 40×.)

The result is a destructive inflammatory process characterized by large areas of necrosis containing aggregates of lipid-laden macrophages or foam cells. These cells impart a yellow color to the involved areas, which often have a soft, pasty consistency. The necrotic soft regions may be confused with tuberculous pyelonephritis on gross inspection. The large numbers of foam cells may be misinterpreted as a renal cell carcinoma by the unwary eye on microscopic examination.

TUBERCULOUS PYELONEPHRITIS

Tuberculous pyelonephritis exhibits tissue changes of a chronic granulomatous nature. The renal involvement is a result of hematogenous spread from a primary site, usually in the lungs. There may be miliary lesions in the cortex consisting of small, epithelioid tubercles with or without central necrosis. A nodular-caseating form also occurs, which results from coalescence of tubercles to form large caseous masses rimmed by epithelioid cells and Langhans' giant cells (Fig. 4–7). Considerable destruction of parenchyma may result. A more detailed discussion is offered in a subsequent chapter.

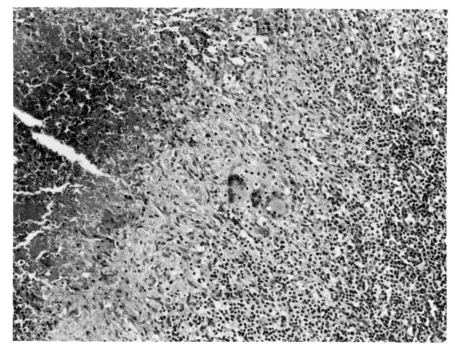

Figure 4–7   The upper left corner exhibits fresh caseous necrosis bordered by a zone of epithelioid cells, Langhans' giant cells, and lymphocytes in a kidney with tuberculosis. (Original magnification 100×.)

RENAL PAPILLARY NECROSIS

This lesion, also known as necrotizing papillitis, is a special variety of interstitial nephritis in which the distal papillae undergo coagulative necrosis and may slough into the renal pelvis and actually be passed in the urine. This potentially fatal affliction is particularly associated with diabetes mellitus, obstructive uropathy, and analgesic (Phenacetin) abuse. The pathogenesis is thought to be related to the already precarious blood supply of the papillae being further compromised by the inflammatory reaction to infection often seen in diabetes or obstructive uropathy. The edema and leukocytic infiltrate produces an increase in interstitial pressure which in turn compromises vessels and results in an infarct of the papillae. In analgesic abuse, a vasculitis or interstitial inflammation may produce a similar reduction in blood supply with resulting infarct.

The lesion appears as a demarcated, pale papilla which fragments easily. Microscopically, the distal papilla appears acellular with only ghosts of tubules and vessels remaining. The inflammatory infiltrate of neutrophils is usually confined to a zone at the base of the papilla at the interface of necrotic and viable tissue.

Vascular Disease

ACUTE TUBULAR NECROSIS

For lack of a better name, acute oliguric renal failure associated with severe trauma, thermal injury, dehydration, or incompatible blood transfusion is designated acute tubular necrosis. Older labels included shock kidney, lower nephron nephrosis, and glomerulonephrosis, to name a few. Although the precise pathogenesis has been the subject of considerable controversy, it is believed by many to result from hemodynamic alterations in the kidney with a subsequent decrease in glomerular filtration and ischemic changes in the tubular epithelium. For this reason, it is classified in the discussion of vascular diseases.

Grossly, the kidney exhibits a pale cortex and a markedly congested medulla. The microscopic morphology is often not in concert with the serious degree of impairment of renal function. The morphologic alterations usually attributed to this condition include glomerular ischemia and degenerative changes in tubular epithelium up to and including frank necrosis. Occasionally one sees an interstitial inflammatory reaction to the necrotic tubules. Foci of extramedullary hematopoiesis have been seen. The renal changes are potentially reversible if the patient can be tided over with peritoneal dialysis or hemodialysis. The author has seen instances, however, in which residual damage has occurred, manifested by patchy tubular atrophy and replacement by interstitial fibrous tissue.

ARTERIOLONEPHROSCLEROSIS

Long-standing arterial hypertension of any cause results in sclerosis of renal arterioles and ischemic glomerular sclerosis. These morphologic changes with the subsequent ischemia perpetuate and accentuate the systemic hypertension, resulting in a vicious cycle.

Grossly, these kidneys are decreased in size and display a uniformly granular subcapsular surface. The microscopic changes in the established case include hyaline sclerosis of renal arterioles with glomerular sclerosis and tubular atrophy. These ischemic atrophic changes occur particularly in the subcapsular cortex and alternate with foci of normal or hypertrophied dilated tubules. Small infiltrates of lymphocytes and interstitial fibrosis are often present in these microatrophic areas. In effect, the foci of atrophy are little valleys between hills of normal or hypertrophied tubules, thus imparting a grossly visible granularity (Fig. 4–3). A mild proteinuria may accompany this arteriolonephrosclerosis, and after many years, there is some compromise of renal function.

It should be emphasized that hypertension is a frequent complication of many renal diseases, and therefore, the morphologic changes of arteriolosclerosis associated with the increase in blood pressure are often present with the other renal diseases described. Chronic glomerulonephritis classically presents a contracted granular kidney contributed to by the ischemic changes resulting from the hypertension.

MALIGNANT HYPERTENSION

When the hypertension is severe and associated with azotemia and Grade IV hypertensive retinopathy, it is designated malignant hypertension or accelerated nephrosclerosis.

If the malignant hypertension arises in a previously normal kidney, the organ is of normal size or may be swollen. The subcapsular surface is smooth and often shows petechial hemorrhages, imparting a so-called fleabitten appearance.

The microscopic changes in malignant hypertension are quite characteristic. There is a striking hyperplastic sclerosis of small arteries and arterioles manifested by fibromuscular proliferation, which imparts a concentric thickening to the vessel. Fibrinoid necrosis of arterial walls and glomeruli may also occur. Erythrocytes are present in tubules. The malignant hypertension may complicate pre-existing renal disease in which case the described vascular changes are superimposed on the characteristics of the pre-existing disorder.

Proteinuria and hematuria are prominent signs during the malignant phase of hypertension. In the untreated patient, renal failure rapidly ensues.

LARGE VESSEL DISEASE

Abnormalities of the renal artery that result in the decrease of renal blood flow may be responsible for the production of renovascular hypertension. The arterial abnormality serves in effect as the vascular clamp, which has enjoyed extensive utilization in the production of experimental hypertension in animals.

In adults, a fortuitous atheromatous plaque in a strategic location can effectively alter blood flow in a renal artery. Thrombus formation and embolization are also possibilities to be considered.

Of special interest are the renal arterial dysplasias. This group of vessel wall abnormalities results from varying degrees of alteration in the amount and distribution of fibrous tissue and smooth muscle in the arterial wall. Three types are recognized, based on the location of the major changes in the media, outer media, or adventitia. Diffuse intimal fibrosis and periadventitial fibrosis also may result in renal arterial stenosis. The fibromuscular dysplasias are characterized by a "string of beads" pattern in the angiogram.

DIABETIC NEPHROPATHY

Diabetes mellitus is a major cause of chronic renal failure and deserves discussion. The renal vasculature is a prime target of the microangiopathy of long-standing diabetes. This condition is manifested as a striking hyaline sclerosis of the efferent arteriole at the vascular pole of the glomerulus. Usually, both afferent and efferent arterioles are thickened, but only the sclerosis of the efferent limb is considered characteristic of diabetes mellitus. One cannot distinguish afferent from efferent arterioles in microscopic sections, so it is necessary to see both arterioles of a glomerulus, and if they both exhibit sclerosis, then obviously the efferent vessel is involved.

The glomeruli of long-standing diabetics often show a net increase in basement membrane and mesangial matrix. This evidence accounts for the glomerulosclerosis, which may be diffuse or nodular. The increase in mesangial matrix contributes to the characteristic nodular variety.

As mentioned earlier, renal papillary necrosis may be seen more frequently in diabetics. The microangiopathy of renal vessels undoubtedly contributes to the vulnerability of the renal papillae.

Alport's syndrome, a form of hereditary nephropathy associated with neural deafness, deserves brief mention. The histologic findings may be those of a mixed glomerulonephritis and interstitial nephritis with characteristic but nonspecific foam cells. A specific electron microscopic finding has recently been defined, consisting of irregular rarefactions in the glomerular basement membranes. This disease may manifest with hematuria and it can progress to terminal renal failure.

The glomerulonephritides, along with pyelonephritis and diabetic nephropathy, are the major causes of terminal renal failure necessitating chronic dialysis or renal transplant.

Neoplasms and Neoplasticlike Lesions

BENIGN NEOPLASMS

The benign neoplasms of the kidney rarely reach the clinical horizon. The medullary fibroma is a small lesion, usually less than a centimeter in diameter, which presents itself to the pathologist as an incidental gray-white nodule in a kidney removed at autopsy or as a surgical specimen removed for another reason. Microscopically, such lesions are interlacing bands of fibrocytes interdigitating with the renal tubules. Some consider them to be hamartomas.

Lipomas occur in renal tissue and, as elsewhere, consist of a circumscribed aggregate of mature fat cells. Rarely do they reach a size to produce symptoms.

The angiomyolipomas are small, mixed mesenchymal masses in either the cortex or medulla, which on occasion are associated with the central nervous system lesion, tuberous sclerosis. The author has seen one of these angiomyolipomas that became a clinically significant renal mass.

Hemangiomas may be a cause of hematuria and usually present in the subepithelial stroma of a calyx.

Leiomyomas probably derive from the smooth muscle of the renal capsule or from venous walls in or beneath the capsule in the cortex.

The cortical adenoma originates from tubular epithelium and usually has a yellow color as a result of the high lipid content. Such lesions are usually less than one centimeter in diameter. There appears to be an association between these lesions and kidneys which are the seat of nephrosclerosis or chronic inflammation. Tubular ectasia that results from these conditions may favor their genesis. The prime significance of the adenoma lies in the belief that renal cell carcinoma, the most common malignant renal neoplasm, originates from it. This concept is supported by the striking resemblance of the adenoma and carcinoma cells along with their chemical similarity that is reflected by a mutually high lipid content.

MALIGNANT NEOPLASMS

Renal Cell Carcinoma. The renal cell carcinoma is the most frequent malignant tumor in the kidney, accounting for at least 80 per cent of renal cancer. Its most common synonym is hypernephroma, which suggests origin from adrenal cortical rests within the kidney. As implied in the earlier discussion about adenomas, this adrenal theory of origin no longer enjoys support.

This neoplasm has a peak incidence after 50 years of age and occurs in males more frequently than females.

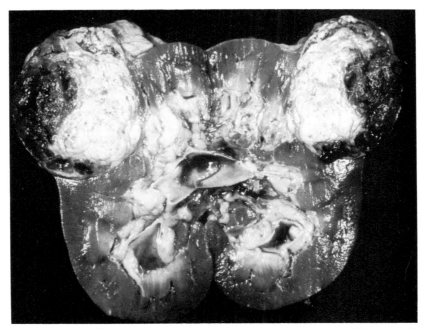

Figure 4–8   Large renal cell carcinoma with extensive hemorrhage in upper pole of kidney which has been bisected.

The renal cell carcinoma usually originates in the cortex of one of the poles of the kidney, and by the time it produces symptoms, it often distorts the organ considerably as a result of extension through the renal capsule and into the renal pelvis (Fig. 4–8). The tendency is to compress rather than infiltrate adjacent parenchyma. Satellite nodules of neoplasm do, however, occur. A distinct border results from this expanding growth, giving the false impression of a true capsule. This neoplasm classically presents a yellow to orange color as a result of the high lipid content. The cut surface often displays white fibrous streaks, foci of hemorrhage and necrosis, and on occasion may be cystic. There is a cystic variant which presents primarily as a large solitary or multiloculated cyst whose true nature is betrayed only by scattered aggregates of clear carcinoma cells in the wall or an occasional papillary projection of clear or solid eosinophilic carcinoma cells into the cyst lumen. Vascular invasion is present at the time of nephrectomy in about one third of the cases.

The microscopic picture often varies considerably from the classic clear polyhedral cells arranged in nests, cords, and tubules (Fig. 4–9). A granular cell variant is common, and one can be completely fooled by the spindle cell type of renal cell carcinoma, which mimics a fibrosarcoma histologically (Fig. 4–10). The cells may be regular in size and shape, or they can exhibit considerable pleomorphism. The arrangement of cells in papillae, nests, trabeculae, or tubules appears to have

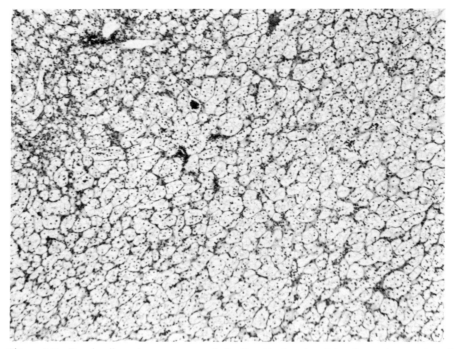

Figure 4–9   Renal cell carcinoma composed of cells with abundant "clear" cytoplasm and small nuclei. (Original magnification 64×.)

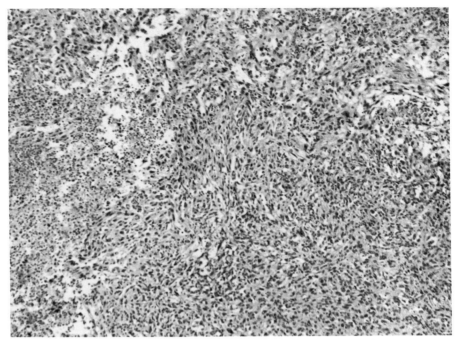

Figure 4-10   Spindle cell variant of renal cell carcinoma. (Original magnification 64×.)

limited biologic significance as far as behavior of the neoplasm is concerned.

Over one half of the patients with renal cell carcinoma exhibit hematuria, and only one fifth actually present with a palpable mass. The systemic sign of fever may be the mode of presentation. Indeed, its symptomatology is as diversified as its microscopic picture. Symptoms from distant metastases may cause the patient to first seek medical care. The lungs are the most popular site for metastasis, but no organ is exempt. Lymph nodes, liver, and bone follow the lung in frequency as sites of secondary tumors.

The probability of five year survival without vascular invasion approximates 50 per cent. With vascular invasion, it decreases to less than 30 per cent.

Wilms' Tumor. Nephroblastoma is the popular synonym for Wilms' tumor. This malignant neoplasm almost exclusively occurs in children. The author has never seen a true adult form of the tumor; however, there are cases reported. These lesions account for 6 per cent of the malignant renal neoplasms. One third of the nephroblastomas appear in infants during the first year of life, and many of these probably developed in utero. Most of the neoplasms develop by the age of five years. It is the second most common malignant neoplasm in children under five, exceeded only by leukemia, and it occurs with nearly equal incidence in both sexes.

The theory which enjoys widest current support places the origin of the neoplasm in the primitive renal blastema. This is a pluripotential tissue which under normal circumstances gives rise to both epithelial and stromal elements in the kidney. When this embryogenesis goes awry and a neoplasm develops, it is not surprising that neoplastic epithelial and stromal components result in a mixed carcinoma and sarcoma which characterizes the Wilms' tumor.

These neoplasms arise in any portion of the renal parenchyma and give the appearance of being encapsulated. Their color varies from gray to yellow with foci of hemorrhage lending a darker hue. Grossly visible cysts are common. Necrosis frequently occurs, imparting a soft friable consistency. They often reach a large volume, accounting at times for one fifth of the weight of the infant. By the time of surgical removal, the neoplasm frequently is much larger than the host kidney.

The microscopic picture mirrors carcinomatous elements typically manifested as tubular or ductal structures in a sea of malignant supporting tissue elements. These latter components may take the form of fibrosarcoma and rhabdomyosarcoma. Chondromatous, osseous, and lipomatous elements may be seen in various stages of maturation. Since only one germ layer is involved in its origin, namely mesoderm, it is considered a mixed tumor and not a teratoma.

Systemic signs of fever and hypertension are frequent. A palpable mass in the child's abdomen is probably the most common herald of Wilms' tumor. Hematuria is less frequently a presenting sign as compared to the renal cell carcinoma. Because of the high degree of vascularity and the tendency for vascular invasion, blood borne metastases are common and increase with the age of the neoplasm. Lungs, liver, brain, and bones are frequently involved, especially the bones of the skull.

Urothelial Neoplasms.   The transitional epithelium of the renal pelvis gives rise to urothelial tumors which have essentially the same growth patterns as those originating in the urinary bladder. They will be discussed in more detail under that organ. Suffice it to say, they account for approximately 8 per cent of malignant renal neoplasms, and 80 per cent of them occur past the age of 40 years. Hematuria and flank pain are the most prominent warnings of such a lesion. Males host this neoplasm about four times more frequently than females.

Sarcoma.   Pure sarcomas comprise only 3 per cent of malignant renal neoplasms. Fibrosarcomas are the most frequent offenders in this category, usually originating in the renal capsule. Leiomyosarcomas likewise are usually of capsular or vascular wall origin and are uncommon. Liposarcomas and osteogenic sarcomas occur even less frequently. The prognosis is generally quite poor for the sarcomas.

Miscellaneous.   The malignant lymphomas may involve the kidney but initial symptomatology is usually related to systemic manifestations or regional involvement elsewhere in the body. The same holds true for plasma cell myeloma, which on occasion can produce renal failure as a result of myeloma protein casts obstructing tubules. Renal amyloidosis may complicate plasma cell myeloma. These are not considered surgical problems.

The kidneys are a frequent site of metastatic carcinoma from primary neoplasms in other tissues. Their affinity for secondary tumors is exceeded only by the liver, lungs, and bones.

Renal Allograft Rejection

Rejection still remains a formidable obstacle to successful renal transplantation in a significant number of recipients of transplanted kidneys.

Transplants from related donors appear to fare better than cadaver grafts, but both types may experience rejection reactions.

Two types of immunologic mechanisms operate in the rejection of the allograft, namely, humoral and cellular. The humoral type of rejection is a rather violent process resulting from circulating antibodies in the recipient to donor lymphocytes. This humoral rejection is also seen in ABO blood group incompatibility between recipient and donor. The recipient's cytotoxic antibodies to donor lymphocytes may result from previous allografts, pregnancies, or blood transfusions. Cellular immunity results from sensitized recipient lymphocytes called immunoblasts. The precise target cell in the allograft which is attacked by the host immunoblasts has not been precisely defined, but much evidence suggests it is the endothelial cell of the donor organ.

The method of antigen exposure which sensitizes the recipient is not entirely clear; however, several possibilities exist, including donor lymphocytes in the allograft, pick-up and delivery of donor antigen by host lymphocytes to the host lymphoid tissue for sensitization, and antigen release into the allograft venous blood which in turn circulates in the recipient.

The reaction patterns can be separated into hyperacute, acute, and chronic.

The humoral immune mechanism is believed to be chiefly at work in the hyperacute rejection. This is manifested by thrombosis of arteries that results in parenchymal necrosis. An infiltrate of immunoblasts is not a feature of this process, although neutrophils may be present. This devastating reaction is rapid and may begin within hours after transplantation. When ABO incompatibility is involved, thrombi may occur within the main renal artery.

The acute rejection may develop in a few days or months after transplantation, and it is the cellular mechanism which is primarily involved. The organ is swollen; histologic changes include: (1) infiltrates around vessels and in the interstitium of mononuclear inflammatory cells previously designated as immunoblasts, (2) striking interstitial edema, (3) focal tubular necrosis, (4) fibrinoid necrosis in glomeruli and small arteries, and (5) focal interstitial hemorrhage. The more severe the reaction process, the less likely is graft survival. The reaction may be modified by immunosuppressive agents.

The chronic rejection reaction may occur weeks to years after transplantation and when advanced, results in a markedly scarred and deformed kidney. Both humoral and cellular immunologic mechanisms are believed to play a role. The characteristic histologic alteration is a striking hyperplastic sclerosis of small and medium sized arteries with a resulting decrease in luminal diameter. The internal elastic lamina of the arteries is multiplied to several strands and there is fibrosis of the intima. The glomeruli exhibit thickening of their capillary walls, and there is tubular atrophy with interstitial fibrosis. The latter changes may result in part from the ischemia due to the marked vascular sclerosis. Focal mononuclear cell infiltrates may be present.

It should be emphasized that the above types of reactions may occur simultaneously in the same allograft, thus combining histologic features.

Glomerular changes in the transplanted kidney may be nonspecific, such as capillary thickening and an increase in mesangium, sometimes referred to as transplant glomerulopathy. It should be remembered, however, that the glomerulus may be the site of recurrent glomerulonephritis, if that was the original disease which led to renal failure. Membranoproliferative or so-called hypocomplementemic glomerulonephritis has a particularly bad reputation for recurring in allografts. A "new" glomerulonephritis, unrelated to any pre-existing disease, of course, may occur.

Finally, it should be noted that acute tubular necrosis secondary to the ischemic insult suffered by the donor kidney in the process of harvesting and transplantation may be responsible for failure of graft function. Both immunologic and ischemic injury may occur in the allograft, making histologic interpretation of the biopsy specimen very difficult. Less commonly, renal grafts fail because of a septic process resulting in a destructive pyelonephritis.

This discussion was concerned with the kidney; however, it should be pointed out that the acute rejection process may affect the ureter with a resulting leak of urine at the anastomotic site.

URINARY BLADDER

INFLAMMATORY LESIONS

Being smooth and glandless and frequently cleansed by urine, the normal mucosa of the urinary bladder affords considerable protection against infectious agents. Nevertheless, infection does occur and may ascend via the urethra, particularly in the female, where the distance is much shorter. Implantation of organisms en route from a primarily infected kidney is a second source of bladder infection. Rarely, direct hematogenous infection may occur. Practically any pathogen may be causative, but the coliform bacillus is the most frequent offender with less common involvement by staphylococci, streptococci, klebsiella, Neisserian organisms, yeasts, and parasites.

In acute cystitis, the mucosa appears edematous and hyperemic. In severe forms, an exudate covers the surface and ulcers and hemorrhage may be grossly visible. The microscopic pattern varies with the severity of the infection. In mild forms, there is edema, congestion, and scattered neutrophils in the lamina propria. As the intensity increases, the number of leukocytes increases to the point where the histologic picture is one of suppuration with extension into muscularis. Ulcers are covered with fibrinopurulent exudate. Blood may be present, as well as a deposit of mineral-laden urinary sediment contributed to by the action of the urea-splitting organisms.

In chronic cystitis, the mucosa harbors many mononuclear cells including lymphocytes, plasma cells, and histiocytes. The amount of fibrous tissue increases and may infiltrate the muscular layer, resulting in a loss of elasticity with a reduction in luminal volume.

SPECIAL VARIETIES

Cystitis cystica is the designation for a lesion which presents a gross appearance of numerous mucosal vesicles measuring from less than 1 mm to over 1 cm in diameter. These vesicles form in the lamina propria from solid aggregates of transitional epithelium known as cell nests of von Brunn, after the person who first described the pathogenesis of the lesion. The nests of cells may become detached from the surface epithelium. Central cells in the nests then become vacuolated, and eventually, as a result of the loss of transitional cells, a hollow cystic structure results that is lined by cuboidal cells. The amount of inflammation in the surrounding lamina propria may be minimal, and the term cystitis is not always appropriate.

When the lining epithelium of the small cysts undergoes a prosoplasia to mucin-forming columnar cells, the condition is designated cystitis glandularis, which is benign in itself but may be a forerunner of adenocarcinoma.

Follicular cystitis refers to a mucosa studded with many grayish nodules which microscopically are lymphoid follicles.

Emphysematous cystitis may be seen in patients with diabetes mellitus. The mucosa is distorted by gas-filled cysts that are probably a result of bacterial or enzymatic action on glucose in the mucosa. Clostridial organisms implanted by instrumentation may produce gas-filled blebs in the lamina propria of the mucosa with very little inflammatory response.

Bullous cystitis is seen in patients with uremia. As a result of the intense edema in the stroma of the lamina propria, the mucosa exhibits a gross polypoid appearance with numerous bullae.

Radiation therapy directed to the uterine cervix or other pelvic structures may produce adverse effects in the urinary bladder. The term radiation cystitis designates these somewhat characteristic changes. In the acute phase, the resulting edema imparts a bullous appearance. Ulcers with fibrinopurulent exudate may be present. The later effects, sometimes appearing years following the therapy, include chronic ulcers in mucosa exhibiting both foci of atrophy as well as hyperplasia, squamous metaplasia, and dysplasia. There is considerable vascular sclerosis. Ectasia of capillaries and venules in a hyalinized stroma is a prominent feature. Bizarre-appearing stromal cells with large hyperchromatic nuclei are reliable indicators of previous irradiation.

Discrimination by the cystoscopist and the pathologist between these atypical epithelial and stromal changes and residual or recurrent neoplasms can be very difficult.

Chronic ulcerating interstitial cystitis, also known as Hunner's ulcer, is a debilitating condition of unknown origin. Both sexes may be affected, but the disease seems to occur most frequently in middle-aged women. The inflammatory process may involve the full thickness of the bladder wall. Although included in the name, ulcers are not always present. There is edema and a chronic inflammatory cell infiltrate with many mast cells in the lamina propria. This condition leads to fibrosis which may extend into the smooth muscle bundles. Any ulcers present are covered with a fibrinous exudate. As the condition progresses and involves a greater area, the volume of the bladder is decreased as a result of the extensive fibrosis which replaces the wall and produces contraction and loss of elasticity. This latter process accounts for the considerable morbidity associated with this disease.

Malakoplakia is a special form of chronic cystitis which occurs predominantly in middle-aged females, but males and children may be afflicted. The gross appearance is one of multiple gray-yellow papules often umbilicated on a background of congested mucosa. The microscopic picture consists of a chronic inflammatory cell infiltrate which fills the lamina propria. The predominant cell is a histiocyte which contains calcospherites. These bear the name Michaelis-Gutmann bodies and are characteristic for this disease. They are composed of a calcium phosphate complex and iron may also be detected in them. These structures may occur free in the lamina propria as well as in histiocytes where it is believed they originate. There appears to be a high association with Escherichia coli infections, and some believe malakoplakia is a variant of lipogranulomatous inflammation which was described under the section on the kidney. Fibrous tissue replaces the granulation tissue as the lesions heal. Malakoplakia is not confined to the urinary bladder; it may involve the ureters and renal pelvis and has been reported in the gastrointestinal tract.

As a result of neoplastic or inflammatory lesions in or adjacent to the urinary bladder, fistulae may form between the bladder and vagina, rectum, colon, or small intestine. Trauma can be an inciting factor in fistula formation. Pyogenic granulation tissue lines the wall of the fistulous tract, and varying degrees of epithelialization may occur. Of course, if the communication is secondary to a neoplastic process, one sees tumor cells in the wall of the tract.

Vesical schistosomiasis deserves brief mention. The adult worms of Schistosoma haematobium, which mature in the liver, migrate against the flow of blood to the veins in and around the urinary bladder and distal ureters. Many eggs are laid in the small veins from which they enter the lamina propria where they incite an intense inflammatory reaction consisting of lymphocytes, plasma cells, and many eosinophils. Epithelioid cells and giant cells accumulate with tubercle formation. The surface may ulcerate, and epithelial hyperplasia may be prominent. Fibrosis of the bladder wall results in a loss of elasticity and a marked decrease in bladder volume. Carcinoma, usually of the squamous type, may be a complication of vesical schistosomiasis.

BENIGN TUMORS

Nonmalignant tumors of the urinary bladder are rare. Those of epithelial type are termed adenomas and are classified as enteric, nephrogenic, and endometrial. The enteric adenoma is of urachal origin and is usually found in the dome in the muscular layer. Adenocarcinoma may, however, develop in these lesions. Nephrogenic adenomas are believed to derive from mesonephric remnants in the bladder wall. They present as nodular or papillary lesions consisting of ductal and tubular structures lined with cuboidal epithelium, which is somewhat reminiscent of renal tubular epithelium. The endometrial lesion is a form of endometriosis that involves the urinary bladder and looks like endometriosis elsewhere in the pelvis. Benign stromal neoplasms of the bladder are extremely rare. Equally uncommon is the extraadrenal pheochromocytoma, which may originate in the vesical wall from sympathetic nervous tissue. Episodic hypertension synchronous with voiding may be the warning of such a neoplasm.

MALIGNANT TUMORS

Urinary Bladder Carcinoma. Carcinoma of the urinary bladder has a peak incidence after the sixth decade and afflicts males three times more frequently than females. Nine thousand deaths a year are attributed to this neoplasm in the United States. Although the origin of this form of carcinoma is unknown in most of these victims, there is an increased risk in certain occupations, such as the printing, rubber, leather, and dye industries. The peak incidence occurs at a lower age in these workers. The following chemicals have been demonstrated to be carcinogenic with respect to carcinoma of the urinary bladder: β-naphthylamine, α-naphthylamine, benzidine, and p-biphenylamine (xenylamine). Medications such as chlornaphazin, used in the treatment of lymphoreticular neoplasms and myeloproliferative disorders, are sus-

TABLE 4–1   Histologic Types of Urothelial Carcinoma and Their Incidence

Type	Per Cent
Transitional cell	90
Squamous cell	7
Adenocarcinoma	2
Undifferentiated cell	1

pected of being bladder carcinogens. Metabolites of the essential amino-acid tryptophan have produced urothelial neoplasms in experimental animals, and excessive tryptophan metabolite excretion has been noted in some humans with urothelial neoplasms. There is also evidence to suggest causative relationships between tobacco smoking and bladder carcinoma.

These carcinomas are of urothelial origin. The urothelium has the potential to develop into transitional epithelium, which is the normal lining of the urinary bladder. It is not limited to that capability, however, but often manifests its potential for producing glandular epithelium as well as squamous epithelium. The previously described cystitis glandularis is an example of the epithelium's former potential, and squamous metaplasia is an example of the latter. Neoplastic counter-

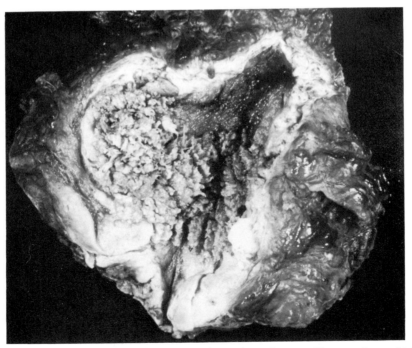

Figure 4–11   The bladder has been opened, revealing a large papillary neoplasm which proved to be a grade II transitional cell carcinoma with squamous metaplasia. There was evidence of superficial infiltration.

TABLE 4–2   Grading of Urothelial Carcinoma According to Degree of Anaplasia°

GRADE	DEGREE
Grade I	Mild anaplasia
Grade II	Moderate anaplasia
Grade III	Severe anaplasia

° From the American Bladder Tumor Registry.

parts of these types of epithelium make up the histologic variants of urothelial carcinoma. (See Table 4–1.)

These carcinomas usually occur in pure form; however, mixtures of the types exist. Approximately 20 per cent of the carcinomas show both transitional and squamous elements (Fig. 4–11).

In geographic areas, such as Africa, where infection with Schistosoma haematobium is a threat, squamous cell carcinoma is the most frequent type seen, while in the United States and Europe most of the bladder carcinomas are of the transitional cell type.

There is considerable biologic significance attached to the cytologic grading of the neoplasm, which is based on the degree of anaplasia manifested as nuclear pleomorphism, number of division figures, hyperchromatism, and nuclear cytoplasmic ratios. (See Table 4–2.) The five-year survival rate for patients with Grade I neoplasms is 80 per cent, whereas for those with Grade III tumors it is only 20 per cent.

Another factor involved in assessing prognosis in a given case is the pattern of growth of the neoplasm. (See Table 4–3.) The in situ and papillary forms generally have a better prognosis than the infiltrating varieties.

Final determinants for prognosis are the depth of infiltration and the presence of metastasis (see Table 4–4), factors which are based on the Marshall modification of the Jewett and Strong classification. This is the system most often used in the United States. As one would expect, Stage O offers a better chance for survival than Stage D_2, with intermediate survivals between the extremes.

As with any neoplastic process, the type and quality of the therapy also influences the prognosis.

Nothing is to be gained from participation in the controversy as to whether a specific papillary lesion is a transitional cell papilloma or a papillary carcinoma, Grade I. The criteria offered by some authorities for a diagnosis of papilloma are arbitrary and, in the author's experi-

TABLE 4–3   Growth Pattern for Urothelial Carcinoma

In situ
Papillary
Infiltrative
Mixed papillary and infiltrative

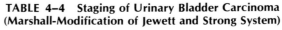

TABLE 4–4 Staging of Urinary Bladder Carcinoma
(Marshall-Modification of Jewett and Strong System)

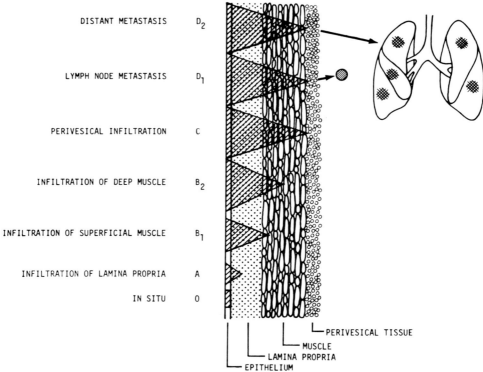

DISTANT METASTASIS	D_2
LYMPH NODE METASTASIS	D_1
PERIVESICAL INFILTRATION	C
INFILTRATION OF DEEP MUSCLE	B_2
INFILTRATION OF SUPERFICIAL MUSCLE	B_1
INFILTRATION OF LAMINA PROPRIA	A
IN SITU	0

PERIVESICAL TISSUE
MUSCLE
LAMINA PROPRIA
EPITHELIUM

ence, impractical, if not impossible, to apply. Such attempts at classification only detract from the important point of which all students of urology must be aware, namely, that any transitional cell papillary neoplasm, no matter how well differentiated, indicates that the patient's urothelium has the propensity for developing a carcinoma in the future. It is impossible to predict with any accuracy which patients will experience recurrence of a papillary neoplasm, which in some instances may even be invasive.

The papillary lesion serves as an indicator to warn the physician of the necessity for continued follow-up of that patient. To ignore this warning may lead to grave consequences. The chief herald of the urothelial bladder neoplasm is hematuria.

Sarcoma. The most important supporting tissue neoplasm in the bladder is rhabdomyosarcoma. This usually, but not exclusively, occurs in children and often displays a polypoid or grapelike gross pattern of growth into the lumen of the bladder. The appellation sarcoma botryoides is used to designate this peculiar gross configuration. Nonspecific mesenchyme associated with the distal portions of the mesonephric duct as it is incorporated in the development of the bladder, ejaculatory ducts, and vasa deferentia is believed to be the tissue of origin for rhabdomyosarcoma.

These tumors arise in the region of the trigone, vesical neck, urethra, and prostate. Histologically, the majority are classified as embryonal rhabdomyosarcomas. A small percentage are pleomorphic rhabdomyosarcomas. The neoplasm consists of nests of primitive myoblasts in a loose, often edematous stroma. Occasionally, more mature myoblasts, some of which have cross striations, are seen. It should be emphasized that the failure to demonstrate cross striations in the neoplastic cells does not necessarily disprove the diagnosis of rhabdomyosarcoma. Less often, an alveolar pattern of myoblasts is seen in urogenital rhabdomyosarcomas.

The prognosis for this tumor is poor; however, it is not uniformly fatal. Other sarcomas including, but not limited to, leiomyosarcoma and fibrosarcoma occur in the bladder.

There is a mixed tumor of the urinary bladder known as carcinosarcoma. As the name implies, both malignant epithelial and stromal elements are present. The epithelial component may be transitional, glandular, or squamous, and the stromal portion can be represented by myosarcoma, osteosarcoma, fibrosarcoma, or any malignant mesenchymal element. These are usually highly malignant neoplasms which present as polypoid masses in the trigone or vesical neck area of the adult bladder.

URETER

For all practical purposes the inflammatory lesions and neoplasms which affect the bladder may involve the ureter, either independently or in continuity. This is particularly true for the urothelial neoplasms. Everything which has been said about these neoplasms in the bladder likewise applies to the ureter and renal pelvis.

The ureter may be the site of metastatic carcinoma or may be involved by the direct extension of both carcinomas and sarcomas from adjacent structures that result in obstruction and the subsequent development of hydroureter in association with hydronephrosis. Carcinoma of the uterine cervix is perhaps the chief offender in this regard.

An inflammatory lesion known as idiopathic retroperitoneal fibrosis encases the ureters, producing obstruction which may result in renal failure. The process is usually but not exclusively bilateral. The triad of hydronephrosis, medial deviation of the ureter, and ureteric obstruction at the level of the brim of the pelvis suggests the diagnosis. The vena cava may be incorporated and infiltrated by the proliferating fibroblasts which characterize the process. This infiltration often results in vena caval thrombosis. Inflammatory in nature, the process terminates as mature, relatively acellular scar tissue encasing the retroperitoneal structures after evolving through a more cellular and exudative phase. In most cases, the origin is unknown; however, the medication, methysergide (a serotonin analogue), is believed to be a causative factor in some cases of retroperitoneal fibrosis. Cases have been associated with carcinoid tumor (serotonin secretor) and with the use of LSD, which is a serotonin antagonist.

Retroperitoneal fibrosis has also been seen in patients with a generalized vasculitis, such as polyarteritis nodosa. A desmoplastic reaction to metastatic carcinoma or a sclerosing lymphoma in the retroperitoneal tissue may mimic this disorder and should be ruled out before a diagnosis of idiopathic retroperitoneal fibrosis is made.

The association in some cases of retroperitoneal fibrosis with mediastinal fibrosis, peribiliary fibrosis, palmar fibromatosis (Dupuytren's contracture), and skin keloids lends support for the new designation, multifocal fibrosclerosis.

PROSTATE

INFLAMMATION

The prostate may be the seat of inflammation. Acute prostatitis manifests histologically as a purulent exudate in the prostatic ducts, glands, and periglandular stroma. Suppuration may occur with the formation of abscesses. Infectious organisms may reach the gland via the urethra as a result of ascending or descending urinary infection. Instrumentation may contribute to this process and on occasion, hematogenous dissemination of organisms from a distant site may be responsible for the prostatic infection. Neisseria gonorrhaea, Escherichia coli, staphylococci, and streptococci are the organisms most frequently incriminated.

Corpora amylacea form from inspissation of the glandular secretions within the prostate. They are present in most prostates, particularly at middle-age and later. These may act as a nidus for mineralization with calcium carbonate and phosphate salts and calculus formation. Intraglandular obstruction with ductal ectasia may then result. Stagnation of secretions under these circumstances is an ideal culture medium for the growth of organisms.

Chronic inflammation allegedly occurs in nearly three quarters of prostates in the sixth decade and older if one considers glands showing focal aggregates of chronic inflammatory cells in the periglandular stroma. It is doubtful that all of these instances of chronic inflammation are clinically significant. This is not to deny that occasional cases of symptom-producing chronic, purulent, or suppurative prostatitis do occur.

A special form of chronic inflammation deserves mention, namely, lipogranulomatous prostatitis. This destructive necrotizing process is comparable to lipogranulomatous pyelonephritis. Chronic inflammatory cells, necrosis, and aggregates of lipid-laden macrophages (foam cells) are seen. Grossly, such a gland is enlarged and may mimic neoplasm or tuberculosis.

Urogenital tuberculosis may involve the prostate, resulting in caseous necrosis and the formation of classical tuberculous granulation tissue. Usually infection spread from the upper urinary tract is responsible, although hematogenous seeding in miliary tuberculosis is possible. Rarely, fungus infections such as histoplasmosis and coccidioidomycosis may involve the prostate. The prostate may harbor Trichomonas vaginalis organisms and serve as a source of repeated infection of a sexual partner.

VASCULAR DISORDERS

The periprostatic venous plexus is commonly the site of thrombi in older men. These thrombi may be the source of pulmonary emboli.

Infarcts occur in the gland as a result of arterial insufficiency, a condition which is usually arteriosclerotic in origin. Compression of vessels by hyperplastic nodules may contribute to focal ischemia, which results in infarcts.

HYPERPLASIA

Hyperplasia and neoplasia are the most common and clinically significant afflictions of the prostate in men over 45 years of age.

The origin of hyperplasia is unknown. Attempts have been made to relate it to an imbalance between androgenic and estrogenic hormones, a process which occurs with aging. Both the glandular and stromal components of the gland may partake in the hyperplasia, which is an increase in glandular epithelial and fibromuscular cellular elements. Often one pattern will predominate. The median and lateral portions of the gland are the seat of the proliferative process. Diffuse enlargement of the gland may occur, but more commonly, a nodular pattern results (Fig. 4–12). The weight of the entire gland may increase from a normal of 20 gm to over 100 gm.

Microscopically, there is an increase in the numbers of glands, and the papillary infolding of the glandular epithelium is more prominent. Enlarged gland fields (lobules) compress the surrounding stroma (Fig. 4–13). When the stroma is involved, nodules of smooth muscle and fibrous tissue are seen, or these components may diffusely increase. Although increased in number, the glands tend to maintain a lobular pattern, and this feature, along with the glands' size and papillary projections, helps to distinguish hyperplasia from carcinoma.

The hyperplastic nodules may compress the intraprostatic ducts and, along with corpora amylacea, may result in ductal obstruction with proximal glandular ectasia. These markedly dilated glands impart a cystic pattern to the cut surface of the hyperplastic prostate. The clinical symptomatology associated with benign hyperplasia is related to the

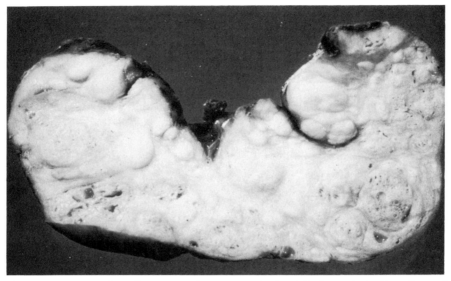

Figure 4–12 Cut surface of a prostate showing a marked nodular hyperplasia. Note the cystic dilatation of glands in the lower portion.

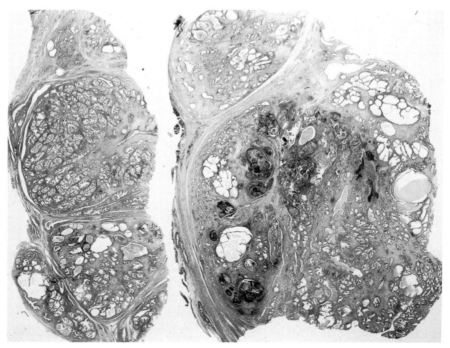

Figure 4–13 Large fragments of an hyperplastic prostate with prominent nodules and adjacent stromal compression. The dark areas in the right fragment are foci of purulent inflammation. (Original magnification 3×.)

obstruction of the urethra, producing a subsequent difficulty in urinating and the retention of urine.

NEOPLASM

Adenocarcinoma.   If one considers the glandular and stromal nodules described above as hyperplastic and not truly neoplastic, then benign neoplasms of the prostate are exceedingly rare.

The most important malignant neoplasm from the standpoint of incidence is adenocarcinoma. This neoplasm is responsible for approximately 18,000 deaths per year in the United States. The older the man, the greater the probability is for him to develop an adenocarcinoma of the prostate. It is estimated that 45 per cent of the patients with adenocarcinoma have extension of the neoplasm beyond the prostatic capsule, and 50 per cent of the patients have metastatic carcinoma when they are initially examined. This neoplasm is to the man what breast carcinoma is to the woman in that it accounts for at least 60 per cent of all metastatic carcinoma in the male skeletal system.

The prostatic glandular epithelium is the major source of acid phosphatase in the male. Neoplastic prostatic epithelium continues to produce this enzyme; however, the quantity produced diminishes as the carcinoma becomes more anaplastic. The elevation of the serum acid phosphatase level generally correlates with the amount of extra-capsular metastatic neoplasm present. Although the serum level of this enzyme is elevated in the majority of patients when metastatic disease is present, it cannot separate patients with local extension beyond the capsule from those patients with bony or distant metastases. It should be emphasized that false-positive elevations of serum acid phosphatase do occur.

Prostatic manipulation, including surgical trauma and prostatic infarcts, may result in the elevation of the serum acid phosphatase level. As measured in most clinical laboratories the serum acid phosphatase is a heterogeneous enzyme. Although the quantity of acid phosphatase in the normal adult prostate exceeds by approximately 1000 times the amount present in other organs, other tissues do produce the enzyme. The liver, kidney, spleen, bone, platelets, and erythrocytes contain acid phosphatase but in quantities much less than contained in the prostate. Disorders of these organs or cells may result in increased serum levels and must be considered in the differential diagnosis.

The wedge-shaped zone posterior to the urethra appears to be the site of origin of most prostatic adenocarcinomas. Let us call this region the posterior zone of the prostate, thereby avoiding the controversy which has arisen over a precise definition of the posterior lobe.

A gross characteristic which is of clinical significance in the diagnosis of prostatic adenocarcinoma is the obliteration of the posterior midline sulcus of the prostate. This increase in volume and change in contour can be readily detected by a careful digital rectal examination.

The texture of the gland involved with adenocarcinoma is also altered. The neoplastic gland is hard and often nodular compared with the resilient normal smooth gland.

The symptoms related to prostatic adenocarcinoma may be those of urethral obstruction due to an increase in the size of the gland as a result of the neoplasm. The neoplasm, however, may be completely asymptomatic locally and only reach the clinical horizon because of the metastasis to the skeletal system which results in pain.

In spite of the facts that specific criteria exist for the diagnosis of adenocarcinoma of the prostate and that it is usually an obvious neoplasm microscopically, cases exist in which the diagnosis is very difficult or cannot be made with certainty.

In the author's experience, the most reliable criteria are the small size of the glands, their proximity to each other without necessarily being "back-to-back," the lack of intraglandular papillae, and their violation of the boundaries of the lobular gland fields (Fig. 4–14). The microscopist is aided more by architectural observations than cytologic changes. Perineural infiltration by carcinoma cells is a confirmatory finding when present; however, in most cases it is certainly not necessary for diagnosis and has no prophetic significance as far as the biologic behavior of the neoplasm is concerned. An intraglandular cribriform pattern is seen in some adenocarcinomas. Various attempts have been made to categorize this neoplasm by histologic and cytologic criteria. The simplest meaningful system recognizes well differentiated

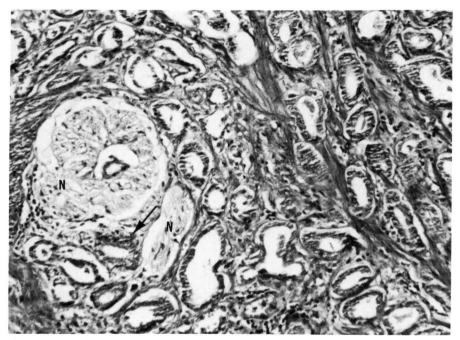

Figure 4–14 Adenocarcinoma of prostate with small acini devoid of papillae. The arrow points to a neoplastic acinus in a perineural space adjacent to nerves (N). (Original magnification 163 ×.)

and undifferentiated carcinomas as opposite ends of the spectrum with one or two intermediate levels of differentiation in between. The patient survival at five years is approximately 10 times greater for the well differentiated neoplasm as compared to the undifferentiated tumor. Staging systems have been developed to facilitate the comparison of the various therapeutic modalities. The so-called American System advocated by Del Regato is depicted in Table 4–5.

The neoplasm readily metastasizes to regional lymph nodes and bones, particularly in the pelvic area and vertebral column where osteoblastic metastases predominate over lytic lesions. At least 75 per cent of the adenocarcinomas are initially androgen dependent and demonstrate a clinical remission when hormonal ablative therapy is instituted. This remission is often heralded by a significant drop in the elevated serum acid phosphatase level.

Microscopically profound changes occur in the carcinoma during remission. The neoplasm appears to undergo atrophy both at the primary and metastatic sites with replacement of bone lesions by neo-osteogenesis. Unfortunately, the remission is not permanent, although

TABLE 4–5   Staging of Prostatic Carcinoma (Modified from Del Regato)

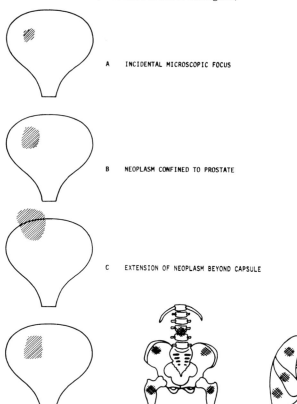

A   INCIDENTAL MICROSCOPIC FOCUS

B   NEOPLASM CONFINED TO PROSTATE

C   EXTENSION OF NEOPLASM BEYOND CAPSULE

D   SKELETAL OR EXTRAPELVIC METASTASIS

it may vary in duration from months to many years. The reactivated neoplasm is apparently independent of hormonal control.

Since both adenocarcinoma and benign hyperplasia are common in older men, it is not surprising that one may see both lesions in the same gland. As mentioned earlier, the carcinoma usually begins in the posterior zone, whereas hyperplasia involves median and lateral zones. The relationship, however, may be more than coincidental. Both prospective and retrospective studies have recently shown a several times higher incidence of adenocarcinoma in men with a previous diagnosis of benign hyperplasia.

A much less frequent carcinoma of the prostate is of ductal origin and accounts for about 3 per cent of prostate neoplasms. This carcinoma originates from ductal epithelium adjacent to the urethra or deeper in the gland. It may often be identified in an in situ phase within the ducts. The pattern is one of transitional carcinoma with occasional glandular components. This neoplasm is not associated with elevations of acid phosphatase and apparently is not under the influence of androgenic hormones. This ductal carcinoma produces symptoms as a result of local growth that tends to extend upward into the trigone area and obstruct the ureters.

Sarcoma. Malignant supporting tissue neoplasms of the prostate are rare, accounting for less than 1 per cent of all fatal prostatic neoplasms. Most of these occur in children or young adults. Clinical symptoms relate to the extensive local invasion and urinary obstruction. The course is usually rapid, with average survival one year or less after diagnosis. Histologically, these may appear as fibrosarcomas, leiomyosarcomas, and rhabdomyosarcomas. The comments made about rhabdomyosarcoma in the urinary bladder also apply to this lesion in the prostate.

MISCELLANEOUS

The entity known as ectopic prostate in the urethra deserves special mention. It is a significant cause of hematuria, particularly in young men. The lesion is found in the prostatic urethra, usually on or near the verumontanum and has a papilliferous or frondlike gross appearance. Microscopically, prostatic acini are seen, and the papillary projections into the urethra consist of a delicate fibrovascular core covered with prostatic glandular epithelium. The prostatic origin of this developmental anomaly has been confirmed by histochemical and ultrastructural studies.

PENIS

INFLAMMATION

The term *balanoposthitis* designates inflammation of the glans penis and the prepuce. It is usually a result of poor hygiene and phimosis. Coliform, staphylococcal, and streptococcal organisms are common infectious agents. Severe or persistent infections may result in scar formation and narrowing of the urinary meatus. In some instances, a systemic disease such as diabetes mellitus or a dermatologic disorder may be the predisposing factor.

Balanitis xerotica obliterans occurs as a scaly lesion on the glans and prepuce. It has a characteristic microscopic pattern with a subepidermal zone of homogenization and edema of the dermal collagen. Beneath this relatively acellular homogeneous band lies a chronic inflammatory cell infiltrate. The overlying epidermis may be either hyperplastic and hyperkeratotic or atrophic. Its relationship to carcinoma is not certain, but some consider this lesion as a precursor of squamous cell carcinoma.

Herpes progenitalis caused by the virus Herpes simplex hominis is characterized by many small vesicles on the glans and prepuce. The vesicles are intraepithelial and may ulcerate. Large eosinophilic intranuclear inclusions are seen in the squamous epithelial cells at the margins of the vesicles. Multinucleated epithelial giant cells are present. The lesions usually heal without immediate complications. In the woman, the labia and uterine cervix are the sites of the vesicles. It is considered to be a venereal infection and is suspected of playing a causative role in the origin of carcinoma of the uterine cervix.

The genital chancre of primary syphilis in the male is usually on the penis. The glans and the prepuce are the most common sites, but occasionally a chancre will locate on the shaft or within the urethra. About one month after the infectious contact, a red hard nodule appears which ulcerates superficially. The lesion is usually painless. Microscopically, there is a pronounced inflammatory cell infiltrate consisting predominantly of plasma cells and lymphocytes. A striking endothelial proliferation is present. Fluid expressed from the ulcer is loaded with the etiologic agent, Treponema pallidum. Examination of this fluid with dark field microscopy is required to visualize the organisms. They can only be demonstrated in histologic sections by the use of special staining techniques such as the Warthin-Starry stain.

The chancre heals in a few weeks, leaving a small scar. If there is no treatment, the manifestations of secondary syphilis may appear. Classically, this is a generalized maculopapular rash which also may involve the genitalia. These lesions are also teeming with Treponema organisms. The serologic tests for syphilis may be nonreactive at the time the chancre appears, but they are virtually always positive at the time the secondary lesions appear.

Syphilis is a systemic disease, and the student is referred to standard medical texts for a more thorough discussion. For descriptions of the less common infectious diseases that produce lesions on or near the genitalia, including chancroid, granuloma inguinale, and lymphogranuloma venereum, the reader is also referred to standard textbooks of medicine and pathology.

NEOPLASMS

Condyloma acuminatum is a neoplastic lesion which occurs on the genitals, the perineum, and perianal areas. The coronal sulcus and inner surface of the foreskin are the sites of predilection for the penile lesions. In reality, they are epithelial papillomas of viral origin, which present as solitary or multiple exophytic lesions having the configurations of a cauliflower.

Histologically, there are fibrovascular cores that result from the marked papillomatosis. These are covered with acanthotic and hyperkeratotic squamous epithelium. Chronic inflammatory cells infiltrate the stroma (Fig. 4–15). The condyloma acuminatum may reach a giant size. The author has seen lesions in the perineum which attained the size of an orange and were partially infarcted, thus creating a foul odor not present in the ordinary lesion. On rare occasions, squamous cell carcinoma may originate in a condyloma acuminatum.

Carcinoma in situ or Bowen's disease is a form of preinvasive carcinoma which may develop in any epidermal or squamous mucosal surface. The penis is no exception. The lesion usually presents on the glans as an erythematous, scaly plaque. Microscopically, the stratified squamous epithelium exhibits dysplasia and a failure to mature as cells approach the surface. The nuclear-cytoplasmic ratio remains large, and division figures are seen even in the superficial layers. Ulcer-

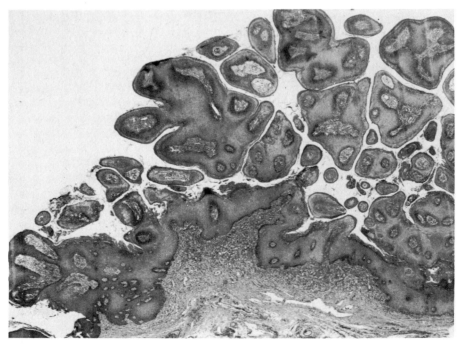

Figure 4–15 Condyloma accuminatum with marked papillomatosis. (Original magnification 12×.)

ation may occur, and eventually, many of these in situ lesions become infiltrative carcinomas.

Erythroplasia of Queyrat is considered by many to be a form of carcinoma in situ. It develops on the glans as a sharply circumscribed, erythematous, velvety plaque. The microscopic picture resembles that of psoriasis somewhat in that there are elongations of rete ridges with acanthosis. The stratum corneum is thinner than normal, and elongated dermal papillae contain dilated capillaries and inflammatory cells. These factors contribute to the redness of the lesion. Division figures may be found near the surface, but the epithelial cells do not exhibit the degree of dysplasia seen in Bowen's disease. This lesion may evolve into infiltrative carcinoma.

Squamous cell carcinoma is the most frequently encountered malignant neoplasm that occurs on the penis. It accounts for approximately 3 per cent of carcinomas in males in the United States, but has a six times greater incidence in the Orient. Most cases occur after middle age. The fact that this neoplasm is virtually nonexistent in men who were circumcised as infants incriminates retained smegma and poor personal hygiene as carcinogenic factors.

The neoplasm tends to originate on the glans or on the foreskin near the corona. The epidermoid carcinoma may present grossly as an elevated fungating mass (papillary neoplasm) or as a sessile lesion. The latter type of lesion exhibits a more aggressive infiltrative growth. Phimosis may initially conceal the neoplasm which develops on the glans or inner foreskin. Ulceration with subsequent secondary infection leads to a purulent exudate and bleeding, which may be the presenting symptoms. The dense connective tissue encasing the corpora spongiosa provides an initial barrier to deep penetration, but once that is violated, the neoplasm has access to the vascular erectile tissue. The papillary exophytic lesions tend to be well differentiated epidermoid carcinomas with superficial infiltration of the subepithelial stroma. They are less prone to metastasize. The sessile lesions are less well differentiated, display more division figures, and behave more aggressively as far as infiltration and metastasis are concerned.

The external iliac, superficial, and deep inguinal nodes are the sites of initial metastatic spread. Distant hematogenous spread may occur in the later stages of the disease.

In spite of the fact that the penis is handled several times a day and is easily accessible for visual inspection, early diagnosis with subsequent adequate treatment is a formidable goal to attain. The mean duration between the initial signs of neoplasm and diagnosis exceeds one year.

MISCELLANEOUS LESIONS

Peyronie's disease is a form of fibromatosis involving the fascia of the penis that results in a plaquelike or nodular induration of the shaft.

This may impart a distinct bend in the penile shaft which tends to curve to the involved side. It may also result in painful erection. As with most forms of fibromatosis, the origin is unknown. A vasculitis has been noted in the loose connective tissue around the corpora in some cases.

Nevi occur on the penis and occasionally give rise to malignant melanomas. Supporting tissue sarcomas and angiosarcomas in the penis are rare.

URETHRA

INFLAMMATION

Urethritis may result from infection with any one of several micro-organisms; however, most cases of urethritis in the United States can be classified as either gonococcal in origin or nonspecific with no organism identifiable. Since gonorrhea is the subject of another chapter, no detailed description will be given here.

In nonspecific urethritis, one sees a purulent exudate presenting at the external meatus, but bacteria are not seen on stained smears and usually cannot be cultured. Reiter's disease is the association of this type of urethritis with arthritis, conjunctivitis, stomatitis, and iritis. Ulcers may appear in the urethra in Reiter's disease as well as on the glans and in the mucosa of the urinary bladder.

Strictures occur predominantly in the bulbomembranous segment of the urethra and result from infections or trauma. Obstetrical injury is the most frequent etiologic factor in women. Gonococcal urethritis, inlying urethral catheters, and instrumentation are the chief predisposing factors in men. Fibrous scar tissue replaces the wall of the urethra and may extend into the adjacent erectile tissue and fascia of the penis. The contraction of this scar tissue with time results in a decrease in the caliber of the lumen and urinary obstruction.

Urethral caruncles occur only in the female and present as sessile or pedunculated red nodular masses at the external meatus. They usually evolve from the posterior margin of the meatus but on occasion appear to originate from the entire circumference. Histologically, they often consist of vascular pyogenic granulation tissue covered with transitional or squamous epithelium. Some exhibit a marked angiomatous pattern while others are predominantly papillomatous with marked hyperplasia of transitional and squamous epithelium. The folds of hyperplastic epithelium often appear to extend deeply into the stroma, mimicking a carcinoma.

Inflammatory polyps may occur in the urethral mucosa. These can be distinguished from the true papillary neoplasms by the broad central core of connective tissue which is infiltrated by chronic inflammatory cells. The surface is covered with transitional epithelium. Fibrous polyps may occur in children and are probably congenital.

NEOPLASMS

Squamous papillomas occur in the urethra and are considered to be condylomata acuminata. Transitional cell papillomas may be seen anywhere in the urethra and have the same connotations as similar papillary neoplasms elsewhere in the urinary tract.

Carcinoma of the urethra is a rare disease which occurs more in women than in men. The neoplasm in males appears to be related to a pre-existing stricture in the cavernous and membranous urethra in the majority of cases. No predisposing factor has been recognized in women. In both sexes, squamous cell carcinoma is the most frequent variety. Adenocarcinoma may spring from Skene's glands in the female or the periurethral glands in the male. Transitional cell and undifferentiated carcinomas also occur.

The carcinomas of the male urethra infiltrate the corpus spongiosum and may present with a fistula in the perineal midline in the case of posterior urethral lesions and on the ventral surface of the penis with anterior urethral lesions.

The clinical signs associated with these neoplasms are purulent discharge, urinary retention, and hematuria. The posterior carcinomas spread to the external and internal iliac lymph nodes, and the anterior urethral tumors metastasize to the inguinal lymph nodes. Those individuals afflicted with urethral carcinomas have a high death rate that is probably related to a delay in diagnosis.

TESTIS AND ADNEXAE

INFLAMMATION

Infectious organisms may reach the testis via the hematogenous route or from other portions of the genitourinary tract via the vas deferens and epididymis. The pyogenic bacteria, including staphylococci, pneumococci, streptococci, and gonococci, may be involved as well as coliform organisms and others. The testis is swollen and painful. Microscopically, the lumens of the seminiferous tubules are filled with neutrophilic leukocytes which may camouflage or displace the spermatogenic elements. Interstitital edema and neutrophilic infiltrates occur. In severe infections, suppuration occurs with the necrosis of tubules and the formation of abscesses. The necrotic foci heal with scar formation and the permanent loss of spermatogenic activity.

One of the most common inflammatory processes in the epididymis is due to infection by the gonococcus as a complication of urethritis. The ducts are filled with purulent exudate, and there may be focal necrosis of the epithelium and disruption of ducts, both of which lead to fibrosis and subsequent sterility.

Several systemic viral infections, including infectious parotitis (mumps), influenza, and smallpox, may result in orchitis. The most common offender in this regard is infectious parotitis, which results in orchitis in about one third of the cases involving postpubertal males. It rarely complicates mumps during childhood. Orchitis may occur without involvement of the salivary glands and may involve one or both testes. The gonad is enlarged and tender due to the intense interstitial edema and inflammatory cell infiltrate. The latter consists of neutrophils, histiocytes, and lymphocytes. Focal necrosis of tubular epithelium may occur, and there is an infiltrate of leukocytes including neutrophils in the tubules. Spermatic activity is disrupted in these foci. Depending upon the severity of the infection and the degree of necrosis, this disease may result in fibrosis of the seminiferous tubules and a permanent loss of spermatogenesis. This residual damage may be diffuse or focal in nature.

Tuberculous orchitis, characterized by caseous tubercles replacing seminiferous tubules, may result from hematogenous spread of organisms from a pulmonary focus of infection, or more commonly, a direct extension from a tuberculous epididymitis.

The testis may be involved in syphilis. Lymphocytic and plasma cell infiltrate and endothelial proliferation characterize lesions of secondary syphilis that result in parenchymal scarring. Gummas with large areas of necrosis may occur in late syphilis.

Granulomatous orchitis refers to a nonspecific inflammatory process in the testis, usually occurring in middle-aged and older men, and apparently of noninfectious origin. The tubules are replaced by an infiltrate of mononuclear cells that include plasma cells, lymphocytes, and epithelioid cells. The outline of the seminiferous tubules remains, but no spermatogenic activity is present (Fig. 4–16). The inflammatory

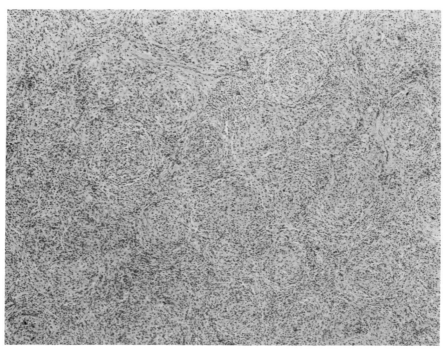

Figure 4–16 Granulomatous orchitis with persistence of outlines of seminiferous tubules and marked chronic inflammatory cell infiltrate. (Original magnification 40 ×.)

infiltrate, which may contain multinucleated giant cells, involves the interstitial area. The exudative phase may subside with residual tubular fibrosis. There is evidence to suggest that this is an autoimmune disease that has a granulomatous response to spermatozoa. Some cases may be associated with trauma, but this relationship is not constant and may be coincidental. Its chief clinical importance is related to its presentation as an enlarged tender testis which closely mimics neoplasm. Microscopically, the polymorphous inflammatory cell infiltrate differentiates the disease from lymphocytic lymphoma. Differentiation of granulomatous orchitis from germinal neoplasms microscopically should not be a problem.

Sperm granulomas occur in the epididymis in response to a leakage of spermatozoa into the periductal stroma as a result of trauma or infection. They elicit an intense inflammatory reaction which initially contains neutrophils. Small granulomas consisting of epithelioid cells, lymphocytes, plasma cells, and eosinophils form around a nidus of necrotic debris and spermatozoa. The lesions heal with scar formation. Grossly, they appear as firm, yellow-white nodules in the epididymis.

VASCULAR DISORDERS

As a consequence of increased mobility or a defective anchoring at the gubernaculum, torsion of the spermatic cord initially produces an intense passive hyperemia, which is the result of prevention of venous return. If the torsion is not corrected quickly, an infarct of the testis results. Microscopically one sees extensive hemorrhage in the interstitium and coagulative necrosis of the seminiferous tubules that leaves only apparitions of the tubules remaining.

Arteriosclerosis of the spermatic artery may result in atrophic changes in the testis manifested by an absence of spermatogenesis and a fibrous thickening of the tunica propria of the seminiferous tubules. Ischemia produced by vascular sclerosis is believed to be the cause of many of the atrophic changes seen in the senile testis.

Varicocele of the internal spermatic vein and pampiniform plexus occurs on the left side owing to a congenital absence or the incompetence of valves at the junction with the left renal vein, which allows a retrograde flow of blood. This situation is exaggerated in the standing position. An important complication of this condition is infertility, which may result even when the varicocele is unilateral. Correction of the varicocele results in a significant improvement in the sperm count as well as in the motility and morphology of spermatozoa in at least 60 per cent of the men treated. The pathogenesis is not understood, and attempts to incriminate temperature elevation in the testes or the presence of abnormally high amounts of adrenal steroids as the product of reflux from the left adrenal vein into the varicocele have not met with much success. Venogram studies have demonstrated the connections between the left and right internal spermatic systems, an observation which could explain why both testes are involved, but the precise mechanism remains a mystery. Also confusing the picture is the fact that some men remain fertile even in the presence of long-standing varicoceles.

CRYPTORCHID

The undescended testis does not produce sperm and is probably at greater risk for the development of a germinal neoplasm. During fetal development, the testes normally reach the scrotum at eight months. Failure of descent results in profound histologic changes which first become apparent when compared to the normal changes that occur in the scrotal gland at about five years of age. During the period from five to nine years when the scrotal gonad shows an increase in tortuosity and in the size of the seminiferous tubules, the cryptorchid lags behind. Spermatogonia are late in their appearance. From ten years of age to puberty, the normal testis undergoes maturation with the appearance of mitoses in the spermatogonia and the development of primary and secondary spermatocytes and spermatids. This process does not occur in the cryptorchid. Although Leydig cells are present in the undescended gland, the tubules remain small and there is some fibrosis of the tunica propria of the tubules. Spermatogenesis does not occur after puberty in the cryptorchid, and as time passes, the tubular sclerosis increases. Islands of immature tubules with indifferent cells (precursors of Sertoli's cells) may be seen in some undescended gonads. From the purely morphologic standpoint, the age of five years is the critical time for surgical placement of the cryptorchid into the scrotum.

The question of increased incidence of germinal neoplasm in the cryptorchid has stimulated considerable controversy. Opinions vary from admitting a possible increased risk to espousing a 40 times greater incidence than in the scrotal testis. Furthermore, the apparent risk appears to remain even after orchiopexy. The interval between orchiopexy and the diagnosis of neoplasm may exceed 25 years with the average about 14 years. Seminoma, embryonal carcinoma, and teratocarcinoma are the neoplasms usually found. Some believe that the younger the patient is at the time of surgical lowering of the testis, the lower the risk is for the development of a subsequent neoplasm; there is apparently no risk for patients whose cryptorchid was brought down prior to the age of six years.

INFERTILITY

It is estimated that 15 per cent of marriages are childless and not by choice; in half of these matings, the husband is the deficient partner as far as fertility is concerned. The problem of the infertile testis has been touched upon in the preceding comments concerning varicocele

TABLE 4–6   Semen: Normal Values

Volume	2.5 ml to 4 ml
Sperm	50,000,000 to 150,000,000 per ml
Motility	At least 80 per cent at initial examination
Duration of motility	At least 12 hours at room temperature
Abnormal forms	Less than 15 per cent

and the undescended gonad, but a more detailed discussion of the spectrum of testicular changes associated with infertility is in order.

Table 4–6 depicts the characteristics of a normal ejaculate.

Abnormalities in the quantity and quality of spermatozoa ejaculated may be produced by extragonadal endocrine disturbances, primary testicular disorders, or abnormalities in the conduit system and accessory sex glands.

The histologic findings seen in testicular biopsies from patients with various extragonadal endocrinopathies are depicted in Table 4–7. In normal postpuberal seminiferous tubules, one sees abundant cellular activity with spermatogonia at the periphery followed by primary and secondary spermatocytes, spermatids, and spermatozoa in the lumen (Fig. 4–17A). The primary spermatocyte is the largest and most conspicuous cell in the series. The Sertoli cell can barely be recognized in the normal tubule, being camouflaged by all of the spermatogenic activity. When spermatogenesis is arrested or diminished (as described below), the Sertoli cell appears as a prominent vacuolated cell in the tubule.

In men with primary testicular abnormality, the morphologic findings can be classified into five groups:

Arrested spermatogenesis, in which maturation is stopped at the same level in all seminiferous tubules, usually at the primary spermatocyte level. All other morphologic features are unaltered (Fig. 4–17B).

Hypospermatogenesis, in which there is a decrease in the number of spermatogonia which go through the maturation process. There are

TABLE 4–7   Testicular Findings in Extragonadal Endocrinopathy

	SERTOLI'S CELLS	GERM CELLS	LEYDIG'S CELLS	TUNICA PROPRIA
Hypopituitarism				
Prepubertal	Immature	Spermatogonia	Immature	Normal
Postpubertal	Present (absent in late stage)	Absent	Atrophic	Sclerosis
Estrogen excess	Present (absent in late stage)	Absent in late stage	Atrophic	Sclerosis
Androgen excess (postpubertal)	Present (absent in late stage)	Absent in late stage	Atrophic (unless due to Leydig tumor)	Sclerosis
Glucocorticoid excess	Present	Arrested or hypo-spermatogenesis	Normal	Normal
Hypothyroidism	Present	Hypospermatogenesis	Normal	Normal

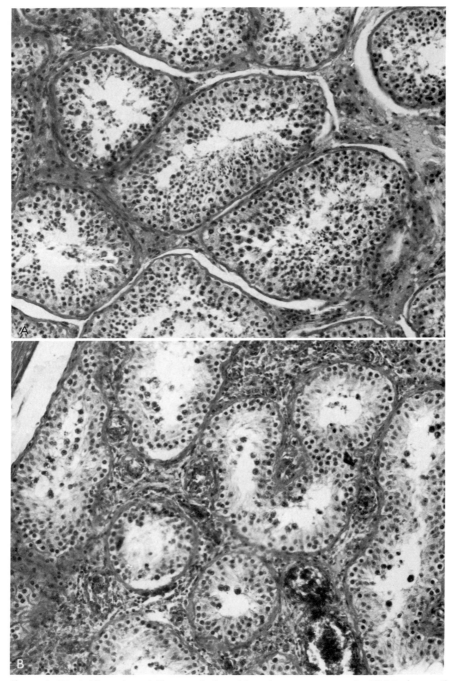

Figure 4–17   *A,* Normal seminiferous tubules with active spermatogenesis. (Original magnification 100×.) *B,* Arrest of spermatogenesis at the primary spermatocyte level. The large cells in the tubular lumens are primary spermatocytes. From a patient with septicemia and azotemia. (Original magnification 100×.)

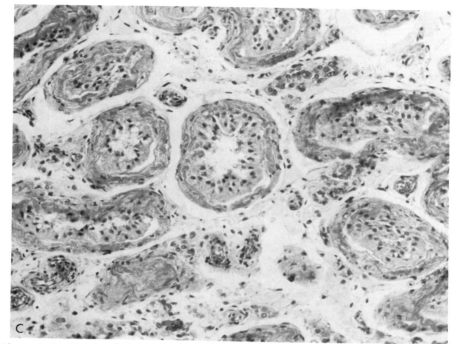

Figure 4–17 *Continued. C,* Seminiferous tubules showing germinal aplasia. Only Sertoli cells are present in tubular lumens. From a patient treated with cyclophosphamide and radiation for Hodgkin's Disease. (Original magnification 100×.)

some spermatozoa formed, but the number is markedly reduced. No other abnormality is noted.

Germinal aplasia, in which there is an absence of spermatogonia. The Sertoli cell is the only occupant of the tubule, which accounts for the synonym "Sertoli cell-only syndrome." There may be some decrease in size of tubular lumens (Fig. 4–17C).

Klinefelter's syndrome, also known as sclerosing tubular degeneration, in which there is an absence of spermatogonia and a marked fibrosis of tubules to the point of obliteration in the fully developed case. There is an accompanying striking hyperplasia of Leydig's cells. Some examples of Klinefelter's syndrome in the early stage show diminished spermatogenic activity. The classic karyotype for these patients is XXY, but several variations of poly X+Y and even mosaic forms such as XXY/XX are recognized. These patients are phenotypic males with a female sex chromatin pattern. The classic syndrome includes sterility, small testes, gynecomastia, female hair distribution, a decrease in facial hair, elevation of urinary follicle stimulating hormone, and delayed puberty. Although many of these individuals have a normal I.Q. and function well in society, approximately one fifth possess subnormal intelligence. The person with Klinefelter's syndrome is at greater risk for developing a nongonadal neoplasm (often multiple) and immunologic disorders.

Postinflammatory testicular atrophy is another cause of primary testicular infertility and may follow severe bilateral orchitis. Mumps is the greatest offender in this regard when it occurs in the postpubertal male. The tubular sclerosis that follows the acute episode is progressive over many years before the end-stage picture is reached. This late stage may be morphologically indistinguishable from the testis of Klinefelter's syndrome (Fig. 4–18). Eliminating the latter possibility requires a sex chromatin evaluation which would show a male pattern in postinflammatory atrophy.

In the first two conditions, the urinary 17-ketosteroids and gonadotropin levels are normal, whereas in germinal aplasia, Kleinfelter's syndrome, and postinflammatory atrophy, there is an elevation of urinary follicle stimulating hormone with normal levels of urinary 17-ketosteroids. The general rule indicates that when there is preservation of germ cells, the urinary gonadotropin levels remain normal.

The underlying causes of the testicular changes noted, excluding those of Klinefelter's syndrome and post-inflammatory atrophy, are poorly understood. One attempt to explain the absence, decrease, or arrest in spermatogenesis likens the seminiferous tubule to bone marrow, which may become hypoplastic or aplastic in response to certain toxins or physical agents such as exposure to radiation. Arrested spermatogen-

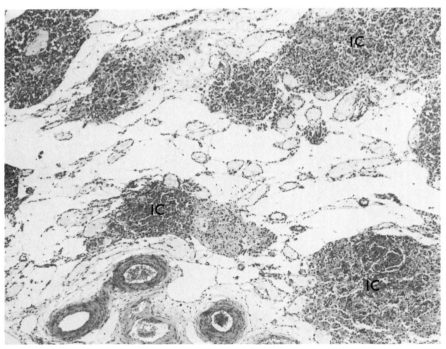

Figure 4–18   Testis from a patient who had mumps many years earlier. There is complete fibrous atrophy of seminiferous tubules associated with large aggregates of interstitial cells (IC). (Original magnification 40×.)

esis may result from febrile illnesses as well as from exposure to high environmental temperatures such as those experienced in working near blast furnaces. The spermatogonia are sensitive to radiation and such exposure accounts for some cases of germinal aplasia. Alkylating agents such as chlorambucil and cyclophosphamide can adversely affect spermatogenesis and may produce germinal aplasia.

Arrested spermatogenesis and hypospermatogenesis may be temporary and reversible in some men. Klinefelter's syndrome and germinal aplasia result in permanent sterility.

The testis may be working at full capacity and producing adequate numbers of high quality spermatozoa, yet the ejaculate is deficient. This situation reflects obstruction in the duct system which is either congenital, postinflammatory, such as gonococcal epididymitis, or acquired, as with vasectomy. If no obstruction in the conduit system exists, the lack of sperms in the ejaculate may result from abnormalities other than obstruction in the epididymis, where the sperm normally take from one to two weeks to complete the journey. Epithelial abnormalities here may adversely affect the sperm. Abnormalities in the accessory sex glands including the prostate, seminal vesicles, and bulbourethral glands may alter the semen to create a hostile medium for sperm transport.

Since the popularity of vasectomy has increased markedly in the past few years, a comment is appropriate concerning the impact of this procedure on the testes. Surprisingly, no adverse morphologic changes have been described. Mild ectasia of seminiferous tubules may be present, but no significant alteration is detected in the germinal epithelium. The epididymal ducts dilate to accommodate the continuous supply of spermatozoa. Phagocytosis of sperms by epididymal cells helps keep the process in equilibrium.

Vasitis nodosa is an inflammatory lesion of the vas deferens characterized by the presence within the wall of small ductal structures and a granulomatous reaction to extravasated spermatozoa. The intramural ductal epithelium of the vas is displaced as a result of vasectomy or a pre-existing inflammation. The irregular ductal structures can be confused with a well differentiated adenocarcinoma by the unwary investigator.

NEOPLASMS

Testicular neoplasms are exceeded only by leukemia, lymphoma, and central nervous system tumors as a cause of cancer deaths in male teenagers and young adults (ages 15 to 34 years). Over 90 per cent of testicular tumors are of germ cell origin; the remainder are derived from the gonadal stroma and rarely, the ducts and supporting tissues of the testes.

Clinically, testicular neoplasms present as an enlargement of the testis that is often, but not always, associated with pain. The more malignant varieties may first present with metastases.

Germinal Neoplasms. Four histologic types of germinal neoplasms are recognized. These include seminoma, embryonal cell carcinoma, teratoma, and choriocarcinoma. These may occur in pure form or in various mixtures in a given testis. A total of 15 combinations is mathematically possible, but these are not necessarily biologically significant. Five groups of histologic types in pure or mixed form emerge which have significance as far as natural history is concerned. They are listed in Table 4–8, along with survival statistics.

The seminoma is the most common of the germinal neoplasms and has its highest incidence between 30 and 50 years of age. These lesions may reach a large size and undergo focal necrosis, but hemorrhage is uncommon. The characteristic gross color is gray-white, and they are usually of a soft consistency. Microscopically, the pattern is typically one of round, polyhedral cells with clear or granular cytoplasm occurring in solid nests associated with a fine stroma. Aggregates of lymphocytes are often present (Fig. 4–19). Some seminomas contain foci of granulomatous reaction or exhibit a marked desmoplastic response. When necrosis occurs, it is usually coagulative in type with ghost cells remaining. The seminoma is subclassified into typical, anaplastic, and spermatocytic types, depending upon the histologic and cytologic appearance. As the name implies, the anaplastic variant exhibits more cellular pleomorphism and division figures and is associated with a higher mortality. Ten per cent of seminomas are of the anaplastic type. The spermatocytic type accounts for approximately another 10 per cent and is characterized by the presence of some cells resembling secondary spermatocytes. Another distinguishing feature is a filamentous pattern of the nuclear chromatin. This tumor is associated with a good prognosis. Seminomas may be seen in an intratubular form and as such are an in situ tumor.

The embryonal carcinoma has its highest incidence during the third decade. It tends to be the smallest of the germinal neoplasms. The gross picture is gray-white with dark foci of hemorrhage and necrosis. The microscopic picture is best described as that of a poorly differentiated carcinoma having a solid pattern or forming poorly de-

TABLE 4–8   Survival in Germinal Testicular Neoplasms*

Histologic Type	Approximate 5 Year Survival (Per Cent)
Seminoma	90
Teratocarcinoma (with or without choriocarcinoma or seminoma)	50
Embryonal carcinoma (with or without seminoma)	35
Teratoma (with or without seminoma)	70
Choriocarcinoma (with or without embryonal carcinoma or seminoma)	0

*Listed in decreasing order of frequency.

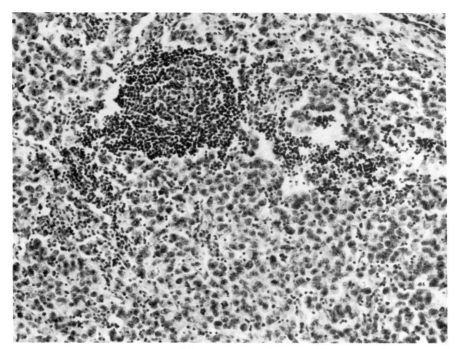

Figure 4–19 Seminoma consisting of fairly uniform cells in a solid pattern with interspersed lymphocytes. (Original magnification 100×.)

fined glandular and papillary structures. Division figures are numerous and there may be elements of primitive neoplastic stroma.

There is a variant of embryonal carcinoma designated as infantile that is the most common testicular neoplasm in children, but it may occasionally occur in adults. There is some evidence to suggest an extraembryonic yolk sac origin of this germ cell neoplasm. It has a distinctly more favorable prognosis than the usual embryonal carcinoma.

The teratoma is a neoplasm made up of components of more than one germ layer, i.e., ectoderm, endoderm, and mesoderm. The components may be represented in a rather primitive state, or they may appear as recognizable tissues. Attempts at organ formation may even occur. These tumors occur in children, where they account for 40 per cent of testicular neoplasms, as well as in young adults. They may reach a large size, and they have a very heterogeneous appearance on a cut surface as a result of the various components. Consistency varies with the presence of epithelial components, cartilage, and bone. Grossly visible cysts may occur. The microscopic picture reflects the myriad of histologic components which may occur in the various stages of maturation. The more mature varieties tend to occur in children. The teratoma has a significant mortality associated with it in adults, but it behaves as a benign neoplasm in children.

Rarely, a teratoma will exhibit complete maturation along one cell line and present as a benign epidermoid cyst or carcinoid tumor in the testis.

The choriocarcinoma is the most malignant of the germ cell neoplasms and fortunately is also the least common. It appears predominantly during the teens and twenties. It tends to be a small primary neoplasm which frequently reaches the clinical horizon with symptoms referable to metastatic spread. This is the most hemorrhagic of the germinal neoplasms. The tumor consists of syncytiotrophoblasts and cytotrophoblasts without true villous structures (Fig. 4–20). The choriocarcinoma in pure form tends to metastasize as such, whereas the other germinal neoplasms may reflect the totipotential nature of the germ cell and present in the metastasis as the primary tumor or as other types of germinal tumor.

The combination of embryonal carcinoma and teratoma is designated teratocarcinoma. Choriocarcinoma or seminoma may be present with it. The presence of the teratomatous elements seems to influence the prognosis favorably as compared to that for embryonal carcinoma or choriocarcinoma in pure forms. Interestingly, the presence of seminoma in combinations with the other germ cell neoplasms does not exert a significant favorable influence, even though it alone is the least malignant. The teratocarcinoma occurs most frequently in the third decade and tends to be the largest of the germinal tumors. Its gross appearance

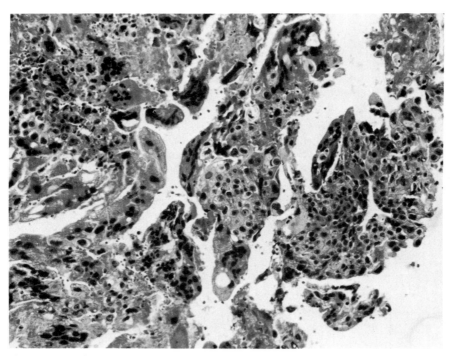

Figure 4–20 Choriocarcinoma with large multinucleated syncytiotrophoblasts and smaller cytotrophoblasts. (Original magnification 100 ×.)

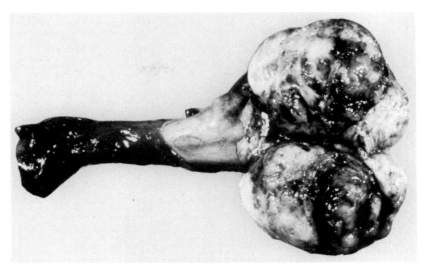

Figure 4-21 Spermatic cord with attached bisected testis replaced by teratocarcinoma. Note dark hemorrhagic foci.

reflects the heterogenous mixture of teratomatous elements in addition to the hemorrhage and necrosis that accompanies the embryonal or choriocarcinoma components (Figs. 4–21 and 4–22).

Most fatalities from germinal neoplasms occur within two years of

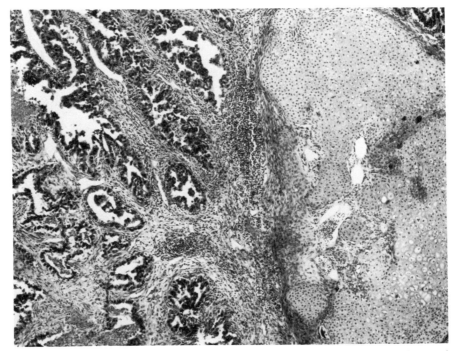

Figure 4-22 Teratocarcinoma exhibiting embryonal cell carcinoma in left portion of photo and cartilaginous component near the right margin. (Original magnification 40 ×.)

diagnosis, and it is unusual for death to occur five years or more following initial treatment. These neoplasms metastasize to lymph nodes, particularly in the retroperitoneal area, but may also appear in nodes above the diaphragm, including the neck. Widespread visceral metastases are common.

There is a marked elevation of urinary chorionic gonadotropin levels in all patients with choriocarcinoma, and occasionally patients with the other germinal tumors will have elevated levels. This elevation either indicates that choriocarcinomatous elements were missed in the initial histologic diagnosis of the neoplasm or that the other tumor types actually produced the hormone.

Several features are associated with a bad prognosis. These include pain at the time of diagnosis, local extension beyond the testis, elevation of urinary gonadotropins, and interstitial cell hyperplasia in the nonneoplastic portions of the testis. Metastases and vascular invasion, as to be expected, also are ominous prognostic signs.

Gonadal Stromal Neoplasms.   The gonadal stroma is believed to be the source of interstitial cells (Leydig's cells), Sertoli's cells, granulosa cells, and theca cells in both the testis and the ovary. These specialized cells have neoplastic counterparts in both sexes and account for 6 per cent of testicular neoplasms.

The most common is the interstitial cell tumor. It occurs in children and adults and is always associated with precocious puberty in children. This is manifested by enlarged external genitals, hirsutism including pubic hair, and a deep voice. The epiphyses of the long bones may undergo premature closure, resulting in short stature.

About one third of affected adult males exhibit gynecomastia. Loss of libido as well as increased libido has been reported. Some men show feminization with a female hair distribution. Many adults with an interstitial tumor may have no symptoms referable to an endocrine disturbance. Endocrine studies have revealed a wide spectrum of hormonal patterns associated with the Leydig cell tumor, including androgens, estrogens, progestational hormones, corticosteroids, or no hormone activity. This neoplasm may be associated with the adrenogenital syndrome, especially when bilateral interstitial cell neoplasms are present. Grossly, the tumors are yellow-brown and sharply circumscribed within the testis. Microscopically, the polygonal or round neoplastic cells tend to occur in solid sheets. The cytoplasm is eosinophilic and occasionally vacuolated. Spindle cell variants occur. Hyalinized fibrous trabeculae may traverse the tumor. Crystalloids of Reinke may be seen in the cytoplasm, helping to identify the cells as interstitial cells. Some students have difficulty in distinguishing this tumor from lymphoma or seminoma. In most Leydig cell tumors, the nuclei appear bland, compared to the very active appearing seminoma nucleus. A good general rule for distinguishing a Leydig tumor is to hold the histologic section stained with hematoxylin and eosin over a white background; the Leydig cell tumor typically appears red, and the seminoma and lymphoma have a blue color as a result of the abundant nuclear material and often clear or sparse cytoplasm. Approximately 10 per cent of interstitial cell neoplasms are malignant and capable of metastasizing.

The other gonadal stromal tumors are rare and deserve only brief mention. They occur in pure form as Sertoli's cell, granulosa cell, or theca cell tumors or in various combinations. Feminization may be a presenting symptom, but a consistent pattern of excess male or female hormone production has not been demonstrated. Most of these tumors are benign, but malignant varieties do exist.

Gonadoblastoma refers to a mixed tumor with both germ cell and gonadal stromal elements. These tumors may be associated with virilization or feminization.

Benign supporting tissue neoplasms, such as fibroma, lipoma, and hemangioma and their malignant counterparts, are extremely rare as primary testicular neoplasms, as are primary carcinomas of the rete testis.

Secondary Neoplasms.   The testis may be the site of metastatic carcinoma, melanoma, or other neoplasms. Malignant lymphoma occurs in the testis, particularly in older men where it is the most frequently occurring gonadal neoplasm. It may manifest in the testis as a tumor prior to other systemic or regional signs.

Adnexal Neoplasms or Neoplasticlike Lesions.   The most common tumor of the adnexal structures is the adenomatoid tumor which is usually found in the epididymis but may occur in the tissue of the testis and the spermatic cord. The inferior pole of the epididymis is the preferred site for this tumor. They usually are without symptoms and are found during palpation of the scrotal contents. These tumors are firm, well-circumscribed and measure up to several centimeters in diameter. They appear to be limited to adults. Histologically, they consist of a stroma of connective tissue and smooth muscle with aggregates of epitheliallike cells arranged in acinar spaces, solid nests, or cords (Fig. 4–23). Often these cells are vacuolated. On occasion, the cells are relatively flat and resemble endothelial or mesothelial cells. The origin of these interesting lesions, which have been misdiagnosed as malignant neoplasms on occasion, is controversial. There have been attempts to relate them to endothelial and mesothelial cells as well as to mesonephric epithelium and müllerian stroma. Ultrastructurally, they resemble mesothelial cells. In the female they occur in the uterus, oviduct, and parovarian tissues.

These are considered benign neoplasms or neoplasticlike lesions which can present as an abnormal solid scrotal mass that the uninitiated pathologist may confuse with adenocarcinoma or sarcoma.

Chronic productive inflammation can result in a diffuse or nodular fibrosis of the testicular tissue, epididymis, or spermatic cord and has been designated inflammatory or fibrous pseudotumor. These tumors may present as suspicious single or multiple scrotal masses in children or adults. Histologically, the picture varies with the age of the process, ranging from young granulation tissue with angioblasts and fibroblasts to hyalinized dense scar tissue. Nearly half of these are seen with

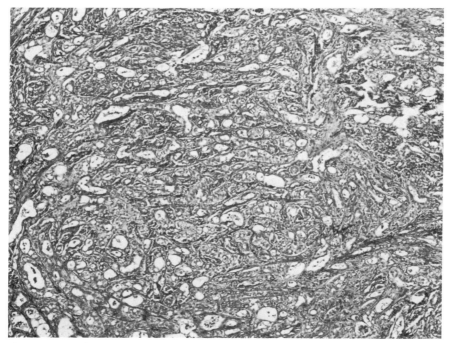

Figure 4–23 Adenomatoid tumor consisting of many gland-like structures in a delicate stroma. Note the resemblance to adenocarcinoma. (Original magnification 40×.)

hydroceles. Trauma or infection may play an etiologic role in some cases.

Various benign and malignant supporting tissue neoplasms may occur in the spermatic cord. The most important of these from the frequency standpoint in children and young adults is the rhabdomyosarcoma.

It is beyond the scope of this discussion, however, to consider these relatively uncommon lesions in detail.

SCROTUM

The scrotal skin is subject to all of the afflictions of skin elsewhere. Epithelial inclusion cysts and pigmented nevi are common lesions.

Squamous cell carcinoma of the scrotum is rare at present but was more common as a neoplasm associated with certain industries several decades ago. Long exposure to hydrocarbons in soot and petroleum products placed certain workers at high risk for this neoplasm. They were usually well differentiated neoplasms which seldom metastasized to sites other than regional lymph nodes.

Supporting tissue neoplasms of the deeper layers of the scrotum are rare.

ADRENAL GLAND

The important lesions of the adrenal gland from the urologic vantage point are cortical hyperplasia and the neoplasms involving the cortex and medulla.

Cortical hyperplasia may result in the adrenogenital syndrome in children. In adults, it can be associated with Cushing's syndrome or cortical hyperfunction, which manifests as obesity, diabetes mellitus, and hypertension. Primary aldosteronism may be associated with hyperplasia of the cortex, with or without cortical nodules. Cortical adenomas may also result in aldosteronism. The distinction between a cortical adenoma and nodule is arbitrary at best, and both lesions are perhaps best classified as adrenal cortical tumors. Carcinoma of the adrenal cortex occurs in children and adults and may or may not be functional. Both the benign and malignant cortical tumors are yellow. The carcinomas are more likely to demonstrate foci of hemorrhage and necrosis as well as capsular and vascular invasion. In some cases, the presence of metastasis is the only convincing criterion of malignancy. The retroperitoneal lymph nodes and the lungs are frequent sites of metastases.

The important medullary tumors include pheochromocytoma, neuroblastoma, and ganglioneuroma. The pheochromocytoma occurs in

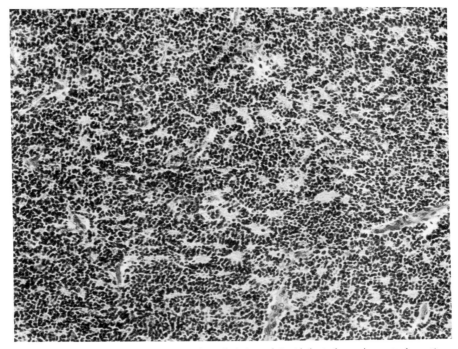

Figure 4–24   Neuroblastoma consisting of small dark nuclei with foci of pseudorosette formation. (Original magnification 100×.)

children and adults and has a higher frequency in patients afflicted with neurofibromatosis. It can be the cause of persistent or episodic hypertension. The tumor may grow to several centimeters in diameter, and a small percentage may metastasize. They are quite vascular and hemorrhagic. The histologic picture is one of solid nests of large cells with amphophilic cytoplasm and pleomorphic nuclei. Pigment granules may be present in the cytoplasm, which typically stains brown when the tumor is fixed in chromate solution.

The neuroblastoma occurs most frequently in young children and is a malignant neoplasm of primitive sympathetic nerve cells. These tumors are subdivided into sympathicogonioma, the most undifferentiated type, and sympathicoblastoma, which is better differentiated. These tumors appear gray-white and often show foci of hemorrhage and necrosis. The characteristic histologic picture is one of small hyperchromatic nuclei with a paucity of cytoplasm and numerous pseudorosettes (Fig. 4–24). These neoplasms have a predilection for hepatic and skeletal metastases, especially to bones of the skull.

The ganglioneuroma occurs at all ages and consists of mixtures of neurofibrils and ganglion cells in various stages of maturity. They usually are benign, but malignant forms exist.

All of the sympathetic neoplasms may occur in extra-adrenal sites associated with sympathetic nerve tissue.

SELECTED REFERENCES

Karsner, H. T.: Tumors of the Adrenal. Washington, D.C., Armed Forces Institute of Pathology, 1950.
  This fascicle covers in detail with excellent illustrations the neoplasms of the adrenal gland.

Lucké, B., and Schlumberger, H. G.: Tumors of the Kidney, Renal Pelvis and Ureter. Washington, D.C., Armed Forces Institute of Pathology, 1957.
  This is a well illustrated authoritative work on the epidemiology and morphology of neoplasms of the upper urinary tract.

Mostofi, F. K., and Price, E. B., Jr.: Tumors of the Male Genital System. Washington, D.C., Armed Forces Institute of Pathology, 1973.
  This is a well illustrated comprehensive fascicle which covers in detail all aspects of the pathology of male reproductive system neoplasms.

Rubin, P.: Cancer of the urogenital tract: Bladder cancer. J.A.M.A., 206:1762, 1775, 2719, 2727, 1968; 207:341, 351, 1131, 1969.
  This series of articles is an excellent review of the incidence, clinical and histologic staging, and etiologic factors in cancer of the urinary bladder. It is an extensive source of references.

Rubin, P.: Cancer of the urogenital tract: Prostatic cancer. J.A.M.A., 209:1695, 1704, 1969; 210:322, 1072, 1079, 1969.
  This series of articles is a superb comprehensive discussion of the pathology, chemistry, staging, and therapy of carcinoma of the prostate.

Wilson, C. C.: Immunologic glomerular injury. Postgrad. Med., 54:157, 1973.
  This is an excellent summary article covering the immunologic and pathogenetic mechanisms of human glomerulonephritis.

Wong, T. W., Straus, F. H., and Warner, N. E.: Testicular biopsy in the study of male infertility – I. Testicular causes of infertility. Arch. Pathol., 95:151, 1973.

Wong, T. W., Straus, F. H., and Warner, N. E.: Testicular biopsy in the study of male infertility – II. Post-testicular causes of infertility. Arch. Pathol., 95:160, 1973.

Wong, T. W., Straus, F. H., and Warner, N. E.: Testicular biopsy in the study of male infertility – III. Pretesticular causes of infertility. Arch. Pathol., 98:1, 1974.

This sequence of three articles classifies and presents with excellent photomicrographs the morphologic findings in the testicular biopsies from infertile males.

REFERENCES

Armenian, H. K., Lilienfeld, A. M., Diamond, E. L., and Bross, I. A. J.: Relation between benign prostatic hyperplasia and cancer of the prostate. Lancet, 2:115, 1974.

Auvert, J., Boureau, M., and Weisgerber, G.: Embryonal sarcoma of lower urinary tract in children. J. Urol., 112.396, 1974.

Butterick, J. D., Schnitzer, B., and Abell, M. R.: Ectopic prostatic tissue in urethra: a clinicopathological entity and significant cause of hematuria. J. Urol., 105:97, 1971.

Caldwell, W. L.: Carcinoma of the urinary bladder. J.A.M.A., 229:1643, 1974.

Cohn, B. D.: Histology of the cryptorchid testis. Surgery, 62:536, 1967.

Comings, D. E., Skubi, K. B., Van Eyes, J., and Motulsky, A. G.: Familial multifocal fibrosclerosis. Ann. Intern. Med., 66:884, 1967.

Conn, J. W.: Primary aldosteronism and primary reninism. Hosp. Pract., 9:131, 1974.

Crocker, D. W.: Renal Artery Stenosis. *In* Sommers, S. C. (ed.): Pathology Annual, New York, Appleton-Century-Crofts, 1968, vol. 3, pp. 187–211.

Deodhar, S. D., and Benjamin, S. P.: Pathology of human renal allograft rejection. Surg. Clin. North Am., 51:1141, 1971.

Gehring, G. G., Rodriquez, F. R., and Woodhead, D. M.: Malignant degeneration of cryptorchid testis following orchiopexy. J. Urol., 112:354, 1974.

Gilbert, D. N., Gourley, R., d'Agostino, A., Goodnight, S. H., and Worthen, H.: Interstitial nephritis due to methicillin, penicillin and ampicillin. Ann. Allergy, 28:378, 1970.

Hinglais, N., Grünfeld, J. P., and Bois, E.: Characteristic ultrastructural lesion of the glomerular basement membrane in progressive hereditary nephritis (Alport's syndrome). Lab. Invest., 27:473, 1972.

Howe, G. E., Prentiss, R. J., Mullenix, R. B., and Feeney, M. J.: Carcinoma of urethra. J. Urol., 89:232, 1963.

Mostofi, F. K.: Pathology and spread of renal cell carcinoma. *In* King, J. S. (ed.): Renal Neoplasia. Boston, Little, Brown and Co., 1967, pp. 41–85.

Smith, B. H.: Peyronie's disease. Am. J. Clin. Pathol., 45:670, 1966.

Smith, B. H., and Dehner, L. P.: Chronic ulcerating interstitial cystitis (Hunner's ulcer). Arch. Pathol., 93:76, 1972.

Sunshine, B.: Malacoplakia of the upper urinary tract. J. Urol., 112:362, 1974.

Chapter Five

NORMAL AND ABNORMAL RENAL FUNCTION

John W. Konnak and Jack Lapides

The purpose of the urinary tract is to aid in maintaining an optimal environment for the efficient functioning of body cells. To accomplish this purpose, the kidney operates through a number of mechanisms. Through the formation of urine, the kidney regulates the extracellular fluid volume and controls electrolyte and acid-base balance; it excretes toxic and waste products while conserving essential substances. In addition, the kidney is an endocrine organ that produces substances such as the enzyme renin and the hormone erythropoietin. It is also a trophic organ which responds to hormones such as aldosterone, antidiuretic hormone, and parathyroid hormone. There is also evidence that the kidney may deactivate substances such as gastrin. Obviously, many of these functions are interrelated.

When the kidneys do not perform their functions in a normal fashion, illness results. Anemia, malaise, nausea, vomiting, hypertension, disorientation, coma, convulsions, renal rickets, weakness, and cardiac abnormalities are some of the manifestations of general cellular dysfunction.

ANATOMY

An understanding of renal anatomy is essential to an understanding of renal function. Each kidney is composed of about 1,000,000 units called nephrons. Each *nephron* (Fig. 5–1) consists of a *glomerulus*, a *proximal convoluted tubule*, an *elongated segment (Henle's loop)*, and a *distal convoluted tubule* which empties into the *collecting tubule* of the nephron. The collecting tubule empties into the *calyx*. From there urine is propelled through the infundibulum into the pelvis, then down

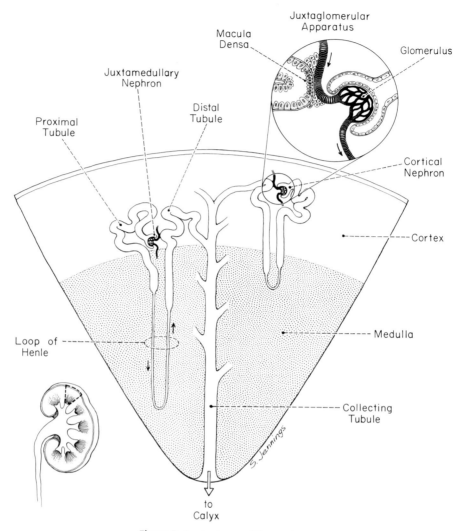

Figure 5–1 Anatomy of the nephron.

the ureter into the bladder. The bladder acts as a storage organ that empties the urine voluntarily at intervals into the external environment. The urologist views the nephron and the urinary collecting system as one long conduit; therefore, an abnormality of the distal part such as the urethra may affect the proximal functioning unit, the nephron.

The *cortex* of the kidney contains the glomeruli and the convoluted tubules; the renal *medulla*, the portion adjacent to the pelvis, contains the elongated tubular segments (Henle's loops) and the collecting ducts. The *juxtamedullary nephrons* are close to the medulla. They have elongated tubular segments which extend deeply into the medulla. The

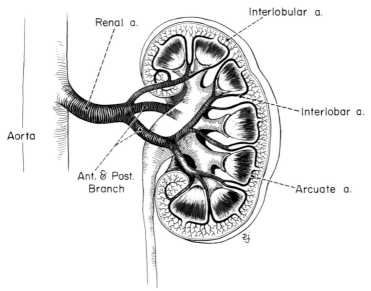

Figure 5–2   Anatomy of the kidney showing the renal blood supply.

nephrons closer to the surface are called *cortical nephrons* and have greatly attenuated Henle's loops.

The renal artery is a short, large caliber vessel that arises directly from the aorta and divides into an anterior and posterior branch as it enters the renal parenchyma (Fig. 5–2). The branches next divide into the interlobar arteries, which course through the renal medulla. At the corticomedullary junction, the interlobar vessels give off the arcuate arteries that in turn branch to give rise to the interlobular arteries in the cortex. The afferent arteriole comes from the interlobular artery and gives off the capillaries of the glomerulus. In the juxtamedullary nephrons, the efferent arteriole from the glomerulus sends extensions into the medulla parallel to Henle's loops; these extensions are called the *vasa recta* (Fig. 5–3). In both superficial cortical and juxtamedullary nephrons the efferent arteriole forms the peritubular capillary network. These capillaries empty into the venous portion of the network, then into the interlobular, arcuate, interlobar, and renal veins and finally into the vena cava. The most proximal portion of the distal tubule contains the macula densa cells. This portion of the tubule lies near the point where the afferent and efferent arterioles enter and leave the glomerulus. Special granular vascular cells in this area plus the macula densa form the *juxtaglomerular apparatus*, which is thought to secrete renin.

COMPOSITION OF BODY FLUIDS

A 70-kilogram adult contains approximately 45 liters of water; 30 liters are in the cells, and 15 liters are extracellular. Of the 15 ex-

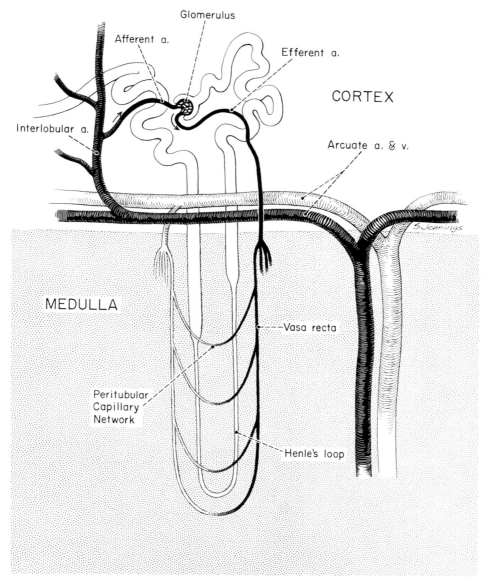

Figure 5–3 Blood supply to the nephron. The efferent arteriole gives off a capillary network surrounding the tubules which is not shown in this illustration.

tracellular liters of water, 11 liters are interstitial (between the cells) and 4 liters are in the cardiovascular system as plasma. The composition of the major body compartments is shown in Figure 5–4. As can be seen, sodium and its anions are the major soluble components of the extracellular fluid. The main difference between interstitial fluid and plasma is the greater concentration of protein in plasma. Because protein does not diffuse freely, a Gibbs-Donnan equilibrium is established

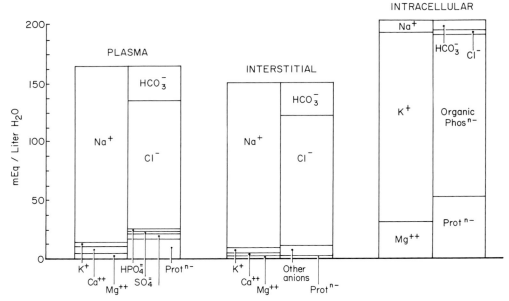

Figure 5–4 The composition of body fluids. (Modified from Gamble, J. L.: Chemical Anatomy, Physiology and Pathology of Extracellular Fluid. 6th ed. Cambridge, Massachusetts, Harvard University Press, 1954.)

between the plasma and interstitial compartments; the negatively charged protein molecules collide with the capillary membrane and are unable to cross into the interstitium, while some of the chloride ions on the other side cross into the plasma. A negative charge is thus built up on the membrane, which slightly favors the movement of sodium from the interstitial fluid into the plasma and anions into the interstitial fluid. Potassium is the major intracellular cation, and organic phosphates and protein are the major anions. This situation exists because there is active transport of sodium out of the cells and potassium into the cells, plus a selective impermeability of the cell membrane to protein and inorganic phosphate. These conditions set up another Gibbs-Donnan system that tends to exclude other anions such as chloride and bicarbonate from the cellular fluid.

Essentially, intravascular hydrostatic and tissue protein osmotic forces tend to promote the movement of water and crystalloid into the interstitial space, while the intravascular protein osmotic pressure (oncotic pressure) and tissue pressure tend to cause material to go from the interstitial fluid into the capillary. The heart provides the energy to generate the intravascular hydrostatic pressure. On the arterial side of the capillary, the sum of the intravascular hydrostatic pressure (30 mm Hg) and the protein osmotic pressure (5 mm Hg) is greater than the sum of the intravascular osmotic pressure (20 mm Hg) and the tissue hydrostatic pressure (10 mm Hg). Therefore, material at the arterial end of the capillary bed tends to move slightly more rapidly from the capillary to the interstitial fluid. The intravascular hydrostatic pressure drops from 30 to 15 mm Hg on going from the arterial end of the capillary to the venous end. Since the other pressures remain constant, material moves here slightly more rapidly from the interstitial fluid into the capillary. The constant size of the plasma and interstitial spaces is determined by this balance of forces.

GLOMERULAR FILTRATION

The glomerulus consists of a capillary network within Bowman's space. Its diameter is approximately 0.2 mm (just visible to the unaided eye). It consists basically of three layers: an endothelium, a basement membrane, and an epithelium consisting of podocytes with foot processes. At the center of the capillary tuft is the mesangium, consisting of mesangial cells and extensions of the basement membrane. About 1000 ml of blood or 600 ml of plasma flows through the kidneys in one minute, and about 120 to 160 ml of plasma is filtered through the 2,000,000 glomeruli in one minute. In the glomerular capillary the intravascular hydrostatic pressure is 75 mm Hg instead of 30 mm Hg as in capillaries elsewhere in the body. The total opposing pressure is 40 mm Hg and consists of the intratubular hydrostatic pressure (10 mm Hg), the interstitial pressure (10 mm Hg), and the intravascular oncotic pressure (20 mm Hg). Therefore, the *effective glomerular filtration pressure* is 35 mm Hg. Knowing this fact, it is not surprising that oliguria and anuria attend shock; a drop in systemic pressure sufficient to lower the pressure in the glomerular capillary by 35 mm Hg may abolish glomerular filtration. Similarly, obstructive uropathies that increase intratubular hydrostatic pressure or pyelonephritis that increases interstitial pressure may decrease glomerular filtration.

The glomerular filtrate is essentially protein-free plasma since the blood cellular elements and most of the protein are not filtered. The pH of the filtrate is 7.4, and its osmolality is about 285 mOs per kg. The glucose concentration is 80 mg per 100 ml, urea nitrogen 15 mg per 100 ml, sodium 142 mEq per liter, chloride 103 mEq per liter, bicarbonate 27 mEq per liter, and potassium 4.5 mEq per liter. Glomerular filtrate also contains many substances besides those listed, such as amino acids, other electrolytes (such as calcium and phosphate), creatinine, and any filterable drugs or chemicals. Approximately 180 liters are filtered in 24 hours. Most of this volume must be reabsorbed.

FUNCTION OF THE TUBULES AND COLLECTING DUCT

The tubule begins with *Bowman's capsule*, which is the thinned-out portion surrounding the glomerulus. Proceeding distally from Bowman's capsule the segments are, in order: the proximal convoluted tubule, (including the thick descending limb of Henle's loop); the thin segment (both the descending and ascending limb); the distal segment consisting of the thick ascending portion of Henle's loop and the distal convoluted tubule; and the collecting tubule.

Tubular function includes all the processes that convert glomerular filtrate into urine. This function includes the reabsorption of most of the filtered water, sodium, chloride, calcium, phosphate, bicarbonate, and amino acids. The volume of the glomerular filtrate is reduced from about 180,000 ml per 24 hours to about 1500 ml per 24 hours. Most unwanted substances either are simply not reabsorbed or are actively excreted. These include potassium, hydrogen ion, ammonia, creatinine, and a host of foreign substances like para-aminohippurate, pyelographic contrast material, penicillin, and sulfonamide compounds.

Reabsorption and Excretion in the Proximal Tubule

ACTIVE TUBULAR REABSORPTION

Tubular reabsorption has been divided into *active* and *passive* types. The active type requires metabolic energy, takes place from a lower to a higher concentration, can be abolished by inhibitors, cooling, or anoxia, and has a limited transport capacity. The limiting transport capacity, or *transport maximum* (Tm), varies from substance to substance and is probably a function of a hypothetical carrier on the lumen side of the tubular cell membrane. Theoretically a substance here binds to this carrier and is transported across the cell membrane. Inside the cell the substance and the carrier disassociate, and the substance passively diffuses through the cell into the peritubular fluid. The carrier is then regenerated, a process which requires energy. If the carrier is saturated, the Tm is exceeded, and the substance escapes in the urine. If substances share a carrier site, competitive inhibition of reabsorption can take place, such as with glucose and fructose. Factors besides Tm may limit reabsorption, such as glomerulotubular balance. Other substances which are actively reabsorbed in the proximal tubule include amino acids, uric acid, lactate, citrate, ascorbic acid, calcium, phosphate, and a host of other compounds. Amino acids are interesting in that similar ones are reabsorbed by the same transport mechanisms. Arginine, histidine, and lysine share one mechanism, while leucine and isoleucine share another; glycine, proline, and hydroxyproline use still another. There is no Tm for sodium; the active transport of sodium will be considered separately.

Sodium and Chloride.   About 80 per cent of the filtered sodium is reabsorbed in the proximal tubule, and with chloride this represents the bulk of the solute reabsorbed here. Although sodium is not transported against a gradient, there is evidence that its transport is active. Chloride is thought to accompany the reabsorbed sodium passively. In addition almost all of the filtered potassium is reabsorbed in the proximal tubule. Despite the reabsorption of all the previously mentioned solutes, the solution in the proximal tubular lumen remains isotonic because about 80 per cent of the filtered water is also reabsorbed. Thus the reabsorption of the major portion of the filtered water is passive and has been termed "obligatory" by Homer Smith.

Although most of the water and solute are reabsorbed in the proximal tubule, some substances are reabsorbed more slowly than water or are not reabsorbed at all. Consequently, these substances increase in concentration. For example, substances such as urea and creatinine increase in concentration in the proximal tubule. The tubular fluid leaving the proximal segment is still isotonic because the remaining sodium salts still provide the major portion of the osmotic pressure, and the loss of glucose and amino acids is equalized by the concentration of urea and creatinine.

FACTORS INFLUENCING SODIUM REABSORPTION IN THE PROXIMAL TUBULE. Adrenocortical steroids, especially aldosterone (second factor), stimulate the reabsorption of sodium in the proximal tubule as well as in the distal segment. The secretion of aldosterone is influenced by the extracellular fluid volume, probably mainly through the renin-angiotensin sytem, and by the blood level of potassium.

Another stimulus which may play a part in the reabsorption of sodium in the proximal tubule as sodium chloride relates to a passive mechanism. Water is reabsorbed from the lumen of the proximal tubule primarily because of the increased colloid osmotic pressure of the fluid of the peritubular capillary network (resulting from the concentration of protein in the blood of the efferent arteriole after the removal of water through glomerular filtration). Following the shifting of fluid from the tubule into the cells and capillaries, there is also a diffusion of sodium and chloride in the same direction in order to maintain isotonicity.

Other factors influencing sodium reabsorption and excretion include the rate of glomerular filtration of sodium (first factor), osmotic diuresis, other diuretics, and a hypothetical "third factor" which inhibits sodium reabsorption on saline loading.

BICARBONATE REABSORPTION IN THE PROXIMAL TUBULE. It has been demonstrated that the excretion of hydrogen ion starts in the proximal tubule and occurs all along the nephron. The partial pressure of carbon dioxide regulates the rate of hydrogen ion excretion. In the renal tubular cell, water and carbon dioxide combine under the influence of carbonic anhydrase to form carbonic acid, which then dissociates into hydrogen and bicarbonate ions. Hydrogen ions pass into the tubular lumen and exchange position with sodium ions of the filtered sodium bicarbonate, forming carbonic acid which slowly decomposes into water and carbon dioxide. The sodium is transported into the cell and combines with the dangling bicarbonate ion to form sodium bicarbonate. In this ion exchange mechanism in the proximal tubule, 90 per cent of the filtered sodium bicarbonate is reabsorbed. Functionally this process is equivalent to the reabsorption of 90 per cent of the filtered bicarbonate. Thus, one of the primary buffer materials has been returned to the body, and in the process excess hydrogen ion has been excreted. As the glomerular filtrate is pushed down the tubule, its pH does not change until all the bicarbonate in the lumen is decomposed.

Calcium and Phosphorus. Most (98 per cent) of the filtered calcium is actively reabsorbed in the proximal tubule. Forty per cent of the serum calcium is bound to protein and therefore is not filtered. Phosphate is also reabsorbed in the proximal tubule, and usually 80 per cent or more of the filtered phosphate is reabsorbed.

Parathyroid hormone influences the reabsorption of both calcium and phosphate. It decreases the reabsorption of phosphate in the proximal tubule, though this effect may be opposed by thyrocalcitonin. There is also evidence that parathyroid hormone decreases the reabsorption of both calcium and sodium in the proximal tubule while increasing calcium (but not sodium) reabsorption in the distal nephron; the net effect of this process is an increased reabsorption of calcium.

There is evidence that the kidney plays a further role in calcium metabolism by converting 25-hydroxyvitamin D to a more active form, 1,25-dihydroxyvitamin D under the influence of parathyroid hormone and other factors. Further discussion of these interactions, however, is beyond the scope of this chapter.

Passive Reabsorption

As the urea concentration in the proximal tubule begins to rise with the loss of water through tubular reabsorption, a concentration gradient is established between the urea in the tubule and the urea in the interstitial space. The urea then moves into the interstitial space. This movement is called *passive reabsorption*, and its rate varies with diuresis and antidiuresis.

FUNCTION OF THE NEPHRON DISTAL TO THE PROXIMAL SEGMENT

As stated previously, the proximal segment of the nephron removes an isotonic solution from the glomerular filtrate, which contains practically all of the filtered glucose, amino acids, bicarbonate, and other essential organic constituents of the extracellular fluid. In addition, 80 per cent of the filtered electrolytes and water are reabsorbed in the proximal tubule. All of the potassium and most of the sodium and chloride are removed. Some hydrogen ions have been added to the glomerular filtrate by tubular excretion. The tubular fluid entering Henle's loop amounts to 20 ml volume in one minute, contains one sixth of the filtered electrolytes, has a pH of 7.4, and an osmolality of 290 mOsm per kg.

To a great extent the processes that occur in the proximal tubule are constant and not too directly related to variations in body function. In contrast, the various activities of the distal nephron are attuned to the momentary needs of the cells of the body. It is in the distal portion of the nephron that the osmolality of the body is adjusted by the concentration and dilution of urine, and the pH is adjusted by the excretion of hydrogen ion.

URINARY CONCENTRATION AND DILUTION

The final concentration of the urine and ultimately the osmolality of the cellular and extracellular fluid is the result of a passive diffusion of water from the collecting tubule into the hypertonic medullary interstitium of the kidney, the process being under the influence of antidiuretic hormone. The maintenance of medullary hypertonicity is the result of the combined functions of Henle's loop acting as a counter-current multiplier and the vasa recta acting as a counter-current exchanger.

In the juxtamedullary nephrons, the thin portion of Henle's loop extends deeply into the medulla and then executes a hairpin turn to form a loop before coursing back to the outer medulla where it joins the thick portion; it then joins the distal tubule in the cortex. The vasa recta of the efferent arteriole also loop into the medulla, parallel to Henle's loops. The blood flow in the vasa recta is 5 per cent of that to the cortex, and the blood in the vasa recta is in contact with a given portion of the medulla for a much longer period of time because it traverses the same tissue in both the ascending and descending limb. This system favors diffusion and concentration of materials.

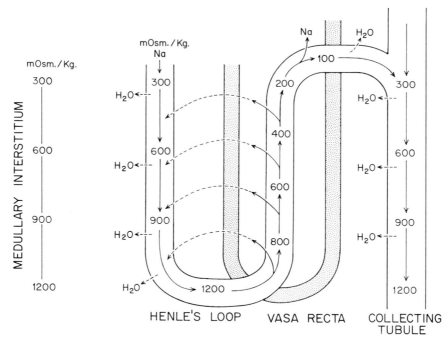

Figure 5–5 The counter-current multiplier in the loop of Henle. Solid arrows crossing membranes indicate active transport; broken arrows crossing membranes indicate passive diffusion.

COUNTER-CURRENT MULTIPLIER IN HENLE'S LOOP

Proximal tubular fluid enters Henle's loop isosmolar to plasma (Fig. 5–5). Sodium may diffuse freely into the descending limb from the medullary interstitium. Sodium is thought to move by an active process into the interstitium from the ascending limb where it diffuses into the descending limb. The fluid in the descending limb becomes increasingly concentrated, both by the diffusion of sodium in and partially by the passive diffusion of water out into the interstitium. As sodium is moved out of the water-impermeable ascending limb, the tubular fluid becomes more hypotonic, until fluid hypotonic to plasma enters the distal tubule. Because of this counter-current multiplier, only a small osmotic gradient needs to be overcome at any portion of the medulla.

COUNTER-CURRENT EXCHANGER IN THE VASA RECTA

Blood enters the vasa recta isosmolar to plasma (Fig. 5–6). As it proceeds more deeply into the hypertonic medulla, water passively diffuses out and solute diffuses in, making the blood hypertonic. Around the loop, as it ascends, solute diffuses out and water diffuses in. The blood

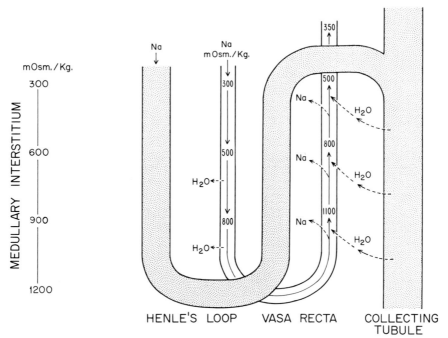

Figure 5–6 Counter-current exchanger in the vasa recta. Solid arrows crossing membranes indicate active transport; broken arrows crossing membranes indicate passive diffusion.

returns only slightly increased in osmolality over plasma (about 325 mOsm per kg). Thus the solute is not washed out destroying the concentration gradient, and the water in the medulla absorbed from the collecting ducts is removed.

Concentration of Urine

It has been demonstrated that the osmolality of the extracellular fluid is monitored continuously by vesicular cells in the supraoptic nuclei. When the osmolality of the interstitial fluid around these cells is increased, the posterior pituitary is stimulated to release antidiuretic hormone (ADH). This is an octapeptide formed by the cells of the hypothalamic supraoptic and paraventricular nuclei and stored at the nerve endings applied to the capillary blood vessels in the neural lobe of the pituitary.

The cells of the distal tubule and the collecting duct are relatively impermeable to water. Antidiuretic hormone increases the permeability of these structures to water. It also increases the permeability of the medullary collecting duct, but *not* the distal tubule, to urea.

When the body is dehydrated, there is a release of ADH. This causes the distal tubule to reabsorb water from the hypotonic fluid from the ascending limb of Henle's loop, allowing it to reach approximate isotonicity with the cortex. Urea does not diffuse freely here and is concentrated. When the tubular fluid has traversed the length of the distal tubule, about 18 or 20 ml of proximal tubular fluid has been reabsorbed. Thus 2 ml of isotonic fluid of an original 20 ml of hypotonic fluid remains. It will be quite obvious at this point that a urine with an osmolality greater than plasma must be formed from a volume of urine less than 2 ml per minute. It is for this reason that no one has ever encountered a person who can excrete a concentrated urine in amounts greater than several liters. If antidiuretic hormone is acting on the collecting duct, water moves out into the interstitial portion of the increasingly hypertonic medulla as the duct courses toward the renal papilla. In this way the tubular fluid becomes concentrated.

ROLE OF UREA IN CONCENTRATION

Urea is progressively concentrated until it reaches the distal collecting duct in the inner medulla and papillary portion of the kidney. Here urea diffuses more freely into the interstitium under the influence of ADH and helps to maintain the medullary osmolality. In the papilla under maximum antidiuresis, urea may account for 40 per cent of the osmolality. Very little of the medullary urea is carried away in the blood because of the low medullary flow and the counter-current exchange mechanism; most of it accumulates in the medullary interstitium and re-enters the tubules by diffusion into the descending portion of Henle's loop. Because of this activity, urea can be concentrated and excreted without the excretion of large amounts of water. Since under ordinary circumstances 30 to 40 per cent of the filtered urea is reabsorbed in the proximal tubule and since reabsorption of urea in the collecting tubule is dependent on water reabsorption, it follows that in water diuresis little urea is reabsorbed and 60 to 70 per cent of the filtered urea is excreted in the urine. In dehydration, much water is reabsorbed in the distal tubule and collecting duct, along with much urea (both because of its increased concentration and the action of ADH), and only 40 to 50 per cent of the filtered urea may be excreted in the urine.

When maximally concentrated, the urine may enter the calyx at the rate of 0.3 ml per minute, or 432 ml per 24 hours with an osmolality of about four times that of plasma, or 1160 mOsm per kg.

Dilution of Urine

On fluid loading, the osmolality of the plasma and extracellular fluid is lowered inhibiting the osmoreceptors, and the secretion of ADH stops. With the fall of the blood level of ADH, the distal tubule and collecting duct regain their impermeability to water. As a consequence the hypotonic fluid from the ascending limb of Henle's loop remains hypotonic despite the isotonicity of the cortical tissue surrounding the distal tubule and the hypertonicity of the medullary tissue surrounding the collecting duct. More sodium may actually be reabsorbed from these structures. From the preceding discussion it is apparent that in diabetes insipidus, a syndrome related to a lack of secretion of antidiuretic hormone, the individual cannot excrete more than 20 ml of urine per minute, 1.2 liters per hour, or 28.8 liters per 24 hours. When renal disease involves the tubules, a copious dilute urine results because the membranes may lose their responsiveness to ADH; and, more important, the counter-current mechanisms may be so affected by disease that the medulla loses its hypertonicity.

From the preceding, it can be seen that the establishment of the medullary hypertonicity by the counter-current mechanisms depends in large part on the active transport of sodium out of the ascending portion of Henle's loop. While the counter-current multiplier of Henle's loop is generally accepted, some experimental models fail to demonstrate the active transport of sodium in the ascending limb. Other theoretical systems dependent on the differential permeability to urea and the active transport of chloride have been proposed. The interested student is referred to the bibliography for further discussion of this controversy. In any event, a dilute urine has its origin in the ascending limb of Henle's loop, and a concentrated urine can be formed only in the collecting tubule.

MAINTENANCE OF A NORMAL pH OF THE BLOOD AND EXTRACELLULAR FLUID

All the processes of normal metabolism are acid producing; 99.99916 per cent of the hydrogen ions produced are transported in buffered form in the blood at a steady pH of 7.43. The main route of excretion of H^+ is in the lung, where about 14,000 mEq H^+ are excreted per day in the form of water vapor. The nephrons contribute their share (about 40 to 60 mEq H^+ per day) by excreting part of the formed volatile carbonic acid and the strong nonvolatile acids such as chloride, sulfuric, phosphoric, and other organic acids. The major strong acid, sulfuric acid, is derived from the oxidation of the sulfur-containing amino acids cystine and methionine; phosphoric acid results from the metabolism of phospholipid and amino acids containing phosphorus.

In order to maintain a pH of 7.4 the body must neutralize these strong acids. The primary buffering occurs from the reaction of the strong acid with sodium bicarbonate to produce the weak volatile carbonic acid and the sodium salt of the strong acid:

$$H_2SO_4 + 2NaHCO_3 \longrightarrow 2NaSO_4 + 2H_2O + 2CO_2$$

The H_2O and CO_2 can be excreted by the lungs; the sodium sulfate is excreted by the kidneys.

If the nephrons excreted unchanged the sodium salts of all the strong acids, the body would soon be depleted of its sodium and its primary buffer, sodium bicarbonate. The renal tubule has an elegant mechanism for excreting the unwanted acid, retaining the sodium, and regenerating bicarbonate. This mechanism has been discussed under the heading "Bicarbonate Reabsorption in the Proximal Tubule." In this discussion it has been mentioned that hydrogen ion exchange

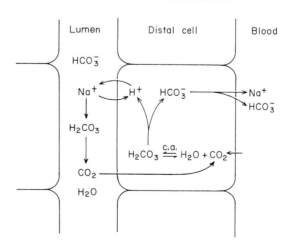

Figure 5–7   Reabsorption of bicarbonate. (Modified from Pitts, R. F.: The Physiologic Basis of Diuretic Therapy. Springfield, Illinois, Charles C Thomas, Pubs., 1954.)

started in the proximal tubule. The main function of the exchange in this portion of the nephron is to conserve the sodium ions of the sodium bicarbonate that has been filtered through the glomerulus. Most of the filtered bicarbonate is reabsorbed in the proximal tubule; about 10 per cent is reabsorbed in the distal nephron (Fig. 5–7).

In addition to continuing to reabsorb bicarbonate, the distal tubule excretes hydrogen ion. It does this in two ways: (1) by the excretion of titratable free acid and (2) by the formation of ammonia. In the excretion of *titratable free acid* (Fig. 5–8), the first step is the same as in the reabsorption of bicarbonate, where CO_2 and H_2O are combined to form carbonic acid. This dissociates to form H^+ and HCO_3^-. The H^+ combines with a neutral salt such as Na_2HPO_4 in the tubular lumen, forming the acid salt NaH_2PO_4. The Na^+ is reabsorbed with the formed HCO_3^-. Formation of this salt reduces the pH of the urine by the acid equivalent of the amount of a strong base required to titrate the urine back to a pH of 7.4.

In the *formation of ammonia* (Fig. 5–9), the deamination of glutamine into glutamic acid and NH_3 is promoted in the tubular cell by the enzyme glutaminase. The ammonia freely diffuses into the tubular lumen where it combines with the hydrogen ion produced from carbonic acid as previously described. The NH_4^- cannot diffuse back and exchanges for the sodium ion of a strong acid salt, which forms the ammonium salt, such as the neutral salt NH_4Cl if the "acid" salt was NaCl. About three fourths of the fixed acid is excreted in this way, and about one fourth is excreted by the formation of titratable free acid. The ammonium ion mechanism permits the body to excrete large amounts of hydrogen ion without making the urine too acid.

Several factors influence bicarbonate reabsorption and hydrogen ion excretion. The glomerular filtration rate and the plasma bicarbonate concentration influence bicarbonate reabsorption. When the plasma

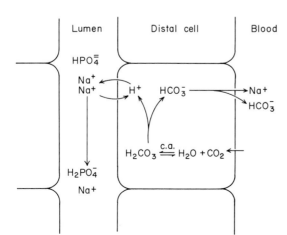

Figure 5–8 Excretion of titratable acid. (Modified from Pitts, R. F.: The Physiologic Basis of Diuretic Therapy. Springfield, Illinois, Charles C Thomas, Pubs., 1954.)

SECRETION OF AMMONIA

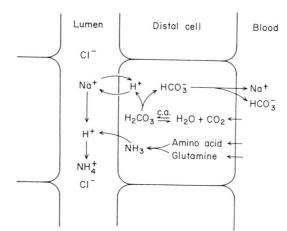

Figure 5–9 Secretion of ammonia. (Modified from Pitts, R. F.: The Physiologic Basis of Diuretic Therapy. Springfield, Illinois, Charles C Thomas, Pubs., 1954.)

bicarbonate is low, the urine is acid and very low in bicarbonate; when the concentration rises to over 28 mEq per liter the excess over this concentration in the glomerular filtrate appears in the urine, stabilizing the plasma bicarbonate at this level. When the plasma bicarbonate falls, titratable free acid is excreted, ammonia is produced, the urine becomes acid, and bicarbonate is regenerated. An increase in the pCO_2 leads to an increase in bicarbonate reabsorption and an increase in plasma bicarbonate. The potassium and hydrogen ions in the tubular cell compete for sodium ion in the tubular lumen. Thus, when there is potassium depletion, excretion of hydrogen ions into the tubular fluid is increased with a resultant increase in the plasma bicarbonate level. On the other hand, an increase in the serum potassium leads to a decreased hydrogen ion excretion and an alkaline urine. Inhibition of the enzyme carbonic anhydrase leads to a decreased secretion of hydrogen ions with a resultant loss in the urine of bicarbonate buffer and sodium ions. Over a period of time this process leads to hyperchloremic acidosis, hypokalemia, and an alkaline urine. A decrease in the glomerular filtration of disodium phosphate as well as sodium bicarbonate also affects hydrogen ion excretion since sodium ions must be present in the tubular fluid in order to effect an exchange between hydrogen and sodium ions.

POTASSIUM EXCRETION

Most of the filtered potassium is reabsorbed in the proximal tubule. The potassium excreted in the urine is secreted by the cells in the distal tubule. The potassium is excreted in exchange for sodium ions in the distal tubular fluid. The rate of potassium secretion is influenced by the amount of potassium in the distal tubular cell, the amount of hydrogen ion in the distal tubular cell, and the amount of sodium ion in the distal tubular fluid. As stated previously, the potassium and hydrogen ion in the tubular cell compete for sodium ion in the tubular lumen. Thus, potassium ion excretion is augmented in hyperkalemia, alkalosis, aldosteronism, and hypernatremia and depressed in hyponatremia, systemic acidosis, Addison's disease, and dehydration.

DIURETICS

Diuretic agents promote the increased excretion of urine by stimulating the nephron to decrease the reabsorption of sodium from the glomerular filtrate by the renal tubular cells and concomitantly the reabsorption of the water and associated anions. Some of the clinical agents commonly used are listed as follows:

Osmotic Diuretics. Mannitol is an osmotic diuretic that is filtered by the glomerulus but is not reabsorbed by the tubule. It osmotically retards salt and water reabsorption. It is used in incipient renal failure and to promote high urine flow in order to prevent clot formation after prostatic surgery.

Carbonic Anhydrase Inhibitors (Diamox). These agents interfere with the production of hydrogen ions from CO_2 and H_2O and thus impede the exchange of hydrogen for sodium ions throughout the nephron. The main effect is in the proximal tubule where normally 80 per cent of the filtered sodium is reabsorbed. There is an increase in the excretion of water, sodium, bicarbonate, potassium, and phosphate. These are low potency diuretics and are ineffective in the presence of acidosis.

Thiazide Diuretics (Chlorothiazide). These drugs inhibit reabsorption of sodium chloride in the cortical portion of the ascending limb of Henle's loop and in the distal tubule, and thus inhibit the dilution of urine without affecting the kidney's concentrating ability. They promote a sodium chloride diuresis. Potassium, bicarbonate, and phosphate are also lost. Clinically, they are used in the treatment of patients with hypertension, a mild cardiac disorder, and in renal failure with edema.

Loop Diuretics (Furosemide and Ethacrynic Acid). They act by blocking the reabsorption of sodium chloride in the ascending portion of Henle's loop and by preventing the concentration and dilution of urine. These are potent natriuretic agents that are effective in renal failure. They also cause a moderate loss of potassium, calcium, and magnesium. Their action is dose dependent. Mercurial diuretics also fall into this class but are seldom used clinically at the present time.

Potassium Sparing Diuretics. Spironolactone is a true competitive inhibitor of aldosterone in the distal tubule. It blocks the reabsorption of sodium at the aldosterone-dependent distal tubular site and prevents its exchange for potassium, thus resulting in potassium sparing. Triamterene blocks sodium-potassium exchange, but not by competitive inhibition of aldosterone. These are mildly effective diuretics and are used where potassium wasting may be a problem.

RENAL FUNCTION TESTS

QUALITATIVE TESTS

A gross estimate of renal fuction may be obtained by routine urine analysis. Albumin and casts indicate damage to the glomerulus. Urine volume is a poor test of renal function, but severe oliguria with volumes below 400 ml per 24 hours indicates a loss of renal function. The urine in renal failure has a low, fixed specific gravity (1.010).

Excretory urography may give a rough estimate of renal function, since modern contrast materials are excreted primarily by glomerular filtration. In the usual doses, there will be little or no visualization of the collecting system if over 75 per cent of the total renal parenchyma is functionally inactive (serum creatinine over 2 mg per 100 ml). A double dose and infusion urography can give visualization at a lesser level of renal function.

QUANTITATIVE TESTS

For laboratory use, the standard renal function tests are those which measure the clearances of inulin and PAH. Inulin is a polymer of fructose which is filtered by the glomerulus and is neither secreted nor reabsorbed by the tubules. The clearance of inulin is therefore a measure of glomerular filtration rate. *Clearance* is defined as the volume of plasma completely cleared of a substance by the kidney. The term is artificial because most substances are not completely cleared by one pass through the kidney. The clearance of inulin may be calculated from the formula

$$C_{inulin} = \frac{\text{urine concentration of inulin} \times \text{urine volume}}{\text{plasma concentration of inulin}}$$

$$\text{or, } C = \frac{UV}{P}.$$

The clearance of inulin is 120 ml per minute or about 180 liters per 24 hours. PAH (para-aminohippurate) is filtered by the glomerulus and secreted by the tubules and, in a small dose, is almost completely removed in one pass through the kidney. The clearance of this substance is a measure of renal plasma flow. Both the inulin and PAH clearances require a loading dose and constant infusion techniques and are more suitable for the laboratory than for clinical practice.

Creatinine is an endogenous product of muscle metabolism. It is produced at a fairly constant rate in a given individual and is cleared primarily by glomerular filtration. The *creatinine clearance* is a practical measure of glomerular filtration and therefore of renal function. The normal creatinine clearance is 140 liters per 24 hours or about 100 ml per one minute. This can be calculated from the standard clearance formula $C = \dfrac{UV}{P}$, or the urinary excretion of creatinine (in grams per 24 hours) may be divided by the serum creatinine (in mg per 100 ml) and multiplied by 100 to give the liters per 24 hours.

The serum creatinine concentration has been correlated with the creatinine clearance, and there is a fairly linear relationship between the two, i.e., a serum creatinine of between 1 and 2 mg per 100 ml in the adult. A serum creatinine of 1.0 mg per 100 ml is correlated with 100 per cent normal creatinine clearance. When the creatinine clearance falls to 25 per cent of normal, the serum creatinine is 2 mg per 100 ml. Therefore, a 7.5 per cent decrease in renal function may be equated with a rise in 0.1 mg per 100 ml of the serum creatinine above 1 mg per 100 ml.

The blood urea nitrogen (BUN) gives a rough estimate of renal function and is elevated when 75 per cent of the total renal mass is nonfunctional. The urea clearance varies with urine flow and also with dehydration, gastrointestinal hemorrhage, liver disease, and catabolic states that often occur in transplant patients on steroids.

The phenolsulfonphthalein test (PSP test) is an estimate of tubular function, and therefore of glomerular function, because it has been shown that the glomerular function can rarely be more impaired than tubular function. An intravenous dose of 6 mg is given, and normal kidneys can excrete 33 per cent of this dose in 15 minutes.

Other tests, such as the concentration test based on the normal kidney's ability to concentrate urine after a period of dehydration, are occasionally used.

RENAL FAILURE

Renal failure is a relative term, since it represents a spectrum between a lack of renal reserve or very mild renal insufficiency and severe renal failure with the uremic syndrome. Minimal renal failure is compatible with a normal life unless the individual is stressed by dehydration or heart failure; severe renal failure with uremia is incompatible with life. Between these extremes is a continuum with progressive impairment of function and increasing disability. Except in the specific disorders of tubular activity, function is usually lost in an orderly manner in progressive renal failure; tubular function is lost in tandem with glomerular function. This gradual process has led to the "all or none" concept wherein whole nephrons are progressively lost in renal failure, leaving a diminishing population of normal nephrons to carry on until their capacity is overwhelmed. Morphologic studies demonstrate marked variability in the patterns of damage to the nephrons. Currently it is generally believed that diseased nephrons contribute to renal function, and responding to the azotemic environment as appropriately as they can, the net effect is an orderly loss of renal function as the disease progresses. The more common renal diseases such as glomerulonephritis, pyelonephritis, hydronephrosis, and hypertensive renal disease tend to present the same clinical and laboratory findings as renal failure becomes advanced.

Whether due to increased intratubular hydrostatic pressure as in hydronephrosis, structural change in the glomerular membrane as in glomerulonephritis and intercapillary glomerular sclerosis, or inflammatory involvement as in pyelonephritis, impairment of glomerulotubular function will lead to the retention of all metabolic end products destined to be excreted from the body primarily by the kidneys. Particularly, the products of protein metabolism, such as phosphates, sulfates, urea, and uric acid, accumulate. When these and other products reach a sufficient level, the uremic syndrome occurs. Clinically uremia is attended by nausea, vomiting, diarrhea, malaise, dyspnea on slight exertion, hyperpnea, twitching, anemia, ease of fatigue, and occasionally by acute abdominal pain and tenderness. This disease may progress to coma, convulsions, and death. Blood chemical studies show an elevation of creatinine, blood urea, and nonprotein nitrogen, a decrease in serum bicarbonate, and an increased phosphate and sulfate concentration. The serum potassium level tends to rise above 5 mEq per liter. As the serum phosphate level rises, the serum calcium level falls. The ionized serum calcium level may remain normal if concomitant acidosis is sufficiently great. Life-threatening uremia usually does not occur until renal function is reduced below 10 per cent of normal.

ACUTE RENAL FAILURE

Acute renal insufficiency has a wide variety of causes. Generally, these fit into three broad categories:

(1) *Defects in renal perfusion*, sometimes called "prerenal" causes, including shock, cardiac failure, dehydration, and bilateral renal embolization.

(2) *Renal parenchymal disorders*, including acute tubular necrosis due to ischemia and toxic nephropathies due to nephrotoxins such as mercuric chloride, carbon tetrachloride, and certain antibiotics such as gentamicin. Acute glomerulonephritis, acute cortical necrosis, and renal failure due to crush injuries and incompatible blood transfusions also fall into this group. Obviously, these etiologic factors tend to overlap.

(3) *Obstructive uropathies*, including bilateral ureteral obstruction and advanced prostatism.

The course of acute renal failure is variable and depends on the cause, the condition of the patient, and the circumstances, but in general, acute renal failure is reversible given proper patient support, treatment of the underlying cause, and management of complications.

Acute tubular necrosis is the most common cause of acute renal failure. The cause falls into two broad categories: *toxic* and *ischemic*. There exists a large and growing list of nephrotoxic materials, including those mentioned previously. In general, the renal lesions produced by nephrotoxic substances are reversible, provided that exposure to the substance is terminated and that the substance has not severely damaged other organs.

Renal ischemia from any cause may produce acute tubular necrosis. Histologically the ischemic form shows a patchy, random distribution of tubular necrosis that includes the basement membrane. Interstitial edema is usually present, and the kidneys are grossly enlarged and edematous. The glomeruli may appear normal. Physiologically there is a marked decrease in the glomerular filtration rate that is associated with an inability to concentrate or dilute urine. Urinary specific gravity is fixed at about 1.010, and the osmolality is within 50 mOsm per kg of serum, or around 300 mOsm per kg. Urine sodium concentration exceeds 20 mEq per liter and is often considerably higher than this.

The important *clinical features* of acute renal failure due to acute tubular necrosis include:

1. *Oliguria during the initial phases.* This is not invariably present, but urine output is usually below 400 ml per 24 hours. The disease seldom produces anuria, and other causes of renal failure such as ureteric obstruction must be considered in the anuric patient.

2. *Deteriorating renal function tests.* The serum creatinine may rise from 1 to 1.5 mg per 100 ml per day with a concomitant rise in the blood urea nitrogen.

3. *Low fixed specific gravity of the urine,* around 1.010 with urinary osmolality of around 300 mOs per kg.

4. *Increased urinary sodium* excretion above 20 mEq per liter.

5. *Increasing serum potassium.*

6. *Symptoms of progressive azotemia and fluid overload.* As time passes (5 to 7 days) the patient may become hypertensive and develop dulled sensorium, vomiting, dyspnea, and progress toward frank uremia.

Recovery usually begins with increasing urine output between the seventh and the fourteenth day. This is called the *diuretic phase.* Improvement in renal function lags behind the increasing output. In some cases the oliguric period is prolonged and may last 30 days or more. In general if recovery has not taken place in six weeks, renal failure may be irreversible. Large amounts of salt and water may be lost during the diuretic phase.

The main *differential diagnosis* is between impaired renal perfusion due to hypotension, dehydration, renal vasospasm as the result of surgery, trauma, or toxic products, and acute tubular necrosis. In the former, the urine sodium is low, usually below 40 mEq per liter, the specific gravity is high, usually around 1.020, and the urinary osmolality is high, perhaps over 1000 mOsm per kg. A provocative test may be helpful in making the diagnosis. Fifty grams of mannitol in solution with 500 ml of normal saline is given over a period of 30 to 60 minutes. If the patient responds with a diuresis, a perfusion defect or dehydration is present. If there is no response, acute tubular necrosis is probably present and further fluids should be restricted. One hundred milligrams (100 mg) of furosemide may also be used as a provocative test.

The rest of the differential diagnosis includes all the other causes of acute renal failure including obstruction. The diagnosis of obstruction is discussed in Chapter 11.

The treatment of acute renal failure is directed at preventing complications of fluid overload, potassium intoxication, uremia, and infection. Fluid is restricted to measured outputs plus the 600 to 800 ml that represent insensible loss in the adult under normal circumstances. If acute renal failure follows surgery, central venous pressure measurements provide a helpful guide to fluid status. Sodium is also restricted to 20 mEq per day in a patient not on dialysis. Daily weights are very helpful in following fluid balance; a patient on a limited caloric intake might be expected to lose 0.5 kg per day. Protein is restricted to prevent a breakdown into nitrogenous wastes and to help limit potassium intake because protein-containing foods are generally high in potassium. Artificial amino acid diets of high biologic specificity which are low in potassium may be used. Dietary potassium is restricted from 0 to 20 mEq per day in a patient not on dialysis, depending on the serum potassium levels. As serum potassium levels rise, the electrocardiogram should be monitered as an index of potassium intoxication.

In order to decrease protein catabolism through gluconeogenesis with the production of sulfate, phosphate, and urea and to decrease the formation of ketone bodies from fat, at least 100 grams of glucose should be given, preferably orally in the form of hard candy.

Electrolyte imbalances are corrected with appropriate parenteral fluids. *Hyperkalemia* may be treated with 8.5 per cent sodium bicarbonate solution to correct acidosis, increase serum sodium, and drive potassium into the cell. Glucose and insulin therapy to promote glycogen formation and storage with potassium in the liver is used with less and less frequency. Ten per cent calcium gluconate infusion may be given to protect the heart from potassium intoxication. A cation exchange resin, sodium polystyrene sulfonate, may be given orally or by retention enema to remove potassium; this substance is administered with sorbitol to promote diarrhea and the expulsion of the resin. Ion exchange resins act relatively slowly and should be given before hyperkalemia becomes an acute problem. One gram of sodium polystyrene sulfonate removes about 1 mEq of potassium, and approximately 200 mEq of total body potassium must be removed to lower the serum potassium 1 mEq per 1.

Asymptomatic acidosis per se without hyperkalemia need not be treated. Blood transfusions generally should not be given to correct a mild or moderate anemia because of the dangers of congestive failure, transfusion reaction, and hepatitis. The patient should be allowed to void on his own, and indwelling catheters should be avoided because of the risks of infection, sepsis, and stricture formation.

During the diuretic phase enough fluid should be given to provide for insensible loss and a urine output of 2000 ml per day. The massive diureses of the past were probably iatrogenic in part due to the belief that the daily insensible loss of fluid amounted to 1000 ml instead of the 400 to 600 ml and thus the patient was given an excess of 500 ml per day during the oliguria phase. If the oliguria lasted 10 days, the individual had an excess of five liters of fluid in his body, which was excreted during the initial part of the "diuretic" phase. The continued diuresis was also iatrogenic in the belief that the patient was being dehydrated by the initial outpouring of urine and needed volume for volume replacement. A mild diuresis will occur due to retained fluid and the diuretic effect of retained urea.

Early dialysis, either peritoneal or hemodialysis, has greatly simplified the management of acute renal failure. On dialysis the patient can be maintained on a near normal diet and only mild fluid restriction. A diet containing 60 grams protein with 60 mEq potassium and 60 mEq sodium per 24 hours with a fluid restriction to 1500 ml would be acceptable on a program of two to three times weekly hemodialysis. Patients on dialysis are much more comfortable and have fewer complications than those not on dialysis.

Despite advances in management, the mortality from acute tubular necrosis remains about 40 to 50 per cent. Most of the deaths are in trauma or postsurgical patients. When these are eliminated, the mortality falls to less than 15 per cent.

CHRONIC RENAL FAILURE

Until relatively recently patients dying from advanced renal disease had no hope for recovery. Now renal transplantation and chronic hemodialysis have permitted the survival of these people for a number of years. Many problems are still present in the use of both methods, but these are gradually being solved. It is anticipated that an ever-increasing number of those dying from renal failure will be restored to a useful, productive status in society in the future.

SELECTED REFERENCES

Papper, S.: Clinical Nephrology. Boston, Little, Brown & Co., 1971.
   This is a well organized text on the structure, function, and medical diseases of the kidney. It has selected references.
Orloff, J., Berliner, R. W., and Geiger, S. R., eds.: Renal physiology. *In* Handbook of Physiology. Baltimore, American Physiological Society and Williams & Wilkins Co., 1973.
   A 29 chapter standard reference text. This text is very comprehensive and deals with all aspects of renal physiology including the research techniques currently in use. It has extensive references. A background in physiology would be useful for the student approaching this volume.
Strauss, M. B., and Welt, L. G., eds.: Diseases of the Kidney. 2nd ed. Boston, Little, Brown & Co., 1971.

A comprehensive standard reference text on nephrology in two volumes with 44 chapters by 59 authors. Contains chapters on renal structure and function as well as on diagnostic methods. This text covers the complete spectrum of medical renal disease. It has extensive references.

Valtin, Heinz: Renal Function: Mechanisms Preserving Fluid and Solute Balance in Health. Boston, Little, Brown & Co., 1973.
A short text on renal physiology, well organized under headings in the margins. Contains standard selected references and problems for the student.

REFERENCES

Frazier, H. S.: Renal regulation of sodium balance. N. Engl. J. Med., 279:867, 1968.

Gombos, E. A.: Acute renal failure, N.Y. State J. Med., 73:2055, 1973.

Jamison, R. L.: Recent advances in the physiology of Henle's loop and the collecting tubule system. Circ. Res., Suppl. I, 34:1, 1974 and 35:1, 1974.

Lapides, J., and Schroeder, K. F.: Urology. *In* Rhoads, J. E. et al.: Surgery: Principles and Practice. 4th ed. Philadelphia, J. B. Lippincott Co., 1970.

Lapides, J.: Use of renal function tests in surgical practice. J. Med. Assoc. Ga., 51:210, 1962.

Steinmetz, P. R.: Excretion of acid by the kidney—functional organization and cellular aspects of acidification. N. Engl. J. Med., 278:1102, 1968.

Chapter Six

URINE TRANSPORT, STORAGE, AND MICTURITION

Jack Lapides and Ananias C. Diokno

Smooth muscle plays an important role in the movement of urine from the nephron to outside the body. Unlike striated muscle, unstriped muscle maintains tension continually without the aid of motor impulses from the central nervous system. It resists extension and will respond to stretch by contracting or shortening and thus increasing its tension. Removal of the stretch stimulus permits the smooth muscle to return to its previous state of resting tension. If the smooth muscle is in the form of a tube, distending the lumen with fluid will evoke a contraction of the muscle of the distended segment so that the fluid will be propelled into the adjacent segment of tube which has the lesser tension of the resting state.

Flaccidity or atonicity of smooth muscle cannot occur immediately following interruption of its extrinsic nerve supply (spinal shock, spinal anesthesia), as is the case with striated muscle. In order to make smooth muscle flaccid, it is necessary to overextend it mechanically for a prolonged period of time. Thus, dilated ureters and atonic bladder are caused by overdistention with urine and not by tonic impulses from the central nervous system having been vitiated. Other factors which may affect the smooth muscle of the ureter are blood supply and toxins (bacterial as well as drugs and chemicals). On a comparative basis, relatively little energy is expended in the performance of work by smooth muscle.

URETER

Glomerular filtration and the flow of glomerular filtrate through the tubule of the nephron are accomplished by the effective glomerular filtration pressure which, it will be recalled, is the result of intravascular hydrostatic, protein osmotic, and intratubular hydrostatic pressures. The urine enters the calyx and distends it under the influence of the effective glomerular filtration pressure. As soon as the smooth muscle of the calyx is stretched, it is stimulated to contract down and propel the bolus of urine into the distal adjacent segment of the collecting system, namely, the infundibulum and thence into the renal pelvis. When the renal pelvis is filled sufficiently with urine from the various calyces and infundibula, it contracts and propels the bolus of urine into the proximal ureteric segment. As it pushes the urine into the segment of ureter, the ureteric muscle in turn is stretched and stimulated to undergo systole. The bolus of urine is thus pushed down into the next segment of ureter, and the process is repeated until the plug of urine is expelled into the bladder lumen. When the rate of formation of urine is low, ureteric peristaltic waves are infrequent. In diuresis, peristaltic waves are shallow and so increased in frequency as to make the ureter appear to be a rigid tube. Recent observations reveal that concomitant with increased contractile activity of the ureter, there is a change in the configuration and size of the ureteric lumen. In order to accommodate increasing rates of urine formation by the kidney, the ureteric lumen markedly enlarges by gradually changing from a stellate shape through a rectangular conformation into an eventual circle or hollow cylinder (Fig. 6–1). This transformation may increase the size of the lumen 22 times. All the peristaltic activity of the calyces, pelvis, and ureter is completely autonomous. It takes place without benefit of motor impulses from the central nervous system, and its normal stimulus is stretch by urine volume. The peristaltic activity of the ureter is so primitive and mechanical in nature that Melick was able to excise a segment of ureter in the pig, reverse the ends of the excised segment, resuture it to the ureter (but in a reversed manner), and have the ureter exhibit perfectly normal peristalsis after healing had taken place.

Increased intravesical and intraureteric pressures will lead to an increase in force of ureteric contractions. Traumatic irritation of the ureter by catheters or calculi can produce large, irregular muscular contractions which are not related to urine volume or intravesical pressure. Transection of the ureter and reanastomosis impair peristalsis temporarily at the site of anastomosis during the period of healing because the neuromuscular transmission of electrical activity is halted at the cut distal end of the proximal portion of ureter. This can be obviated during the immediate postoperative period by spatulating or "ellipticizing" the ends of the ureters being anastomosed so that the mechanical activity of the most distal tongue of the proximal ureter will stimulate the most proximal slip of the distal ureter which faces it across the ureteric lumen, and start a peristaltic wave down the distal ureter. When healing is completed, perfectly normal ureteric function is resumed unless marked scar tissue formation occurs at the site of suturing.

There are no motor nerves to the smooth muscle of the calyces, infundibula, pelvis, and ureter. Sympathetic fibers to the ureter control

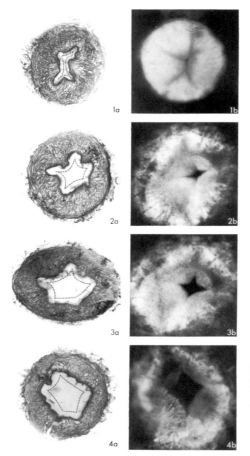

Figure 6–1 Cross-sections of ureter instantaneously frozen during peristalsis (1a, 2a, 3a, 4a) and photographs of lumen of ureter during activity (1b, 2b, 3b, 4b).

Legend continued on the following page

its vascular elements. Afferent fibers traveling with the vascular motor fibers carry sensory impulses from the ureter to spinal segments T-11, T-12, L-1, and L-2. Painful stimuli from the ureter are perceived along the area of distribution of the ilioinguinal, iliohypogastric, and genitofemoral nerves. Since tonicity and peristalsis of the ureter are autonomous, no adrenergic, cholinergic, sympatholytic, or parasympatholytic drug in a physiologic dose will influence, immediately and directly, muscular activity of the ureter. Parenteral histamine has been shown to increase ureteric muscular activity in the dog. There is no therapeutic drug which will cause relaxation or dilatation of the ureter.

A number of articles have appeared in the literature suggesting that ureteric peristalsis can be influenced by stimulation of the autonomic nerves and central nervous system and by adrenergic and cholinergic drugs. The pharmacologic agents and ureteric responses listed in recent studies are similar in nature to those observed during the early part of the twentieth century by Satani, Henderson, Lucas, and many others. Despite all the evidence marshaled to date, it still remains to be

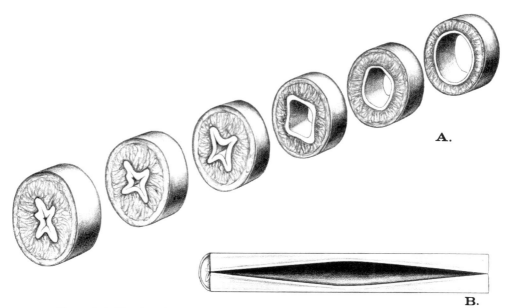

A.

B.

Figure 6–1 *(Continued)* Diagrammatic representations of ureteral configuration (A, B). (From Woodburne, R. T., and Lapides, J.: The ureteral lumen during peristalsis. Am. J. Anat. *133*:255–258, 1972. Copyright by The Wistar Press. Reprinted by permission.)

demonstrated that the ureter in the intact human is influenced in more than a *modulatory degree* by the autonomic nervous system, central nervous system, or drugs in a physiologic dose.

Dilated or hydroureter occurs when there is overdistention of the ureteric muscle for a period of time. This implies that the kidney must be producing urine in order to stretch the ureter and, secondly, that there must exist an abnormality along the course of the ureter which prevents the ureter from emptying itself in a normal fashion. The disease may be an intrinsic or extrinsic narrowing of the ureter anywhere along its course, up to and including its meatus; an obstruction within the lumen of the ureter such as stone or tumor; an involvement of the wall of a segment of ureter by inflammation or some process preventing normal peristaltic activity of that segment without necessarily narrowing the lumen of the ureteric segment; a distended bladder due to urethral obstruction or neurogenic involvement; or voiding with abnormally high intravesical pressures.

When a ureter ceases its normal function either because its kidney has undergone nephrectomy or because disease has impaired renal function, its smooth muscle becomes atrophic whereas the epithelium and lumen remain essentially unchanged.

URETEROVESICAL VALVE

In the normal individual ureteric peristalsis is initiated at the proximal end of the ureter and is propagated distally through its intrinsic neuromuscular mechanism until the urine is propelled into the bladder. The urine is stored in the bladder until the individual decides to empty the bladder voluntarily at a suitable time and in an appropriate place. During storage as well as micturition no urine flows back grossly from the bladder into the ureters or refluxes. Everyone is agreed that the occurrence of reflux or gross regurgitation of urine is an abnormal finding and may be due to some disturbance of the valvular mechanism located in the region of the intravesical portion of the ureter or that segment which is in the wall of the bladder.

Although the exact mechanism of action of the ureterovesical valve in preventing gross regurgitation is not wholly agreed upon at present, experimental and clinical evidence suggests that it acts in the form of a flap-valve. The distal ureter, devoid of its circular layer of muscle, passes obliquely through the seromuscular layer of the bladder wall and then courses submucosally for a variable distance. It is believed that intravesical pressure (and perhaps intrinsic ureteric elongation via muscle fibers coursing from the ureteric meatus to attachments in the posterior urethra) compresses the intramural portion of the ureter so that reflux is prevented but efflux is permitted.

Any disease process or iatrogenic procedure which makes rigid the ureteric orifice and intramural ureter, shortens the submucosal length of the ureter, markedly enlarges the ureteric orifice, weakens the vesical muscular backing of the intramural ureter, or promotes a marked increase in intravesical pressure may lead to ureteric regurgitation. Ureteric reflux has been found in children and adults of both sexes, and it has been associated in many instances with obstructive uropathy at the vesicourethral junction and distally. The obstructions include vesical neck contracture, prostatism, urethral valves, urethral stricture, and meatal stenosis. Functional obstruction, as observed in patients with neurogenic bladders who cannot open the urinary sphincter adequately during micturition, cannot relax the periurethral striated muscle reflexly, or demonstrate a spastic contraction of the periurethral striated muscle and therefore must void with increased intravesical pressures, is often associated with ureteric reflux. A high incidence of urinary tract infection is found in patients with ureteric backflow. Some cases of reflux are discovered in conjunction with abnormal development of the ureter or the ureterovesical junction such as in bladder exstrophy, ectopic ureter, and duplication anomalies. Operative procedures which enlarge the ureteric orifice may lead to ureteric reflux.

Ureteric regurgitation is diagnosed by x-ray examination of the urinary tract following instillation of radiopaque material into the bladder. The best techniques include voiding cystourethrogram and cineradiography. Backflow of contrast material from the bladder up the ureters confirms the diagnosis.

The significance of ureteric reflux is highly controversial and perhaps overemphasized at the moment. As stated previously, ureteric regurgitation is a sign of incompetence of the ureterovesical valve mechanism. The incompetence in many cases is produced by obstructive uropathy with its associated facets of increased voiding pressures and urinary tract infection. Thus, ureteric reflux is another sign of lower urinary tract abnormality, particularly obstructive uropathy, and suggests to the physician that a thorough search should be made for the primary cause.

Treatment should be aimed toward alleviating the obstructive uropathy or primary cause. In many cases, elimination of the obstruction will result in disappearance of the high intravesical voiding pressures and recurrent or persistent urinary tract infection. The ureteric reflux will disappear in many instances or, if persistent, will be of no more significance than bladder trabeculation, cellule formation, or diverticula which empty.

It should be noted that bladder contents under normal conditions probably enter the ureteric lumen and ascend continually. On the basis of hydrodynamic principles, Shapiro has demonstrated that bulk reflux is inherent in peristaltic pumping regardless of the competency of the ureterovesical valve. Thus, urine or bacterial particles from the bladder cross the ureterovesical junction into the ureter without necessarily producing harmful effects.

There are numerous reports in the literature attesting to the fact that patients can maintain normal anatomical configuration and function of the kidneys over a period of years despite the presence of ureteric reflux. Lalli and Lapides reported on the long-term follow-up of ureteroneocystostomy by the "fish-mouth" technique in a series of patients and showed unequivocally that normal renal function and structure can coexist with ureteric reimplantation not utilizing an antireflux technique.

There is no question that reflux associated with unrecognized or undiagnosed lower urinary tract dysfunction and infection will predispose the patient to more frequent and severe bouts of pyelonephritis than would occur without ureteric regurgitation. Thus it is extremely important for the physician to pinpoint and treat the lower urinary tract abnormality so that reflux and pyelonephritis do not occur or disappear with conservative measures. The attitude that reflux is primary and congenital and that its treatment consists of ureteric reimplantation into the bladder without a thorough workup of the lower urinary tract is to be condemned, for such a procedure has led to the loss of many kidneys and some lives. Ureteroneocystostomy is often attended by complications and, more importantly, reflux cured with successful reimplantation will soon recur if the underlying lower urinary tract disease persists.

BLADDER AND URINARY SPHINCTER

When distended with fluid, the bladder is shaped like a round-bottomed flask in that it is composed of a spherical portion called the

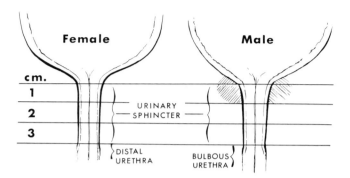

Figure 6–2 The urinary sphincter in both the young adult male and female is the proximal 3 cm of the posterior urethra.

fundus and a cylindrical part commonly known as the posterior urethra. In the young adult male and female the posterior urethra is approximately 3.0 cm long. The male posterior urethra includes the prostatic and membranous portions, whereas in the female it is the proximal three fourths of the entire urethral length (Fig. 6–2).

The fundus and posterior urethra should be considered as one unit both anatomically and functionally. Embryologically, both are derived from the vesicourethral sac of the urogenital sinus, and both possess smooth muscle and elastic tissue in their walls. Parasympathetic fibers coursing in the pelvic nerve supply identical motor impulses to the fundus and urethra. The smooth muscle of the bladder can be considered as a sheet of muscle in the form of a reticulum or webwork which extends without interruption down into the urethra as the muscular wall. There is a particularly heavy concentration of elastic connective tissue fibers in the wall of the urethra (Fig. 6–3).

This bladder unit consisting of a sphere and a cylinder has certain intrinsic properties which are completely independent of any nervous

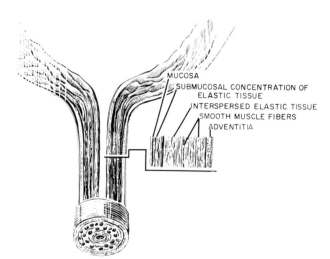

Figure 6–3 The urinary sphincter or posterior urethral wall has a particularly heavy concentration of elastic fibers in the submucosal layer and interspersed among the smooth muscle fibers.

regulation from the central nervous system. As stated previously, the smooth muscle and elastic tissue exert continuous tension in an autonomous fashion and with a negligible expenditure of energy. When the bladder fundus is being distended with fluid, the smooth muscle fibers of the bladder wall are first stretched and in turn are caused to contract and increase their tension. Thus, measurement of intravesical pressure will demonstrate an initial increase on filling of the bladder with fluid, but then, as filling continues, the intravesical pressure will remain approximately constant until bladder capacity is reached (Fig. 6–4). At capacity, the intravesical pressure will start to rise sharply in the form of a straight-line relationship. The ability of the bladder fundus to maintain a relatively low intravesical pressure with distention is due to its vesicoelastic properties and is called accommodation. It serves an important function in that it permits the ureters to pump urine into the bladder without excessive effort. The sharp rise in pressure at capacity is believed to be due to the stretching of connective tissue in the bladder wall.

Fluid present in the bladder fundus is prevented from leaking out through the urethra by the proximal 3.0 cm of the urethra or the tubular part of the bladder unit. The urethra accomplishes this by virtue of the continuous intrinsic autonomous tension exerted by the smooth muscle and connective tissue in its wall. These tissues keep the urethra compressed so that its lumen is sufficiently obliterated to prevent urine from flowing out of the bladder fundus under low or moderate pressures.

When high intravesical pressures occur as a result of increased intra-abdominal pressure such as in coughing, straining, or exercising, urinary incontinence would ensue if given only the proximal urethra or urinary sphincter per se to stop it. Under conditions of high intravesical pressure, the efficiency of the urinary sphincter must be enhanced to maintain continence. The organism accomplishes this feat with the aid of the voluntary striated muscle surrounding the posterior urethra.

The muscle of the urogenital diaphragm and levator ani surround the urethra and are in contact with it for about 2.0 cm. In the female, it

Figure 6–4 When the bladder is filling with urine, the intravesical pressure remains constant until bladder capacity is reached. Distending the bladder beyond capacity results in a marked increase in intravesical pressure.

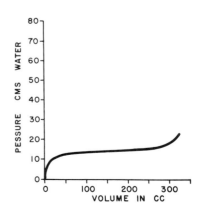

is the mid 2.0 cm of urethra, and in the male it is the corresponding distal prostate and membranous portions of urethra which are contiguous with the periurethral striated muscle (Fig. 6–5). These muscles increase the efficiency of the urinary sphincter by compressing the urethra circumferentially and elongating it by pulling it cephalad. The striated muscle can act on a voluntary basis, or contraction can take place reflexly. One can willfully compress the urethra and prevent urinary incontinence when the bladder is full and the patient has an urgent desire to urinate. Or the urinary sphincter can be compressed and elongated reflexly when assuming the erect posture or in coughing, straining, and filling of the bladder (Fig. 6–6). The striated muscle is supplied by motor fibers emanating from motor neurons in the ventral horn of the upper sacral segments and carried in the pudendal nerve. It is important to note that the urinary sphincter is the intact urethra and that the striated muscles surrounding the urethra are of secondary importance since they can increase the efficiency of the urinary sphincter but cannot substitute for it. The striated muscles serve also to interrupt urination rapidly (one to two seconds) when there is an urgent need, by compressing and elongating the urinary sphincter until the vesical smooth muscle stops contracting (10 to 20 seconds).

The basic bladder unit can store urine under moderate pressure autonomously, but it cannot evacuate its contents without the aid of motor impulses from the central nervous system. The bladder (fundus and urethra) is supplied by sensory and motor fibers. The afferent fibers

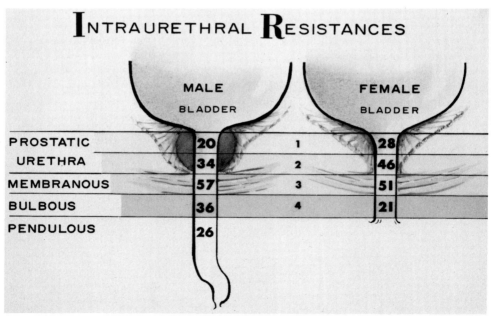

Figure 6–5 The periurethral striated muscle (levator ani and muscle of the urogenital diaphragm) is contiguous with the mid 2 cm of the female urethra and its counterpart in the male—the distal part of the prostate and membranous portions of the urethra.

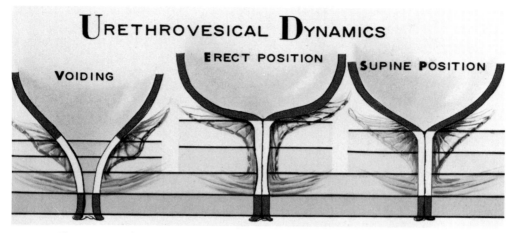

Figure 6–6 When the patient assumes the erect position or contracts the periurethral striated muscle, the urethra is elongated and compressed. During micturition the periurethral striated muscle is relaxed. In addition, the urethrovesical junction is pulled open into a funnel-shaped structure by active contraction of the vesicourethral smooth muscle sheet. The net result is a functional shortening and widening of the posterior urethra.

carry pain, temperature, and proprioceptive (desire to void and fullness) sensations and travel primarily in the pelvic nerve. The motor neurons supplying the musculature of the bladder are situated in the lateral horns of the sacral spinal cord at the levels of S-2, S-3, and S-4. The motor fibers extend from the motor neuron to the wall of the bladder and posterior urethra where ganglionic synapses and postganglionic fibers are situated. The motor pathways are parasympathetic in nature and also form part of the pelvic nerve (Fig. 6–7).

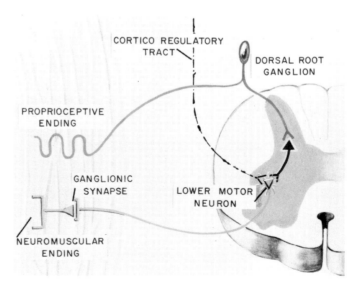

Figure 6–7 The spinal reflex arc concerned with micturition is found at the level of sacral spinal cord, segments 2, 3, and 4.

In the infant, micturition takes place in an uncontrolled fashion and by virtue of a simple spinal reflex arc synapsing in the sacral spinal cord. The limbs of the reflex arc have been described in the previous paragraph. Although the motor side of the reflex is part of the autonomic nervous system and has ganglionic synapses, for purposes of clarity the reflex arc can be considered in exactly the same light, reflexwise, as the simple, skeletal segmental reflex arc. As the bladder fills with urine and is stretched, proprioceptive endings in the wall are stimulated to send sensory impulses to the sacral spinal cord. In the infant spinal cord, the motor neurons to the bladder are activated by the proprioceptive impulses, and motor impulses are transmitted to the bladder muscle to cause it to contract. The bladder may exhibit several weak contractions with small volumes of urine without expelling any urine, but then with increased stretching a strong detrusor contraction will occur with resultant emptying of the bladder.

Measurement of intravesical pressure during normal micturition indicates that pressures varying between 25 and 50 cm of water obtain at the height of urination. Yet, when the bladder is at rest and storing urine, it may require intravesical pressures of greater than 150 to 250 cm of water to overcome the resistance of the posterior urethra or urinary sphincter so that urinary flow occurs. We have already discussed the fact that the urinary sphincter maintains urinary continence during stress by virtue of being elongated and compressed by the periurethral striated muscle. During urination, it is preferable to have low intravesical pressures obtaining, since high pressures, as seen in obstructive uropathy, predispose to infection, dilatation of the urinary tract, and renal deterioration.

How does the urinary sphincter decrease its resistance during urination? The posterior urethra accomplishes this in a most simple fashion. First, there is relaxation of the periurethral striated muscle either reflexly or voluntarily. This results in some decrease in length of the urethra and tension of the urethral wall against its lumen. *A further decrease in length of the urethra and increase in caliber of the urethral lumen is effected by active contractions of the smooth muscle of the bladder and urethra.* When the bladder begins to contract down upon a bolus of urine, the urethrovesical junction and proximal portion of the urinary sphincter are pulled open by active contraction of the muscle sheet which is continuous from the bladder into the posterior urethra (Fig. 6–8). The urinary sphincter does not open by passive relaxation but by active contraction of the vesicourethral muscle fibers.

The urinary sphincter is a tube, not a ring, with its greatest resistance in the midposterior urethra and its least resistance at the vesical outlet or urethrovesical junction. It can be readily discerned that any pathologic entity which prevents a widening of the urethral lumen, a shortening of its length, and a decrease in tension of its walls against the lumen during initiation of urination will lead to the complications of obstructive uropathy just as certainly as will an obstructing prostate, occluding calculus, or pinpoint stricture. A urethrovesical junction which appears quite adequate on urethroscopy during the storing phase

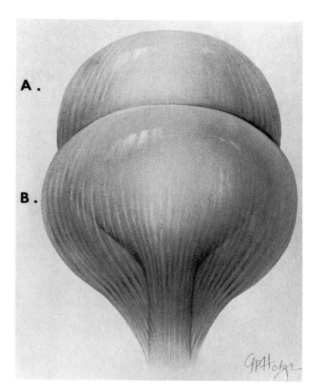

Figure 6–8 When the detrusor muscle contracts down upon a bolus of urine, the urethrovesical junction is *pulled open* by the muscle sheet and the vesicourethral configuration changes from a flask with a long narrow neck in *A* to a squat bottle with a short wide neck in *B*.

of the bladder might be entirely inadequate during micturition because a wide-caliber rigid ring at the urethrovesical junction prevents the pulling-open of the vesical outlet, shortening of the urethra, and increase in its caliber. Similarly, a bladder with involvement of its lower motor neurons and with a resultant inability to contract fully its muscle sheet will be unable to open the urinary sphincter and permit voiding at low intravesical pressures.

The normal urinary sphincter can maintain continence in the infant between voidings, but it cannot prevent the reflex voiding contractions. Thus, the normal baby will not dribble urine continuously but will wet at intervals during forceful bladder contractions. Voluntary control of urination is gained or the child becomes "housebroken" as soon as the corticoregulatory tract begins to function. The corticoregulatory tract (Fig. 6–9) runs from the motor cortex to the lower motor neurons and can stimulate the lower motor neurons to discharge motor impulses or can inhibit the lower motor neurons from discharging in response to afferent impulses from the bladder and elsewhere. Thus, the individual with normal voluntary control is able to urinate with only a small volume of urine in the bladder by having the higher centers stimulate the lower motor neurons; or one can urinate with a large volume of urine in the bladder by removing the inhibitory influence from the higher

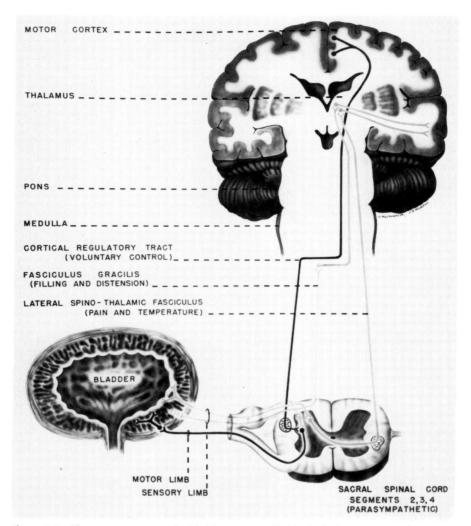

Figure 6–9   The motor neurons to the bladder are controlled by the higher centers via the cortico-regulatory tract.

centers and permitting the lower motor neurons to become activated by proprioceptive impulses from the stretched bladder wall.

In addition to the descending corticoregulatory tract, there are sensory tracts ascending to the higher centers. Pain and temperature are carried to the brain via the lateral spinothalamic tracts, whereas proprioceptive sensation ascends by way of the posterior columns.

The exact function of the sympathetic or adrenergic system in urination is unknown at present. Studies have shown that alpha and beta adrenergic receptors are present in both the bladder and the urethra. When the presacral or hypogastric nerve is stimulated in the male, the urethrovesical junction closes and the posterior urethra contracts with resultant seminal emission; during this time the detrusor initially contracts and then relaxes.

It is probable that the sympathetic nervous system relates primarily to sexual function and affects the urinary bladder indirectly in carrying out this activity, i.e., inhibiting detrusor contraction during ejaculation. Since, in the male, urination, continence, and ejaculation utilize the posterior urethra, it is apparent that the several functions must be highly coordinated in order to avoid urinating during intercourse or ejaculating during urination. This concept is supported by recent studies demonstrating a close relationship among the hypogastric, pelvic, and pudendal nerves to the bladder, urethra, and periurethral striated muscle.

The urethral wall not only possesses smooth muscle which is a continuation of the detrusor meshwork into the posterior urethra responsive to cholinergic stimulation and involved in storage and evacuation of urine, but has the smooth muscle layer just mentioned which is influenced by the sympathetic or adrenergic system and is related to sexual function. Although the layer of adrenergic sensitive smooth muscle is activated primarily during orgasm, it can affect continence and micturition in patients with neurogenic bladder and other disorders of the lower urinary tract.

Cystometric Apparatus

Bladder function is evaluated by a series of diagnostic procedures which include endoscopy, urography, cystometry, and electromyography. The instrument used in measuring various modalities of bladder function is called the cystometer. There are various types of cystometers in use, but we prefer the simple, inexpensive water type (Fig. 6–10), consisting of a graduated reservoir, a Murphy drip, a screw clamp to regulate the rate of flow of fluid, a water manometer (meter stick with attached glass tubing), rubber tubing to connect the Murphy drip and water manometer to a glass Y tube, and a hemostat to start and stop the flow of fluid. It will be noted in Figure 6–10 that the top of the manometer is made level with the Murphy drip in order to permit the flow of fluid from the reservoir even with high intravesical pressures. The cystometer is made ready for use by filling the reservoir and tubing with sterile water so that all the air bubbles are removed from the system except in the Murphy drip chamber. The zero mark on the manometer is made level with the subject's bladder. The cystometric apparatus can be used most efficiently by being hung on a parenteral fluid stand.

Method of Cystometry

The cystometric examination is initiated by requesting the patient to void and observing the time required to initiate micturition; the size, force, and continuity of stream; the amount of straining during urina-

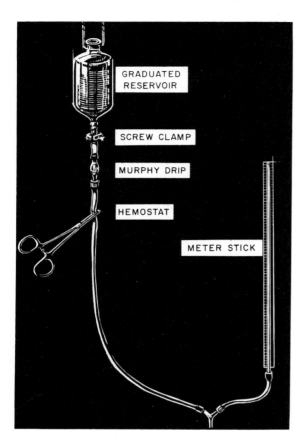

GRADUATED RESERVOIR

SCREW CLAMP

MURPHY DRIP

HEMOSTAT

METER STICK

Figure 6–10 The water cystometer is a simple, extremely reliable apparatus for evaluating bladder function.

tion; and the terminal dribbling. The male is requested to void in the erect position and the female in the erect or sitting posture. After the patient has completed voiding and assumed the lithotomy position, a No. 16 or No. 18 French retention catheter is passed through the urethra into the bladder and left in place. The volume of residual urine is measured. Through the catheter 60 ml of cold and then 60 ml of warm water are instilled to test exteroceptive sensation.

The urethral catheter is then connected to the water manometric cystometer, and water is instilled into the bladder at a rate of about 1 ml per second; this rate is obtained by adjusting the screw clamp so that the flow of fluid is just beyond the drop stage or a slow stream. The patient is requested to inform the examiner when the first desire to urinate occurs and again when the bladder feels quite full. The intravesical pressures and volumes are plotted on a cystometrographic sheet.

When the subject's bladder is full, the urethral catheter is removed and the patient is requested to cough in the lithotomy position. After observing the individual for evidences of stress incontinence, the patient is again requested to void and the micturition pattern is noted.

The patient then resumes the lithotomy or supine position and is recatheterized. A second volume of residual urine is obtained and the Urecholine supersensitivity test performed. Fluid is instilled into the bladder from the cystometric apparatus at a rate of 1 ml per second. When the volume of fluid in the bladder reaches 100 ml, the intravesical pressure is recorded and the flow of fluid stopped. After repeating the control run several times, the adult patient is given 2.5 mg of Urecholine subcutaneously and the cystometric runs are repeated 20 and 30 minutes after Urecholine administration. In children, the Urecholine dosage is calculated in accord with their weight, assuming the average adult to weigh 150 pounds. Thus, a 25-lb child would receive 25/150 or 1/6 of 2.5 mg Urecholine or 0.41 mg; a 50-lb child, 50/150, 1/3 of 2.5 mg or 0.8 mg; a 75-lb child, 75/150, 1/2 of 2.5 mg or 1.75 mg.

INTERPRETATION OF CYSTOMETRIC EXAMINATION

An individual with normal micturition starts voiding within several seconds after request if the bladder is full and the patient has an intense desire to urinate. On the other hand, if the bladder contains a small volume of urine, it may take 20 to 30 seconds before micturition is initiated; some individuals may be unable to begin urination at all in the presence of the examiner. The urinary stream is of good caliber and force and uninterrupted. The normal male is able to project his stream at least several feet beyond the urethral meatus and in a straight line. At the termination of urination, the stream is interrupted for a short period of time as efforts are made to empty the urethra with forceful contractions of the periurethral striated musculature. On completion of urination, the volume of residual urine is less than 30 ml.

The normal subject is able to perceive cold and hot water, has the first desire to void somewhere between 175 and 250 ml volume, and feels full between 350 and 450 ml volume.

When fluid is first instilled into the bladder, there is a rather sharp rise in intravesical pressure during the first 50 ml volume to between 5 and 25 cm of water, and then the intravesical pressure remains approximately constant until bladder capacity is reached. At a volume of 350 to 450 ml, the patient complains of bladder distention and the intravesical pressure begins to increase in a straight line relationship with the volume. No uninhibited voiding contractions of the detrusor are observed at any time during filling of the bladder, even at capacity when the subject is uncomfortable. After distending the bladder to capacity and the catheter has been removed, no urine is propelled through the urethra on coughing. Micturition with a full bladder conforms to all the characteristics previously outlined.

The intravesical pressure rise in the Urecholine supersensitivity test is less than 15 cm of water over that of the control in the normal subject. The cystometrograph and cystometric findings of the normal bladder are depicted in Figure 6–11.

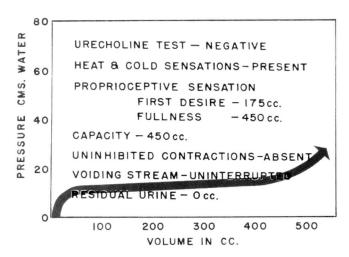

Figure 6–11 Cystometrograph of normal bladder.

URECHOLINE SUPERSENSITIVITY TEST

As stated previously, when bladder muscle is stretched by fluid flowing into the lumen of the bladder, it responds by contracting and increasing the intravesical pressure (Fig. 6–12). The stretch response of bladder muscle is a phenomenon localized to the muscle fibers; it is not mediated by acetylcholine, and it is completely independent of the central nervous system. Normal, atonic, and neurogenic bladders dem-

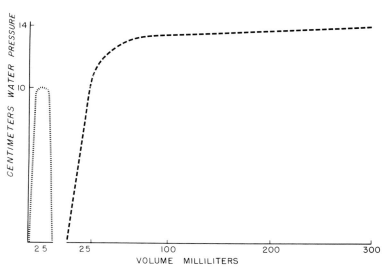

Figure 6–12 When 25 ml of fluid is instilled into the bladder, the detrusor muscle is stretched and stimulated to contract and produce a rise in intravesical pressure. On cessation of stimulation, the smooth muscle of the bladder resumes its previous resting tension. A continuous flow of fluid into the bladder will result in a sustained increase in intravesical pressure.

onstrate essentially the same response to stretching, i.e., they all exhibit an intravesical pressure varying from 5 to 18 cm of water in response to a flow rate of 1 ml per second at a volume of 100 ml.

When 2.5 mg of Urecholine is administered subcutaneously to an adult with a normal bladder, the intravesical pressure response to stretching is increased by 2 to 15 cm water over that of the control. The maximal response is observed usually 20 to 30 minutes after injection of the Urecholine. Differential blocking of the motor limb of the reflex arc indicates that the Urecholine stimulates primarily at the neuromuscular junction and to a slight degree at the ganglionic synapse. It should be emphasized that every normal bladder responds to Urecholine and stretch with a rise in intravesical pressure never greater than 15 cm over the control with the exception of the uremic or azotemic patient.

If 2.5 mg of Urecholine is administered subcutaneously to an adult with significant detrusor denervation, the intravesical pressure response to stretch will always be greater than 15 cm over that of the control. The motor and sensory paralytic bladders show the greatest sensitivity at the neuromuscular junction and the ganglionic synapse respectively (Figs. 6–13 and 6–14).

In the patient with an uninhibited neurogenic bladder, the lower motor neuron is supersensitive while the ganglionic synapse and

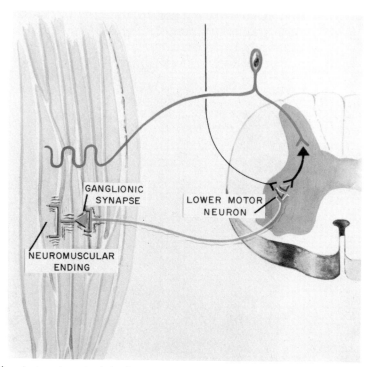

Figure 6–13 A chronic impairment of the lower motor neuron or nerve fiber will result in denervation supersensitivity of the neuromuscular ending and ganglionic synapse.

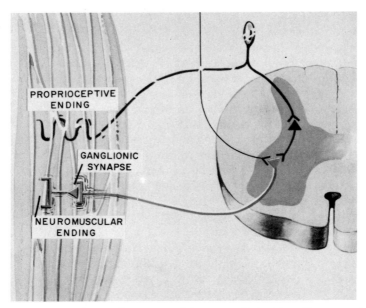

Figure 6–14 Chronic denervation of the sensory limb of the reflex arc results in supersensitivity, primarily of the ganglionic synapse and to a lesser degree of the neuromuscular ending.

neuromuscular junction retain their normal sensitivity (Fig. 6–15). Thus, the patient having a bladder with involvement of its upper motor neurons demonstrates supersensitivity to Urecholine by exhibiting an uncontrolled voiding contraction of the bladder at a smaller volume than during the control run. The response to Urecholine is variable in patients

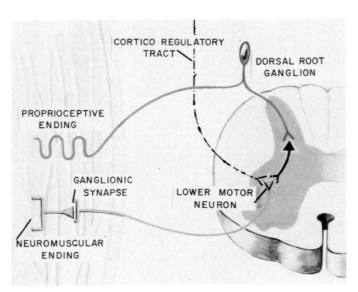

Figure 6–15 Destruction of the corticoregulatory tract leads to denervation supersensitivity of the lower motor neuron.

with uninhibited neurogenic bladders because not all patients with this type of bladder will exhibit an uninhibited bladder contraction at a bladder volume of 100 ml with 2.5 mg Urecholine.

In clinical practice, one uses the stretch response test according to the following regimen. The usual cystometric examination is performed. Several control bladder stretch response tests are obtained, using a flow rate of 1 ml per second and recording the intravesical pressure at 100 ml volume. The adult patient is given 2.5 mg of Urecholine subcutaneously and stretch response tests are obtained at 10, 20, and 30 minutes after administration. If the greatest intravesical pressure rise over that of the control is less than 15 cm of water, the patient does not have significant chronic neurogenic disease in the sacral spinal cord area or the lower reflex arc. If the patient demonstrates a pressure response greater than 15 cm over that of the control and is not uremic, the patient definitely has a neurogenic bladder which may be due to chronic involvement of the corticoregulatory tract, the sensory limb of the lower reflex arc, the motor limb of the segmental reflex arc, or any combination of the three. The method of differentiating the various types of neurogenic bladder will be discussed in the following sections of this chapter.

ELECTROMYOGRAPHY OF THE UROGENITAL DIAPHRAGM

Because micturition and continence depend upon the closely coordinated activity of the bladder, urethra, and periurethral striated muscle, it is essential to know the dynamics of the levator ani and especially the muscle of the urogenital diaphragm during the storage and evacuation phases of the bladder. A large share of the urinary difficulties encountered by the patient with spinal cord disturbances stems from the lack of coordination between the detrusor and the periurethral striated muscle.

Measurement of the striated muscle contraction or relaxation can be readily accomplished by inserting an electrode into the urogenital diaphragm and observing the action potentials via an electromyographic machine; the examination is performed in conjunction with the cystometric study. The technique for proper placement of the electrode is relatively simple but does require some experience. With the female in the lithotomy position and a guiding index finger in the vagina, the fine needle electrode is pushed gently through the epithelium of the urethral perimeatal tissue at approximately 11 to 2 o'clock and about 3 to 5 mm lateral to the meatus. The needle point is moved deeper in millimeter steps, for the muscle is often quite superficial. In the male a guiding finger is placed in the rectum and the needle is inserted in the midperineum. The electrode point is then moved gently toward the region of the membranous urethra. Proper placement is indicated by the appearance of discrete action potentials on the machine's sound system and the oscilloscope screen.

The normal individual, tense because of the test situation, will demonstrate a barrage of motor impulses as the electrode needle is first inserted into the muscle. As the patient relaxes, the tempo of the electrical activity will gradually subside to a slow discharge of one to two motor units or complete absence. Upon request to "tighten his or her bottom" the subject can contract the striated muscle surrounding the urethra as indicated by a burst of sustained action potentials.

During cystometry the continuous filling of the bladder with fluid or air will stimulate a progressive increase in the number of motor units firing until capacity is reached (Fig. 6–16). If the patient attempts to void, the electrical activity will disappear regardless of the onset of an actual detrusor contraction, i.e., just thinking of voiding without having the bladder contract will silence the muscle of the urogenital diaphragm (Fig. 6–16). Motor impulses will return as soon as the patient ceases thinking of urinating or actually finishes urinating.

NEUROGENIC BLADDER

Interference with the normal conduction of nerve impulses over one or more of the nerve tracts concerned with urination produces dysfunction of the bladder. Bladders so affected are called neurogenic bladders and can be one of several different types or combinations thereof.

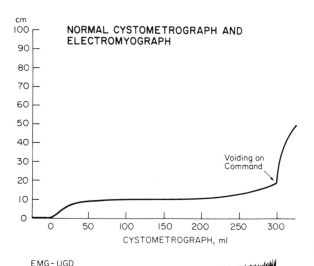

Figure 6–16 The motor impulses to the urogenital diaphragm increase as the bladder reaches capacity and stop abruptly when urination is considered or performed.

GROUP 1: THE UNINHIBITED NEUROGENIC BLADDER

Etiology.   The primary cause of the uninhibited neurogenic bladder is a defect in the corticoregulatory tract. The lesion may be at the upper end of the tract in the region of the upper motor neurons and may be produced by paresis, cerebrovascular accident, or a brain tumor. In the spinal cord, the tract may be involved by tumor, trauma, multiple sclerosis, and congenital anomalies such as spina bifida and myelomeningocele (Fig. 6–17).

In some patients with uninhibited neurogenic bladders, no other neurologic deficit can be demonstrated. It is suggested that, in these people, there has been a failure in the normal development of the integrating centers concerned with micturition, a type of motor apraxia.

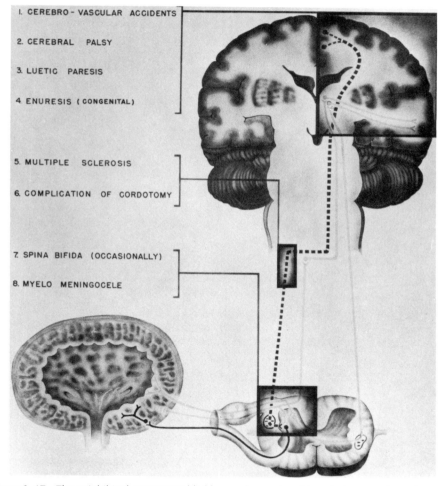

1. CEREBRO - VASCULAR ACCIDENTS

2. CEREBRAL PALSY

3. LUETIC PARESIS

4 ENURESIS (CONGENITAL)

5. MULTIPLE SCLEROSIS

6. COMPLICATION OF CORDOTOMY

7. SPINA BIFIDA (OCCASIONALLY)

8. MYELO MENINGOCELE

Figure 6–17   The uninhibited neurogenic bladder can be produced by a lesion anywhere along the corticoregulatory tract.

Signs and Symptoms.   The most frequent complaint voiced by the patient with an uninhibited neurogenic bladder is that of increased frequency of urination, urgency, and incontinence *not* associated with dysuria. The patient states that as soon as a desire to urinate arises, he or she must rush to the urinal, for a short delay may result in soiling of clothing. The patient is unable to prevent the onset of urination for very long once the desire to micturate becomes apparent.

In patients with multiple sclerosis, one of the earliest signs of the disease is hesitancy in the initiation of urination. The patient will reveal that, instead of one or two seconds for urine to start flowing, one or two minutes may elapse before the bladder begins to contract. The hesitancy in urination may precede the onset of uninhibited contractions by several months or more.

When the uninhibited neurogenic bladder occurs in a child, the picture is that of a youngster who has not been completely toilet-trained.

Dysuria and a decrease in size and force of stream do not present in patients with the uninhibited bladder unless the patient has, in addition, obstructive uropathy, urinary tract infection, or bladder neoplasm.

Because some of the symptoms of prostatism can be frequently observed in elderly patients with uninhibited bladder developed as a result of cerebrovascular accidents and subsequent involvement of its upper motor neurons, the unwary physician may be misled into performing an unnecessary prostatectomy.

Diagnosis.   *A positive diagnosis can be made only by performing a cystometric examination.* Perception of temperature, filling, and distention is intact. On filling the bladder with fluid, uncontrolled contractions of the bladder will occur (Fig. 6–18). There may be many small contractions of the detrusor before a strong, sustained voiding contraction occurs, or there may be no small contractions and just one vigorous

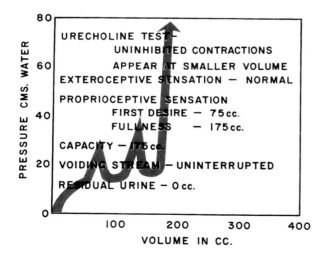

Figure 6–18   Cystometrograph of the uninhibited neurogenic bladder.

voiding contraction at several hundred milliliters of volume. *A normal bladder never demonstrates any voiding contractions even at bladder capacity.*

On occasion, difficulty may be encountered in attempting to differentiate between a small capacity, inflamed spastic bladder, and an uninhibited neurogenic bladder. One can obviate this problem by giving the patient 100 mg of Banthine (methantheline bromide) intravenously and repeating the cystometrograph. If the patient has an uninhibited neurogenic bladder, the cystometric curve will show disappearance of the uninhibited contractions and a marked increase in bladder capacity (Fig. 6–19). However, if it is a small inflamed bladder, the cystometrograph will be unchanged by the anticholinergic agent. The differential Banthine test is based on the fact that the small inflamed bladder is caused by a noncholinergic localized muscle spasm while the small uninhibited neurogenic bladder is produced by uncontrolled motor impulses conducted along parasympathetic motor fibers and is susceptible to blockade by anticholinergic agents such as Banthine and atropine (Fig. 6–20).

The Urecholine supersensitivity test elicits a variable effect in the patient with an uninhibited neurogenic bladder. In the individual with a lesion of the corticoregulatory tract, the lower motor neuron is supersensitive whereas the ganglionic synapse and neuromuscular junction retain their normal sensitivity. Thus, the patient will demonstrate supersensitivity to Urecholine by exhibiting an uncontrolled voiding contraction of the bladder at a smaller volume than during the control run. The response is said to be variable because not all patients

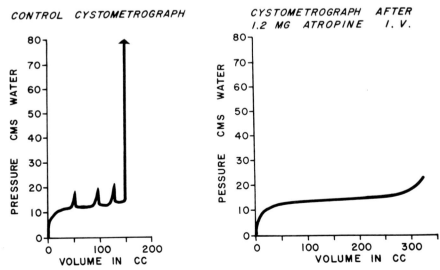

Figure 6–19 The uninhibited neurogenic bladder can be differentiated from the spastic, inflamed bladder by giving the patient 1.2 mg atropine or 100 mg of Banthine intravenously. The anticholinergic agent will suppress the uninhibited contractions of the neurogenic bladder and increase its capacity but will have no effect on the small, spastic, inflamed bladder.

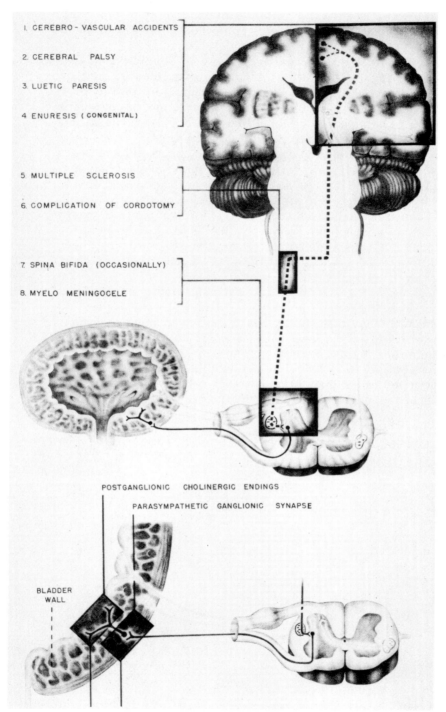

1. CEREBRO-VASCULAR ACCIDENTS

2. CEREBRAL PALSY

3. LUETIC PARESIS

4. ENURESIS (CONGENITAL)

5. MULTIPLE SCLEROSIS

6. COMPLICATION OF CORDOTOMY

7. SPINA BIFIDA (OCCASIONALLY)

8. MYELO MENINGOCELE

POSTGANGLIONIC CHOLINERGIC ENDINGS

PARASYMPATHETIC GANGLIONIC SYNAPSE

BLADDER WALL

Figure 6–20 Banthine blocks motor impulses at the ganglionic synapse and neuromuscular ending.

with this type of bladder will exhibit an uninhibited bladder contraction at a bladder volume of 100 ml with 2.5 mg of Urecholine subcutaneously.

Electromyography in the patient with an uninhibited neurogenic bladder has disclosed that three patterns of periurethral striated muscle activity may be encountered. In the first type normal function occurs; the patient can contract or relax the urogenital diaphragm at will and the striated muscle acts in a coordinated reflex fashion with the detrusor, i.e., in a tonic contracted state when the bladder is storing urine and in a completely relaxed state when the bladder is evacuating urine. In essence the individual has partial control over micturition in that detrusor contraction cannot be inhibited, but the urethra can be "clamped off" by voluntary contraction of the striated muscle encircling the urethra. *In our experience, this combination of functions is the most common mechanism for recurrent urinary infection in young girls.*

As discussed previously in the chapter on urinary infection, the most common causes for cystitis are entities which lead to marked increases in intravesical pressure or vesical overdistention with resultant decreased blood flow through the bladder wall. The impairment of circulation lessens host resistance to bacterial invasion because of a decrease in available hematogenous antibacterial elements and the deterioration of local tissue immunity provided by structural integrity.

When the bladder of a child of the type just described (uninhibited bladder with a normally controlled urogenital diaphragm) fills with urine, uncontrolled contractions of the detrusor occur in association with a desire to void. If the child voids immediately, intravesical pressures remain low and no urinary infection occurs. But should the child attempt to prevent urination and hold her urine, a marked rise in intravesical pressure will occur. The increase in intravesical pressure develops because the bladder muscle is contracting forcefully and involuntarily in an attempt to evacuate the bladder while simultaneously the child is trying to prevent incontinence by voluntarily contracting the periurethral striated muscle. Under these circumstances trabeculation of the bladder wall, diverticula, urinary tract infection, ureteric reflux, or hydroureter may develop.

The second type of urogenital diaphragm function found in association with the uninhibited bladder is the uncontrolled, reflex coordinated one. The primary symptoms of these patients are day and night urgency, pollakiuria, and urge incontinence. These children do not develop urinary infection because their bladder function is exactly that of the infant. When the bladder is filled to the volume wherein an uncontrolled detrusor voiding contraction occurs, the periurethral striated muscle simultaneously relaxes because of coordinated reflex inhibition, and the child voids with a strong, full stream at low intravesical pressures. *This category is the most common cause for urinary incontinence in the child.*

The third type of periurethral striated muscle action seen, rarely with the pure uninhibited bladder but quite commonly with the reflex and mixed neurogenic bladders, is the uncoordinated, involuntary spastic contraction. In these individuals the urogenital diaphragm is in a state of spastic contracture regardless of detrusor muscle shortening, and so when the patients void, their bladders work against a urethral lumen closed by encircling spastic striated muscle. They are the people who demonstrate poor urinary streams, large postvoiding residual volumes, urinary infection, and reflux.

Endoscopy reveals no obvious abnormality of the bladder and urethra in the patients with uninhibited bladders associated with an uncontrolled, reflexly coordinated urogenital diaphragm. However, the individuals with uninhibited bladders and either normally functioning or spastic urogenital diaphragms may have bladders with all the hallmarks of obstructive uropathy.

Treatment. Infrequently, in adults, an uninhibited neurogenic bladder may revert to normal following removal of a tumor of the central nervous system, recovery from a cerebrovascular accident, or subsidence of edema occurring after chordotomy. In most adult patients, however, the uninhibited bladder can be expected to be permanent. On the other hand, the majority of children will develop cortical control of the bladder on reaching puberty. It is interesting to note that full control of micturition is not attained by most children until after puberty. This observation is based on the finding that Urecholine stimulation will cause uncontrolled contractions of the detrusor muscle in many children whose cystometric curves are perfectly normal prior to cholinergic stimulation. Normal adults do not show uncontrolled bladder contractions with 2.5 mg of Urecholine.

Therapy, in general, is palliative in that the physician attempts to decrease the number of uninhibited detrusor contractions and to enlarge bladder capacity by judiciously blocking uncontrolled motor impulses with Banthine or atropine preparations. Treatment is begun with a moderate dose of the drug and the amount is gradually increased until the desired effect is obtained. With propantheline bromide (Pro-Banthine) the initial oral dose is 15 mg q.i.d. and with tincture of belladonna 20 drops q.i.d. Other anticholinergic agents which can be used are atropine tannate, atropine sulfate, and homatropine. It should be noted that some patients do not absorb methantheline bromide very well from the gut and thus may show no response even to high doses of the drug. The eventual dose will be the one which abolishes increased frequency of urination, urgency, and incontinence without causing partial or complete urinary retention. Not infrequently, in the elderly man with an uninhibited neurogenic bladder, urinary retention occurs even with low doses of Pro-Banthine. On examination, this type of patient is found to have prostatism and requires prostatectomy before he can be placed on an adequate dose of anticholinergic drug. Occasionally, the severity of the uninhibited neurogenic bladder may be markedly decreased by prostatectomy alone. The patient should discontinue the anticholinergic drug at intervals to determine whether or not he can get along without the drug and also to minimize any tendency to become resistant to the effects of the medication.

Another approach to the problem of nocturnal enuresis, in both children and adults, involves regimens designed to keep the patient from falling into too deep a sleep and thus being more receptive to the sensations warning him of impending micturition. *d*-Amphetamine sulfate in a dose of 10 mg at bedtime or ephedrine sulfate in a 25 to 50 mg amount has been used to convert enuretics into light sleepers. Many types of electrical apparatus have been devised to awaken the patient as soon as wetting of the bed occurs. If one uses this particular method over a period of time, it is anticipated that the patient will eventually be able to awaken before urinary incontinence takes place. It is postulated that with a regulated fluid intake prior to bedtime, a patient's bladder will be full at a certain time each night and will empty itself if the patient is in the depths of slumber. If the apparatus stimulates the patient to awaken at the same hour each night because of enuresis, after a brief period the subject will find that he or she is sleeping lightly prior to the sounding of the alarm and thus will be able to perceive the desire to micturate before incontinence actually ensues.

If a patient with an uninhibited neurogenic bladder harbors a urinary tract infection, treatment of the cystitis may alleviate the urgency and incontinence.

The girls and women with recurrent urinary infection associated with an uninhibited neurogenic bladder are best treated with a regimen of prompt and frequent voiding, initial antibacterials, and anticholinergic medication in the severe cases.

GROUP 2: THE REFLEX NEUROGENIC BLADDER

Etiology.   This type occurs in transverse myelitis in which both the sensory and motor tracts to and from the higher centers are interrupted above the level of sacral spinal segments 2, 3, and 4. Trauma, multiple sclerosis, neoplasms, atrophy, and meningitis may involve the spinal cord sufficiently to give rise to a functional transection. Extensive brain lesions may occasionally cause a reflex neurogenic bladder. Figure 6–21 depicts the type of lesion resulting in a reflex neurogenic bladder.

Signs and Symptoms.   Micturition is reflex and involuntary. The patient cannot initiate or stop micturition in a normal way. Some patients may learn to start micturition through stimulation of the reflex arc (through the gamma efferent system) by pinching the skin in various parts of the body and prodding the bladder by tapping the abdomen.

All specific sensation associated with the bladder is lost. The patient cannot feel heat, cold, or distention. Many patients, however, learn to detect a full bladder through the reflexes activated by distention of the bladder such as sweating, spasticity of the lower extremities, and headache because of elevated blood pressure, or by a vague visceral sensation such as fullness of the abdomen.

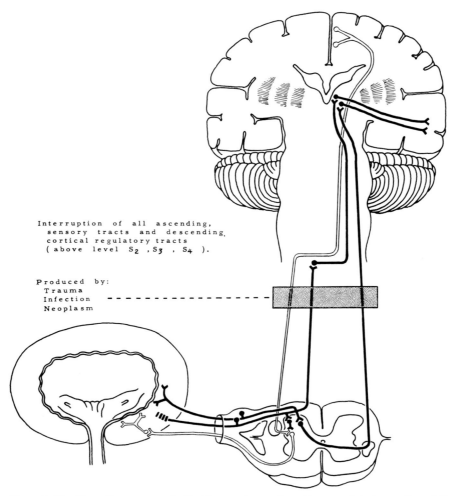

Interruption of all ascending,
sensory tracts and descending,
cortical regulatory tracts
(above level S_2 , S_3 , S_4).

Produced by:
  Trauma
  Infection
  Neoplasm

Figure 6–21   The reflex neurogenic bladder can be produced by complete transection of the spinal cord above the sacral level.

Autonomic hyperreflexia is a phenomenon frequently observed in quadriplegics with lesions above the outflow of the splanchnic nerves or about T-6. Pathologic autonomic reflexes are manifested by bradycardia, paroxysmal hypertension, sweating of the forehead, severe headache, and "goose-flesh." Distention of the bladder and of the rectum are the most common causes of hyperreflexia. In the normal individual, afferent impulses from the bladder wall travel to the spinal cord and then to the higher centers via the lateral spinothalamic and fasciculus gracilis tracts. While traversing the spinal cord, these afferent impulses set off sympathetic reflexes, resulting in arteriolar spasm of the skin and splanchnic bed vessels.

As a result of the vasoconstriction, the blood pressure begins to rise. Pressure receptors in the carotid and aortic sinuses perceive the blood pressure rise and attempt to keep the individual normotensive by sending afferent impulses to the vasomotor center in the brain. The vasomotor center decreases the blood pressure by slowing the heart via efferent vagal impulses and by dilating the skin and splanchnic vasculature through the sympathetic pathways of the cord.

In the patient with a high spinal cord lesion, only one of the two regulatory mechanisms of controlling hypertension is operating and that is the slowing of the heart via the tenth nerve. Vasodilatation cannot occur because efferent impulses emanating from the vasomotor center cannot be conducted beyond the area of the lesion in the cord. Thus, the patient will exhibit bradycardia and hypertension.

Aside from the disagreeable symptoms produced by the hyperreflexia, the phenomenon may threaten the patient's life with the complications of severe hypertension such as cerebrovascular accidents and renal failure. Some patients adapt to their situation so that in six to eight months they are not affected by bladder or bowel distention.

However, during the initial phase it may be necessary to control the autonomic hyperreflexia, and this can be accomplished temporarily with drugs or permanently by rhizotomy or neurotomy. Any agent which will prevent the vasoconstriction will be efficacious, and thus one may use Banthine, Arfonad, hexamethonium, spinal block, or spinal anesthesia.

Diagnosis. Physical examination will reveal a transverse myelitis with a level higher than S-2, S-3, and S-4. The bulbocavernosus reflex is hyperactive and saddle anesthesia is present. Cystometric examination reveals completely absent exteroceptive and proprioceptive sensation and the presence of uninhibited contractions of the bladder (Fig. 6–22). Similar to the uninhibited neurogenic bladder, the reflex neurogenic bladder may show many small detrusor contractions and then a strong voiding contraction, or there may occur only one large

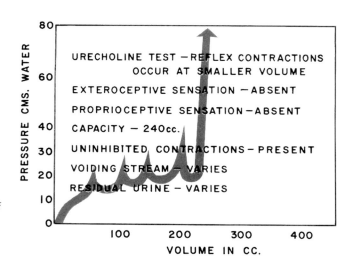

Figure 6–22 Cystometrograph of the reflex neurogenic bladder.

voiding contraction at functional capacity. The Urecholine supersensitivity test will demonstrate a variable response at 100 ml bladder volume. However, in all cases, 2.5 mg of Urecholine subcutaneously will elicit voiding contractions at smaller volumes than the control when the bladder is filled beyond 100 ml.

Electromyography of the periurethral striated muscle in patients with reflex neurogenic bladders discloses, in general, two types: namely, the coordinated and the uncoordinated.

In the case of the coordinated urogenital diaphragm, the bladder empties itself with a good stream and rather completely because, as in the normal bladder, the periurethral striated muscle shows an abrupt and total electrical silence when a reflex detrusor contraction occurs, indicating complete relaxation.

The urogenital diaphragm which is not in synchrony with the detrusor voiding contraction will show electrical activity and muscle contraction as the bladder attempts to empty itself. The persistent uncoordinated contraction of the periurethral striated muscle may be clonic or tonic in type and will result in high intravesical pressures, high residual urines, a poor stream, and recurrent urinary infections.

Treatment.   The theoretically ideal method of dealing with reflex neurogenic bladders would be to restore normal nerve function. This has been accomplished in those patients whose spinal cord activity has been impaired only temporarily. However, most cases of spinal cord injury result in permanent impaired function.

Since the ideal method of therapy is not obtainable at present, other less satisfactory forms of treatment are being utilized. Before discussing specific therapeutic methods, it would be well to designate the problems to be overcome by therapy. The problems can be divided into two main categories, namely, the mental and physical. The mental concerns itself with urinary continence. It is obvious that the paraplegic will have mental difficulties if he becomes a social outcast because of a foul-smelling body due to urinary incontinence. On the physical side can be listed renal insufficiency, which is the major cause of death in these patients. Renal insufficiency, in turn, is directly related to pyelonephritis, hydronephrosis, and nephrolithiasis, which are produced to a great extent by abnormal micturition involving increased intravesical voiding pressures or vesical overdistention.

Most patients with transverse myelitis experience a varying period of complete nonfunctioning of the spinal cord caudad to the level of injury before a particular permanent type of neurogenic bladder emerges. This inactive period is called spinal shock and is associated with detrusor areflexia and urinary retention. Appropriate treatment during this phase involves drainage of urine from the patient's bladder so that bladder overdistention and increased intravesical pressure do not occur. Ideally, intermittent catheterization is probably the best method, but if it is not feasible, an inlying urethral catheter can be utilized over a short period of time.

If the male patient develops a pyogenic urethritis with fever while on an inlying catheter, it is best to institute vesical diversion either by cutaneous vesicostomy or suprapubic cystostomy until reflex activity of the detrusor has fully developed. At that time, intermittent self-catheterization can be instituted or reinstituted and the vesicostomy or cystostomy closed.

When reflex activity of the bladder begins to return, a number of methods for handling continence and preventing cystitis or pyelonephritis are available to the physician, depending upon the patient and bladder function.

Clean, intermittent self-catheterization at intervals regular and frequent enough to prevent wetting and vesical overdistention is an excellent way of urine disposal in patients of all ages and both sexes. Anticholinergic agents are employed to control reflex detrusor activity in the interval between catheterizations. It is obvious that the method is not suitable for patients with small capacity or spastic bladders and for quadriplegics with limited or no hand function.

In the male with vigorous, coordinated detrusor urogenital diaphragm reflex activity, no special treatment is necessary, other than the use of a condom type urinary collecting device. The patient can be taught to willfully set off reflex contractions of the detrusor in order to empty the bladder by forceful blows to the suprapubic area overlying the bladder. Thus the individual can select the time and place to void, empty the bladder, and optimally maintain a sterile urine.

When there is increased urethral resistance by virtue of spasticity and dyssynergia of the periurethral striated muscle, and urinary retention with high intravesical pressures obtain, then transurethral sphincterotomy is necessary. This procedure produces a defect in the wall of the posterior urethra so that urine drips from the bladder through the urethra constantly and the bladder is thus kept relatively empty with decreased spastic reflex activity. A penile incontinence device is a necessity after sphincterotomy; and, of course, this form of therapy is not suitable in the female because of the unavailability of an effective incontinence apparatus.

For the quadriplegic female patient who cannot catheterize herself or the male patient who refuses sphincterotomy, cutaneous vesicostomy or supravesical diversion, e.g., cutaneous ureteroileostomy or ureterosigmoidostomy, is preferred.

GROUP 3: THE AUTONOMOUS NEUROGENIC BLADDER

Etiology.   This type is produced when both limbs of the reflex arc which controls the bladder are destroyed. Figure 6–23 indicates the site of the lesion which may be located in the sacral spinal cord, the conus or cauda equina, or the motor and sensory roots in the sacral plexus. Etiologic factors include *traumatic lesions*, such as a gunshot wound, auto accident, occupational injury, and extensive operative procedures in the pelvis (combined abdominal-perineal resection); *in-*

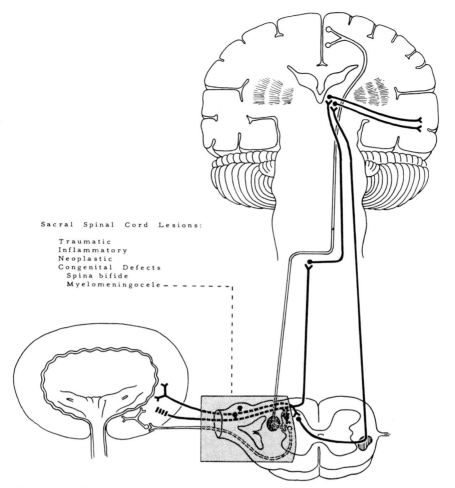

Sacral Spinal Cord Lesions:

Traumatic
Inflammatory
Neoplastic
Congenital Defects
 Spina bifide
 Myelomeningocele

Figure 6–23 The autonomous neurogenic bladder is produced by a lesion involving both limbs of the reflex arc.

flammatory lesions, such as intra- and extradural abscess, chronic arachnoiditis, and radiculitis; *neoplasia;* and *congenital anomalies,* such as spina bifida and myelomeningocele.

It should be noted that spinal shock, which follows immediately most injuries of the spinal cord, produces an autonomous neurogenic bladder. The autonomous neurogenic bladder persists throughout the period of spinal shock. When the spinal cord regains function, the bladder will change its function in accord with the absence or presence of a permanent lesion. Spinal anesthesia involving the innervation of the bladder will also produce a transient autonomous neurogenic bladder.

Signs and Symptoms. The patient cannot perceive bladder fullness and cannot initiate micturition in a normal fashion. In the individual who has a chronic lesion and has not had medical advice or care (e.g., the child with a congenital lesion of the sacral cord), one may observe that the subject has learned to void by applying external force to the bladder. The pressure is applied either by contraction of the body muscle lining the abdominal cavity, which increases intra-abdominal and thus intravesical pressure, or by applying manual pressure directly to the bladder in the suprapubic region (Credé's maneuver). Thus, one can almost make the diagnosis by observing the act of urination. On request to void, the patient will take in a deep breath and strain. During the straining, urine will be expelled from the urethra but will stop as soon as the patient becomes short of breath and needs to inspire again. This process is repeated until urine no longer can be expressed from the bladder.

These patients will tend to be incontinent on coughing, straining, and distention of the bladder beyond a certain volume (varying with the individual patient). The incontinence is due primarily to paralysis of the periurethral striated muscle, which cannot compress and elongate the urinary sphincter when intravesical pressure is markedly elevated. Intravesical pressure in these patients will vary not only with exertion but with the state of the bladder wall. A small inflamed spastic bladder will develop a high pressure at a low volume, whereas an atonic bladder may not develop the same pressure until it is filled with a liter or two of fluid. In some patients there may also be a constant dribbling of urine due either to chronic stretching of the smooth muscle and elastic tissue of the urinary sphincter with resultant atonicity and dilatation, or to overflow incontinence. Residual urine in the autonomous neurogenic bladder will vary from 0 ml to large volumes, depending on the patient's ability to squeeze the bladder, tonicity of the bladder wall, and resistance of the urinary sphincter.

Diagnosis.   The history of straining to void and the finding of saddle anesthesia and absent bulbocavernosus reflex on physical examination will be highly suggestive of a lesion in the sacral spinal cord area.

Cystometric examination (Fig. 6–24) will reveal a bladder with complete absence of sensation, varying residual urine, and varying capacity. No voluntary or involuntary voiding contractions of the detrusor are observed during cystometrography. The Urecholine supersensitivity test will be markedly positive. The combination of absent uninhibited contractions and positive Urecholine supersensitivity test unequivocally denotes a lesion involving only the lower segmental vesical reflex arc.

Prior to the use of the supersensitivity test one could arrive at the diagnosis of an autonomous neurogenic bladder only by exclusion. The presence of a neurologic deficit in the sacral cord area as determined by physical examination and electromyography and the absence of obstructive uropathy on endoscopy would suggest the autonomous bladder. Now the supersensitivity test actually makes the diagnosis regardless of endoscopic and physical findings.

Electromyography of the periurethral striated muscle may demonstrate two patterns in accord with the extent of denervation. One type

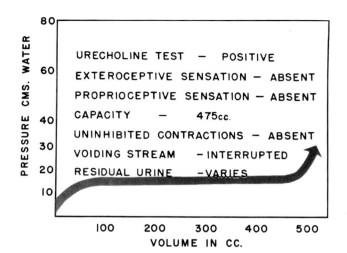

Figure 6–24 Cystometrograph of the autonomous neurogenic bladder.

reveals complete absence of normal motor units with associated fibrillation potentials. These patients can empty their bladders at low intravesical pressures with Credé or Valsalva maneuvers and are usually incontinent.

The second group of patients will exhibit minimal to moderate motor activity of the urogenital diaphragm, which cannot be relaxed voluntarily or involuntarily. Thus bladder emptying is impeded with resultant high intravesical pressures during voiding attempts and large residual urines.

Treatment.   In the patient with a completely denervated bladder and urogenital diaphragm, voiding is accomplished by teaching the individual to apply external pressure over the bladder with the hands (Credé's maneuver) or by using Valsalva's maneuver. Urinary incontinence is controlled by moderately increasing urethral resistance with an alpha adrenergic drug such as ephedrine sulfate in a dose of 10 to 50 mg orally q.i.d.

Clean, intermittent self-catheterization is the treatment of choice for people with the spastic urogenital diaphragm or incomplete bladder emptying.

When urinary incontinence cannot be controlled by drugs and self-catheterization, particularly in the female, the physician can implant an artificial urinary sphincter. The Scott-Bradley-Timm apparatus is a hydraulically activated sphincter mechanism which can be made to open or close at will by squeezing one of two bulbs buried beneath the skin. The device is new and partially tried but to date has been quite successful in a number of patients.

In order to use the sphincter in the group of patients with spastic urogenital diaphragms, it is necessary to decrease urethral resistance prior to the implantation. Transurethral sphincterotomy or widening of the urethra will accomplish this task.

Urinary diversion is used as a last resort when conservative measures have failed. If the diversion is at the bladder level, the urethra must be transected and closed to establish continence.

GROUP 4: THE SENSORY PARALYTIC BLADDER

Etiology. Any disease process which interrupts the sensory limb of the lower reflex arc or the long afferent tracts to the brain (Fig. 6–25) may give rise to the sensory paralytic bladder. It has been observed most commonly in tabes dorsalis and pernicious anemia, and occasionally in multiple sclerosis, diabetes mellitus, syringomyelia, and progressive muscular atrophy.

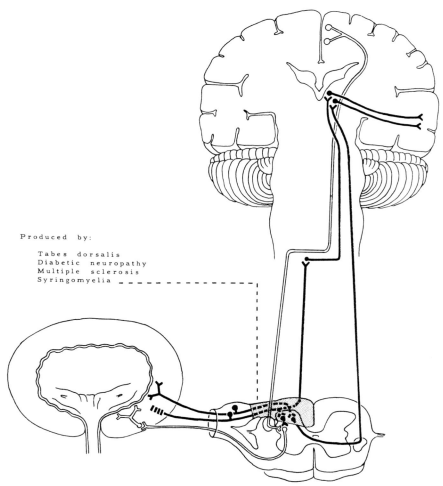

Produced by:

Tabes dorsalis
Diabetic neuropathy
Multiple sclerosis
Syringomyelia

Figure 6–25 Any process which interrupts the sensory limb of the lower reflex arc or the long afferent tracts to the brain may give rise to the sensory paralytic bladder.

Urinary difficulties arise in these patients because of the insidious development of atonicity and decompensation of bladder muscle. The flaccidity of the detrusor, in turn, is due to mechanical overdistention of the bladder by retained urine because of a lack of sensation and desire to void. Periodic studies of the bladder in tabes dorsalis have shown that the earliest change is one of diminished sensation with normal capacity and complete emptying. As the disease advances with the slow insidious loss of sensation of fullness, it is observed that the patient's bladder must be filled with gradually increasing amounts of urine before the desire to void is apparent. After a certain point, the bladder begins to decompensate and residual urine appears.

Signs and Symptoms.   There are no complaints which are typical of the patient with a sensory paralytic bladder. When the bladder begins to decompensate, there will be difficulty in starting urination, a decrease in size and force of the stream, terminal dribbling, and pollakiuria and dysuria if infection supervenes. Overflow incontinence may occur with advanced disease when urinary retention of large volumes of urine is present.

On physical examination the individual may demonstrate sensory deficits, the stigmata of tabes dorsalis, and absent bulbocavernosus reflex.

Diagnosis.   Cystometric examination (Fig. 6–26) reveals diminished to absent sensation, no uninhibited contractions, a large-capacity bladder, and varying amounts of abnormally high residual urines. The Urecholine supersensitivity test is markedly positive. Tests for neurosyphilis may be positive if the patient has tabes dorsalis. There are no characteristic findings on endoscopy.

The electromyogram of the urogenital diaphragm will usually show synchrony between detrusor and striated muscle, i.e., the periurethral striated muscle will relax with detrusor contraction. However, if the

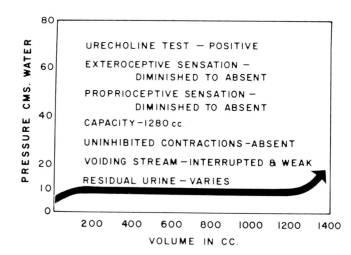

Figure 6–26   Cystometrograph of the sensory paralytic bladder.

bladder is large and decompensated, the recruitment of action potentials during bladder filling will not begin until the volume is quite large and the bladder is distended enough to stimulate the sensation of fullness.

Treatment.   Most sensory paralytic bladders can be completely rehabilitated, provided that the bladder muscle has not been impaired permanently. The primary aims in treating these patients are therapy of the generalized disease such as syphilis or pernicious anemia, restoration of normal bladder tonicity, and prevention of future decompensation once normal detrusor tone has been regained. If the diagnosis is made prior to the appearance of abnormal postvoiding residual urine volumes, the patient is instructed to void every 2 to 3 hours by the clock and several times at night. When decompensation has taken place, Urecholine and Myocholine (bethanechol chloride) have been found to be extremely valuable.

Urecholine Regimen for Rehabilitating Atonic Bladders. On the basis of numerous experimental and clinical observations the following regimen for the use of Urecholine in rehabilitating atonic bladders has been established. After the urinary bladder has been thoroughly evaluated, the patient's urethral catheter is removed, or if a suprapubic tube is present, it is clamped. Urecholine is administered to the adult patient subcutaneously in a dose of 10 mg every four hours around the clock. If the patient is somewhat decrepit, the starting dose can be decreased to 7.5 mg subcutaneously. In children, the dose is determined on a weight basis, using 150 lb or 70 kg as the average adult weight. Thus, the initial dose of a 50-lb child would be one third of the 10-mg 150-lb adult dose, or 3.3 mg subcutaneously.

With this dose it is usual for the patient to perspire profusely. In an occasional patient mild abdominal cramping and diarrhea may also be present. The patient's urinary function is evaluated by noting the volume voided per micturition and time of micturition as related to the time of drug administration. The patient is catheterized approximately 24 hours after start of drug therapy and immediately following the voiding induced by the last injection of Urecholine (about 20 to 30 minutes after administration). The bladder is drained and the residual urine noted. In most patients, micturition will be induced by the drug dosage advocated and the residual urine after 24 hours will be reduced.

The 10-mg subcutaneous dose of Urecholine every four hours is continued until the residual urine is reduced to less than 30 ml and is maintained at that level for three days. Anywhere from three days to several weeks of therapy may be needed to attain this objective. After reaching this goal, the subcutaneous dose of Urecholine is reduced to 7.5 mg every four hours. On reducing the dose, some patients may start to develop a residual urine, whereas others will continue to have none. Irrespective of the residual urine, the lower dosage level is continued until the patient again demonstrates no residual for three days. At this point, the subcutaneous dose is reduced to 5 mg every four hours and the observations continued. After attaining complete bladder emptying for three days with the 5-mg dose, the Urecholine is changed from the subcutaneous to the oral form of administration in a dose of 50 mg q.i.d. This dose is continued until the patient demonstrates efficient urination and then it is stopped. The patient is watched carefully for a few days following cessation of therapy to make certain that urination continues in a satisfactory manner.

In most patients the undesirable effects of Urecholine are markedly minimized when the dosage is finally reduced to 5 mg subcutaneously. No side effects are usually observed with the 50-mg oral dose. It will be noted that after the patient has been on therapy for a few days, urination will begin to occur in the interval between doses, rather than 10 to 20 minutes after each subcutaneous administration. Infrequently,

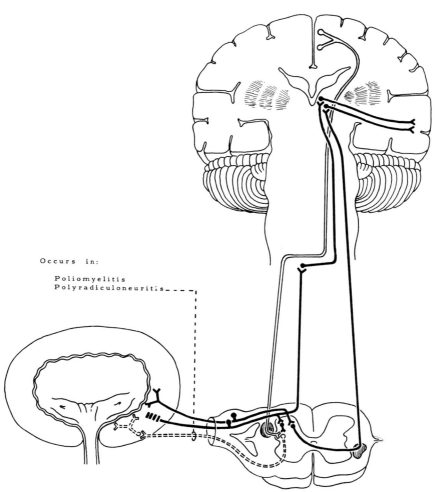

Occurs in:

Poliomyelitis
Polyradiculoneuritis

Figure 6–27 The motor paralytic bladder is frequently associated with poliomyelitis and poly-radiculoneuronitis; it is the result of involvement of the lower motor neurons or motor fibers.

one will encounter a patient with a bladder which responds partially to Urecholine but which cannot be weaned completely from cholinergic therapy. Should the cholinergic medication and program of frequent, periodic voiding fail to rehabilitate the decompensated bladder, then clean, intermittent self-catheterization is utilized.

GROUP 5: THE MOTOR PARALYTIC BLADDER

Etiology. This abnormality obtains when the motor neurons or nerves that control the bladder are impaired (Fig. 6–27). If left alone, the bladder in this condition distends and decompensates, but sensation is normal. The atony observed clinically so often in these cases is due to urinary retention and overdistention of the detrusor; it can always be prevented by early and adequate drainage.

Poliomyelitis, polyradiculoneuronitis, tumor, trauma, and congenital anomalies are some of the disease processes which may produce the motor paralytic bladder. The abnormal bladder may be a temporary affair as in some cases of infection, tumor, and trauma or it may become permanent. Also, the motor paralysis may be partial or complete.

Signs and Symptoms. In the acute cases the patient will complain of painful distention of the bladder and an inability to initiate urination. The chronic case with partial involvement may give exactly the same history as the individual with obstructive uropathy, namely, difficulty in starting micturition, a decrease in size and force of the stream, interrupted stream, straining to void, and recurrent episodes of urinary tract infection. This type of case in children is occasionally misdiagnosed and the patient subjected to unwarranted operative procedures.

Diagnosis. Cystometric examination (Fig. 6–28) reveals perfectly normal exteroceptive and proprioceptive sensation and a normal cys-

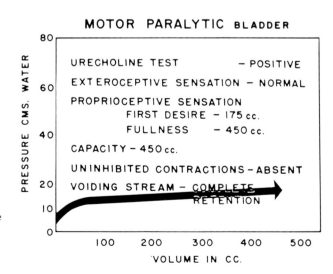

Figure 6–28 Cystometrograph of the motor paralytic bladder.

tometric curve. The patient cannot initiate micturition and no involuntary contractions of the detrusor are observed. The residual urine and bladder capacity will vary with each individual. The Urecholine supersensitivity test will be markedly positive in the chronic case and absent in the acute case. Saddle sensation is normal. The bulbocavernosus reflex may or may not be present. Endoscopic examination is negative for obstructive uropathy in the uncomplicated case. Electromyography of the periurethral striated muscle will vary with the extent of denervation and show activity varying from complete paralysis to spasticity and coordinated to asynchronous.

Treatment. Most of the patients with poliomyelitis and a motor paralytic bladder are best treated by prompt urethral catheter drainage since they regain normal bladder function within a short period of time after onset of paralysis provided that the bladder musculature has been protected by drainage. The return of function can be determined by cystometric examination and is indicated by the occurrence of voiding contractions of the bladder.

The chronic case with partial motor paralysis responds quite satisfactorily to Urecholine therapy. If the bladder is atonic, the complete Urecholine regimen for rehabilitating decompensated bladders (as outlined under the heading Sensory Paralytic Bladder) is employed. All the patients who respond to Urecholine will have to be maintained on the parasympathomimetic agent for the rest of their natural lives. These individuals have a permanent deficit of motor function which can be made more efficient with the use of a supplementary extrinsic cholinergic drug.

Urecholine is useless for stimulating urination in patients who have a complete motor paralysis of the bladder; it is helpful only in those patients who have some degree of motor activity. Clean, intermittent self-catheterization is the treatment of choice for these patients. Ephedrine sulfate is added to the program if urinary incontinence is present.

EVALUATION OF CYSTOMETROGRAPHY

It should be borne in mind that the cystometric examination is a procedure which is used in conjunction with other methods, e.g., pyelography, cineradiography, voiding cystourethrogram, endoscopy, and urethral resistance measurements, in arriving at a diagnosis. It cannot and should not be used in a manner similar to that employed by the cardiologist in reading an EKG. The electrocardiogram is entirely objective in nature, whereas the cystometric examination is both subjective and objective. Furthermore, the actual cystometrograph in a particular type of neurogenic bladder may vary, depending upon existing conditions. For example, the motor paralytic bladder may show a capacity of 450 ml if the patient is catheterized shortly after the onset of urinary retention; if the patient is not catheterized for a period of days, the capacity may be 1000 ml.

Frequently, one must perform endoscopy in addition to the cystometric examination in order to arrive at a diagnosis. For example, a middle-aged male with undiagnosed poliomyelitis may present himself with a complaint of acute urinary retention. Cystometrography may disclose normal sensation and normal bladder capacity but no evidences of bladder contraction, either voluntary or involuntary. These are exactly the findings one frequently observes in patients with acute urinary retention due to an enlarged prostate. Thus, urethroscopy must be performed in addition to the cystometric examination in order to arrive at a correct diagnosis.

However, the cystometric examination, which now includes the Urecholine supersensitivity test, is the only objective method for specifically pinpointing a lesion of the corticoregulatory tract or the lower segmental reflex arc involving bladder function. All other tests are suggestive in that lesions of the sacral cord or corticoregulatory tract may be diagnosed, but it is the cystometric examination which shows that the bladder per se is involved. For example, an individual may have hyperactive reflexes, ankle clonus, and positive Babinski signs, but this does not definitely mean that the bladder is an uninhibited neurogenic type until the cystometric curve denotes uncontrolled contractions of the bladder. On the other hand, a positive diagnosis of uninhibited neurogenic bladder can be made on cystometrography alone — irrespective of the absence or presence of any other neurologic deficits. We have found the same to be true of the Urecholine supersensitivity test. When it gives a positive response, the patient has a lesion of the lower segmental reflex arc regardless of any other findings. It is extremely important to comprehend these concepts, for we have found a number of cases of neurogenic bladder with absolutely no other sign of neurologic deficit — indicating that the diagnoses in these cases would have been missed completely if one were depending solely on a complete neurological and electromyographic examination to make the correct diagnosis.

TYPES OF URINARY INCONTINENCE

The most common error made in the diagnosis and treatment of urinary incontinence in children is the assumption that most of the cases observed are on a psychogenic basis. Experience indicates that a large number of children with urinary incontinence suffer from obstructive uropathy, sacral spinal cord lesions, upper motor neuron defects, and developmental anomalies of the urinary tract. It is obvious that urinary incontinence of the "physiologic type" does not alarm the physician or parents until the child is about three years old. At this age one expects most children to be toilet-trained; complete urologic investigation is necessary if incontinence persists beyond the age of three.

Urinary incontinence of a type other than the physiologic, i.e., a weak, dribbling stream, should be studied as soon as possible, irrespective of the age of the child. The incontinence may be indicative of a progressive process which is endangering the life of the individual, as, for example, in obstructive uropathy. Since the various types of urinary incontinence occur in both the child and adult, no attempt will be made to discuss them separately.

URINARY RETENTION WITH OVERFLOW INCONTINENCE (PARADOXICAL)

Etiology.   When the bladder is unable to empty itself and becomes overdistended, the intravesical pressure increases and eventually overcomes the resistance of the urinary sphincter, thus resulting in a dripping type of incontinence. It has been labeled paradoxical incontinence because with a constant leaking of urine from the bladder, the uninformed observer would expect the bladder to be kept empty rather than full.

The inability of the bladder to empty may be due to obstruction to the outflow of urine, atonicity of the bladder muscle and elastic tissue, impaired detrusor contraction, or uncoordinated activity of the periurethral striated muscle. In the child, some causes of obstructive uropathy are strictures of the urethra, its meatus, and urethral valves; large ureteroceles; ectopic ureteric orifices in the urethra; and, rarely, vesical neck contracture. In the adult male, vesical neck contracture, prostatic carcinoma, benign prostatic hyperplasia, and urethral stricture are some of the more frequent conditions leading to urinary retention.

Adult onset of urinary retention in the female is associated most frequently with a long history of infrequent voiding and detrusor decompensation. Urethral and vesical outlet obstruction are rare, being present primarily with neoplasm and stricture.

As we have noted in a previous discussion, both children and adults with neurogenic bladders often experience urinary retention with overflow wetting. The sensory paralytic, motor paralytic, autonomous, and mixed neurogenic bladders may be responsible. Common etiologic disease entities include myelomeningocele, spina bifida, tumors, infectious myelitis, and injury.

Signs and Symptoms.   The patient leaks urine constantly from the urethra and is unable to initiate and maintain a good urinary stream. Examination of the abdomen reveals a distended bladder. In cases with involvement of the sacral spinal cord, the bulbocavernosus reflex will usually be absent, and varying degrees of saddle anesthesia will be apparent.

Diagnosis.   The medical history, physical examination, laboratory studies, excretory urography, endoscopy, cystometry, and electromyography may all be needed to clearly define the kind of incontinence and its cause. All types of overflow incontinence will have in common urinary retention, impaired emptying of the bladder, and an unceasing constant or intermittent dribbling of urine.

Treatment. In general, relief of the urinary retention is required to alleviate the paradoxical incontinence. Thus, operative removal or correction of obstructive factors, recompensation of the detrusor, institution of physiologic voiding habits, intermittent self-catheterization, and urinary diversion operations are some of the therapeutic measures which may be indicated.

ECTOPIC URETER

Etiology. During the course of development of the ureters from wolffian duct buds, two ureters may arise on one side (ureteric duplication). The orifice of the ureter draining the upper portion of the renal collecting system will be located medial and inferior to the orifice of the ureter draining the lower segment of the kidney. Occasionally, the orifice of the ureter draining the upper segment of the kidney will open into the vas, seminal vesicle, ejaculatory duct, or prostate in the male, and the urethra, vestibule, vagina, uterus, or uterine tube in the female. The ureter with an orifice located in an abnormal position is termed an ectopic ureter.

An ectopic ureter is frequently associated with disease such as hydronephrosis, pyelonephritis, and urinary incontinence. The incontinence is seen primarily in the female because the ectopic ureter may be located outside the sphincter of the urinary tract, such as in the vestibule or vagina. If the ectopic ureteric orifice is in the distal portion of the urethra, incontinence will be present because the resistance in the distal urethra to urinary flow will be much less than the resistance of the midportion of the urethra. The male with an ectopic ureter will usually be continent because the ectopic ureteric orifice opens or empties into the prostatic urethra, which presents less resistance to urinary flow than the membranous portion of the urethra; thus the urine will flow into the bladder rather than through the distal urethra.

Signs and Symptoms. The female patient with urinary incontinence due to an ectopic ureter will present with a micturitional history pathognomonic of the condition. She will state that since infancy she has had constant leaking of urine which is present day and night. In addition, the patient will relate that she voids normal amounts of urine at regular intervals.

Examination of the patient may reveal urine dripping from the urethral meatus, from an abnormal opening in the vestibule, or from the vagina. Frequently the ectopic orifice is difficult to find and may require prolonged observation of the vestibule and genitalia before the orifice is located.

Diagnosis. Cystometric examination is perfectly normal. Endoscopy of the urethra and vagina may be necessary to locate the ectopic ureteric opening. Excretion pyelography may demonstrate duplication anomalies of the ureter and renal collecting system. The upper segment of kidney may be hydronephrotic, atrophic, or so involved with disease that it may not visualize at all. Occasionally it is necessary to color the urine with a parenterally administered dye such as methylene blue, in order to aid in the localization of the ectopic ureteric meatus.

Treatment. If the ectopic ureter and its associated renal segment are markedly dilated and the remaining ureters and renal tissue are normal, partial nephrectomy and occasionally complete ureterectomy are indicated. An ectopic ureter of normal caliber may be reimplanted into the bladder or anastomosed to its associated ureter. The necessity for conservation of renal tissue is a prime factor in selecting the type of operation to be employed.

TOTAL INCOMPETENCE OF THE URINARY SPHINCTER

Etiology. When the entire urethra in the female or the prostatic and membranous urethra in the male is compromised, a constant dripping type of incontinence will result. In the child, congenital failure of the urethra to close properly, epispadias, will result in urinary incontinence. In the female adult, trauma during parturition may produce a defect in the urethral musculature along its entire length (but with an intact mucosa) and resultant leaking of urine. A similar type of defect may be created iatrogenically during repair of procidentia, cystocele, urethral diverticulum, vaginal hysterectomy, and transurethral resection of the urethra.

In the male, radical prostatectomy and, at times, simple prostatectomy may be associated with disruption of the integrity of the urinary sphincter remaining in the region of the membranous urethra, with resultant dripping incontinence.

Signs and Symptoms. The chief complaint will be that of leaking of urine per urethra especially in the erect or sitting positions. Palpation and percussion of the bladder will reveal no evidence of distention.

Diagnosis. Cystometric examination will demonstrate a normal bladder with no residual urine and an inability to maintain continence for more than several minutes (with contraction of the periurethral striated musculature). Electromyogram studies of the muscle of the urogenital diaphragm will reveal normal activity coordinated with detrusor function. On urethroscopy, a defect in the wall of the urethra may be seen. Intraurethral resistance measurements may demonstrate abnormally low pressures.

Treatment. The principle upon which therapy is based involves reconstruction of the urinary sphincter, posterior urethra, or true bladder neck. In the case of epispadias, this implies closure of the urethra to form a muscular tube at least 3 to 4 cm in length as in Young's procedure.

Incontinence in the male following prostatectomy is extremely difficult to treat. Until recently most surgical procedures employed to correct this distressing complication have met with failure. Scott, Bradley, and Timm have just devised an artificial, plastic sphincter which can be implanted into the human body and which encircles the urethra. The hydraulic mechanism is dynamic so that the sphincter can be tightened or relaxed by repetitively compressing one of two plastic balls buried just under the scrotal (or labial in the female) skin. A considerable degree of success has been attained, but final evaluation will need further trial.

When there is a longitudinal defect along the floor of the female urethra, continence may be restored by excising the urethral defect and reapproximating normal urethral wall.

STRESS INCONTINENCE (PARTIAL INCOMPETENCE OF THE URINARY SPHINCTER)

Etiology. Urinary incontinence on coughing, straining, flexing, and lifting has been designated as stress incontinence. It is seen infrequently in males following prostatectomy and in paralysis of the periurethral striated muscles. It is, however, a common occurrence in females.

Studies of the mechanics of the normal urinary sphincter in women reveal that the urinary sphincter or urethra is a mobile structure whose length varies with the type of activity. A young, nulliparous woman under spinal anesthesia may demonstrate a urethral length of 3.8 cm. If she is perfectly relaxed in the supine position, the urethral length will still be 3.8 cm without anesthesia. Voluntary contraction of the levator ani muscles will lengthen the urethra to 4.3 cm. Reflex contraction of the levator ani, as in changing from the supine to the erect position, will also increase urethral length to 4.3 cm. The urethral length of 35 normal women without urinary incontinence varied from 3.0 to 4.5 cm, with an average of 3.8 cm both in the supine and standing positions.

It is interesting to note that intraurethral resistance to the retrograde flow of fluid is increased every time the urethra is lengthened; and the urethra is elongated when the periurethral striated muscles are stimulated to contract as in coughing, straining, sneezing, and sudden voluntary interruption of urination.

Intravesical pressure in the normal individual varies also with type of activity. In the supine position, the average intravesical pressure in the female is approximately 17 cm of water. On standing, the pressure is increased to 32 cm, and on straining it is elevated to 60 cm. A portion of the intravesical pressure in the relaxed, supine position and the increases beyond that pressure observed on standing, straining, or coughing are due entirely to contraction of the striated muscle surrounding the body cavities.

When normal females cough or strain, a "beak" or "infundibulum" of bladder fluid contents enters the proximal third of the urethra and then returns to the bladder after cessation of exertion. Apparently the urinary sphincter cannot keep the urine confined entirely to the fundus of the bladder when intravesical pressure is increased abruptly; urine is pushed into the lumen of a portion of the urinary sphincter.

The basic lesion common to female patients with stress incontinence was found to be an abnormally short urethra when the patient assumed the standing position or strained. The urethral length in the supine position in these patients was frequently within normal limits, but on assuming the standing position there was a shortening or telescoping of the urethra to an average length of 2.3 cm, as contrasted with 3.8 cm in the normal patient. It is evident that if the length of the urinary sphincter or urethra is decreased sufficiently, stress incontinence will result—particularly when it is known that stress forces urine part way down the urethra in the normal female. A 3-cm urethral length in the standing position seems to be the critical length at which transition from continence to incontinence occurs.

An abnormally short urethra is not invariably associated with stress incontinence, and a normal length urethra in the standing position is not a guarantee against stress incontinence. Other factors such as intravesical pressure, status of the urethral epithelium, and tonicity of the muscle and elastic tissues in the wall of the urethra play a part in determining the effectiveness of the urinary sphincter in maintaining urinary continence.

On occasion, the patient may have scar tissue replacing a portion of the normal muscular and elastic tissue of the urethral wall. Urethral length in these patients may be within normal limits in both the supine and standing positions, but the individual may still exhibit stress incontinence. Under these circumstances the actual length of the urethra or sphincter is normal, but the functional length has been decreased by the dimensions of the segment of scar tissue; *adequate tension of the urethral wall requires normal muscle and elastic tissue around the entire circumference of the urethra.*

A decrease in the functional length of the urinary sphincter or urethra can be produced by a urethrovaginal fistula. Again, there is inadequate resistance by the urethral wall because of an opening in its circumference. In some patients, the urethral length is decreased in addition to the functional shortening caused by scar tissue or fistulas.

In our experience, fibrous tissue formation has been produced by electroresection of the urethra for various reasons, inadequate repair of urethrovaginal fistulas, and iatrogenic trauma to the urethral floor during transvaginal operative procedures. Intravesical pressure is an important factor in the apparently mysterious appearance and disappearance of stress incontinence under certain conditions. It has been shown that patients with large cystoceles and hernias do not develop high intravesical pressures on exertion. This is apparently due to the fact that a high pressure requires a compression of the body cavity by all the striated muscles surrounding the cavity. If there is a weak area in the muscular wall of the perineum or abdomen, the pressure will be dissipated by the bulging of the hernia or cystocele. Thus a patient who is a potential candidate for stress incontinence because her urethra shortens abnormally in the erect position may not show stress incontinence if she has a large cystocele. When the cystocele is repaired with resultant increase in intravesical pressures on exertion, incontinence makes its appearance. The reverse has been found to be true also in that some patients with stress incontinence have demonstrated marked improvement in urinary control with the development of a large cystocele or uterovaginal descensus.

Signs and Symptoms. Loss of urine on straining is the chief complaint of patients with stress incontinence. The exertion may be slight, such as in stooping and bending over, or it may be considerable, producing increased intra-abdominal pressure, as in lifting a heavy object. The patient may state that she remains dry despite exertion if she does not permit her bladder to become distended. Permitting the bladder to become too full may result in incontinence even while the patient is supine and relaxed.

Diagnosis. Cystometric examination reveals a normal bladder except for the patient's inability to maintain continence on straining. The Urecholine supersensitivity test is negative. In most patients, the urethral length will be less than 3.0 cm in the erect position. The urethral length is determined by placing the patient in the lithotomy position and catheterizing her with a No. 16 Fr. calibrated retention catheter (5 ml balloon and graduated in centimeters for a distance of 5 cm from the balloon). The catheter balloon is inflated and gently snugged against the vesical outlet, and the urethral length is measured. The bladder is distended to capacity with fluid, and the patient assumes the standing position with the catheter clamped and still in the bladder. The urethral length is measured again; the catheter is removed; the patient is requested to cough or strain, and she is observed for urinary leakage.

Endoscopy reveals no abnormalities in most patients, but in an occasional patient defects or scarred areas will be observed in the urethral wall.

Abnormal bladders frequently misdiagnosed as cases of stress incontinence include the uninhibited neurogenic bladder, the motor paralytic bladder, the autonomous neurogenic bladder, and combinations thereof. Occasionally, stress incontinence and an uninhibited neurogenic bladder may coexist. The correct diagnosis and appropriate therapy may be difficult if a thorough examination is not done.

On the other hand, the examiner may not infrequently make a positive diagnosis on the basis of the patient's history and a simple test readily performed in the office. With the patient in the lithotomy position, the bladder is filled with water through a catheter. The catheter is removed and the patient is requested to cough. A positive test is obtained when the bladder fluid is propelled beyond the urethral meatus, and then is prevented by inserting the index finger along the lateral wall of the vagina and holding the urethrovesical junction in place.

Treatment. The milder cases of stress incontinence can initially be treated conservatively by perineal exercises involving isometric contractions of the periurethral striated muscles and by the use of drugs producing sustained tonic contracture of urethral adrenergic smooth muscle, e.g., ephedrine sulfate 25 to 50 mg q.i.d. or Ornade, one spansule b.i.d. In patients not responding to medical therapy or in those with severe incontinence, it is necessary to operate and fix the urethrovesical junction with the urethra in a lengthened position. This can be readily accomplished by suturing the anterior wall of the urethra or urethrovesical junction to overlying rectus fascia; this procedure is called anterior urethropexy.

When stress incontinence is due to a functional loss in length of the urethra by virtue of an area of scar tissue in the floor of the urethra, the urethra is approached transvaginally, and the scar tissue is excised so that normal muscle can be approximated to normal muscle. Sometimes there is not only scar tissue or a defect in the wall of the urethra but also an actual decrease in length of the urethra in the erect position. In this type of situation it is necessary to utilize both procedures, namely, transvaginal urethral repair and suprapubic anterior urethropexy.

UNINHIBITED NEUROGENIC BLADDER

See the section on Neurogenic Bladder for a full discussion.

URINARY FISTULAS IN THE FEMALE

Etiology. Operative trauma, neoplasms, auto accidents, and gunshot wounds may result in the establishment of a tract conducting urine from the ureter, bladder, or urethra into the vagina.

Signs and Symptoms. The complaint of leaking of urine from the vagina is common to all members of this group. The method by which the patient loses urine through the vagina may vary. The leaking of urine may be constant or it may occur at intervals not associated as well as associated with micturition.

Diagnosis. Cystometric examination may be normal or it may reveal a small capacity bladder. Pyelography usually discloses ureteric injuries with evidence of hydroureter and hydronephrosis above the site of trauma and puddling of radiopaque medium in the region of the ureteric disruption. Endoscopic examination of the bladder and urethra may demonstrate the fistulous opening. Examination of the vagina will frequently reveal the vaginal end of the fistulous tract. Methylene blue given intravenously may aid in defining the fistulous meatus in the vagina.

Congenital anomalies, such as ectopic ureter producing leaking of urine from the vagina, must be distinguished from the fistulas. Occasionally, partially fused labia minora in the young child may deflect urine ejected from the urethral meatus into the vagina and produce postmicturitional leaking from the vagina. (This situation can be corrected readily by separating the labia minora.)

Treatment. Excision of the fistulous tract and closure of the openings in the urinary tract and perhaps the vagina is the indicated therapy if feasible. Vesicovaginal fistulas can be handled quite nicely by approaching the area suprapubically and performing the procedure popularized by O'Conor. The method of handling a ureteric defect must be tailored in accord with the needs of the individual case.

PSYCHOGENIC INCONTINENCE

Etiology. Some cases of incontinence in children and in adults arise as the result of conflicts in the relationship between patient and environment. The author does not feel qualified to discuss in detail the psychiatric aspects of these cases. Suffice it to say that the patient develops urinary incontinence in an attempt to solve some difficult personal problem.

Signs and Symptoms. The urinary incontinence is usually of an intermittent type and simulates the picture of the uninhibited neurogenic bladder. These patients, however, do not complain of increased frequency of urination and urgency. *Their primary manifestation is bed-wetting and soiling of clothes with urine.* In his questioning, the physician may uncover obvious evidence of an unfavorable home environment, e.g., separation of the parents or sibling rivalry.

Diagnosis. The endoscopic and cystometric examinations will be entirely normal. No objective evidence of defects in the sphincter mechanism or innervation of the bladder will be found. Some physicians will object to making a diagnosis of psychogenic incontinence by exclusion; however, in many of the cases when there is an abnormality of the urinary tract or its innervation to account for the enuresis, the etiology may be difficult to determine because of friction which may have arisen between parent and child due to the incontinence.

Treatment. The patient with a presumptive diagnosis of psychogenic incontinence should be referred to the psychiatrist for examination, advice, and treatment if indicated. Since there are a myriad of situations causing psychogenic urinary incontinence, the psychiatrist may choose to treat the patient or the parents, or merely refer them in turn to a child guidance clinic or social service.

MIXED TYPES OF INCONTINENCE

For the sake of completeness and accuracy, it would be well to mention that not all cases of incontinence are strictly of one pure type or another; many different combinations can occur. For example, in children one may encounter urinary incontinence which may be both uninhibited and psychogenic in type. Failure to recognize the presence of both types may drive the urologist to distraction if he is treating the patient for an uninhibited neurogenic bladder, or may drive the psychiatrist wild if he is treating the child for psychogenic incontinence.

In the elderly male, overflow incontinence due to obstruction as well as an uninhibited neurogenic bladder due to an upper motor neuron lesion may be present simultaneously. The female with stress incontinence may also be plagued by an uninhibited neurogenic bladder.

The diagnosis of a mixed type of urinary incontinence can be made without too much difficulty, provided that a complete examination is performed.

For alleviation of the incontinence, one must treat each of the types involved.

CAUSES AND MANAGEMENT OF PEDIATRIC ENURESIS

Since urinary incontinence in the child is so important from both the physical and mental health aspects, it would be well to reiterate certain pertinent facets. The child with involuntary loss of urine and an associated urinary infection or a weak, dribbling stream should be referred immediately for urologic consultation; these cases often involve spinal cord disease, urethral valves, and other congenital anomalies which may have already resulted in kidney damage.

Most of the girls and boys subject to "benign" bed wetting owe their difficulties to delayed development of higher center control or to excessively sound sleeping; few are psychogenic in origin. Such anticholinergic agents as Pro-Banthine, Atratan, and tincture of belladonna can be used for the uncontrolled bladder due to delayed cortical maturation, while the mild nervous system stimulating agents ephedrine sulfate, Tofranil, and Ornade are effective in hypersomniacs.

SELECTED REFERENCES

Bors, E., and Comarr, A. E.: Neurological Urology. Baltimore, University Park Press, 1971.
  A superb reference source for almost any noteworthy contribution to the field of neurogenic bladder written by two outstanding authorities who have devoted their lives to patients with transverse myelitis.
Boyarsky, S.: Neurogenic Bladder. Baltimore, Williams and Wilkins Co., 1967.
  A symposium devoted to a discussion of both the basic and clinical aspects of bladder physiology and physiopathology as viewed in the year 1965. The experts participating in this outstanding meeting update Langworthy's efforts.
Diokno, A. C., Koff, S. A., and Bender, L. F.: Periurethral striated muscle activity in neurogenic bladder dysfunction. J. Urol., 112:742, 1974.
  This is the first report of research correlating the function of the urogenital diaphragm with that of the detrusor in patients with normal and neurogenic bladders. The material is of great importance in the future diagnosis of micturition problems.
Hinman, F., Jr.: Hydrodynamics of Micturition. Springfield, Ill., Charles C Thomas, Publisher, 1971.

A summary of the discussions of primarily urologists and engineers interested in urination from the hydrodynamic viewpoint. The workshop illustrates quite vividly the great need for closer interdisciplinary effort and the tremendous benefit to be derived therefrom.

Langworthy, O. R., Kolb, L. C., and Lewis, L. G.: Physiology of Micturition. Baltimore, Williams and Wilkins Co., 1940.

An excellent summary of the research and knowledge concerning urination from the beginnings of organized investigation to 1940. This is a splendid reference for many of the basic principles and pertinent bibliography.

Lapides, J.: Symposium on neurogenic bladder. Urol. Clin. N. Am., 1:1, 1974.

The latest information on both the basic and clinical aspects of the normal and neurogenic bladder.

REFERENCES

Donker, P. J., Ivanocici, R., and Noach, E. L.: Analysis of the urethral pressure profile by means of electromyography and the administration of drugs. Br. J. Urol., 44:180, 1972.

Kiil, R.: The Function of the Ureter and Renal Pelvis. Philadelphia, W. B. Saunders Co., 1957.

Lapides, J.: Physiology of the intact human ureter. J. Urol., 100:441, 1948.

Lapides, J.: Micturition and the adrenergic system. Urologists' Letter Club, May, 1974, p. 48.

Lapides, J., and Lovegrove, R. H.: Urinary vesico-vascular reflex. J. Urol., 44:397, 1965.

Pfau, A.: The influence of the adrenergic system on the lower urinary tract. Urol. Digest, May, 1974, p. 15.

Schulman, C. C.: Electron microscopy of the human ureteric innervation. Br. J. Urol., 46:609, 1974.

Scott, F. B., Bradley, W. E., and Timm, G. W.: Treatment of urinary incontinence by implantable prosthetic sphincter. Urology, 1:252, 1973.

Chapter Seven

PHYSIOLOGY OF THE MALE GENITAL SYSTEM

William C. Baum

THE DETERMINATION OF SEX

Any consideration of the physiology of the male genital system is best initiated by a review of current concepts that are relative to the determination of sex.

Most agree that the primitive gonad, like the internal and external genital apparatus whose function it eventually influences, is basically bipotential with respect to sexual identification. The initial directional decision is undoubtedly chromosomal, modified, in all probability, by embryonic gonadal organizers that arise within the primitive structure.

The human karyotype consists of 46 chromosomes, or 23 pairs of chromosomes, one member of each pair having its origin from each parent. Of the 23 pairs, 22 are homologous and 2 are sex chromosomes, heterologous (XY) in the male and homologous (XX) in the female.

In the process of gametogenesis, the male and female gamete divide into two, with a 50 per cent reduction in sex chromosomes (Fig. 7-1). Both sex and somatic chromosomes are reduced from the diploid number 46 to the haploid number 23. Thus each gamete eventually possesses either an X or Y chromosome. Each female gamete invariably has an X chromosome.

The Y chromosome is one of the smallest of the human chromosomes, but it contains a very powerful male determinant. In clinical entities involving abnormalities of chromosomal constitution, its presence in an XXXY pattern still leads to testicular differentiation. There are undoubtedly several different genetic loci on the Y chromosome concerned with male differentiation, for should structural abnormality of this chromosome occur through a partial deletion of the Y, incomplete male differentiation results.

In contrast, the X chromosome is a large human chromosome and

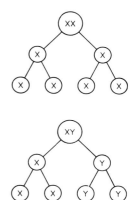

Figure 7–1   The process of gametogenesis.

GAMETOGENESIS

contains 5 per cent of the total DNA content of the haploid set (X + 22 autosomes). It handles genetic coding for functions of almost every body system. Barr (1949) was the first to identify the presence of a chromatin mass at the periphery of a ganglion cell in laboratory animals and then in the cells of most mammals. This identification technique has been used since as a means of assessing the presence and numbers of X chromosomes in patients who have errors of sexual differentiation. The biologic function of the X chromosome is most complex. Interested students are referred to the reviews of Grumbach and Van Wyk (1974) and Lyon (1972) for more detailed information.

The gonads of both sexes arise from anlagen located on the urogenital ridge. Until the 12 mm stage of embryologic development, these structures are morphologically similar and could potentially differentiate as either testis or ovary. By this time primordial germ cells migrating from the posterior endoderm of the yolk sac have invaded the undifferentiated gonad and exist as potential spermatozoa or oogonia.

After an investigation of early embryos, Jost (1972) and Jirosek (1971) came to the conclusion that ovary and testis are derived from a common source, the primitive gonad. It is their belief that there is an inherent tendency for the primitive gonad to develop into an ovary, provided that germ cells are present and persist. This inherent tendency is negated in the intended male fetus by the existence of testis determiners on the Y chromosome. Jost and Jirosek were able to demonstrate the onset of testicular differentiation in intended males as early as the 12 mm stage, with regression of primitive müllerian ducts by the 30 mm stage. In the gonad destined to become an ovary, a lack of differentiation persisted to the 80 mm stage, when primordial germ cells were seen to enlarge and become oogonia for the first time.

Jost (1972) has theorized from studies conducted in freemartins that testicular differentiation and the possible inhibition of ovarian differentiation are the result of a nonsteroidal humoral influence unrelated to androgen. The long period of latency before ovarian development can take place readily explains why patients with an XXY chromosomal constitution develop testes rather than ovaries. Evidently, prior differentiation of testes by action of the genes on the Y chromosome precludes later differentiation as an ovary.

The bipotential character of the genital system is mirrored in the subsequent development of the duct system. The müllerian ducts serve as anlagen of the uterus and fallopian tubes. The mesonephric or wolffian ducts have the potential to develop into epididymis, vas deferens, and seminal vesicles. During the third month of gestation, the persistence of one system and involution of the other occur simultaneously, depending on the intended sex. Jost has clearly shown that secretions from the fetal testis are the directional determinants. In the presence of the testis the müllerian system involutes, and the wolffian system completes its intent. In the absence of the testis the wolffian ducts are resorbed, and the müllerian system matures. Evidently, female development does not depend on the presence of an ovary, for the equally satisfactory development of uterus and tubes can occur if no gonad is present.

Jost (1972), in a brilliant series of experiments on the rabbit fetus, demonstrated that the influence of a fetal testis on duct development is exerted locally and unilaterally. If one testis is removed at an early stage of growth, the oviduct develops normally on that side, whereas müllerian involution occurs on the side of the remaining testis. Jost's findings have been confirmed by a number of investigators in tissue culture studies and in studies on humans with varying forms of hermaphroditism. These researchers feel that the fetal testis secretes a macromolecular, androgen-independent, nonsteroidal material that is responsible for müllerian involution. However, the stimulation of primitive wolffian ducts to develop into epididymis, vas deferens, and seminal vesicles does require androgen. Concentrations of androgen that are required for male duct stimulation appear to be higher than the concentrations needed for masculinization of the external genitalia and derivatives of the urogenital sinus. It is possible that this effect is due to a testosterone binding protein found in the wolffian ducts which is similar to that found in adults for concentrating testosterone at germ cell and ejaculatory duct sites. Another interesting observation on male duct differentiation is that these tissues lack the 5 α-reductase necessary to convert testosterone to dihydrotestosterone, in contrast to the urogenital sinus and genital tubercle which acquire this enzyme even before the testis has developed the capacity to synthesize testosterone. This difference may explain why the latter tissues are sensitive to systemic androgen whereas this is not true for wolffian derivatives.

More evidence for the bipotential character of embryonic sexual development is to be found in the external genitalia. At the 30 mm stage the external genitalia are identical. The genital tubercle, urethral folds, urogenital slit, and labioscrotal swellings are common to both sexes. The genital tubercle may become the glans penis or clitoris. The urethral folds may close to form the penile urethra or may remain open as labia minora. The labioscrotal swellings may form the labia majora or scrotum.

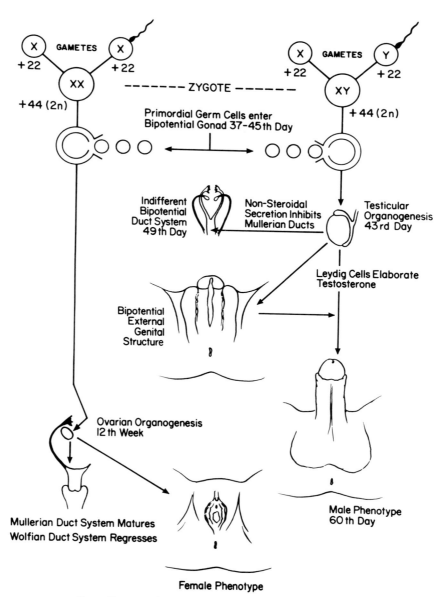

Figure 7-2   Mechanisms influencing the determination of sex.

As in the gonad and genital ducts there is an inherent tendency for the external genitalia to feminize independent of hormonal influence. Male differentiation occurs only if androgenic stimulation occurs during gestation. The fetal Leydig cells proliferate at the 30 mm stage, and the testosterone secreted is converted to dihydrotestosterone, which in turn binds to cytosol androgen receptors in the target cells. After fetal Leydig cells have completed intrauterine functions, they again revert into mesenchymal cells to lie dormant until puberty, when they again return to a mature state under the influence of the pituitary gland.

Thus, it is evident that the determination of sex is primarily a chromosomal responsibility triggering, as it does, the directional influence on the homologous bipotential primitive gonad (Fig. 7–2). Once oriented, this structure in turn elaborates its own influences in the male that subsequently cause the bipotential duct system and external genitalia to move toward masculinity, or in the female, in the absence of androgen, permits the normal tendency to feminization to evolve. Disturbances in this normal pattern that result in clinical problems commonly grouped under the general heading of "intersexuality" must have their origin prior to birth, either at the chromosomal level in the primitive gonad through disturbances in its secretory function, or by reason of exogenous influences of an endocrine nature in the embryo or its maternal environment.

As Bunge (1970) points out, chromosomal errors responsible for disturbances in sexual determination may arise from a faulty replication of germ cells during spermatogenesis or oogenesis or from a faulty mitotic division of cells in the zygote after fertilization.

Each species is characterized by a certain number of chromosomes in its basic cell. Cells with chromosomal numbers different from normal are termed *aneuploid*. Aneuploidy may occur as a result of nondisjunction (Fig. 7–3) in either the meiotic or mitotic division. If a member of a pair of homologous chromosomes fails to separate during anaphase, one daughter cell receives an extra chromosome while the other receives

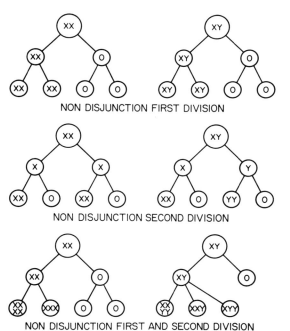

NON DISJUNCTION FIRST DIVISION

NON DISJUNCTION SECOND DIVISION

NON DISJUNCTION FIRST AND SECOND DIVISION

Figure 7–3 Aneuploidy as a result of nondisjunction.

none and is thus in deficit. Aneuploidy may also result from anaphase lag. Improper orientation of one chromosome at the equatorial plate during metaphase may cause a loss of a chromosome from one or both daughter cells. If only one member of the chromosomal pair is lost, the descendant from one daughter cell is normal while the other lacks a chromosome. If both chromatids are lost, both daughter cells have one less chromosome.

If an error in mitosis occurs after fertilization, an individual may develop with two or more cells differing in chromosomal constitution. Embryos that are developed from gametes of abnormal chromosomal makeup are prone to additional errors of replication. The resulting condition is termed *mosaicism* and accounts for many of the paradoxes between genotype and phenotype. The sex chromosome constitution in mosaics may vary in different tissues and even in different areas of the same tissue, making investigation for purposes of identity very difficult.

A similar situation may occur in individuals with more than one cell line. Unlike patients with mosaicism, in whom different cell lines have the same genetic origin, these patients have more than one cell line, each of which has a different genetic origin. Possible explanations for this phenomenon, termed *chimerism,* are double fertilization of a binucleate ovum, the fusion of two complete zygotes before implantation, or the fertilization by separate spermatozoa of an ovum and its polar body.

Chromosomal errors may also arise from disturbances in structure as well as in number. Short arm, long arm, deletions, isochrome formation, duplication, and translocation are all possible variations in structure. Many such abnormalities are compatible with fertilization and may be transmitted in Mendelian fashion.

Clinical entities that involve disturbances of sexual differentiation are not limited to errors of chromosomal intent. Endocrine disorders of embryonic or maternal origin and genetic mutation all contribute to abnormalities that are found. Recent advances in the understanding of these disorders have made reclassification of errors in sex differentiation imperative. Grumbach and Van Wyk (1974) have recently proposed a logical modification of the older Klebs categorization. To the categories of true hermaphrodite, female pseudohermaphrodite, and male pseudohermaphrodite have been added disorders of gonadal differentiation that include much of the recently contributed information on disturbances of gonadal organogenesis and chromosomal genetic intent. Admittedly, there are overlapping situations inherent in the nature of the classification, but it is a workable one for the clinician. The review of Grumbach and Van Wyk is exhaustive and up-to-date and needs no reiteration.

The contemporary physician armed with those diagnostic aids available to him should be able to identify the nature of the entity involved and direct reasonable therapy accordingly. The infant who presents with sexual ambiguity should have the benefit of an accurate determination of the X chromatin pattern or karyotype analysis. If the X chromatin pattern is positive, consideration should be given to a differential diagnosis of female pseudohermaphroditism, true hermaphroditism, or seminiferous tubular dysgenesis (Klinefelter's syndrome).

The female child who presents at birth with obvious sexual ambiguity and whose clinical course shortly after birth is marked by vomiting and dehydration with associated hyperkalemic acidosis and hyponatremia should be suspected of having congenital adrenal cortical hyperplasia. Discovery of an elevated 17 α-OH-progesterone level should confirm the diagnosis and establish the need for immediate use of cortisone, salt, and salt-retaining steroids. If adrenal cortical hyperplasia is excluded and a reliable history of maternal ingestion of androgens or progestational hormones during pregnancy can be elicited, it may be logically assumed that this was the source of virilization. These patients usually feminize at puberty, and early treatment is not needed. Should examination indicate the presence of gonadal structures in the inguinal canals or labial folds, true hermaphroditism may be present. Pelvic examination, urethroscopy, x-rays with contrast material, and eventually laparotomy with identification of gonadal intent by biopsy may be required. The assignment of sex should be based on an assessment of the presenting genitalia, i.e., on function. Extirpation of heterologous gonadal tissue is desirable when possible or total gonadectomy when not (bilateral ovi-testes.) Seminiferous tubular dysgenesis, or Klinefelter's syndrome, is seldom diagnosed at birth, the child presenting as a male phenotype. A karyotype analysis, if done by chance, can demonstrate an XXY constitution. Immediate therapy is not indicated.

If the X chromatin pattern is negative, the patient may be a male pseudohermaphrodite, i.e., one whose genital duct system or external genitalia is ambiguous, exhibiting in one or more respects the female phenotype, but whose gonads are testes. Such patients are chromatin-negative.

The patient may be a true hermaphrodite, i.e., possessed of both ovarian and testicular gonadal tissue. About 30 per cent of true hermaphrodites are chromatin-negative. Thirdly, the patient may manifest one of the syndromes classified under gonadal dysgenesis, i.e., Turner's syndrome and its variants; at least 80 per cent of these patients are chromatin-negative. Investigation of these patients should include a karyotype analysis, x-rays, urethroscopy, and possibly laparotomy. The most difficult decision involves those chromatin-negative patients who present with a microphallus and whose gonadal androgenic potential at puberty remains in question. All clinicians agree that a decision on the sex of rearing is highly desirable before 18 months of age. If reconstructive surgery is to be done, it should be accomplished by 2½ years of age at the latest. After this period of time serious psychiatric disorders can be expected in the child and equally serious social problems can be predicted for the family involved. Gonadal function can be tested by giving human chorionic gonadotropin. Grumbach recommends 500 to 1000 I.U. daily for seven days with frequent monitoring of testosterone levels. This procedure provides objective evidence of Leydig cell capacity to secrete testosterone, and it demonstrates phallic growth potential. Trial administration of testosterone ethanate in patients with micropenis, 50 mg intramuscularly every two weeks for eight weeks, will provide evidence of penile growth capacity. If penile growth does not take place to a significant degree and the external and internal genital ambiguity is severe, i.e., strongly favors the female phenotype, a reversal of sex is preferable to any attempt to create a male compatible with chromosomal intent but who in adulthood will be totally incompatible with the sex of rearing from the functional standpoint.

Plastic reconstructive surgery will provide functionally acceptable external and internal genital structures once the directional decision is made and can be supported by appropriate hormonal substitutional therapy, if required, after puberty. In patients with incomplete forms of the testicular feminization syndrome and in patients with male pseudohermaphroditism who are best reared as females from the functional standpoint, gonadectomy should be carried out to prevent the possibility of virilization at puberty. In patients with the complete syndrome of testicular feminization, gonadectomy may be delayed until puberty in the hope that testicular estrogens will bring about feminization. However, considering the possibility of tumor formation in these patients and the necessity for ultimate gonadectomy, it may be advisable to carry out the procedure early and provide estrogen substitution therapy after puberty.

PREPUBERTAL SEXUAL DEVELOPMENT

Once normal sexual differentiation is established, the male embryo is faced with two great developmental tasks, namely, somatic growth and the maintenance of the continuity of the germ plasm. The latter goal is accomplished by the appearance of the primordial germ cell in the primitive gonad and its subsequent cellular organization into cords later to become the seminiferous tubules. Banking the walls of these tubules are large stem cells, or potential spermatogonia, that are destined to lie quiescent awaiting the chain reaction which is initiated by the pituitary gland at the time of puberty. In the meantime neighboring somatic cells move ahead with the other primary task, which is to build the body that will house this sexual cellular potential. This conservation of reproductive power until such time as the individual is not only physically capable of propagating the species, but also able to maintain the product of conception in a relatively hostile environment, is an intriguing protective mechanism of nature that has reached a high degree of specialization in the human. Interestingly, this mechanism is paralleled in many ways in lower forms of life as well.

In addition to its role as guardian of the germ cell, the gonad must also effect union with the degenerating mesonephros, which is no longer needed by the kidney, and thus provide itself with a conducting system for sperm that will be formed later. The epididymis and vas deferens, so formed, provide a link between the testis and the urethra and are situated in such a fashion as to allow the prostate gland and seminal vesicles to provide the major fluid portion of the ejaculate by an associated duct system. The link is necessary because of the physiologic intolerance of the testes in their intra-abdominal position. Perhaps fleeing the heat of the abdominal cavity, the testes descend at the third month of gestation from their retroperitoneal position in the midabdomen and, as the embryo grows and straightens out from its original flexed intrauterine position, finally come to rest in the scrotal sac by the eighth month of development. There is considerable evidence to indicate that this process, as well as being a mechanical one, is also of an endocrine nature. The anterior lobe of the pituitary gland is responsible for an internal secretion that certainly plays a major role in this migratory activity, for it is known that its administration to cryptorchids in whom there is no structural impediment often results in descent. Further support is given this observation by the knowledge that the testes of rodents, normally intra-abdominal in position except during rutting, can be made to descend out of season by the administration of pituitary hormone, while on the other hand hypophysectomy will in itself prevent seasonal migration of the rat testes.

In the normal situation, the gonads are suspended in the scrotal sac by the spermatic cord, surrounded by the fascial and muscular envelope encountered in their trip through the abdominal wall, and possessed of an efficient thermoregulating mechanism. Reference has already been made to the descent of the testes in terms of escape from body temperature. From the standpoint of preservation of the species it would seem illogical to expose the gonads to the danger of trauma as they exist in their normal adult position, but the cellular activity of the organ is so arranged that it can function only at temperatures existing in the extra-abdominal position. It is interesting to note that prolonged increases in temperature of as little as 1.5 to 2.0°C above normal are suf-

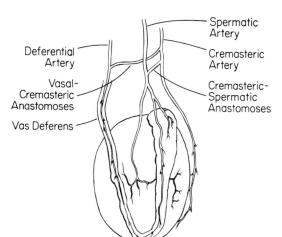

Deferential Artery

Vasal–Cremasteric Anastomoses

Vas Deferens

Spermatic Artery

Cremasteric Artery

Cremasteric–Spermatic Anastomoses

Figure 7–4 Arterial supply to testis and epididymis.

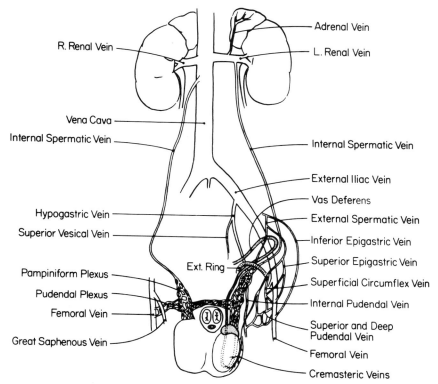

Figure 7–5 Venous drainage systems of the testis and epididymis.

ficient to bring about degeneration of the germinal epithelium after puberty.

Thermoregulation involves several mechanisms, including the contraction and relaxation of the cremaster muscle, increased surface area for heat loss provided by the rugal folds of the scrotum, and perhaps most important of all the design of the circulatory system of the testis. Three arterial vessels supply the testis: the internal spermatic, the deferential branch of the inferior vesical artery, and the cremasteric artery from the deep epigastric (Fig. 7–4). They anastomose freely and spread out over the surface of the testis sending penetrating branches into the parenchyma. Blood returns by the veins of the pampiniform plexus (Fig. 7–5). It is felt that the venous collection actually precools the arterial blood by a counter current exchange that reduces the temperature of arterial blood by at least 3°C. The returning blood passes by two sets of veins into the vena cava. There are at least three intercommunicating venous channels which cross the midline, establishing connections between the right and left testis. Hotchkiss (1967) and others have demonstrated these cross channels by venogram and feel that the existence of these channels explains the bilateral disturbance in testicular function often observed in patients with unilateral varicocele. Studies by Tessler and Krahn (1966), however, tend to negate the validity of this explanation. Recently it has been theorized that blood carrying relatively high concentrations of toxic metabolites such as steroids, which are known depressors of spermatogenic function, from the left adrenal and left renal veins can enter directly and in an undetoxified state into the left internal spermatic vein, thus materially affecting spermatogenesis.

Unilateral or bilateral failure of testicular descent is a common clinical entity. The potential damage to spermatogenesis that is inherent in the cryptorchid state and the recognized increase in the incidence of testicular carcinoma in the testis so involved pose a therapeutic challenge to both pediatrician and urologist.

A small percentage of these retained testes may be ectopic; i.e., they are normally developed, have passed through the inguinal canal, but are thwarted in attaining their scrotal goal for reasons not well understood. Their spermatic cord is usually of normal length, and germinal epithelium is potentially good. Orchiopexy is indicated as soon as the diagnosis is established and certainly well before puberty.

The true cryptorchid retains his testis or testes in the inguinal canal, possesses a short spermatic vasculature (a manifestation of testicular dysgenesis), and, although opinion varies widely in this regard, such testes are probably potentially inferior with respect to future spermatogenic potential. Most surgeons agree that salvage of the true cryptorchid testes is most likely if orchidopexy is performed before the age of six years.

Children commonly present with migratory testes or pseudocryptorchidism. These testes retract on stimulation and at puberty usually assume their scrotal position without interference. Prognostication in this instance and differentiation from true cryptorchidism may be accomplished by the administration of human chorionic gonadotropin (4000 I.U.) three times weekly for three weeks. If migratory the testes may descend permanently or may descend, then retract again, and finally descend at puberty. .

Since many clinical entities that involve sexual failure, such as Klinefelter's syndrome, male pseudohermaphroditism, and hypogonadotropic eunuchoidism, may present with associated cryptorchidism, these syndromes should be kept in mind and ruled out in differential diagnosis.

PREPUBERTAL SEXUAL FUNCTION

The following consideration of sexual function is divided into three chronologic life periods: pubertal, adult, and senescent. The preceding discussion of the determination of sex, gonadal organogenesis, and certain aspects of prepubertal somatic development as related to sexual function has provided a background for the further perusal of the relationship of the testis as target organ to its related endocrine glands.

The prepubertal testis shows little evidence of the physiologic ac-

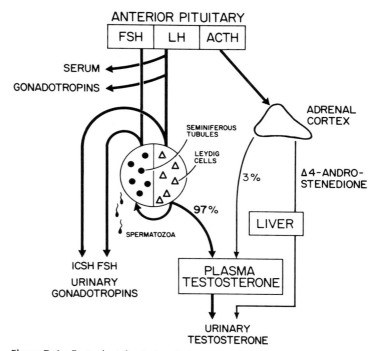

ANTERIOR PITUITARY

Figure 7–6   Postpubertal anterior pituitary–sexual target organ relationships.

tivity that will characterize its function after the age of 12 to 14 years. Histologically its cellular components show differentiation into three potentially functional units: (1) the germinal epithelium lining the seminiferous tubules, (2) the interstitial cells of Leydig, and (3) the sustentacular cells of Sertoli. These units lie dormant until awakened at the time of puberty by the secretions of the anterior lobe of the pituitary gland (Fig. 7–6). At this time the hypophysis elaborates a follicle stimulating hormone (FSH) and an interstitial cell stimulating hormone (ICSH). Interstitial cell stimulating hormone acts on the Leydig cell, causing it to secrete androgen and estrogen. Radioactive label studies show that the ICSH localizes in the Leydig cell and in the peritubular membranous cells. Pituitary FSH acts on the seminiferous tubules to induce and maintain spermatogenesis. Label studies also show testicular binding for FSH, but the precise localization is in doubt. It is possible that the Sertoli cells are the target. The maturing germ cell does not concentrate FSH. Some investigators feel that FSH is synergistic to the action of ICSH on Leydig cell steroidogenesis. At present most feel that the mode of action for ICSH on the seminiferous tubules is one of stimulation of endogenous testosterone secretion. It is felt that testosterone is an important element in the regulation of human spermatogenesis.

As in many endocrine functions, the target organ (testis) is also involved in a balanced regulatory function in its relationship to the pituitary gland, a so-called negative feedback by means of the hormones it produces. Thus, if Leydig cells through disease or injury produce less than the normal amount of androgen, the pituitary tropic ICSH increases in titer in the serum. By contrast, if Leydig cells produce greater amounts of androgen, the pituitary output of tropic hormone (ICSH) is inhibited, and the serum titer will be less than normally expected. Theoretically, the seminiferous tubules should produce a separate hormone with similar functional capacity. McCullagh suggests that such a hormone exists and terms it "Inhibin." Del Castillo theorizes that the Sertoli cell produces an estrogen that controls FSH output from the pituitary gland. A welter of theoretical suggestions have been offered by many investigators to explain the mechanisms of FSH secretion and its reciprocal balance. To date the information remains purely theoretical.

The production of testicular androgen is explained by the direct action of ICSH on Leydig cell adenylyl cyclase. Cholesterol, the basic precursor, is synthesized near the smooth muscle endoplasmic reticulum. It is then transported to the mitochondria where pregnenolone is generated and then converted to progesterone, 17 α-hydroxyprogesterone, Δ^4-androstenedione, and finally testosterone. Testosterone is transported in the venous circulation and lymphatics as a beta globulin. About 97 to 99 per cent of circulating testosterone is bound; the remaining 1 to 3 per cent is a free component and is assumed to be the metabolically active portion.

Testosterone acts on the target accessory sex glands, the prostate gland, and the seminal vesicles, stimulating them to cellular function. At this level an enzyme, 5 α-reductase, transforms testosterone to dihydrotestosterone, and this substance is attached to a specific binding protein. Testosterone has a generalized somatic effect on the growth of facial hair, body hair, muscular development, and the growth of the external genitalia. It also brings about the cessation of long bone growth. This is evidently a direct effect and is not due to dihydrotestosterone since many of these tissues do not possess the enzyme 5 α-reductase.

It is of interest that tissues other than the Leydig cell, such as the seminiferous tubules and epididymis, have the ability to transform steroid precursors such as acetate and cholesterol into testosterone. The rationale would seem to be one of assurance of high local concentrations of testosterone rather than a contribution to the systemic androgenic pool.

Testosterone and dihydrotestosterone are broken down into various metabolites, mainly, 17-ketosteroids. Following this reduction, the 17-ketosteroids are conjugated with glucuronic and sulfuric acid and then are excreted in the urine. Of the total urinary 17-ketosteroid production, the testis accounts for approximately 30 per cent and the adrenal cortex the rest. Androsterone, etiocholanolone, and epiandrosterone are derived from testosterone metabolism. Dehydroepiandrosterone is derived primarily from the adrenal cortex. The metabolic interconversions between testicular and adrenal androgens and nonandrogenic 17-ketosteroids make the original source of any urinary 17-ketosteroid impossible to determine. Testosterone is also converted to the estrogens estradiol and estrone. This accounts for a relatively small fraction of overall androgen metabolism, and the clinical significance of this fact is a matter of conjecture.

SPERMATOGENESIS

The second major cellular function of the testis is that of spermatogenesis. Microscopic inspection of the seminiferous tubules reveals a primitive stem cell of type A spermatogonium. This cell divides to perpetuate its kind and in addition gives rise to spermatogonia specifically committed to become mature spermatozoa. These cells, or type B spermatogonia, differentiate by further mitotic divisions to produce a new generation of germ cells, the primary spermatocytes. Once formed they go immediately into an interphase or resting stage, then divide again with a reduction of the number of chromosomes from the diploid to haploid number. In this division there is a duplication of the amount of DNA followed by a long prophase that involves the rearrangement of the chromatin threads in which the nuclei now progress through the leptotene, zygotene, pachytene, and diplotene stages to form the secondary spermatocytes. Each secondary spermatocyte is haploid and has only one sex chromosome, an X or a Y.

The secondary spermatocytes have a short life and divide by meiosis, each giving rise to two smaller daughter cells or spermatids. Each spermatid undergoes a metamorphosis called spermiogenesis that transforms it to spermatozoa. During this process a nuclear cap is elaborated, the nucleus is condensed, and a flagellum is added. During spermiogenesis the spermatids embed themselves in the Sertoli cells. The bulk of the spermatid cytoplasm with its contained RNA is released and taken up by the Sertoli cell, and as a result sperm are devoid of RNA. In all, this process of maturation from spermatogonium to sperm takes about 74 days. The process of spermatogenesis results in the accumulation of sperm at the central lumen of the seminiferous tubule. From here by a continuous process, sperm pass through the rete testis and efferent ductules, a passive process accomplished by the smooth muscles in the walls of the seminiferous tubules. Transfer through the rete testis and efferent ductules is by cilia. The collecting tubules unite to form the epididymis, some 20 feet of coiled structure, which joins with the vas deferens, itself some 15 feet in total length.

Spermatozoa undergo a process of maturation within the ductus epididymis, acquiring full functional competence. Mature sperm are stored in the tail of the epididymis and vas deferens until ejaculation. Longevity of stored sperm may be as great as 30 to 70 days, but aging changes occur which affect fertilizing capacity. Ejaculation after prolonged abstinence usually results in a high percentage of dead sperm. Removal of the sperm in the absence of ejaculation is not well understood but probably occurs through pyknotic degeneration and absorption.

Survival of sperm in the epididymis is directly dependent on the functional integrity of the epididymal cell and it in turn on the endocrine activity of the Leydig cell. In humans, sperm require 21 days to pass through the epididymal system. There is evidence to show that failure of Leydig cell activity during this transport may lead to poor sperm motility.

The third cellular component, the Sertoli cell, lines the basement membrane of the seminiferous tubule. The cells provide a supportive or nutritive role for the germinal epithelium. Ultramicroscopic studies show a close relationship between germ cells in varying degrees of maturation and the Sertoli cells, enclosing as they do the primary spermatocytes, spermatids, and spermatogonia. A hormone secreting role has been suggested for the Sertoli cell that is supported by ultramicroscopic investigation, which shows the presence of organelles usually attendant on such function.

PREPUBERTAL SEXUAL FAILURE

Most clinicians interested in an orderly classification of prepubertal sexual failure feel that it is best based, for purposes of etiologic localization, on the relationship of the pituitary gland as a producer of tropic stimulating hormone and the target organ as recipient and reciprocal producer of a pituitary regulating material. Thus, syndromes may be described as hypogonadotropic or hypergonadotropic with respect to this relationship.

Hypothalamic prepubertal sexual failure occurs infrequently and is secondary to extensive involvement of the hypothalamic-pituitary tracts or nuclei, such as might be found with suprasellar cysts or gliomas. Interference with the ability of the pituitary to produce tropic hormone would result in sexual failure through a lack of stimulation of the target organ. Other pituitary functions are usually concomitantly involved, such as growth and adrenal and thyroid function. By reason of the nature of the process, these individuals seldom constitute therapeutic problems at the clinical level but must be considered in differential diagnosis.

Panhypopituitarism, or failure of all anterior lobe function, is a rare syndrome whose clinical features include hypothyroidism with myxedema, adrenal insufficiency with Addisonism, dwarfism, and hypogenitalism. Obesity may or may not be present, depending on whether the primary disease involves the hypothalamus as well. Gynecomastia is never present. These unfortunate individuals do not show the characteristic changes expected at puberty; they lack sexual potency, are infertile, and exhibit a very low gonadotropic titer. They have a poor prognosis and also do not constitute a significant clinical problem.

HYPOGONADOTROPIC SYNDROMES

Delayed puberty constitutes a fairly common example of the failure of pituitary gonadotropic stimulus. Patients so involved have evident retardation of the outward signs of adolescence. The entity is familial in nature. The presenting sexual underdevelopment poses a diagnostic challenge, for the investigating physician must separate these patients from those with true hypogonadotropic eunuchoidism. Although the majority mature without substitution therapy, the social and psychologic problems involved in the afflicted child make therapy advisable. A 12 week course of human chorionic gonadotropin 4000 I.U. intramuscularly three times weekly followed by a 12 week wait is often of value. If no response is noted, an additional course may be given. If, after three such courses, improvement is followed by regression, it must be assumed that the patient has hypogonadotropic eunuchoidism.

Hypogonadotropic eunuchoidism is an inherited autosomal dominant disorder whose basic defect lies in the hypothalamus rather than in the pituitary gland. The involved gonadotropic hormones are completely or partially deficient. Patients are usually taller than average and exhibit eunuchoidal features, with testes of prepubertal size and consistency. Thyroid and adrenal functions are not disturbed. Congenital anomalies such as cryptorchidism, deafness, craniofacial asymmetry, anosmia, harelip, and cleft palate are commonly associated. Testicular biopsy reveals immature seminiferous tubules, an absence of Sertoli cells, and a few well-defined Leydig cells. Urinary gonadotropins are low or absent. Serum ICSH and FSH levels are well below normal range. Plasma testosterone levels are in the female range.

If studies are borderline or inconclusive, clomiphene citrate may be administered as a test of pituitary-hypothalamic responsiveness. The classic entity will not respond. Since the defect is hypothalamic and the pituitary is theoretically capable of being stimulated, the use of ICSH release hormone seems a logical form of therapy. Success has been reported on an experimental basis, but the agent is not available for general clinical use. Chorionic gonadotropin is recommended, 200 to 400 I.U. intramuscularly three times weekly. Prolonged use will permit maturation. The addition of menopausal gonadotropin 150 units three times weekly may be needed to achieve testicular maturation, this material being rich in FSH. Expense is considerable, and ultimately a switch to testosterone replacement therapy is indicated.

HYPERGONADOTROPIC SYNDROMES

Seminiferous tubular dysgenesis, or Klinefelter's syndrome, was first described in 1942 by Klinefelter, Reifenstein, and Albright. Their patients were characterized by eunuchoidism, azoospermia, gynecomastia, and mental retardation associated with elevated serum levels of FSH and ICSH. Later, the application of Barr's chromatin analysis found them chromatin-positive. Still later, karyotype analysis found them possessed of an XXY chromosomal constitution. In the variants of the syndrome the presenting abnormalities seem to be influenced by the presence of patterns other than the usual XXY. Thus, if more than two X chromosomes plus a Y chromosome are present, the changes are more severe. Evidently, the presence of abnormal numbers of X chromosomes in testicular tissue is the focal point for seminiferous tubule and Leydig cell changes observed in this entity. Clinically, these patients show little change except for excessive long bone growth in the lower extremities prior to puberty. After puberty, findings may vary from subtle variations of normal to the classic features of the disease. Variants of the syndrome include an XXXXY disorder and an XXXY disorder accompanied in each instance by cryptorchidism, mental retardation, asthenia, prepubertal testicular damage, and osseous growth abnormalities. In individuals with mosaicism who have a normal stem cell line (XY), less severe changes are seen, with mental retardation sometimes being the only presenting feature. Treatment of the syndrome is limited to correction of the androgen deficiency. The existing infertility is not amenable to treatment. Gynecomastia, if present, lends itself to reconstructive plastic surgery.

Germinal cell aplasia is a rather uncommon entity characterized by azoospermia associated with an elevated FSH, but normal ICSH titer. Androgen production is normal. The presenting complaint is usually one of infertility, and testicular biopsy will show germinal aplasia. Leydig cells are present, as are Sertoli cells. An XXY chromosomal pattern has been found in a few cases but the cause remains obscure. Treatment is of no avail.

XYY syndrome is a rare entity that demonstrates evidence of varying degrees of infertility with associated personality disorders of an aggressive sort. Serum FSH and ICSH titers are usually normal but occasionally are elevated if testicular damage is severe. Testicular biopsy will show abnormalities varying from spermatogenic arrest to germinal aplasia. There is no available therapy.

Reifenstein's syndrome is a hereditary disorder marked by eunuchoidism, gynecomastia, hypospadias, azoospermia associated with seminiferous tubular hyalinization, and Leydig cell deficiency. Unlike those afflicted with Klinefelter's syndrome, these patients have an XY chromosomal complement with a chromatin-negative buccal smear. Urinary androgen levels are decreased and urinary gonadotropin levels elevated. Treatment consists of androgen substitution therapy and reconstructive surgery for hypospadias and gynecomastia.

Prepubertal castrate syndrome is also a rare clinical entity that involves patients born without recognizable testicular tissue. The patient presents with a male phenotype and it must therefore be assumed that failure of testicular organogenesis occurred after the seventh to fourteenth week of fetal life. In other instances the syndrome may involve those persons devoid of functioning testes by reason of bilateral testicular torsion with infarction, or loss by reason of trauma and disease. In the absence of testicular tissue, puberty will fail to occur. If untreated, sexual failure will persist and a hypergonadotropic serum titer will be found. Androgen replacement therapy should be instituted at puberty.

Eunuchoidal patients requiring androgenic substitution need larger doses of testosterone to attain full sexual maturation than those required for maintenance alone. The long acting cyclopentyl propionate esters of testosterone are preferable; 200 mg given intramuscularly every two weeks for two to three years followed by 100 to 200 mg every two to three weeks for maintenance is recommended. Testosterone pellets may be used instead. Six 75 mg pellets may be placed subcutaneously with a pellet injection gun every four to six months. Cost and danger of infection are factors mitigating against this form of administration. Oral preparations include methyl testosterone as a languet 25 to 30 mg daily or fluoxymesterone 5 to 10 mg daily. These agents will produce a reasonably good response but are nowhere nearly as effective as the long acting deep injectable form.

Eugonadotropic syndromes are forms of selective pituitary gonadal insufficiency that present not because of developmental abnormalities, nor by reason of androgenic failure, but rather because of infertility. In normal male habitus, possessed of normal androgenic and gonadotropic serum titers, the only deficit is spermatogenic. Semen analysis usually shows an oligospermia of varying degree. This entity may well represent a defect in the normal interaction between pituitary FSH secretory mechanisms and the testicular target cell responsible for spermatogenesis. Therapy to date has been disappointing since there is no available substitute for the defect.

SEXUAL PRECOCITY

While pituitary and testicular deficiency are not uncommon during the prepubertal phase of existence, the converse, sexual precocity, is a clinical rarity. Nevertheless, it is important that the physician be acquainted with the common causes for premature masculinization in order that he may effectively organize a program for differential diagnosis and therapy when this condition does come to his attention in practice.

Four basic causes of precocity in the male demand consideration: (1) genetic or constitutional tendencies, (2) cerebral or hypothalamic disorders, (3) testicular hyperfunction, and (4) adrenal cortical overactivity.

Constitutional Sexual Precocity

The majority of cases of precocious sexual development are, on investigation, found to be free of demonstrable organic disease. Within this group a small percentage of individuals will be found whose premature physical attainment has a genetic or hereditary basis. Careful history will usually reveal a family tendency in this direction. Children so affected will show early growth patterns. In the female, menstruation occurs and pregnancy is possible under 14 years of age. In the male, adult sexual activity may be noted at this relatively early period of life. These patients do not, interestingly enough, show abnormal titers of androgen, and as a rule live normally when maturity of mind parallels the prematurity of body.

Cerebral Disorders

Intracranial lesions on the floor of the third ventricle or near the pineal gland may involve a theoretical "sex center" in the posterior hypothalamus, or secondarily stimulate the anterior pituitary to increase secretion of gonadotropins by contiguous pressure and thus produce evidences of excessive maleness at an age not usually associated with such changes. Such lesions produce associated signs and symptoms of increased intracranial pressure such as nausea, vomiting, internal hydrocephalus, failing vision, and headache, of all which make the diagnosis an obvious one.

Testicular Abnormalities

Hypertestoidism is usually secondary to an abnormality of growth and function of the Leydig cell. The basic pathologic evidence may be simply interstitial cell hyperplasia, or it may be neoplastic in the form of adenoma or carcinoma. Whatever the cause, these patients show clinical evidences of virilism. The genitalia are large, accessory sex glands show hypertrophy and hyperfunction, muscular development is augmented, acne is present, and the hair pattern is that of an adult. Precocious libido is evident. Premature fusion of the epiphyses may permanently stunt the patient's growth. From the metabolic standpoint these patients have an increased output of 17-ketosteroids, the adrenal cortical metabolites (dehydroisoandrosterone, 11-oxygenated steroids, active corticoids). Careful palpatory examination of the testes is mandatory in all cases of precocity. Large, hard testes are characteristic of hyperplasia, while tumor is usually palpable as an isolated hard nodule, often with atrophy of the contralateral gonad. Testicular biopsy is not recommended in the case of suspected neoplasm, but surgical exposure and orchiectomy is both diagnostic and therapeutic in such cases. However, biopsy is an aid in the diagnosis of hyperplasia.

Adrenal Abnormalities

The term *adrenogenital syndrome* is applied descriptively to those cases of sexual precocity or heterosexual abnormality secondary to adrenocortical dysfunction.

For purposes of discussion these entities will be divided into two groups on the basis of the time of onset, i.e., pre- or postnatal.

PRENATAL ADRENOGENITAL SYNDROME

Congenital Virilizing Adrenal Hyperplasia.   At least six forms of congenital adrenal hyperplasia (Fig. 7–7) have been described in the literature, all with a common etiologic deficit inherent in the enzymatic biosynthesis of cortisol. The defect in cortisol output activates the reciprocal servomechanism that regulates hypothalamic pituitary adrenocortical function, thus causing an excessive output of ACTH with resultant adrenal cortical hyperplasia and an accelerated synthesis of adrenal cortical steroids. Precursors of cortisol accumulate behind the enzymatic blockade and are secreted. Synthetic pathways that lead to androgen production are not blocked and result in a rise in measurable output.

Of the six forms known, only three are predominantly virilizing. A partial C-21–hydroxylase defect leads to simple virilism. A complete C-21 defect leads to virilization with an associated salt-losing syndrome and impaired aldosterone secretion. Death in early infancy is common owing to the mineral cortical crises. These two entities account for 90 per cent of patients with adrenogenital syndrome.

A defect in hydroxylation at the C-11 position leads to virilization and hypertension with increased secretion of 11-desoxycorticosterone and 11-desoxycortisol plus excessive adrenal androgens.

The other defects involve a 3 β-hydroxysteroid-dehydrogenase defect with male or female pseudohermaphroditism and adrenal insufficiency, a 17 α-hydroxylase defect leading to male pseudohermaphro-

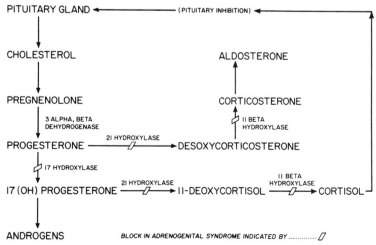

Figure 7–7   Disturbances in steroid biosynthesis in the adrenogenital syndrome.

ditism, sexual infantilism, hypertension, and hypokalemic alkalosis and finally a desmolase complex defect that produces sexual infantilism and adrenal insufficiency.

Patients with a predominantly virilizing syndrome have elevated levels of the 17-ketosteroid, 3 α-, 17 α-, 20 α-pregnanetriol in the urine with an associated elevation of plasma 17 α-hydroxyprogesterone.

Secretion of androgens postnatally leads to accelerated growth, stunting due to premature closure of the epiphyses, and masculinization of the female. Girls with the C-21–hydroxylase defect, in addition to being salt losers, are the most severely masculinized and are usually mistaken for males, having a penis and associated labioscrotal fusion. If only partial block of C-21-hydroxylase occurs, less masculinization is evident. Patients with the 11 β-hydroxylase defect exhibit only equivocal evidences such as clitoral enlargement. All have a common urogenital sinus with normal tubes and ovaries.

Males with adrenal hyperplasia show normal sexual development at birth, but pronounced virilism is soon evident, and if untreated, the high levels of circulating adrenal steroids suppress the release of gonadotropins, which cause the testes to remain infantile. Bone age is accelerated, and epiphyses fuse prematurely with stunting.

Diagnosis. The problem in diagnosis lies in the difficulty in differentiating the sexual ambiguity present in the newborn with adrenal cortical hyperplasia from that caused by genetic intersexuality. Physical examination, roentgenographic and urologic endoscopic examination alone are not sufficient to establish diagnosis. The physician must resort to chromosomal karyotype analyses, nuclear chromatin pattern, documentation of elevated urinary 17-ketosteroids, and abnormal urinary metabolites characteristic of the particular enzyme deficiency involved. It is essential to show that this abnormal output of metabolites can be suppressed by the administration of dexamethasone, confirming the fact that the adrenal lesion is due to hyperplasia and not neoplasm.

Differentiation of congenital adrenogenital syndrome must be made from the rare instance of infant virilization caused by an androgenic tumor in the mother that exists during pregnancy or from the mother's ingestion of androgenic agents (progestins) during pregnancy. These infants have normal urinary steroid levels.

In the male infant a Leydig cell testicular tumor may produce a virilizing syndrome. The tumor is usually palpable, and excretion of pregnene steroids is normal. Androgen producing adrenal neoplasms in the male, like the female, produce large amounts of 17-ketosteroids, mainly dehydroepiandrosterone. This abnormal steroid output is characteristically not suppressed by dexamethasone administration.

Treatment. The goal of therapy is to suppress adrenal activity by supplying cortisol or other glucocorticoids which inhibit corticotropin output, thus preventing secretion of adrenal androgens. Initial doses of 10 to 20 mg of cortisol per day for infants and 20 to 40 mg per day for children is desirable. Maintenance doses are then established on the basis of measured response of urinary ketosteroids, growth rates, and osseous development. Treatment must be continued through life in girls and withdrawn in late adolescence in males. There is some evidence to indicate a higher incidence of adrenal cortical carcinoma in untreated cases.

Infants with salt-losing syndromes demand prompt therapy with salt replacement intravenously plus 2 to 5 mg of 11-desoxycorticosterone intramuscularly. Cortisol succinate should be administered intravenously in 25 mg doses over the first 24 hours.

POSTNATAL ADRENOGENITAL SYNDROME

The most common cause of postnatal virilization in the female that is due to adrenal cortical overactivity is a tumor, usually malignant. Patients so involved show normal genital development at birth, but virilization is rapid in onset with both corticosexual and corticometabolic (Cushing's syndrome) presentation. The output of 17-ketosteroids is high, and urinary dehydroepiandrosterone is elevated. Pyelography, tomography, and selective angiography may aid in diagnosis.

Other causes of feminine virilization must be considered in the differential diagnosis. Ovarian arrhenoblastoma produces an identical clinical picture but without the corticometabolic abnormalities. Lipoid ovarian tumors, by contrast, often show characteristics of Cushing's syndrome, but muscular development is good, strength is preserved, and both urinary cortisol and urinary corticosteroids are normal. The level of 17-ketosteroids may be normal or slightly elevated. Urinary androgens are not elevated by administration of ACTH nor suppressed by dexamethasone.

FEMINIZING ADRENOGENITAL SYNDROME IN THE MALE

This entity is invariably the result of an adrenal tumor. It usually occurs in the twenties or thirties, but the author has seen one six-year-old patient with the abnormality. Patients usually have bilateral gynecomastia, testicular atrophy, loss of libido, obesity, and feminine hair distribution. The tumors are usually large and thus are detectable by radiographic techniques. Diagnosis is made by the discovery of high levels of urinary estrogens. The level of 17-ketosteroids is usually increased as well as metabolic end products of steroid metabolism. Stimulation with ACTH or suppression with dexamethasone is usually unrewarding.

Treatment involves radical surgical extirpation with supportive corticosteroid therapy postoperatively because of atrophy of the contralateral adrenal gland. The outlook is guarded when malignancy is present.

SEXUAL FUNCTION IN THE ADULT

The transition brought about by the onset of puberty leads directly to a consideration of the adult phase of sexual function. The function of the target organ with respect to spermatogenesis and androgen production has been discussed. The effect of androgen on the accessory sex glands has been mentioned and is further elaborated here.

PROSTATE GLAND

The prostate gland of the adult lies like a flattened cone with its base at the neck of the bladder in front of the rectum and its apex suspended by the urogenital diaphragm. It is pierced by the urethra and ejaculatory ducts and is enclosed in a firm fibrous capsule. While no attempt is made in this chapter to give the details of its anatomy and embryology, both of these factors play a considerable role in the prostate gland's physiology and so are considered briefly together here. The spatial relationships of the prostate, divided as it is into five lobes, is best understood by visualizing the urethra and duct systems as they are associated with the gland. Embryologically, this musculoglandular structure arises from the urethra as five distinct groups of evaginating buds that soon form tubules and separate into the five lobes. Each tubular system lies in a bed of fibromuscular stroma, and in the adult stage no actual distinct barrier can be noted between lobes except the posterior, which remains distinct and may actually have a separate function from the others. The posterior lobe lies below the ejaculatory ducts and utricle, the lateral lobes are placed on each side, the anterior above the urethra, and the median between the urethra and the ejaculatory ducts. The gland system is really of two types: those external or peripheral in the substance of the gland, made up of folliclelike tubules, each with an excretory duct opening into the urethra; and those internal or periurethral in location. Both systems have a layer of smooth muscle surrounding the gland and its duct for purposes of emptying. Supplied by the hypogastric plexus, the terminal nerve fibers have been said to possess sensory, secretory, and motor functions.

The prostate shows only gradual growth during the prepubertal phase of male existence, but at puberty the organ greatly increases in size and all lobes, except the anterior, are affected to the same degree. There is a thickening of the muscular tissue surrounding the tubular elements and an increase in the amount of interlobular and intralobular connective tissue. Active secretion commences at this time and is the specific function of the columnar acinar epithelium under endocrine stimulus, which is supplemented by chemical and nervous stimuli. The fluid is formed and excreted in small amounts daily in a phase described by Huggins (1946–47) as the "resting secretion," usually totaling 0.5 to 2.0 ml per day. This material is removed during acts of urination, with the individual unaware of its formation.

The resting phase is greatly augmented during ejaculation by parasympathetic stimulation, with the production of 3 to 5 ml of opalescent fluid that makes up about 80 to 85 per cent of the volume of the ejaculate. This stimulus appears to result in two separate intracellular processes: a washing out of material already formed within the cell, largely citrate and protein, and an active increase in the secretion of chlorides and certain enzymes. The response to such stimuli is variable. The experiments of Huggins suggest that there are strong and weak secretory glands, a factor of importance in evaluating the sexual function of the individual. Fatigue effects are observed when ejaculation occurs at very short intervals with marked reduction of fluid volume and protein content. The normal 4 to 5 ml quantity may be reduced to as low as 1.0 ml if ejaculation is repeated within an hour; it returns to 2.0 ml if two hours elapse between orgasms, and resumes normal levels within 24 hours. Some of the strong secretory glands show very little evidence of fatigue on repeated ejaculation. It is known that secretory volume is adversely affected by starvation, systemic illness, chronic prostatic infection, and the withdrawal of either pituitary or testicular sources of stimulation. Androgen administered to the normal adult has little effect on secretory output but if given to the prepubertal male or castrate a definite increase in the mass of the glandular cell results, followed by active mitosis and increased secretion.

In animals the same quantitative response is obtained from 5 mg of androgen as is obtained with 25 mg, suggesting that there is a maximum response with a definite amount of the hormone beyond which no further activity is obtained despite an increase in the dose of the drug used. Withdrawal of androgens by orchiectomy in the adult causes a measurable decrease in secretion within 24 hours and cessation of all activity by 7 to 23 days after the procedure. Orchiectomy is associated with marked prostatic gland cell reduction and reduction in epithelial height, nuclear size, and acinous diameter. The epithelium becomes pseudostratified and the nuclei become pyknotic. This change is reversible through the administration of androgen once again. Estrogens produce a similar response through pituitary secretory depression. Huggins has shown that 0.4 mg of diethylstilbestrol effectively neutralizes 10 mg of testosterone propionate as measured by prostatic secretory activity. Under the influence of estrogen, cytologic changes occur in the gland characterized by metaplasia of the columnar epithelium of the ducts, posterior urethra, and utriculus to stratified squamous cell type. This is also a reversible process should androgen be allowed to resume its normal role in function.

Stimulation of the nerve supply to the gland causes increased secretion, as do parasympathomimetic drugs. Sectioning of the nerve supply has no adverse effect on the hormonal response.

Thus, as a result of the androgenic stimulus brought on by puberty, the prostate engages in an active secretion of chemical origin known as the resting secretion. This is augmented by parasympathetic nervous stimulation which occurs during erotic arousal, producing a fluid of a different chemical nature that is subject to the fatigue of overactivity and dependent on the inherent secretory "strength" of the gland. Both forms of secretion are materially affected by debility, inanition, the withdrawal of androgens, and the administration of estrogens.

The product of secretory activity is delivered from the urethra in a liquid state. It coagulates on standing, only to undergo subsequent liquefaction within 10 to 15 minutes of ejaculation. This latter process is due to the presence of the proteolytic enzyme fibrinolysin. It in turn is rapidly inactivated by fibrinogenase, which is also present in the gland. The prostatic fluid has a pH of 6.4, is 93 to 98 per cent water, and contains cations of sodium, potassium, calcium, and a concentration of zinc higher than that contained in any other tissue fluid. Castration and estrogens reduce the uptake of radioactive zinc by the prostate, but the administration of testosterone will reverse this effect. It is felt that zinc plays a very important role in sperm metabolism. The anions are chiefly chloride and citrate. Sugars are present in remarkably small amounts compared to the high concentration of fructose in seminal vesicular fluid, which again is a factor in sperm metabolism.

Prostatic fluid contains large amounts of the polyamines spermine and spermidine, as well as water soluble choline derivatives. Lipids are present as cephalin and as cholesterol. The enzyme β-glucuronidase is found in prostatic fluid, and it may represent a concentrating mechanism for hormones in target organs since sex hormones are believed to circulate in the blood stream largely as soluble glucuronides.

Another enzyme, acid phosphatase, is found in large amounts. In the prepubertal male as little as 1.5 King-Armstrong (KA) units per gram of tissue can be isolated, while at puberty this increases to 73 KA units per gram and in the adult is present in amounts ranging from 522 to 2284 KA units per gram. Alkaline phosphatase is also present but in small amounts (0.25 to 3.4 KA units per gram). The cellular distribution of these enzymes has been shown by Gomori to be quite different. Alkaline phosphatase occurs chiefly in the walls of capillaries, while the acid phosphatase is present only in the glandular epithelial cell or in the secretions within the lumina of the acini. Active secretions of the enzymes occur during sexual stimulation. The acid phosphatase contained in prostatic fluid obtained after ejaculation in man ranges from 1890 to 3950 KA units while that obtained by digital expression was 117 to 1192 KA units. The secretion of acid phosphatase is then one of the functions of the acinar epithelial cell. Alkaline phosphatase on the other hand was found to be present in amounts of 2.25 KA units after sexual stimulation and 27 KA units during resting secretion, or that obtained by digital expression. Active secretion evidently washed out only small amounts of alkaline phosphatase as would be expected from its cellular location, mentioned above. As yet, no definite function can be ascribed to acid phosphatase other than the fact that it has been found to hydrolyze the phosphorylcholine produced by the seminal vesicles, thus liberating choline and inorganic phosphorus. Normally, acid phosphatase does not enter the bloodstream from the prostate in any appreciable amount. This is not true in prostatic carcinoma, a factor to be considered further under the discussion of involutional changes. Another enzyme, aconitase, is found in large amounts in the prostate and is responsible for the conversion of *cis*-aconitic acid to citric acid. Citric acid is present in high concentrations in prostatic tissue and may function in the accumulation of calcium and possibly the precipitation of calcium salts within the gland.

From this brief discussion it is evident that the prostate is not the simple structure that it was formerly thought to be but is rather a highly complex gland whose chief function is to provide a suitable fluid means of transport for the sperm. Probably other activities and effects exist, but these are as yet unknown. The presence of numerous enzyme systems and the high concentrations of ions present suggest a nutritive function with respect to the sperm and possibly some specific action on the metabolism of this tiny, independently active unit.

SEMINAL VESICLES

The seminal vesicles intimately share in the endocrine changes mentioned in the above discussion of prostatic physiology. They, too, are dependent on androgen stimulation for growth and function and are adversely affected by specific and generalized disease, the withdrawal of androgen, or the administration of estrogen. Anatomically these structures lie as symmetrically lobulated pouches behind the bladder and above the prostate. They join with the ampulla of the vas deferens to form the ejaculatory ducts which in turn penetrate the prostate gland and open at the verumontanum on each side of the prostate utricle. Their internal structure consists of a convoluted tubular pattern divided by septa made up of folds of mucosa. The glands are surrounded by a fibromuscular stroma and are supplied by nerves from the hypogastric plexus. Secretion occurs as a continuous process, the contents of the gland being forcibly ejected during ejaculation. It is not known whether there is a resting and active secretory phase similar to that found in the prostate. The glandular product is a yellow viscid substance of tapiocalike consistency with a pH of 6.7. Huggins and Johnson have shown it to contain a large amount of reducing substance, probably the greatest source of sugar so essential to the life of the sperm outside of the seminal tract. Miller and Bauguess have demonstrated that most of the potassium, sodium, and total nitrogen of the ejaculate are produced by this structure. These findings tend to refute the older teaching that the seminal vesicles are primarily storehouses for sperm.

GLANDS OF COWPER AND LITTRE

The two other accessory sex glands, Cowper's and Littre's, have minor functions but are also representative of gonadal activity. Cowper's glands are situated as two small compact pea-sized lobules within the substance of the external vesical sphincter and on ejaculation or sexual stimulation produce a clear mucoid secretion rich in albumin. The glands are emptied by the contraction of this sphincter. Situated along the course of the urethra, the glands of Littre provide a fluid of similar consistency.

Integrated Ejaculatory Response

The cellular process of spermatogenesis and the endocrine secretory function of the accessory sex glands would be of little use without an integrated nervous system control.

There are three primary responses to erotic stimuli: (1) a general response motivated by the autonomic system, (2) an erectile response, and (3) an ejaculatory response (Figs. 7–8 and 7–9).

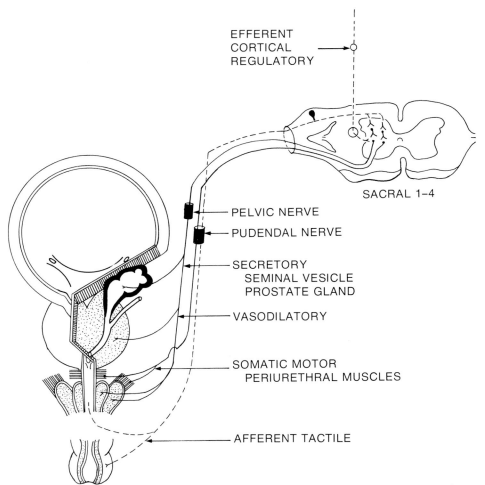

EFFERENT
CORTICAL
REGULATORY

SACRAL 1–4

PELVIC NERVE

PUDENDAL NERVE

SECRETORY
SEMINAL VESICLE
PROSTATE GLAND

VASODILATORY

SOMATIC MOTOR
PERIURETHRAL MUSCLES

AFFERENT TACTILE

Figure 7–8   Integrated functional nervous system connections in the processes of erection and ejaculation.

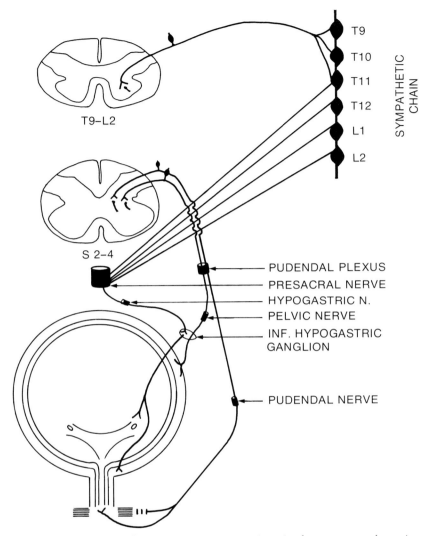

T9
T10
T11
T12
L1
L2

SYMPATHETIC
CHAIN

T9–L2

S 2–4

PUDENDAL PLEXUS
PRESACRAL NERVE
HYPOGASTRIC N.
PELVIC NERVE
INF. HYPOGASTRIC
GANGLION

PUDENDAL NERVE

Figure 7–9 Integrated functional nervous system connections in the processes of erection and ejaculation.

The general autonomic reaction is marked by an increased pulse rate, a rise in blood pressure, an increased peripheral blood flow, and a diminution of auditory and visual senses.

The erectile response may be a basic lower motor neuron reflex arc phenomenon of no sexual significance, such as is seen in the child or adult with a full bladder, or it may have erotic origin through tactile afferent stimuli arising from the genitalia. These stimuli are mediated over the pudendal nerve to sacral segments 2, 3, and 4 and then via parasympathetic pathways (pelvic nerve), which are vasodilatory to the penile corporal arterial supply, producing an erection which is maintained by the opening of arteriovenous shunts and the concomitant inhibition of venous outflow. The erectile response may also have its origin in higher centers mediated over corticospinal pathways at the same time as facilitory stimuli to the lower motor neuron sacral reflex arc centers duplicate the process of erection. One of the penalties of evolutionary sophistication of the nervous system has been the addition of the phenomenon of erectile inhibition, which again arises in the higher centers, is often subconscious, and is mediated over the same corticospinal pathways with a resultant loss of erection by reversal of the process.

The ejaculatory response is more complex and while it may follow erection, it is independent of it. Sexual arousal, whether tactile lower motor neuron sacral reflex arc or upper motor neuron facilitory in origin, produces not only erection but also parasympathetic secretory activity of the gland cells of the seminal vesicles and prostate gland, creating an "active" secretion. On reaching summation, sympathetic stimuli by way of the upper lumbar communicating rami 1, 2, 3, and the hypogastric nerve permit closure of the bladder neck that prevents retrograde ejaculation, stimulates forward propulsion of spermatozoa from the testes through the ductule efferentes and epididymis into the vas deferens, and finally promotes contraction of smooth muscle of the seminal vesicles and prostate in order to evacuate the contents of their accumulated active secretions that are now mixed with spermatozoa into the posterior urethra.

The stimulus of this bolus of seminal fluid in the posterior urethra sends afferent stimuli via the pudendal nerve to the sacral cord 2, 3, and 4 and via efferents over the same nerve to the striated musculature of the perineum (ischiocavernosus, bulbocavernosus, and transverse perinei). The tetanic contraction and relaxation of these muscles force the bolus of semen from the urethra to complete the process of ejaculation. Conscious awareness of this activity constitutes the orgasm.

In summary there exists a complex phenomenon involving sympathetic, parasympathetic, and central nervous systems, upper and lower motor neuron coordination, secretory activity, vasodilatory effect, and the utilization of both smooth and striated muscle to accomplish a single purpose. Its complexity places the physician in a position of awe and provides some insight with respect to the problems faced when the orderly process goes awry.

Functional Aspect of Sexual Outlet

Discussion of this aspect of sexual function, once the limited sphere of the textbook and consultation room, has become so commonplace that few individuals, regardless of age, can plead ignorance of the procreative act. The newsstand, radio, television, and lecture hall have replaced the poolroom as the source of information on a topic once considered restricted, and the public, as recipient, has exhibited a degree of enthusiasm that would do credit to a thwarted Victorian adolescent.

It is not the purpose of this section to comment on the social aspects of the sexual revolution of the past twenty-five years. It is worthwhile, however, to point out that the welter of information available on the subject has created an emphasis on one aspect of bodily function in excess of its psychologic and physiologic importance to the individual and to society as a whole and presents the physician with a dilemma in his role as advisor. It has become increasingly difficult for the physician to establish a point of reference with respect to sexual function. What is normal? What is abnormal? What is acceptable? What is unacceptable? Who is an expert? It is both dangerous and unwise for a physician to use his own experience as an example, for at best it must be considered limited.

Recognizing this fact, biologic statisticians have employed the techniques of Mr. Gallup to poll the public in order to obtain a broad spectrum of behavior characteristics for purposes of comparison. The results, while open to interpretation, have provided information of value.

As an example, frequency of sexual outlet has been studied and the experience of thousands from adolescence to old age recorded. As expected, average sexual outlet varies according to certain biologic factors such as age, metabolic rate, nutritional status, hereditary pattern, and psychologic conditioning. The frequency of sexual outlet is further modified by environment and social factors of the particular segment of society in which the individual lives. The variation in any group chosen at random is remarkably high; so much so, that it is difficult to say what is normal or abnormal with respect to frequency of sexual outlet.

Kinsey and co-workers (1948) state that over 75 per cent of the population have intercourse from one to six times per week, while nearly a quarter (22.3 per cent) may be classified as in the extremes of over- or underactivity. Of those questioned by him, 7.6 per cent had as many as seven experiences per week, a few as high as 20 to 30 per week, and some as little as two to three times a year. E. J. Farris of the Wistar Institute has made an extensive study of the use of artificial insemination in problems of barrenness and has noted that his donors, all young males in good health, require at least three to five days between donations before the ejaculate returns to normal in all components. Of hundreds examined, only a few have shown the capacity for frequent ejaculation without reduction in cell count and volume, and even they show appreciable changes after three days of consecutively delivered specimens. Considering the average then, it would appear that frequency of two to three times a week would be the most physiologic from the standpoint of satisfying the demands of fertility. This does not imply that rates higher than this are abnormal, nor that fertilization is the sole purpose of sexual activity. The physician should recognize that the variations mentioned do occur, and that if they suit the needs of the individual, they can hardly be considered beyond the limits of normal.

In his role as advisor, the physician is seldom confronted with problems of function in excess of normal, and whenever he is, the facts usually reveal a misconception of role and a misunderstanding of what was expected. While modern education has dispelled some of the myths surrounding performance in the young adult, there is no doubt that tales of sexual accomplishment, particularly with regard to frequency of outlet, are usually far in excess of practice. The inexperienced individual, cognizant of such tales, may find it a bit of a shock when he fails to measure up. In this instance reassurance that he falls within the norm and is not doomed to a life of sexual failure is all that is required. Occasionally the role of sexual athlete is found to be a coverup for an underlying personality disorder and as such falls within the sphere of psychotherapy.

By contrast, performance less than normally expected may indicate severe underlying organic disease. The previous discussion of prepubertal sexual failure is pertinent. In the adult diseases of the central nervous system that affect erectile and ejaculatory function, diseases of the vascular system and entities producing general debility may seriously affect sexual function. A careful history and physical survey as well as indicated laboratory studies usually serve to pinpoint the existence of such factors. Trauma or disease involving the spinal cord may destroy the function of erection if the sacral segments, cauda equina, and pelvic parasympathetic plexuses are involved. Absence of erection in these instances is usually associated with a loss of the bulbocavernosus-rectal reflex, a patulous anal sphincter, and autonomous vesical dysfunction. If spinal cord trauma is above the sacral segments, erectile function may return after recovery from spinal shock, but unfortunately it is frequently uncontrolled and uninhibited. It may accompany massive reflex activity in the lower extremities and may be abnormally sustained, particularly in high cervical lesions.

Ejaculation is a more complex spinal segmental reflex function that involves the parasympathetic secretory stimulation to the accessory sex glands, the sympathetic smooth muscle expulsive capacity of the same structures, including closure of the vesical neck to prevent retrograde ejaculation, and finally somatic striated muscle activity via the pudendal nerve and sacral arc to forcibly expel semen from the urethra. Any discussion of disturbances of ejaculation must therefore consider all three nervous systems. In brief, it may be said that ejaculation is abolished by cord damage between the sixth thoracic and third lumbar segments. To abolish the ejaculatory response effectively, damage must be extensive within these limits. Patients subjected to sympathectomy with complete removal of lumbar one to three bilaterally experience ejaculatory impotence. If the ganglia are removed to L_1 on one side and D_{12} on the other, the process is not disturbed. Trauma is seldom this selective. In addition, the second step in the ejaculatory response must also be considered, namely the stimulus set off by the bolus of semen in the posterior urethra with efferents synapsing in the sacral cord, returning via the internal pudendal nerve to the periurethral striated muscles in order to set up the forces of seminal expulsion. Loss of the sacral cord and cauda equina will abolish this aspect of ejaculation.

Far more common than the organic causes for sexual failure are those of psychic origin. It is safe to say that 90 per cent of patients who present with a primary problem of impotence have as a basis for the complaint some disturbance in facilitation mediated over corticospinal pathways. At one point in man's evolutionary development his main concern at the time of sexual intercourse, other than the pure enjoyment of the act, was that he might be attacked by a predator in this relatively defenseless position. The rapid ejaculatory response characteristic of lower forms is said to be a reflection of this basic insecurity. Such fundamental evolutionary concerns have been replaced in modern times by a more diverse set of interfering stimuli, ranging from the unexpected return of the husband of the lady seduced, to conscious or subconscious consideration of the effects of a falling stock market on the estate of the performer. Whatever form the inhibitory stimulus may assume, its effect is equally devastating. Erectile impotence, once experienced, creates a lasting problem. The insecurity introduced by failure makes further attempts at facilitation at the next effort even more difficult. Thus, negative reinforcement compounds the problem as impotence, complete or partial, becomes a way of life. Interruption of the cycle may be attained through counsel. Insight and reassurance may be all that is required; if impotence is sustained, psychiatric therapy may be advisable. The common practice of administering androgen to these individuals is to be decried. Except for its supportive empirical role, such therapy is worthless, for the defect is not organic, and no amount of androgen therapy will alter the situation. Ejaculatory impotence is far less common than erectile but does occur. Fear of impregnation may be an etiologic factor in many men. Premature ejaculation is far more common and is an accompaniment of the immature personality, the overresponder whose trigger mechanisms are set at a much lower level than normal for many body functions. Enuresis is a common accompaniment of the disorder. Therapy ranging from anesthetic jellies to psychiatrist's counseling may be required, usually with negative results.

Senescent Phase of Sexual Function

In contrast to the rather abrupt cessation of reproductive capacity in the female, the male experiences a gradually diminishing erotic response with declining years. The frequency of erection, the speed with which it is attained, and the duration prior to ejaculation are all affected. Sexual capacity reaches a peak in adolescence and from that period on shows a gradual decline paralleling similar changes in other cellular metabolic functions, as evidenced by a decreased capacity for work and expenditure of nervous energy.

The capacity to reach repeated climax is lost early in adult life, being rarely present after 40 years of age. The mean frequency of sexual outlet falls from two to three times per week in early adulthood to one time per week at 65 years and less by 75. Complete cessation of sexual activity is experienced by only 5 per cent of patients under 65, but by 75 years at least 50 per cent are so affected.

Interestingly enough, plasma testosterone levels usually remain within normal limits throughout old age. In those instances in which Leydig cell activity does decline, symptoms similar to the female climacteric may be evident. Since symptoms such as these may accompany other entities in the aging process, differentiation by androgen assay is helpful. The use of LH assays is not of benefit, since many men after 45 experience an increase in serum LH titers despite normal testosterone levels. If levels are below 0.15 microgram per liter, substitution therapy is indicated. Improvement in sexual function seldom occurs, but the benefits to be gained from a correction of negative nitrogen balance make such treatment worthwhile.

The prostate gland, like the testis, must bear its share of the burdens induced by the degenerative changes of age. Nodular glandular hyperplasia of the prostate gland displaces normal tissue, affecting not only the physiology of the gland itself but also, by reason of the outlet obstruction produced, threatening the very existence of the individual through the loss of vesical and renal function. In addition, 20 per cent of men so involved have carcinomatous changes within the glandular tissue that constitute a threat of even greater magnitude by reason of obstructive uropathy and eventual metastases to distant sites.

It is worthy of mention that palliative control of prostatic carcinoma was made possible through an understanding of the endocrine dependency of the prostate gland gained from the investigations by Charles Huggins and many others in the early 1940s. It is ironic that the endocrine dependencies of normal cellular physiology that are present to the benefit of man can reverse roles to participate in his destruction. The disappointment in the palliative rather than curative nature of Huggins' discovery is lessened perhaps by the knowledge that at this late stage of life man has completed a generation of sexual activity, has participated in the propagation of the species, and now must face the inevitable conclusion that life is ultimately finite. The contention of Alfred Scott Warthin that man's true immortality lies in the continuity of his germ plasm may be worthy of more than passing consideration.

SELECTED REFERENCES

Jones, H. W., and Scott, W. W.: Hermaphroditism, Genital Anomalies and Related Endocrine Disorders. 2nd ed. Baltimore, Williams & Wilkins Co., 1971.

Paulsen, C. A.: The Testis. *In* Williams, R. H. (ed.): Textbook of Endocrinology. 5th ed. Philadelphia, W. B. Saunders Company, 1974.

Robbins, S. L.: Pathologic Basis of Disease. Philadelphia, W. B. Saunders Company, 1974.

REFERENCES

Barr, M. L., and Bertram, E. G.: A morphological distinction between neurones of the male and female behavior of the nucleolar satellite during accelerated nucleoprotein synthesis. Nature (Lond.), *163*:676, 1949.

Brown, J. S., Dubin, L., Becher, M., and Hotchkiss, R. S.: Venography in subfertile man with varicocele. J. Urol., 98:388, 1967.

Bunge, R. G.: Intersexuality. *In* Campbell, M. F., and Harrison, J. H. (eds.): Urology. 3rd ed. Philadelphia, W. B. Saunders Company, 1970.

Grumbach, M. M., and Van Wyk, J. J.: Disorders of Sex Differentiation. *In* Williams, R. G. (ed.): Textbook of Endocrinology. 5th ed. Philadelphia, W. B. Saunders Company, 1974, pp. 423–496.

Huggins, C. B.: The Prostatic Secretion. The Harvey Lecture Series. XLII, 1946–7, pp. 148–193.

Jirosek, J.: Development of the Genital System and Male Pseudohermaphroditism. Johns Hopkins University Press, 1971.

Jost, A.: A new look at the mechanisms controlling sex differentiation in mammals. Johns Hopkins Med. J., *130*:38, 1972.

Kinsey, A. C., Pomeroy, W. B., and Martin, C. E.: Sexual Behavior in the Human Male. Philadelphia, W. B. Saunders Company, 1948.

Lyon, M. F.: X-chromosome inactivation and developmental patterns in mammals. Biol. Rev., *47*:1, 1972.

Tessler, A. N., and Krahn, H. P.: Varicocele and testicular temperature. Fertil. Steril., *17*:201, 1966.

Chapter Eight

URINARY INFECTION

Jack Lapides

BACILLARY AND ENTEROCOCCAL INFECTIONS

Physiopathology

HOST RESISTANCE

Except for acute staphylococcal and tuberculous infections of the kidney, most cases of bacterial pyelonephritis begin at the bladder level as a cystitis. Thus, it is most important to clearly define the basic physiopathologic mechanisms involved in the genesis of cystitis and the clinical conditions which trigger these mechanisms.

In general, invasion of body tissues by bacteria is determined by the interaction of the microorganism and the resistance of the host. When the resistance of the host is inadequate, the germ will gain a foothold in the tissue and multiply. On the other hand if the host resistance is sufficient, the organism will not damage the tissue. Numerous illustrations of the latter can be readily observed in the presence of pathogens on the skin, oropharynx, colon, or vagina of the healthy individual. Experimentally, Hinman introduced pathogens into the urinary bladder of healthy humans and found that they disappeared within 48 hours without producing a cystitis.

If host resistance is the determinant of infection, what impairs it insofar as the urinary tract is concerned? Without delving into minutiae it can be stated that tissue integrity and blood supply are major factors in protecting body tissues from the onslaught of the ubiquitous bacterium. A breakdown in the surface of the lining of the bladder is often the result of erosion caused by the presence of an indwelling catheter, the action of a mobile calculus with a roughened, irregular exterior, the growth of an exophytic neoplasm, or invasion of the tissue by a parasite (e.g., schistosomiasis). All of these conditions often are associated with pyuria and bacteruria.

However, the majority of urinary tract infections follow ischemic episodes that involve the bladder and are caused by overdistention of the bladder and high intravesical pressures. In the female child, delayed development of voluntary control over detrusor contraction is the most common entity leading to cystitis and pyelonephritis. High pressures in these children occur when they attempt to prevent urination. The mechanism is described in detail under the heading "Uninhibited Neurogenic Bladder" in Chapter Six. Essentially, the little girl does not develop control over the bladder at the time of toilet-training but does attain voluntary activity over the periurethral striated muscle. Thus, when her bladder is filled with urine to the point where a reflex contraction of the detrusor is set off and she is not in a situation appropriate to emptying or she chooses not to void, she prevents urine from being propelled through the urethra by constricting it through the voluntary contraction of the encircling periurethral striated muscle. The final effect of a healthy detrusor contracting against a closed urethra is to raise the intravesical pressure to levels ranging from 100 to 250 cm of water. Contrast this pressure to the normal voiding pressures of 15 to 40 cm and one can readily comprehend the ischemia, bladder trabeculation, vesical diverticula, and ureteric reflux which ensue when the situation is not corrected. The phenomenon can be reproduced by merely having a normal patient initiate a voiding contraction of the bladder without being able to expel the fluid from the bladder and recording the intravesical pressure with a manometer through an inlying catheter.

On a physiopathologic basis, it is readily apparent that the disease process can be reversed by simply having the child void as soon as the uncontrolled contraction begins, which is heralded by the almost simultaneous onset of the desire to urinate. Another approach involves regular periodic voiding by the clock that is frequent enough to empty the bladder before the uninhibited contraction occurs. A third remedy entails the use of anticholinergic drugs such as Ditropan (oxybutynin chloride), Pro-Banthine, or tincture of belladonna to suppress the uncontrolled motor impulses and frequent voiding.

With this concept fresh in mind, consider the high intravesical pressures which occur with urethral obstruction, e.g., vesical neck contracture, prostatic hyperplasia, prostatic carcinoma, posterior urethral valves (in boys), and urethral strictures. In these individuals the neuroregulatory apparatus is normal in that they can initiate a voiding contraction at will, inhibit the onset of a voiding contraction when the bladder is full, and stop urination abruptly. However, their trouble occurs when they voluntarily set off an emptying contraction of the bladder but cannot expel the fluid from the bladder because of a structural impediment somewhere along the urethra. As in the case of the little girl who constricts her urethra volitionally in an attempt to prevent propulsion of urine through the urethra when an uncontrolled detrusor contraction occurs, the bladder muscle contracts against a closed system, and its energy is used to produce tension and high intravesical pressures rather than to dissipate the energy by contracting down and propelling urine through the urethra. This action is known as isometric rather than isotonic contraction of the detrusor fibers.

The disease process in the structurally obstructed patient can be cured by the removal of the prostate gland, correction of the stricture, or incising the urethral valve and allowing the bladder to contract isotonically rather than isometrically.

A second major pathophysiologic way of decreasing host resistance and inducing cystitis is overdistention of the bladder. The voluntary inhibition of urination for prolonged periods of time is by far the most common cause for recurrent urinary infection in adult women; it occurs to a lesser extent in girls and males. This infrequent voiding has been found to be associated with the relative unavailability and uncleanliness of public female urinals, undergarment styles, types of occupation, and the attitudes of school teachers and employers. Infrequent voiding not only leads to recurrent urinary infection but is the main reason for the majority of atonic, decompensated bladders with partial or complete urinary retention that are observed in women. In the early stages therapy is directed toward having the patient institute a regimen of voiding every two to three hours during the day and from one to two times at night regardless of the sensation of fullness and desire to void. The more advanced cases may need a cholinergic drug like bethanechol chloride to stimulate the detrusor and an alpha adrenergic blocker such as Dibenzyline to decrease urethral resistance. Women with the permanently decompensated bladders may need to be on a regimen of self-catheterization.

Sexual intercourse, bubble-baths, cleanliness of the female perineum, and vaginal flora are believed to be of no significance in the occurrence of urinary infection in the female.

BACTERIAL INVADER

Practically all of the urinary infections are caused by gram-negative organisms derived from the patient's own intestinal tract. The most common causative bacterium is Escherichia coli; other frequently found germs include pseudomonas, proteus, aerobacter, klebsiella, and streptococcus faecalis.

The bacteria can reach the bladder by way of the blood stream, lymphatics, or urethra. The most common route is unknown for patients not on an inlying catheter. *As mentioned previously, recognition of factors that decrease host resistance is much more important in the treatment of urinary infection than is the determination of the pathway of invasion of the microorganism.*

BACILLARY PYELONEPHRITIS

Most bacillary inflammations of the kidney follow infections of the bladder, which spread to the upper tracts by way of the ureteric lumen, blood vessels, and lymphatic channels. Incompetence of the uretero-vesical valve that leads to a regurgitation of bladder contents up the ureter to the kidney is a common cause for acute pyelonephritis in little girls, with recurrent urinary infection due to the uninhibited neurogenic bladder. It is extremely important to note that the ureteric valve incompetence and the reflux are rarely primary but secondary to the recurrent cystitis and high intravesical pressures. The cure is treatment of the uninhibited neurogenic bladder and not solely the ureteric reimplantation into the bladder. Pyelonephritis can be readily controlled by simply solving the lower urinary tract problem.

In some cases bacillary pyelonephritis may be primary in the kidney wherein host resistance has been decreased by the presence of a calculus, growth of a neoplasm, infection by an acid-fast or staphylococcal organism, congenital anomaly causing hydronephrosis, or trauma. Obviously, the gram-negative organisms must have reached the kidney by way of the transient bacteremias, which occur repeatedly in the daily living of the normal individual. Again, eradication of the pyelonephritis in these patients requires restoration of normal host resistance by removing the calculus or performing a ureteropyeloplasty.

Diagnosis

The determination of the presence of a urinary tract infection, like any other disease process, involves a complete workup of the patient that includes a history, physical examination, and laboratory studies as a minimum effort. However, from a practical viewpoint the urinalysis is the major determinant of the final diagnosis, and thus a discussion of the examination of the urine is essential. Strictly speaking, the presence of bacteria in the *uncontaminated* urine specimen, regardless of colony count, indicates a urinary infection. The requisite that there must be a bacterial colony count of at least 100,000 per cubic ml before a diagnosis can be made is a popular misconception derived from a distortion of a practical method for estimating urinary infection in mass public health surveys. It has been determined that a physician would make the correct diagnosis in approximately 88 per cent of cases with urinary infection if the sole criterion was a colony count of 100,000 or more on culture. The microscopic examination of the urine, including the sediment stained with methylene blue, is at least as accurate as the culture and has the advantages of immediacy and economy.

URINE SURVEY

Urinalysis.   The urine should be examined for pH, specific gravity, albuminuria, glycosuria, red blood cells, leukocytes, and bacteria. A normal, clean, voided urine is negative for sugar and protein on routine testing; and microscopy of the centrifuged sediment reveals no more than an occasional leukocyte, erythrocyte, or bacterium per high power field. The presence of some bacteria or white blood cells in every high power field is indicative of a urinary infection.

Culture.   The culture is a useful method for determining the type of organism and its sensitivity to antibacterial medication after diagnosis has been made with the microscope.

Clinical Picture

Cystitis.   The patient with acute bacterial invasion of the bladder wall complains of increased frequency of urination (pollakiuria), burning and discomfort during urination (dysuria), and urgency. In severe cases the individual may manifest urinary incontinence and strangury. The patient may have noted a bloody, cloudy, or malodorous urine.

Physical examination may disclose suprapubic tenderness on palpation of the abdomen. The urethra and bladder often are painful to touch per vagina or rectum. Fever is present in the severe, acute case.

The urinalysis reveals the presence of bacteria and leukocytes, and culture is positive.

In the uncomplicated case, the excretory urogram shows normal kidneys, ureters, and bladder. On cystoscopy the epithelial lining of the bladder appears inflamed, edematous, and perhaps may bleed on examination.

Pyelonephritis.   The patient with acute pyelonephritis usually appears quite ill with fever, chills, nausea, and complains of flank pain in addition to the findings of cystitis. On examination of the back, pain will be elicited by prodding the costovertebral angle area. The urine is infected, and the excretory urogram may show delayed visualization because of the interstitial and tubular involvement of the parenchyma by the organism, and hydroureteronephrosis due to impairment of peristalsis of the calyces, pelvis, and ureter. These structures are also invaded by the microorganisms and their function affected by the toxins produced as well as by the inflammatory response.

When the cause for the acute pyelonephritis is not determined and repeated episodes occur, chronic pyelonephritis ensues. Chronic involvement of the kidneys can occur insidiously in that the acute episodes may be minimal, without symptoms or signs of renal infection, or, for that matter, of cystitis. As mentioned previously, when repeated episodes of cystitis lead to incompetence of the ureterovesical valve and reflux begins, further bouts of cystitis or the persistence of cystitis will inevitably cause first, acute, and then chronic pyelonephritis.

The clinical course of chronic pyelonephritis is one of low grade, progressive renal deterioration that is usually associated with persistent or recurrent cystitis. In the author's experience if the lower urinary tract problem can be solved, the kidneys can be readily cleared of active infection and the loss of renal function arrested. Only the decreased renal function tests and roentgenographic evidence of changes of chronic pyelonephritis will remain as residua of the previous active involvement.

The detailed pyelographic changes are discussed in Chapter Three. Suffice it to state that the infection, necrosis, and scarring that occurs in the kidney results in shrinking the size of the kidney, an irregular parenchymal surface or kidney outline, and an abnormal configuration of the collecting system. Some parts of the collecting system appear constricted while others are dilated; the calyces are bulbous and the infundibula may be narrowed. Frequently only a portion of the kidney, such as an upper or lower pole, may undergo changes while the rest remains normal.

IDENTIFICATION OF THE FACTOR IMPAIRING HOST RESISTANCE

By far the most important facet in the diagnosis of urinary infection is the determination of the weak spot in the patient's defense which permitted invasion by the pathogen. Thus, the physician needs to evaluate each part of the urinary tract, and this scrutiny may require endoscopy, cystometry, and urography, including excretory or retrograde pyelography, voiding cystourethrogram, arteriography, and laminagraphy. If the primary diagnostic tests reveal a neurogenic bladder, more detailed neurologic examinations may be required, and discovery of a calculus necessitates a battery of laboratory tests to seek the cause for the formation of the stone.

As previously proposed, the most common entities that decrease host resistance in the female are the uninhibited neurogenic bladder and infrequent voiding. In the young female child, the most frequent cause is the uninhibited or infantile bladder and to a lesser extent the infrequent voider, while the reverse is true in the adult. In the male infant and young boy, stenosis of the urethral meatus and posterior urethral valves commonly precipitate urinary infection, while obstructive uropathy in the prostatic urethra is the leading cause in the adult male.

A myriad of diseases of the genitourinary system can lead to urinary infection but to a lesser extent than those previously mentioned. Some of these are bladder exstrophy, epispadias, ureterocele, ectopic ureter; carcinoma of urethra, bladder, ureter, and pelvis; prostatic, vesical, ureteric, and kidney calculus disease; intersex problems; enterovesical fistulas; supravesical urinary diversion; urethral diverticula; condyloma acuminata of the urethra; interstitial, radiation, and cancer chemotherapy cystitis; polycystic kidney disease.

Because recurrent urinary infection in the older male is often misdiagnosed as chronic prostatitis, it is well to note that true chronic prostatitis is an infrequent entity, rarely symptomatic, usually secondary to urethrocystitis, and easily eradicated provided host resistance factors can be corrected. Primary chronic prostatitis can occur with prostatic calculi and prostatic neoplasm.

Many of the men with recurrent urinary infection have early obstructive uropathy as the basis for their infection. The prostatism is often not recognized because the patient still has a fair stream and no residual urine. Despite these minimal findings, the bladder muscle may have undergone considerable hypertrophy with a marked increase in the intravesical voiding pressure because of the prostatic obstruction. The abnormally elevated intravesical voiding pressure leads to ischemia of the bladder wall and increased susceptibility of the vesical tissue to invasion by bacteria. If this situation is misinterpreted as chronic prostatitis and treatment consists only of antibacterial medication, the immediate episode of infection may be cleared, but without any doubt the infection will recur because the basic factor decreasing host resistance has not been corrected, namely, prostatectomy for the prostatic obstruction.

There are a number of adult males who have been diagnosed as having chronic prostatitis on the basis of symptoms of perineal discomfort, inguinal aching, scrotal pangs, and impotence. These individuals have no abnormal findings on physical, laboratory, endoscopic, or urographic examination and should be given psychotherapy rather than antibacterials and prostatic massage.

Treatment

The basic principles involved in the therapy of urinary infection include (1) identification and removal of the factor decreasing host resistance and (2) eradication of the invading organism with appropriate antibacterial medication. From the foregoing discussion, it is apparent that a rather wide range of operative procedures and medical regimens are necessary to rejuvenate host resistance, e.g., pyelolithotomy, urethroplasty, repair of vesicovaginal fistula, prostatectomy, resection of bladder tumor, incision of urethral valves, drug treatment for tuberculosis or schistosomiasis, and alkalinization of urine for uric acid and cystine stone formers.

In most of the girls and women with recurrent urinary infection, a program of voiding frequently enough to avoid overdistention and elevated intravesical pressures can cure the repeated episodes of cystitis. On a normal intake of food and fluids, urinating every two to three hours during the day and once or twice at night handles the situation very well. When the patient has a desire to void more frequently, she should respond to the urge for no harm results from too frequent urination, while definite deleterious effects invariably occur with infrequent voiding. In the child and adult with the uninhibited neurogenic or infantile bladder, the urge to void may be so frequent that it will be necessary to alleviate the desire with the use of anticholinergic agents such as Pro-Banthine, tincture of belladonna, Ditropan, or atropine tannate.

If the patient has ureteric reflux as a result of multiple previous infections of the bladder or ureteropyelonephritis, it may often disappear after the patient has been placed on a good voiding regimen and her infection dissipated with antibacterial medication. Ureteroneocystostomy is indicated in the event that ureteric reflux associated with recurrent episodes of pyelonephritis cannot be controlled with an appropriate voiding program.

When an infection develops in a space and results in a cavity filled with pus under high pressure, such as is seen in carbuncles, perinephric abscesses, pyohydronephrosis, and cystitis with urinary retention, two general effects are noted. The patient becomes septic and remains unchanged despite vigorous antibacterial medication *until the pressure within the cavity is relieved by drainage.* The decompression can be accomplished by incision and drainage of the carbuncle and perinephric abscess or by catheterization of the bladder in retention. The infected hydronephrosis can be drained surgically or by ureteric catheterization if feasible.

The virtues of the decompression vividly illustrate that increased intraluminal pressure disseminates bacteria into the blood stream, and that the infection cannot be controlled until the pressure within the cavity is lowered so that blood flow to the walls of the space is increased enough to permit the natural antibacterial elements to reach the microorganisms and eradicate them. Again, host resistance is of primary importance in the prevention and eradication of infection. Antibacterial drugs help but are usually ineffectual if nothing is done to improve host resistance.

At the present time, the physician has a rather extensive array of antibiotic and chemotherapeutic drugs for treatment of the various types of urinary infection. These include the oral preparations containing sulfonamides, penicillin, nitrofurantoin, tetracyclines, cephalosporin, chloramphenicol, and nalidixic acid. Some of the popular commercial products are Polycillin, Gantanol, Macrodantin, Keflex, NegGram, and Bactrim. Most initial infections are caused by the Escherichia coli group and can be easily overcome with most of the oral preparations.

Nitrofurantoin, in the form of Macrodantin capsules for those who can swallow pellets and as the oral suspension of Furadantin for children and adults who cannot ingest pills, is widely used because it is effective in most of the initial and uncomplicated lower urinary tract infections; and, of equal importance, germs do not tend to become resistant as often to Macrodantin as to some of the other medications. The latter aspect is of great importance in the intermittent or continuous long term therapy of young girls during the period of improving host resistance by indoctrinating good voiding habits, i.e., frequent and prompt urination. The dose administered in adults is 100 mg three times daily for 7 days and then 100 mg twice daily for 14 more days. A good long term regimen is 200 mg a day. The amount for children is calculated on a weight basis using 150 pounds as the average adult standard.

The common practice of using a number of drugs one after another, without seeking and treating the factor decreasing host resistance, is to be condemned, for it not only develops resistant bacteria but frequently creates untoward reactions in the patient so that only parenteral, often nephrotoxic, agents remain as a last resort therapy.

On occasion it is necessary to turn to parenteral administration of antibacterial agents to contain and eradicate rampant or resistant urinary infections. Effective drugs include aminoglycosides (kanamycin, gentamicin, streptomycin), polymyxins (polymyxin B, colistimethate), penicillins (ampicillin, penicillin G, carbenicillin), and cephalosporins (cephalothin, cephaloridine). A combination of parenteral drugs which has been shown to be highly effective for most severe urinary and systemic infections includes kanamycin 0.5 gram intramuscularly twice a day and penicillin G 30 to 40 million units intravenously over 24 hours for a period of 3 to 10 days. This combination is particularly useful in patients admitted as emergency cases or for inpatients without culture and sensitivity studies.

STAPHYLOCOCCAL INFECTIONS*

Acute staphylococcal infections of the kidney were common in the preantibiotic era but are now quite rare. However, when it is encountered, the condition may not be recognized because of its ill-defined early signs and symptoms, and treatment may be delayed until its complications of renal carbuncle and perinephric abscess are quite florid.

Etiology

Albarran, who first described this lesion, suggested that the route of infection was probably hematogenous. Subsequent investigators have established this to be a fact. The Staphylococcus aureus is the most frequent infecting organism although any of the other staphylococcal strains may be responsible. The portal of entry for the invader is commonly the skin and mucous membranes. Furuncles and carbuncles of the skin are the commonest foci while upper respiratory infections are the most frequent mucosal sites of entry. Any suppurative process of the body may be the focus for hematogenous spread of staphylococci which become filtered out in the kidney. Likewise, urethral instrumentation occasionally accounts for the introduction of organisms into the blood stream which eventually are filtered out in the kidney to produce this lesion. Defloration followed by chill has been observed in our clinic in three different instances as the etiologic factor in producing staphylococcal infection of the kidneys. In many instances, however, no primary lesion can be demonstrated, a fact which strongly suggests that the portal of bacterial invasion may be insignificant in size.

Pathology

This lesion, like the initial lesion of renal tuberculosis, is situated in the cortical zone of the kidney where the vascular supply of that organ is most

---

*The description of this infection by Reed M. Nesbit in his text *Fundamentals of Urology* (1942) is a classic and so, with his permission, the author has taken the liberty of reproducing the chapter in its near entirety for the present work. The following excerpt from Dr. Nesbit's work also appears in Chapter IV, pages 37–41 of the fourth, revised edition, published in 1953.

abundant; a fact which no doubt accounts for the high incidence of early and complete healing which occurs in this type of infection since the majority of cases heal spontaneously and get well without extensive destruction of the kidney. Grossly the kidney is enlarged from congestion and edema; multiple small areas of suppuration are disseminated throughout the cortex. These small abscesses may enlarge to varying degrees and occasionally may involve the entire parenchyma. The more extensive suppurative processes have been described by many authors who have applied to them the terms "abscess of the kidney," "septic infarct," and "renal carbuncle."

Progress of the Lesion

The microscopic sized minute areas of suppuration throughout the cortex almost invariably resolve—heal, and leave little behind to reveal any evidence of serious damage to the renal parenchyma.

The minute areas may coalesce to form larger areas of suppuration becoming macroscopic sized abscesses of varying size. Rarely the entire kidney is destroyed by a diffuse suppurative process.

Spread of the infection to the perinephrium may occur by either of two routes; by direct extension from a small cortical abscess rupturing through the capsule of the kidney into the perinephric fat; by lymphatic extension from the infected renal cortex. Once suppuration is established in the perinephric fat, it encounters an ideal medium for extension with a minimum of vascular supply as a defense. Thus, perinephric abscess generally starts within the perirenal fat capsule and it may remain well localized in its extent, although it generally involves the entire perirenal capsule within a relatively short period of time. As it spreads and develops it produces a rapid destruction of the perirenal fat. If perinephric abscess extends beyond the confines of Gerota's fascia, it may point in several directions. A common site is Petit's triangle where it eventually may produce a fluctuant swelling. Perinephric abscess can also follow downward along the course of the ureter in the retroperitoneal space, and may eventually come to the surface at the external ring or it may extend downward into the pelvis, and patients have been seen in whom such abscesses had eventually come to the surface in the perineum by way of the ischiorectal fossa; or in rare instances rupture of perinephric abscess through the floor of the bladder has occurred. Another direction in which perinephric abscess occasionally points is upward toward the diaphragm. In this situation the infection may spread directly through the diaphragm and produce a reaction in the parietal pleura with some thickening and exudation. Investigations have disclosed that 16 per cent of all perinephric abscess cases seen in the University Hospital showed x-ray evidence of pleural or lung involvement. In these patients there was pleural thickening and varying amounts of effusion. Eventually adhesions may form between the visceral and parietal pleura and in a few rare instances, the abscess ruptures through the diaphragm into the substance of the lung, producing a suppurative pneumonitis; and this in turn ruptures into a bronchus thus providing drainage. The patient who has this type of perinephrobronchial fistula develops a productive cough and purulent sputum. Basilar suppurative pneumonitis should always arouse suspicion on the part of the physician, regarding the presence of perinephric abscess as a etiological factor. Primary suppurative lesions occurring above the diaphragm do not penetrate that structure but subdiaphragmatic infections frequently spread upward; in fact the pulmonary complications of an undiagnosed perinephric abscess may be the first localized symptoms of the patient's disease and if then the physician unwittingly overlooks the primary lesion, the patient may eventually succumb to an inadequately drained abscess and chronic suppurative pneumonitis. Simple drainage of the perinephric abscess results in prompt cure of the pulmonary lesion.

It is to be here noted that perinephric abscess has been listed as one of the complications of acute staphylococcal infection of the kidney. But—while some perinephric abscesses develop in this fashion, there are other causes for perinephric suppuration: tuberculosis of the kidney, advanced pyelonephritis, calculus pyonephrosis, rupture of the kidney, and gangrenous retroperitoneal appendix.

Symptoms and Signs—of acute staphylococcal infection of the kidney. The disease is generally unilateral clinically although the lesion may be bilateral.

In general, the symptomatology and progress of the disease run a characteristic course. The onset is usually abrupt, generally with a chill.

A high fever is the rule. Most patients have temperatures ranging between 103 and 105°F. immediately after the onset of the disease and the temperature chart runs a septic course during the acute phase of the disease, lasting 5 to 10 days.

Pain is constant from the onset. It is renal in its location and the patient complains of its presence either in the upper quadrant anteriorly or in the costo-vertebral region; and sometimes the pain is so severe as to simulate renal colic and may require the use of opiates for relief.

Costo-vertebral tenderness is always present. True costo-vertebral tenderness is elicited by pressure with a single finger just beneath the twelfth rib and just lateral to the long back muscles. In eliciting the sign of costo-vertebral tenderness, the examining physician should be scrupulously careful not to confuse tenderness of the back muscles with costo-vertebral tenderness. These are two separate anatomical points. In acute staphylococcal infection of the kidney, true costo-vertebral tenderness is always present.

Constitutional symptoms of infection are practically always present—weakness, loss of appetite, prostration, sweating,—in fact, the entire catalogue of constitutional symptoms always associated with sepsis.

Bladder irritation is uncommon, a fact which frequently causes the physician to overlook the possibility of urinary tract infection. The medical profession as a whole have long associated the symptoms of bladder irritation with urinary tract infection, and, for that reason, the absence of bladder irritation all too frequently causes the physician to overlook the possibility of a kidney or urinary tract lesion when considering the differential diagnosis of a patient who is acutely septic. The patient with acute staphylococcal infection of the kidney almost never has increased frequency or burning on urination during the early stages of the disease. During the later stages of the disease, as will be pointed out later, bladder irritation may occur.

Leucocytosis—tends to be high, the average leucocyte count running about 10,000. It is not at all uncommon to find a leucocyte count of 12,000 to 15,000 in this condition and we have seen cases with a leucocytosis as high as 33,000.

The urine—is usually negative except for the presence of staphylococci. Occasionally microscopic hematuria is seen and on rare occasions a gross hematuria may accompany the onset of the disease. A trace of albumin is occasionally present! In all instances the staphylococcus can be demonstrated in the urine by staining the centrifuged sediment. Organisms may not appear in the urine until 2 or 3 days after onset of the disease; and they are to be found in the urine for varying periods of time. In some instances the bacteria disappear in 48 to 72 hours while in others they may persist in the urine for 90 days or longer. The rapid disappearance of organisms from the urine often leads to confusion in the diagnosis, not only of staphylococcal infection of the kidney, but also of its serious complications. During the acute phase of the disease, pus cells rarely if ever are present in the urine. It should be remembered that the lesion is situated in the cortical zone of the kidney and involves the glomerulus and it is natural to understand that pus which forms in the tiny lesions of that area does not escape from these lesions into the urine. Thus it is evident that a complete examination of the urine including staining of the dried sediment is essential to the diagnosis. The author, on numerous occasions, while seeing patients suspected of having acute staphylococcal infections of the kidney, in the University Hospital, has been informed by the student or intern that the urine is normal; the inquiry has then been made, "In what way is the urine normal?" The reply, "A microscopic examination failed to disclose any pus so the urine was considered normal." After such a reply had been made, a request for a urine specimen was made and staining of the sediment performed on the spot. Disclosure of staphylococci on the stained sediment invariably accomplished two purposes: it established the diagnosis and it emphasized the importance of staining the urinary sediment in all cases suspected of infection. One cannot assume under any circumstances that a urine is normal when it is free from pus cells. Another interesting phenomenon has been observed in cases of this type. Many cases in which staphylococci can be demonstrated upon staining the urinary sediment have failed to give positive culture of organisms on the usual laboratory media. For this reason a simple culture of the urine may fail to establish a diagnosis while an ordinary stained sediment will establish it. It is thought by some bacteriologists that the organisms are so devitalized by their passage through the kidney that they will not grow in the ordinary culture media.

Secondary invasion of the urinary tract in coccal infections has been long observed and commented upon. In about 50 per cent of the cases a secondary invasion with the colon bacillus occurs during the second week of the disease. The exact portal of entry or method of invasion by the colon bacilli in these cases is unknown. Some investigators have suggested that the kidney in overcoming the primary invader, lays itself open to attack by the secondary invader. When the secondary invasion by the colon bacillus occurs, one frequently finds that the cocci disappear from the urine or can be found only by painstaking search. The bacillary invader takes over the entire picture. Coincident with bacillary invasion, pus appears in the urine for the first time. When bacillary infection of the urine takes place there usually occurs bladder irritation, with symptoms of increased frequency, burning, and dysuria, and the patient then becomes aware of a urinary tract disturbance. In the light of the fact that about 50 per cent of all cases with staphylococcal infection undergo this secondary colon bacillus invasion during the second week of the disease, one is led to speculate as to whether many cases of so-called primary bacillary urinary tract infections have had their origin in acute staphylococcal infection of the kidneys that pass undiagnosed and unsuspected.

Clinical Course of the Disease

Acute staphylococcal infection of the kidney usually runs a stormy though self-limiting course with a high fever, pain, and costo-vertebral tenderness, all of which persist for several days and then gradually subside so that the important symptoms and signs have run their course in from 7 to 14 days. Usually by the 14th day the temperature has returned to normal and the patient is free from pain or tenderness. If secondary invasion of the urinary tract by B Coli takes place during the second week, it generally produces some degree of bladder irritation. Some patients show a slight recurrence of fever on being allowed out of bed after their symptoms have disappeared. This is nearly always a transient rise and usually subsides in 24 to 48 hours.

If the symptoms and signs of the acute disease persist more than 10 to 14 days, one of the complications of staphylococcal infection of the kidney must be suspected. Likewise, any accentuation of symptoms or signs during the course of the disease suggest the occurrence of complications. Uncomplicated cases end in a complete recovery, except for cortical scars which probably have no importance insofar as renal function is concerned.

A typical example of an uncomplicated case seen in the University Hospital demonstrates some of the classical diagnostic features of this disease. A 30 year old male complained of severe left flank pain of 24 hours duration. Onset was abrupt and was followed by nausea, vomiting, and fever. There were no urinary symptoms. His health had been excellent except for a recent severe upper respiratory infection.

On examination he appeared septic, showing evidence of moderate dehydration and perspiring profusely. There was a marked left costo-vertebral tenderness and moderate left upper abdominal tenderness. The temperature was 99.6°F. on admission but reached 101.2 degrees F. a few hours later. The urine contained occasional leucocytes and many staphylococci were found on the stained sediment. The following day the urine was normal and it remained so during the remainder of the patient's hospitalization. Upon admission there was a leucocytosis of 12,500. Pyelograms were negative. He was treated by rest in bed, fluids, and sulfanilamide, and was entirely free from pain and tenderness in 48 hours. The temperature and blood count were normal by the fifth day when he was allowed out of bed. He was discharged on the tenth day, feeling well.

In this case it is noteworthy that pain and costo-vertebral tenderness, so acute and severe during the first 48 hours, were entirely lacking thereafter. It is also of interest and importance that cocci were present in the urine for only a 24 hour period. The fever and leucocytosis persisted for 5 days. Had this patient been first examined 48 hours after the onset of his illness, the precise diagnosis could not have been made because the urine was then normal and remained so upon subsequent examinations.

Differential Diagnosis

Acute Appendicitis. Differential diagnosis in atypical cases is sometimes difficult. The lesion that most commonly causes confusion is acute appendicitis. The absence of nausea, vomiting, and muscle spasm and the presence of costo-vertebral tenderness and high leucocytosis generally suffices to make the differentiation possible even though cocci have not yet appeared in the urine.

Occasionally the differential diagnosis between acute appendicitis and acute coccal kidney cannot be clearly established. In the event that the urine is entirely normal or contains a few cocci and the physician has reason to suspect the imminence of appendiceal rupture, he is justified in performing appendectomy.

Acute hydronephrosis must be ruled out in some instances. Several cases in our series complained of extremely severe pain which suggested the presence of acute ureteral obstruction, but excretory pyelograms effectively settle this point.

Acute cholecystitis has been difficult to differentiate in a few instances. One spectacular example which we have observed is noteworthy. The case summary is as follows: a 22 year old graduate nurse was admitted to the hospital during an attack of excruciating right upper quadrant pain radiating to the back, with associated nausea and vomiting. She was extremely toxic with a temperature of 103°F. and had two severe chills. There were no urinary symptoms. Examination revealed exquisite tenderness and extreme muscle spasm in the right upper quadrant of the abdomen. There was also acute right costo-vertebral tenderness. The leucocytosis rose from 11,000 to 33,000 in 48 hours with a corresponding increase in all symptoms and signs. Repeated urinalyses were negative. Although coccal kidney was strongly suspected the diagnosis of acute empyema of the gall bladder could not be ruled out, and a laparotomy was performed on the third day of the illness. All abdominal viscera were found to be normal. The kidney was found to be enlarged when examined by palpation through the peritoneum, and on the second postoperative day, showers of staphylococci appeared in the urine confirming the diagnosis of acute staphylococcal kidney. All symptoms and signs cleared up by the 14th postoperative day although the urine contained organisms for approximately one month.

Complications

During the course of pneumonia, a failure of clinical response within the expected period or a marked accentuation of symptoms and signs suggest the complications—lung abscess or empyema; and similarly, a failure of expected clinical response in acute staphylococcal kidney or a marked increase in symptoms or signs during conservative treatment suggest the occurrence of its complications—perinephric abscess or carbuncle of the kidney. These complications occur in about 10 per cent of cases and the attending physician must realize the possibility of their development and recognize their appearance should they occur. The occurrence of either of these complications is heralded by an increase in tenderness or pain. The muscle spasm overlying the lesion becomes more pronounced and a general constitutional reaction to a profound degree of sepsis becomes evident with chills, drenching sweats and weakness. There may even develop a slight bulging in the flank if a perinephric abscess is forming. In the event that the physician sees the complication, i.e., perinephric abscess or carbuncle of the kidney only after it is fully developed and has not had the opportunity to follow the patient from the onset, he may be confronted with one who has been suffering from sepsis for a considerable period of time and who is not only profoundly septic but also dehydrated and anemic and in a poor state of nutrition. In such cases the physical signs are fairly constant and include a sign which was discovered by Dr. Clifford Keene, previously a resident on the Surgical Service in the University Hospital, i.e., that all cases having perinephric abscess or carbuncle of the kidney show rales at the base of the lung on the affected side. A normal urine should in no way interfere with the establishment of the diagnosis in suspected cases. At least 50 per cent of all cases having perinephric abscess or carbuncle of the kidney are found to have normal urine at the time of diagnosis.

Roentgen ray studies are often helpful in making the diagnosis of perinephric abscess or carbuncle of the kidney.

In perinephric abscess, the typical x-ray findings are: obscuration of psoas shadow on the affected side, lateral curvature of the spine with concavity toward the lesion, and fixation of the kidney on the affected side as demonstrated by pyelographic films made during respiration. It is important that the kidney on the uninvolved side demonstrate motion during respiration in obtaining this sign.

When carbuncle of the kidney is present there may be in addition to the above signs, a characteristic deformity of the kidney demonstrated by pyelogram.

SELECTED REFERENCES

Brumfitt, W., and Asscher, A. W.: Urinary Tract Infection. London, Oxford University Press, 1973.
   Recent researches conducted in England on urinary tract infection in the human are recorded in this volume, a collection of the papers and associated discussions given during the Second National Symposium held in London in 1972. The subjects cover diagnostic methods, the natural history of infection in the child and adult, bacterial resistance, pathogenesis, and treatment. When some of the findings and remaining problems are viewed in the light of the material presented in our chapter, the pieces begin to fall into place.

Kass, E. H.: Progress in Pyelonephritis. Philadelphia, F. A. Davis Company, 1965.
   Almost every aspect of urinary tract infection known in 1964 is discussed by a group of international authorities during the Second International Symposium on Pyelonephritis and published in this compendium. The contents include epidemiology, ecology, and pathophysiology of urinary infections as well as the cause and treatment of pyelonephritis. One can obtain a good overview of the ideas regarding urinary infection prevalent at that time.

Kunin, C. H.: Detection, Prevention, and Management of Urinary Tract Infections. Philadelphia, Lea and Febiger, 1972.

The author, a nephrologist, has written this work with the intention of having it used as a practical guide in the handling of urinary tract infection by physicians, nurses, and allied health personnel. All of the material is presented in a concise and lucid fashion. The handbook is divided into five sections under the headings of An Overview of Urinary Tract Infections, Guides to Examination of the Urine and Evaluation of Renal Function, Principles of Urinary Bacteriology, Care of the Urinary Catheter, and Management of Urinary Tract Infection.

Lapides, J.: Pathophysiology of Urinary Tract Infections. Univ. Mich. Med. Center J., 39:103, 1973.

This article reviews the evidence supporting the concept that host resistance is the primary factor in urinary tract infection. The material ranges from that published in the early 20th century to research presently being conducted. The viewpoint is from that of a physiologist.

Stamey, T. A.: Urinary Infections. Baltimore, Williams & Wilkins Company, 1972.

Some of the prevalent ideas regarding urinary infection stem from the influence of the author's publications. The volume describes in great detail the investigations which led to Stamey's views on chronic prostatitis and urinary infection in the female. The viewpoint is from that of a bacteriologist.

REFERENCES

Altemeier, W. A.: The significance of infection in trauma. Bull. Am. Coll., (Feb.), 1972.

Andriole, V. T., and Lytton, B.: The effect and critical duration of increased tissue pressure on susceptibility to bacterial infection. Br. J. Exp. Pathol., 66:308, 1965.

Beeson, P. B.: Factors in the pathogenesis of pyelonephritis. Yale J. Biol. Med., 28:81, 1955.

Cabot, H.: The doctrine of the prepared soil: a neglected factor in surgical infections. Can. Med. Assoc. J., 11:610, 1921.

Cabot, H., and Crabtree, E. G.: The etiology and pathology of nontuberculous renal infections. Surg. Gynecol. Obstet., 23:495, 1916.

Cox, C. E., and Hinman, F., Jr.: Experiments with induced bacteriuria, vesical emptying and bacterial growth on the mechanism of bladder defense to infection. J. Urol., 86:739, 1961.

Lapides, J., Costello, R. T., Jr., Zierdt, D. K., and Stone, D. E.: Primary cause and treatment of recurrent urinary infection in women: preliminary report. J. Urol., 100:552, 1968.

Lapides, J., and Costello, R. T., Jr.: Uninhibited neurogenic bladder; a common cause for recurrent urinary infection in normal women. J. Urol., 101:539, 1969.

Lapides, J., and Diokno, A. C.: Persistence of the infant bladder as a cause for urinary infection in girls. J. Urol., 103:243, 1970.

Lapides, J., Diokno, A. C., Lowe, B. S., and Kalish, M. D.: Follow-up on unsterile, intermittent self-catheterization. J. Urol., 111:184, 1974.

Nesbit, R. M., Lapides, J., and Baum, W. C.: Fundamentals of Urology. 4th ed. rev. Ann Arbor, Michigan, J. W. Edwards, 1953.

Chapter Nine

GONORRHEA

Karl R. Herwig

Gonorrhea is the second most common communicable disease in the United States, outranked only by the common cold. It is usually venereal in its spread, that is, transmission is by sexual contact, although neonates can contract the disease at birth and prepubertal females can contract it from infected towels and bed linen. Asymptomatic carriers, both male and female, represent an important reservoir of the disease and have allowed gonorrhea to reach epidemic proportions. Gonorrhea is an egalitarian disease that affects all people equally, although the incidence varies with the age of the patient population. Persons aged 15 to 24 years have a higher infection rate than those in any other age group.

ETIOLOGY

Neisseria gonorrhea causes gonorrhea. It is a gram-negative, non-motile diplococcus that does not grow well in the normal atmosphere. It requires special media for culturing, such as Thayer-Martin media, and an atmosphere of 10 per cent carbon dioxide. Differences in sugar fermentation reactions and fluorescent antibodies separate the gonococcus from the other *Neisseria* that infect humans. Humans are the only naturally known reservoir of the organism.

PATHOLOGY

Gonorrhea can be readily innoculated in the conjunctiva, urethra of either sex, and the female genital passages. Less commonly it is found in the oral pharynx and the anal canal. The type of mucosa of the particular area of the genitourinary tract determines the susceptibility of that tissue to infection. Columnar epithelium that lines the urethral glands, prostatic ducts, Skene's glands, endocervix, and fallopian tubes furnishes fertile sites for growth of the bacteria. Transitional epithelium is only slightly susceptible and will not support the gonococcus for long. Squamous epithelium does not support growth at all. The bacteria elicit an intense inflammatory reaction with an outpouring of white cells and the disruption of normal cells.

After the initial lesion occurs, the infection may be completely eradicated, either spontaneously or as the result of therapy; it may spread locally to involve other organs of the genitourinary tract; it may remain hidden in the genital mucosa and be asymptomatic; or it may invade the blood stream and cause endocarditis, arthritis, or perihepatitis. The end result, even for those cured, is usually scar tissue formation which can lead to obstruction of the genitourinary passages.

MANIFESTATION

In the male, the gonococcus causes acute anterior urethritis. Symptoms develop after a short incubation period of two to seven days. The initial symptoms consist of tickling and itchy irritation of the urethral meatus that is usually associated with a slight watery discharge. The discharge soon becomes copious with a thickened yellowish mucopurulence. Burning and pain upon urination develop, but there is usually no frequency or urgency unless the posterior urethra is involved. Acute gonococcal urethritis can cause urinary retention because of fear of voiding through the inflamed urethra. If allowed to go untreated, the discharge and the symptoms can persist, or other organs, such as the prostate gland, epididymis, or blood stream can become involved.

In females, 80 per cent or more remain asymptomatic after contracting the disease. Some complain of slight dysuria or a transient vaginal discharge. The diagnosis becomes evident with the development of pelvic inflammatory disease (P.I.D.) or with endocervical culture of suspected contacts.

DIAGNOSIS

The diagnosis of gonorrheal urethritis is suspected from obtaining a history of exposure, eliciting the typical signs and symptoms, and finding intracellular gonococci in the stained white cells of the urethral discharge. The staining can be done with methylene blue, gram stain, or fluorescent antibody technique. The final diagnosis, however, can only be made from positive culture of the organism. This fact should be borne in mind in any case where litigation is suspected, since attorneys have learned that the microscopic appearance of an organism does not constitute definitive identification. The special medium, Thayer-Martin or Transgrow, is reliable for culture and identification of the gonococcus and should be used in all suspected cases.

Stains and smears of the endocervical canal and urethra are inadequate for diagnostic purposes in the female. Suspected patients should have cultures taken from the endocervical and anal canals for positive confirmation. Some advocate routine culturing of the endocervical and anal canals for positive confirmation. Some advocate routine culturing of the endocervical canal of all females between the ages of 15 and 45 years when performing a pelvic examination. In addition to culture of the urethra, endocervix, and anus, oral pharyngeal culture should be taken from suspected patients, especially homosexuals.

COMPLICATIONS

In males, the common complications include acute prostatitis, epididymitis, arthritis, urethral stricture, and nonspecific urethritis. Nonspecific urethritis frequently follows successful treatment for gonorrhea. It probably represents overgrowth of bacteria in the urethra from decreased resistance. Urethral stricture, a late complication, results from the reparative process with scar formation. It can cause significant impairment of the urinary tract.

In females, pelvic inflammatory disease, a local peritonitis, sterility from tubal obstruction, and pelvic abscess constitute the common complications.

THERAPY

The gonococcus is sensitive to almost all antibiotics if given in adequate amounts.

RECOMMENDED TREATMENT

PARENTERAL. Men and women should receive 4,800,000 units of aqueous procaine penicillin G divided into two doses, given as two intramuscular injections at one visit, together with 1 gram of probenecid given orally at least one-half hour prior to injection.

ORAL. Men and women should receive 3.5 grams of ampicillin and 1 gram of probenecid administered simultaneously.

ALTERNATIVE TREATMENT FOR PATIENTS WHEN THE RECOMMENDED THERAPY IS CONTRAINDICATED

PARENTERAL. Men should receive 2 grams of spectinomycin dihydrochloride pentahydrate in one intramuscular injection. Women should receive 4 grams of spectinomycin dihydrochloride pentahydrate in one intramuscular injection.

ORAL. Men and women should receive tetracycline hydrochloride, 1.5 grams in an initial dose followed by 0.5 gram four times a day until a total dose of 9 grams has been administered.

This therapy may be repeated if the initial treatment fails; however, the initial treatment is successful in over 95 per cent of the patients treated. Serologic tests for syphilis should be obtained at six and twelve weeks after treatment so that any masked syphilis will be uncovered, although the dosage of penicillin in the recommended regimen is adequate for primary syphilis. Spectinomycin appears to have no therapeutic effect upon syphilis.

PROPHYLAXIS AND IMMUNITY

Exposure to gonorrhea affords a very slight, insignificant immunity to reinfection. Attempts are being made to improve this immunity with an antigonococcal vaccine that would help control gonorrhea among highly susceptible populations. In an effort to detect the asymptomatic carriers, radioimmunoassays to determine the presence of gonococcal antibodies are being developed. High titres of these antibodies suggest the presence of the organisms, and it is hoped that they should aid in the battle to stop the gonorrhea epidemic.

SELECTED REFERENCES

Center for Disease Control. Morbidity and Mortality Weekly Reports, Atlanta, Georgia.
In an area undergoing rapid change, periodicals offer more current information than textbooks. This is the weekly communication from the national center. It contains current and authoritative reports, especially in the therapeutic and epidemiologic areas.

Holmes, K. K., and Beaty, H. N.: Gonococcal infections. *In* Wintrobe, M. M. et al. (eds.): Harrison's Principles of Internal Medicine. 7th ed. New York, McGraw Hill Book Company, 1974, pp. 788–792.
This is a concise overview of gonorrhea, its pathophysiology, and manifestations.

REFERENCES

Armstrong, J. H., and Wiesner, P. J.: The need for problem-oriented venereal disease clinics. J. Am. Venereal Dis. Assn., *1*:23, 1974.
Beware male asymptomatic gonorrhea. World Medical News, *13*:4 (April), 1972.
Ellner, P. D.: Diagnosis of gonococcal infection. Clinical Medicine, *78*:16, 1971.
Owen, R. L., and Hill, J. L.: Rectal and pharyngeal gonorrhea in homosexual men. J.A.M.A., *220*:1315, 1972.
Pederson, A. H. B., Wiesner, P. J., Holmes, K. K., Johnson, C. J., and Turck, M.: Spectinomycin and penicillin G in the treatment of gonorrhea. J.A.M.A., *220*:205, 1972.
Schroeter, A. L., Turner, R. H., Lucas, J. G., and Brown, W. J.: Therapy for incubating syphilis. J.A.M.A., *218*:711, 1972.
The doctor's role in gonorrhea control. World Medical News, *13*:20 (Feb.), 1972.
VD meeting: How close is an antigonococcal vaccine? Hosp. Pract., *7*:35(Aug.), 1972.

Chapter Ten

GENITOURINARY TUBERCULOUS INFECTION

Cheng-yang Chang

Since the advent of chemotherapy in 1946, the primary treatment for genitourinary tuberculosis has been medical rather than surgical. Many nephrectomies have been obviated because of modern combined therapy. The incidence of genitourinary tract tuberculosis has declined in recent years, but the rate of decrease is not compatible with that of pulmonary tuberculosis. This lag may be due to the late onset (sometimes 10 to 20 years) of genitourinary tuberculosis as a complication of pulmonary tuberculosis.

The insidious onset of genitourinary tuberculosis can make diagnosis difficult. White blood cells in the urine may be the only sign at the onset of the disease, and the patient is frequently asymptomatic otherwise. For this reason, every abacterial pyuria patient should be suspected of having a tuberculous infection until tests for acid-fast bacilli have proved negative.

PATHOGENESIS

Renal or genitourinary tuberculosis has to be considered as a local manifestation of a generalized tuberculosis infection. The portal of entrance of mycobacterium tuberculosis is usually pulmonary but could be the intestine or genitalia.

There are many theories regarding the pathogenesis of renal tuberculosis. The most acceptable concept is as follows.

A hematogenous dissemination of tubercle bacilli occurs from a primary focus situated either in the lungs or infected parabronchial, mediastinal, or mesenteric lymph nodes. Lymph node foci may have harbored quiescent lesions for long periods and may have only recently broken down to discharge a shower of infected material into the systemic circulation. Such cases often demonstrate no evidences whatever of pulmonary disease when examined by x-ray of the lungs. Blood-borne tubercle bacilli are carried to both kidneys and may be arrested in the capillary tufts of the glomeruli, where a tubercle develops.

The primary lesions occur in the glomeruli and are situated in the cortical zone of the kidney where the vascular supply and the mechanisms of defense and repair are most abundant. Medlar has demonstrated that the cortical lesions of renal tuberculosis frequently heal. He studied 100,000 serial sections made from the kidneys of patients who died of pulmonary tuberculosis, but who had no clinical evidence of renal involvement. Medlar's investigation demonstrated that bilateral kidney involvement was constant and that the majority of the lesions were situated in the cortical zone; 71 per cent of the lesions showed healing, although some were broken down and caseating.

Tubercle bacilli and pus mix with the glomerular filtrate and pass down the tubular system to the medullary loop. The organisms may become arrested in the narrow loop of Henle and find favorable soil for growth because of the sluggish flow of urine at this point; also, the medullary zone is relatively avascular and is more vulnerable to destructive inflammatory processes than the cortical zone.

The medullary lesions enlarge and have less of a tendency to heal than the cortical lesions; these are the lesions the clinician eventually recognizes as chronic renal tuberculosis; the primary renal lesion is frequently overlooked. In fact, it may be entirely healed at the time the kidney is examined in the operating room or at postmortem examination.

PATHOLOGY

The characteristic lesion of chronic tuberculosis seen by the surgeon is situated in the medullary portion of the parenchyma. By a process of tissue destruction, it extends in all directions within the lobules. The process extends along the course of the tubules and through the lymphatics until it ruptures into the pelvis, generally at the tip of the papilla or near that point. When the infection reaches the renal pelvis, it spreads along the submucosa and mucosa, producing widespread tuberculous pyelitis which, in turn, allows retrograde extension into other portions of the kidney; a rapid involvement of the entire renal parenchyma may develop from this type of spread. The infection in the submucosa often extends downward along the course of the ureter with the ureteric wall thickening irregularly, depending upon the extent and the degree of its involvement. Ulceration of the mucosa may take place, and occasionally complete stenosis of the ureter occurs, cutting off any exit for pus and urine, an event which rapidly accelerates the destruction of the kidney.

Bladder involvement occurs as a complication of renal tuberculosis in the majority of cases. This develops in two ways: (1) the tubercle bacilli in the urine produce inflammation of the bladder mucosa. In the early stages this inflammation is situated only in the neighborhood of a ureteric orifice. From this point, the process spreads in all directions and may eventually involve the entire bladder. (2) A second way in which lesions of the bladder may occur is by direct submucosal extension from the infected ureter. Either type of tuberculous cystitis is progressive and, if allowed to advance unchecked, may eventually result in a permanent contraction of the bladder with gross ulcerations throughout.

Genital infections occur in about two thirds of all men who have renal tuberculosis and involve the prostate gland, the seminal vesicles, the vas deferens, and the epididymides. This involvement usually occurs by direct contamination from the infected urine passing through the prostatic urethra. The infection of the prostate gland may develop insidiously or rapidly. If the infection develops insidiously, the process is one of chronic tuberculosis of the prostate gland with a tendency towards fibrosis and nodularity. If it runs a rapid course, an abscess of the prostate may develop with early caseation and rapid destruction. Tuberculous infection of the epididymis generally occurs by retrograde extension along the vas deferens, which becomes inflamed and nodular because of localized caseating lesions along its course. The lower pole of the epididymis is usually involved first in this type of extension, and the process usually develops slowly, although rapid and fulminating epididymitis may occur. When epididymitis occurs on one side, an extension to the other side often follows by way of the vas.

Tuberculous urethritis in the male, although fortunately rare, is a complication of the first magnitude. It is an ulcerative process that involves the mucosa as well as the underlying corpus spongiosum and produces extensive stricture of the urethra. Manipulative treatment frequently results in periurethral abscess or hematogenous dissemination.

SYMPTOMS AND SIGNS

Symptoms are nonspecific. Constitutional symptoms that include general fatigue, loss of body weight, low grade afternoon fever, malaise, and night sweating are occasionally present, but not as frequently as in pulmonary tuberculosis.

Pyuria may be the only finding when the tuberculous lesion is limited to the kidney. Hematuria is a fairly common symptom in renal tuberculosis if the lesion ulcerates into a blood vessel. If an obstruction of the infundibulum, ureteropelvic junction, or ureter occurs owing to scar contracture, then flank pain or sepsis may develop. However, most of the symptoms are dependent upon tuberculous involvement of the bladder, and these symptoms are burning on urination, pollakiuria both day and night, suprapubic pain, occasional strangury and hematuria. Hugh Cabot once stated, "the kidney is an inarticulate organ; its vocal cords are the bladder." This statement is especially apropos of renal tuberculosis, for virtually the only telltale symptoms are those arising from bladder complications.

Symptoms and signs of epididymitis are common in adults, but rare in children. They include swelling and tenderness of the epididymis and thickening or beading of the vas deferens. Prior to chemotherapy, draining scrotal sinuses were a common complication of tuberculous epididymitis. Induration or nodularity of the prostate and thickening of seminal vesicles suggest an acid-fast bacterial involvement.

DIAGNOSIS

History. The history of exposure to tuberculous infection in one's family, professional contact such as working in a sanitarium, or pulmonary tuberculosis in the past is very important. Genitourinary tuberculosis may occur anywhere from 10 to 20 years after the primary lesion has healed.

Skin Test. The P.P.D. (Protein Precipitated Derivative) or O.T. (Old Tuberculin) skin test should be done.

Urine. Most cases of renal tuberculosis present a characteristic urinary picture. The urinary pH is acid, and the urine shows a trace of albumin, a few red cells, many pus cells, and no microorganisms by the usual staining methods. Any time that a complete examination of the urine discloses these characteristic findings, tuberculosis must be suspected until disproven. However, other infections may coexist with urinary tuberculosis. For this reason, all refractory cases of urinary infection should be suspected of having tuberculosis.

In suspected cases, Ziehl-Neelsen's technique for staining acid-fast bacilli is employed in examining the urinary sediment. In addition, a 24-hour urine or the first voided morning specimen is screened for the tubercle bacillus by guinea pig inoculation and culture. Because the tubercle bacilli are spilled intermittently from tuberculous lesions of the kidney, a single urine culture and inoculation test may not be adequate. To be reliable, a minimum of three consecutive specimens should be collected from each patient.

X-ray Studies. A routine chest roentgenogram is helpful when it shows an old scar of tuberculosis infection; but even if it is negative, renal tuberculosis cannot be ruled out.

A scout film of the abdomen may demonstrate opaque shadows in the region of the kidneys secondary to calcification of necrotic renal parenchyma.

Excretory urography may reveal the typical moth-eaten appearance of involved calyces, dilated calyces due to stricture of infundibula (Fig. 10–1), or parenchymal caseation necrosis; hydroureteronephrosis that is due to ureteric stricture (Fig. 10–2); irregularity and filling defect of the ureter caused by ureteritis cystica; or a functionless kidney (Fig. 10–2).

Retrograde catheterization of the ureters is used to delineate the strictured segment of a nonfunctioning kidney and its ureter, as well as to collect urine specimens for acid-fast studies.

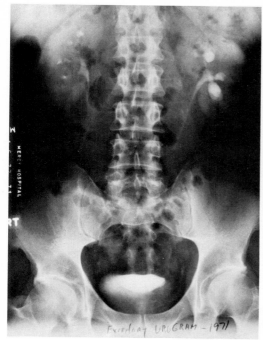 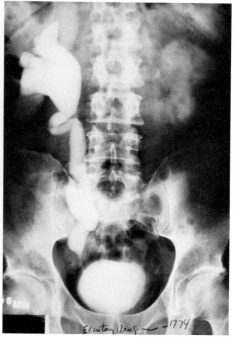

Fig. 10–1   **Fig. 10–2**

Figure 10–1 An upper and lower infundibular stricture with associated distortion of adjacent collecting system of left kidney.

Figure 10–2 Patient was not treated for his tuberculosis, and three years later repeat excretory urograms showed nonvisualization of the left kidney and hydroureteronephrosis of the right kidney secondary to stricture of the distal ureter.

Endoscopy. The bladder mucosa in tuberculous cystitis demonstrates multiple small yellowish-white opaque nodules surrounded by zones of erythema, especially in the periureteric and trigonal areas. Some of the lesions may be ulcerated and on biopsy will reveal the typical chronic infective granuloma of tuberculosis. The ureteric orifices may be gaping and retracted in chronic tuberculous ureteritis. Not infrequently, the bladder capacity is reduced, and cystoscopy is difficult.

TREATMENT

Prior to the advent of streptomycin therapy for tuberculosis in 1946, nephrectomy was used frequently to eradicate unilateral renal disease. Now medical regimens are of primary importance. However, surgical procedures are still employed in selected cases, such as

(1) Partial nephrectomy for localized renal lesions not responding to medication.

(2) Nephrectomy for far-advanced renal disease as in pyohydronephrosis or marked cavitation.

(3) Supravesical urinary diversion (cutaneous ureterostomy, cutaneous ureteroileostomy) for markedly contracted bladders.

(4) Urethroplasty for urethral stricture.

Medical Therapy

Triple therapy is advised in various combinations; most doctors use the following:

Isoniazid (I.N.H.) 100 mg three times a day.

Sodium para-aminosalicylate (Sod. P.A.S.) 5 grams three times a day.

Streptomycin 1.0 gram I.M. twice a week.

Pyridoxine (Vitamin B_6) 50 mg two times a day.

Oral triple therapy has proved as effective as injection, usually using rifampin 600 mg daily, cycloserine 250 mg twice daily, or ethambutol 1 gram daily as substitutes for the streptomycin. Ethionamide can be used as a substitute if the patient cannot tolerate one of the medications (i.e., gastrointestinal disturbance from Sod. P.A.S.). Liver function should be monitored because of the hepatotoxic side effects of this drug, especially in alcoholics.

Under special conditions, such as the development of drug-resistant bacteria or for surgical preparation, pyrazinamide or kanamycin can be added to the program.

The minimum duration of therapy is two years. Ample rest is advised with cessation of strenuous work for at least six months; sedentary work and light housework can be permitted.

Caution should be used in disposing of urine until the culture and animal inoculation tests are converted to negative.

Intravenous pyelograms, urine culture, and urine analysis should be repeated every four months in the first year, every six months in the second year, and then followed by yearly check-ups.

Surgery

Nephrectomy is indicated under certain special conditions, such as a nonfunctioning kidney with secondary infection, hypertension, or inability to rule out tumor.

Partial nephrectomy has been used in local caliectasis secondary to stricture of infundibula. Urinary diversion is indicated in patients with severe, long-standing bladder or ureteric disease.

Cutaneous ureterostomy is useful in patients with severe strictures of the ureter and also in poor-risk patients who cannot tolerate a major diversionary procedure. Ileal or colonic conduits are sometimes used. Bladder capacity may be increased using a cystoplasty in which a segment of ileum or colon is sutured to the bladder.

PROGNOSIS

Most cases of genitourinary tuberculosis, when detected early enough, can be treated by triple-drug therapy with excellent results and will thereafter yield consistently negative cultures for acid-fast organisms. Some late cases need to be treated with a combination of surgery and antituberculous medication. Prognosis for life is usually good under proper treatment and close followup.

SELECTED REFERENCES

Ehrlich, R. M., and Lattimer, J. K.: Urogenital tuberculosis in children. J. Urol., *105*:461, 1971.
   A very good account of childhood tuberculosis.

Hanley, H. G.: Conservative surgery in renal tuberculosis including renal cavernotomy. Br. J. Surg., 48:415, 1961.
   Observations on the operative techniques for renal tuberculosis.

Lattimer, J. K., Uson, A. C., and Melicow, M. M.: Tuberculous infections and inflammations of the urinary tract. *In* Campbell, M. F., and Harrison, J. H., (eds.): Textbook of Urology. 3rd ed. Philadelphia, W. B. Saunders Company, 1970, vol. I, p. 443.
   A complete account of urinary tract tuberculosis by men who have been major active participants in the development of the modern concepts of therapy.

Medlar, E. M., Spain, D. M., and Holliday, R. W.: Post-mortem compared with clinical diagnosis of genito-urinary tuberculosis in adult males. J. Urol., *61*:1078, 1949.
   Classic description of the pathogenesis of genitourinary tuberculosis.

REFERENCES

Cooper, H. G., and Robinson, E. G.: Treatment of genitourinary tuberculosis: Report after 24 years. J. Urol., *108*:136, 1972.

Gow, J. G.: Genito-urinary tuberculosis: A study of 700 cases. Lancet, 2:261, 1963.

Hanley, H. G.: The indications for surgery in renal tuberculosis. Br. J. Surg., 45:10, 1957.

Kerr, W. K., Gale, G. L., and Peterson, K. S.: Reconstructive surgery for genitourinary tuberculosis. J. Urol., *101*:254, 1969.

Nesbit, R. M., and Bohne, A. W.: A present day rationale for the treatment for urinary tuberculosis. J.A.M.A., *138*:937, 1948.

Nesbit, R. M., and Thirlby, R. L.: Results of streptomycin therapy in urinary tuberculosis. Trans. Am. Assoc. Genitourinary Surg., *43*:48, 1951.

Vasquez, G., and Lattimer, J. K.: Danger to children of infection from exposure to urine containing tubercle bacilli. J.A.M.A., *171*:29, 1959.

Wyrens, R. G.: Indication for extirpative renal operation for tuberculosis. J. Urol., 87:1, 1962.

Chapter Eleven

OBSTRUCTIVE UROPATHY — URETEROHYDRONEPHROSIS

William J. Butler

Ureterohydronephrosis defines a specific and interrelated structural and functional change in the ureter and kidney that is the result of an obstruction to the normal flow of urine from the kidney to the bladder. The cause of the obstruction may be a mechanical or functional impediment to the transport of urine. The resultant increase of the intrarenal pelvic pressure initiates the distinctive morphologic pattern of hydronephrosis that is characterized by increased intraluminal and interstitial renal pressures with ischemia, parenchymal atrophy, and a simultaneous loss of renal function. Relief of the obstruction with a reduction of the intrarenal pelvic pressure permits a degree of repair with the improvement of renal function and the reversal of the ureteric changes. Ischemia and urinary stasis predispose to bacterial invasion and calculus formation.

Hydronephrosis and hydroureter are terms that have been traditionally used to describe the individual elements of obstructive uropathy in the upper urinary tract. Unfortunately, these terms are also loosely used to indicate lesions of similar physical appearance without the implied obstructive origin. Examples of this usage are the urographic appearance of pyelocalyectasis that results from destructive inflammatory disease, calyces of broad dimensions, and large caliber ureters of unknown origin. The scope of this chapter is limited to a concise presentation of ureterohydronephrosis as defined above, its origin, pathogenesis, pathophysiology, diagnosis, and treatment. Anatomy and pathology are covered in Chapters One and Four; pathogenesis and pathophysiology are amplified in Chapters Five, Six, and Eight.

ETIOLOGY

A diverse variety of diseases and pathophysiologic states have been identified as causes for ureterohydronephrosis. Most of them constrict or occlude the ureter. Congenital muscular deficiencies of the ureter may obstruct by acting as a barrier to the orderly transmission of peristalsis. Congenitally abnormal intramural ureterovesical segments may permit a ready reflux of urine from the bladder up the ureter, with the direct transmission of higher vesical pressures. Similar ureterovesical urinary reflux occurs in neurogenic bladders and decompensated bladders, producing ureterohydronephrosis. The following outline presents the more commonly encountered obstructions to the ureter. For further information see Chapters Two, Ten, and Twelve through Fifteen.)

   I. Calculi
  II. Ureterovesical obstruction from lower tract disorders
     A. Vesical neoplasm
     B. Prostatic neoplasm
     C. Neurogenic bladders
     D. Decompensated bladder
     E. Chronic cystitis
 III. Extrinsic masses or neoplasms
     A. Invasion from contiguous neoplasm
     B. Tumors of broad ligament
     C. Pregnancy
     D. Retroperitoneal granuloma or fibrosis
     E. Aneurysms of aorta or iliac artery
     F. Renal masses or cysts displacing ureter
  IV. Trauma
     A. Iatrogenic
       1. Ligatures, clamps, packs
       2. Previous ureteric surgery with stricture
       3. Impacted calculi causing severe ureteritis or secondary scarring when the calculus is removed
     B. Penetrating wounds
     C. Irradiation with periureteric scar
     D. Delayed periureteric cicatrix following initial trauma
     E. Recent ureteric anastomosis
   V. Congenital lesions
     A. Ureteric stenosis at any level (length of segment may vary)
     B. Aberrant renal vessels may constrict ureter
     C. Abnormally thick fascial bands around ureter
     D. Ectopic ureteric stoma below bladder neck (urethra or seminal vesicle)
     E. Abnormal vesical ureteric junction with reflux of urine
     F. Ureterocele
     G. Ureteric valve or redundant mucosal fold
     H. Adynamic ureteric segment (muscular deficiency)
  VI. Intrinsic ureteric neoplasms
     A. Epithelioma
     B. Benign fibromuscular polyps

VII. Ureteric stricture from inflammatory disease
    A. Tuberculosis
    B. Nonspecific chronic ureteritis (usually with chronic pyelonephritis)

PATHOGENESIS AND PATHOPHYSIOLOGY

Occlusion of the ureter produces a prompt dilatation proximally with progressive atrophy of the renal parenchyma, simultaneously blunting and distending the renal pelvis and calyces. Longstanding partial obstruction may produce an enormously ballooned cystic kidney with a mere shell of cortex in which a few nephrons continue to secrete urine. The intrapelvic hydrostatic pressure, at first elevated with acute obstruction (50 to 70 mm Hg) falls to normal levels with chronic obstruction (5 to 15 mm Hg). Calculus formation is a frequent complication, either in the form of primary renal calculi aided by a relatively static pool of urine, or secondary to urease-producing bacteria. Ischemia, anoxia, and urinary stasis predispose to bacterial invasion. The complication of pyelonephritis produces added renal damage that is often severe and, in addition, poses the continued threat of septicemia. Chronic infection with inflammation in the pelvis and ureteric wall interferes with peristalsis, produces fibrosis, and reduces the potential reversibility from the dilated state. Pyonephrosis describes hydronephrosis with purulent contents in the renal pelvis and ureter.

With complete occlusion, the wall of the ureter becomes dilated and atrophic with diminished or no peristalsis. However, with partial occlusion the ureteric muscle undergoes hypertrophy, although the peristalsis of the distended ureter exhibits less force and amplitude. Ureteric decompensation is a term used to describe the greatly dilated hypertrophied ureter with weak ineffective peristalsis.

Hydronephrosis of pregnancy apparently reflects a degree of ureteric compression at the inlet of the bony pelvis by the enlarging uterus and disappears after parturition. It appears in the second trimester, may be unilateral or bilateral, and often partially diminishes in the third trimester.

Release of the ureteric obstruction permits recovery of the surviving nephrons and the improvement of their functional capacity. The ureteric dilatation and hypertrophy are inclined to reverse, unless infection or fibrosis has produced permanent damage.

Compensatory hypertrophy of the contralateral kidney follows when the ipsilateral kidney is obstructed. Simultaneous with a decrease of renal blood flow to the obstructed kidney is an increase in renal blood flow to the nonobstructed kidney. Compensatory hypertrophy is believed to be a true growth process, which is produced when an increased work load exists and is observed whenever contralateral renal function is impaired. Such a kidney can produce 70 to 90 per cent of the estimated total renal function.

A large body of experimental studies and clinical data has accumulated in the literature of this century, but as yet most of the pathophysiologic explanations of the hydronephrotic process remain theoretical. Micropuncture techniques have demonstrated the direct transmission of increased intrapelvic pressures to intratubular, precapillary, and interstitial spaces. Renal blood flow in acute ureteric occlusion is at first transiently increased but within hours exhibits a marked decrease which persists throughout the chronic state, with atrophy of the renal arteries. Venous congestion is prominent early and persists. Tissue studies indicate a shift from aerobic to anaerobic metabolism, gluconeogenesis to glucolysis, and interference with free fatty acid metabolism. Traditional theory envisions an imbalance of urine secretion by the kidney against higher intrapelvic pressures that is caused by the inability to rapidly transport urine to the bladder. The increased renal intratubular and interstitial pressures contribute to ischemia and further cellular atrophy. Mechanisms such as pyelolymphatic and pyelovenous back flow of the urine provide a form of compensation. Thus it is possible to reach a stable compromise so that the average volume of urine secreted by the kidney matches the transport capabilities of the obstructed ureter. If the obstruction to urine flow is severe, the renal atrophy is severe.

Renal function is reduced in the hydronephrotic kidney and is improved by release of the obstruction. A variable pattern of renal deficits is observed, as defined by function tests such as the excretion of dyes, inulin, para-aminohippurate, concentration, and dilution. The reduced function of a unilateral hydronephrosis presents no problem when the contralateral kidney is normal. When the disease is bilateral or in a solitary kidney, the reduced renal function can be classified clinically either as renal insufficiency or as renal failure, depending on whether normal values of serum creatinine, urea, and phosphates exist in the presence of a normal intake. Adequate relief from the obstruction permits an immediate conversion from a state of relative oliguria (or anuria) to a state of relative polyuria. A diuresis frequently ensues, usually augmented by a previous accumulation of body water, electrolytes, and metabolites. The state of renal failure may thus convert to a state of renal insufficiency with return of near normal serum values for electrolytes, creatinine, urea, and phosphates. Persistence of the state of renal failure may be further complicated by anemia, hypertension, congestive heart failure, and pyelonephritis. Disturbances of calcium metabolism may appear, leading to renal rickets, osteodystrophy, and hyperparathyroidism.

DIAGNOSIS

The diagnosis of ureterohydronephrosis is arrived at by adhering to the fundamentals of clinical diagnosis that include a careful history and physical examination, urinalysis, and serum creatinine. Since the lesion is often asymptomatic, there is no substitute for a low threshold of suspicion on the part of the examining physician. The following outline

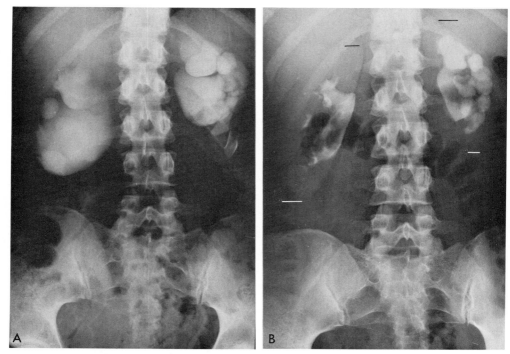

Figure 11–1 *A,* An excretory urogram of a female, age 26, who experienced intermittent flank pain. The bilateral hydronephroses were interpreted as probably congenital ureteropelvic junction obstructions with more hydronephrotic atrophy in the left kidney. Retrograde pyelograms proved the diagnosis correct, and Figure 11–1, *B* demonstrates the appearance three months after bilateral pyeloplasty. The right renal parenchyma suggests some compensatory hypertrophy, while that on the left remains atrophic as outlined by the marks at the upper and lower poles of the kidneys.

presents pertinent points that should point toward the existence of ureterohydronephrosis.

    I. Presenting complaint
       A. Flank pain (intermittent or constant)
       B. Dysuria (when infection is present)
       C. Hematuria
       D. Sepsis (may be fulminating)
       E. Unexplained gastrointestinal symptoms
       F. Symptoms of uremia
       G. Osteodystrophy or rickets
   II. Past history
       A. Urinary calculus
       B. Pelvic irradiation
       C. Transurethral surgery
       D. Urinary vaginal fistula
       E. Previous renal trauma
       F. Urinary tuberculosis

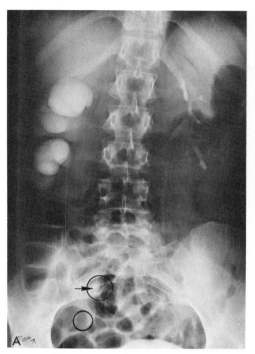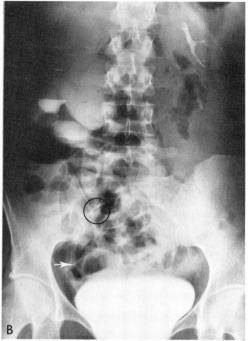

Figure 11–2   *A,* An excretory urogram of a female, age 33, with a history of four operations for renal calculi on both sides, persistent proteus mirabilis urinary infection, and recurrent pain in the right flank. The contrast material is being slowly excreted by the large right ureterohydronephrosis, but the renal pelvis and ureter is not yet well filled. The lowermost shadow outlined in the pelvic portion suggests a calculus in line with the ureter. Another suspicious shadow lies just medial to the right sacroiliac joint and could also be a calculus. This film was obtained with the patient elevated 30 degrees from horizontal. Figure 11–2, *B* illustrates the x-ray film obtained in the upright position, taking advantage of the high specific gravity of the excreted contrast medium which flows down filling the widely dilated ureter to the suspected calculus at the sacroiliac joint marked by the upper arrow. The arrow indicates the course of the ureter from this point downward as being of relatively normal caliber even where it flows by the lower calculus identified by the arrow in *A.* Note the layering effect of the contrast media in the calyces and the filling of the renal pelvis accomplished by placing the patient in the upright position. At operation, an ureterolithotomy, the diagnosis based on the excretory urogram, was confirmed.

    G. Ureteric surgery
    H. Recurrent urinary infection
III. Physical findings
    A. Palpable flank mass (which may transilluminate in infants and youths)
    B. Other abdominal masses
    C. Retroperitoneal lymphoma or neoplasm
    D. Aneurysm of aorta or iliac artery
    E. Intrapelvic mass
    F. Chronic urinary retention
    G. Carcinoma of urinary bladder or prostate
    H. Carcinoma of rectum or colon
    I. Spinal cord disease and congenital myelodysplasia (neurogenic bladder)

J. Constant urinary leakage from urethra in infants and children (urethral valves in the male and ectopic ureter in the female)

IV. Laboratory findings
  A. Routine urinalysis
    1. Pyuria
    2. Hematuria
    3. Bacteriuria
  B. Elevated serum creatinine
  C. Azotemia
  D. Neoplastic cells in urine

Identification of ureterohydronephrosis is accomplished by obtaining an excretory urogram. (See Figs. 11-1, 11-2, 11-3, and 11-4.) Delay of excretion in the affected kidney may require repeated exposures over three to six hours in order to obtain sufficient opacification of the dilated collecting system and to identify the point of obstruction. The thickness of the renal parenchyma can be measured to provide an estimate of the degree of atrophy. The presence or absence of a hypertrophied contralateral kidney can be observed. With knowledge of the serum creatinine, or creatinine clearance, a fairly accurate estimate of relative renal function may be made. The amount of parenchymal atrophy provides some prognosis about the potential function of the obstructed kidney.

If the cause of the obstruction is unclear or if the kidney fails to excrete the contrast material, additional and more sophisticated urologic and radiographic techniques may be necessary. These include cystoscopy, retrograde pyelography, cystometry, antegrade pyelography, selective angiography, cystourethrography, and sonography (refer to Chapter Three).

In the case of intermittent hydronephrosis, the urogram may be normal, except when the patient is experiencing pain. Emergency urography during pain may be necessary to identify the obstructed kidney. Hydration urography is also utilized to serve a similar purpose.

THERAPY

The treatment of a specific clinical patient with ureterohydronephrosis is inseparably tied to the treatment of the cause, whose character and prognosis influence the selection of therapy. It is therefore important that the probable cause be identified in order to plan rational therapy. Unfortunately, this course of action is not always possible for a variety of reasons. The patient may present with a life-threatening septicemia that does not permit time to investigate the cause. The cause may be obscure, especially in infants in whom only a limited investigation may be possible. Other important variables that enter into the therapeutic decision are the age of the patient, the personality and lifestyle,

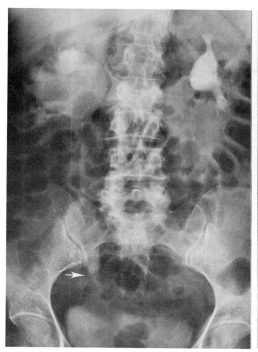 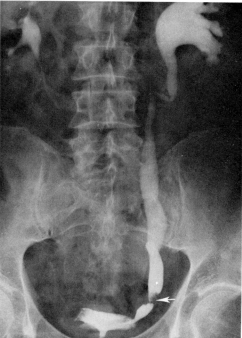

Fig 11–3   Fig. 11–4

Figure 11–3 An excretory urogram obtained ten days following abdominal hysterectomy because urine began to drain from the vagina. A large right ureterohydronephrosis is demonstrated with the dilated ureter ending abruptly just below the bony pelvis as indicated by the arrow. This is presumed to be the point of ureteral trauma and extravasation of urine. A cystoscopy and right retrograde ureterogram demonstrated a complete block just below this point and confirmed the impression obtained from the initial excretory urogram.

Figure 11–4 The x-ray demonstrates ureterohydronephrosis above a filling defect in the lower left ureter. The patient is a male, age 59, with a history of recurrent transitional cell carcinoma of the bladder, Grade II. He presented with left renal colic and the urine sediment revealed red blood cells and neoplastic cells. A cystoscopy ruled out neoplasm of the bladder or urethral epithelium. A presumptive diagnosis of ureteral carcinoma was made and proven at operation.

the systemic state, and the degree of renal and ureteric functional impairment.

The age of the patient, life expectancy, and the presence of systemic disease modify therapy. For example, a congenital hydronephrosis discovered in childhood would be appropriately reconstructed, whereas the same lesion discovered in the sixth decade of life might be just as appropriately treated expectantly, if it is asymptomatic and the total renal function is adequate. The lifestyle of the patient must be considered, especially when urine collecting devices are contemplated in the therapeutic plan. The mental, emotional, and manual capability to manage such a device must be present.

The lesion may be bilateral or unilateral. If unilateral, the presence or absence of a healthy contralateral kidney obviously bears heavily upon the therapeutic decision. Advanced hydronephrotic atrophy may raise doubts about preserving the kidney if it alone will not support life. In that case a nephrectomy would be the more conservative operation. A dilated decompensated ureter might require a prolonged period of decompression to recover function, so that a form of prolonged urinary diversion must be planned. The presence of complications significantly alters management. The more common complications are pyelonephritis, pyonephrosis, septicemia, and calculi. When hydronephrosis is bilateral or in a solitary kidney, total renal function is reduced so that a clinical state of either renal insufficiency or renal failure exists. Relief of the obstruction abruptly changes the clinical picture from that of a relative oliguria to that of a relative polyuria. This requires a shift of therapy from a restriction of water, electrolytes, and metabolites that require renal clearance to an expanded intake. Laboratory measurements of serum creatinine, sodium, and potassium with documentation of urinary output will monitor the degree and rate of improvement of the renal function. Persistence of renal failure requires appropriate dietary management and treatment of the complications. Progression to a state of terminal renal failure may require hemodialysis or renal transplantation.

Ureterohydronephrosis is most frequently encountered in a clinical setting that is not immediately life-threatening and, as such, permits careful evaluation and formulation of a plan of treatment. However, there are two circumstances, fulminating sepsis and anuria, which may require prompt action to prevent mortality prior to establishing an accurate diagnosis of the cause.

Severe pyelonephritis complicating hydronephrosis may present with fulminating sepsis. Adequate treatment requires prompt reduction of the elevated intrarenal pressure by urinary diversion with or without removal of the obstruction (i.e., calculus). Systemic toxicity and circulatory collapse may only permit the introduction of a nephrostomy catheter through a small incision or trocar. This maneuver may be life-saving, providing drainage of purulent urine and permitting sepsis to subside. Simultaneous management of renal failure, antibacterial therapy, circulatory and cardiopulmonary support, correction of anemia, and treatment of intercurrent disorders such as diabetes may be necessary to attain recovery. Investigation of the cause and consideration of more permanent solutions can usually await systemic improvement.

The patient who presents with anuria from an unknown origin (and with an empty bladder) is a candidate for cystoscopy and retrograde pyelography in order to diagnose the cause and possibly to provide relief of the obstruction. The procedure also serves to differentiate nonobstructive anuria, such as renal artery thrombosis, acute glomerulonephritis, and acute tubular necrosis. Introduction of a ureteral catheter above the point of obstruction may provide sufficient temporary diversion of the urine to permit time for diagnosis and to better prepare the patient for definitive surgery if indicated. If the obstruction cannot be successfully bypassed with this maneuver, the institution of peritoneal dialysis or hemodialysis will provide the necessary life support to allow time for further investigation of the cause and to arrive at a decision about surgical intervention. Similarly, anuria immediately following a retroperitoneal or pelvic operation should arouse suspicion of ureteric obstruction. Prompt fluid restriction, cystoscopic investigation, and surgical correction are indicated. If edema is present, dialysis may be necessary to remove excess body water prior to the operation. The availability of dialysis in recent years has significantly altered the management and prognosis of patients who are anuric because of complete ureteric obstruction.

The majority of patients with ureterohydronephrosis are observed in a clinical setting that permits a more deliberate and thoughtful approach to the problem. Management may take the path of prevention, expectant therapy, or planned surgical treatment. Preventive measures include early recognition and treatment of neurogenic bladders, awareness of the risks and the complications of transurethral and retroperitoneal surgery, and the complications of irradiation therapy. Expectant management with follow-up urograms will document the emergence of ureteric obstruction and the rate of change. Minimal to moderate ureterohydronephrosis, such as relatively stable asymptomatic congenital ureteropelvic obstructions in adults or moderate dilatation following irradiation for carcinoma of the cervix, may in some instances be properly treated expectantly. Interval urograms, serum creatinine, and urinalysis serve to monitor the progress. Emergence of symptoms of pain, declining renal function, or the development of urinary infection may require reevaluation of the therapeutic course.

Surgical Techniques

Surgical solutions generally fall into two categories: (1) removal of the cause with the reestablishment of functional continuity of the urinary tract or (2) permanent urinary tract diversions. A classic example of the first category is the removal of an obstructing calculus. Reconstructive surgery for adynamic ureteric segments, segmental muscular hypertrophy, benign ureteric polyps, fibrotic ureteric stenosis, and compression by blood vessels or fascial bands are examples of lesions that lend themselves to treatment in the first category. The surgical operations that are used to accomplish these ends are ureterolithotomy, pyelolithotomy, ureteroplasty, pyeloplasty, ureterovesical anastomosis, segmental excision with reanastomosis of ureter, and primary anastomosis of ureter with surgical accidents.

The Foley Y-V pyeloplasty for correction of ureteropelvic stenosis is a classic example of this first category of surgery (Fig. 11–5). A Y-incision is mapped on the inferior aspect of the dilated pelvis with the stem of the Y extended down the ureter through the stenosis. The apex of the pelvic flap (marked A) is sutured to the apex of the ureteric incision (marked A'), with the remaining edges evenly proportioned and sutured to produce a widely funneled ureteropelvic outlet. Nephrostomy drainage may be incorporated for temporary decompression.

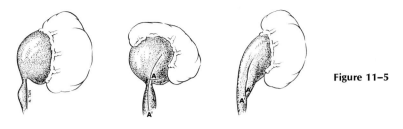

Figure 11–5

FOLEY Y-V PYELOPLASTY

Isolated enteric segments and tubes constructed from the bladder to bridge gaps in the ureter are also utilized in these reconstructive techniques (see Figs. 11–6,*B* and 11–6,*C*), although the reestablishment of urinary tract continuity for long endopelvic ureteric defects may present a serious surgical challenge. Lesions that involve only the lowermost ureter can usually be managed by dividing the ureter above the obstruction and anastomosing it to the side of the bladder. When the entire endopelvic ureter is functionally damaged as high as the bony pelvic inlet, a crossed ureteroureteral anastomosis can be performed (Fig. 11–6,*A*). For ureteric obstruction at slightly lower levels, the bladder flap method of Ockerblad may be successful (Fig. 11–6,*B*).

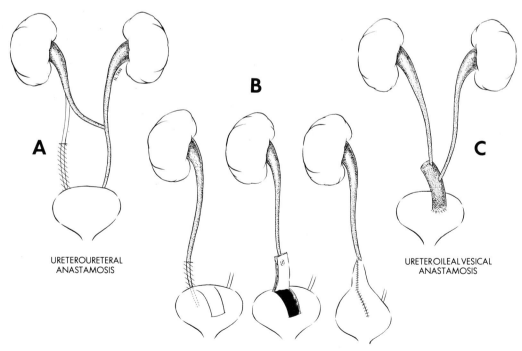

URETEROURETERAL ANASTAMOSIS

URETEROILEAL VESICAL ANASTAMOSIS

REIMPLANTATION OF URETER INTO A BLADDER FLAP

Figure 11–6

When the ureteric lesions are bilateral and extensive, a segment of ileum may be utilized to connect the ureters to the bladder (Fig. 11-6, C). Nephrostomy drainage is frequently employed simultaneously with these procedures.

Permanent urinary diversions are selected when the urinary bladder is removed by surgical operation or if its functional capacity is destroyed. Severe fibrotic contracture associated with chronic bacterial infection, irradiation necrosis, contracted neurogenic bladder, and vesical neoplasms are examples of lesions that would require permanent supravesical diversion of the urine. Ureteroileal cutaneous anastomoses (Fig. 11-7,A) and ureterosigmoid cutaneous anastomoses are examples of permanent urinary diversions, both utilizing an isolated enteric segment as a conduit from the retroperitoneum to the anterior abdominal wall. In recent years the use of colonic segments in children has been found superior to the ileum because the stoma tends to remain patent and does not require frequent revision during the growing years. These operations permit minimal interruption of the ureteric vasculature during the technical performance of the operation and utilize the mobility of the mesenteric blood vessels to place the enteric stoma at a preplanned spot on the abdominal wall for the most efficient attachment of the urinary stomal collecting device. Cutaneous ureterostomy (Fig. 11–7,B) is also in this category but carries a higher risk of interference with the ureteric blood supply. In general, it is preferred when the ureter is enormously dilated and hypertrophied. Cutaneous ureterostomy is also a less traumatic operation than ureteric enteric cutaneous diversions and may therefore be preferable when the patient is a poor surgical risk.

Some surgical techniques for diversion of the urine above the bladder do not interrupt the continuity of the urinary tract and may be maintained indefinitely. This continuity is maintained by decompressing the dilated upper urinary tract. Nephrostomy catheter drainage, which has wide applications, is also used in conjunction with corrective

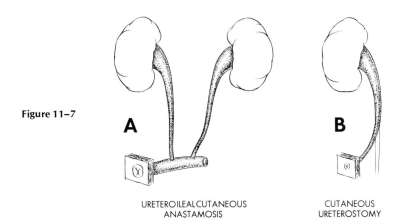

Figure 11–7

A

B

URETEROILEALCUTANEOUS
ANASTAMOSIS

CUTANEOUS
URETEROSTOMY

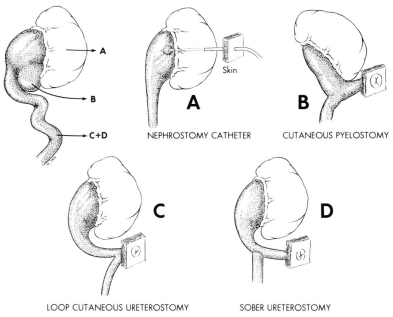

Figure 11–8

procedures to ensure adequate decompression of the renal pelvis (Fig. 11–8,*A*). Cutaneous pyelostomy (Fig. 11–8,*B*) and loop cutaneous ureterostomy (Fig. 11–8,*C*) are employed primarily in children with greatly dilated ureters and pelves. The Sober ureterostomy is applicable to greatly dilated and tortuous ureters and possesses the advantage of not requiring an extensive secondary closure as does the loop cutaneous ureterostomy (Fig. 11–8,*D*). Vesicostomy at the bladder level is also in this category and provides urinary decompression while preserving continuty of the urinary tract. All of these operations can be discontinued if the cause of the obstruction is resolved.

As mentioned above, nephrostomy catheter drainage is often used in conjunction with reconstructive surgery and is important because it protects the kidney from the adverse effects of increased urinary pressures postoperatively until the urinary transport system recovers adequate function. Introduction of urographic contrast media through the nephrostomy catheter permits easy recognition of this event, and the catheter can simply be withdrawn. In event of delay or the persistence of ureteric obstruction, such drainage can be maintained indefinitely by changing the catheter at regular intervals. The presence of the catheter in the kidney presents the disadvantage of contributing to the continued presence of bacteria and the formation of calculus deposits. It is for this reason that the establishment of cutaneous stoma for permanent urinary diversion is desirable. On the other hand, nephrostomy catheter drainage can be established in large dilated kidneys with minimal surgical trauma and is without peer as the operative choice when the accompanying severe systemic disorders make the patient a poor surgical risk.

After diversion of the urine has been accomplished, the patient must be followed expectantly with urography, serum creatinine, and urinalysis since stenosis of the cutaneous stoma or stenosis of the ureteric anastomoses may again contribute to the reappearance of ureterohydronephrosis.

An enterostomal therapist can be of invaluable assistance to the physician and the patient, providing expert advice regarding the various devices and skin adhesives, preparing the patient psychologically, and in the postoperative management of the stoma. This continual attention minimizes complications and helps the patient experience a more comfortable stomal life.

SELECTED REFERENCES

Campbell, M. F., and Harrison, J. H.: Urology. Philadelphia, W. B. Saunders Company, 1970.
The following chapters deal with ureterohydronephrosis: Chapter 2: Merrill, J. P.: Treatment of renal failure. Chapter 3: Kiil, F.: Physiology of the renal pelvis and ureter. Chapter 9: Hinman, F., Jr.: The pathophysiology of urinary obstruction. Chapter 21: Rusche, C., and Morrow, J. W.: Injury to the ureter. Chapter 33: Lapides, J.: Neuromuscular vesical and ureteral dysfunction.

Crabtree, E. G.: Urological Diseases of Pregnancy. Boston, Little, Brown and Co., 1942.
A textbook of historical interest, reflecting the emerging concept of a long term relationship of pyelonephritis and nephritides with hypertension and the cardio-renal-vascular complex.

Emmett, J. L.: Clinical Urography. 3rd ed. Philadelphia, W. B. Saunders Company, 1971.
Beautifully illustrated categories of radiography in obstructive uropathy are presented by a urologist.

Flocks, R. H., and Culp, D. A.: Handbook of Operative Surgery. 3rd ed. Surgical Urology, Chicago Yearbook Medical Publishers, Inc., 1967.
A surgical manual illustrated by master surgeons.

Glenn, J. F.: Urologic Surgery. 2nd ed. Hagerstown, Md., Harper and Row Publishers, 1975.
Chapter 6 by J. H. DeWeerd is a superb and concise presentation of surgery of the renal pelvis and ureteropelvic junction for congenital hydronephrosis.

Kiil, F.: The Function of the Ureter and Renal Pelvis. Philadelphia, W. B. Saunders Company, 1957.
Merrill, J. P.: The Treatment of Renal Failure. 2nd ed. New York, Grune and Stratton, 1967.
Nowinski, W. W., and Guss, L. J.: Compensatory Renal Hypertrophy. New York, Academic Press, 1969.
Scott, R., Sr.: Current Controversies in Urologic Management. Philadelphia, W. B. Saunders Company, 1972.
Scott concisely presents the current national controversy over the selection of types of permanent urinary diversions, pyeloplasty, surgical solutions to large ureteric defects, and the subject of ureterovesical reimplantation. Adversarial presentations by numerous authors are included.

REFERENCES

Agusta, V. E., Panko, W. B., and Gillenwater, J. Y.: Changes in the in vivo metabolism of hydronephrotic canine kidney. Invest. Urol., *11*:379, 1974.

Bricker, N. S., Shwayri, E. I., Reardan, J. B., Kellog, D., Merrill, J. P., and Holmes, J. H.: An abnormality in renal function resulting from urinary tract obstruction. Am. J. Med., *23*:554, 1957.

Butcher, H. R., Jr., and Sleator, W., Jr.: The effect of ureteral anastomosis upon conduction of peristaltic waves: An electrourographic study. J. Urol., *75*:65, 1956.

Engel, R. M.: Complications of bilateral ureteroileal cutaneous urinary diversions: A review of 208 cases. J. Urol., *101*:508, 1969.

Gillenwater, J. Y., Vaughn, D., Jr., Shenasky, S. H. II., Agusta, V. W., Middleton, G., and Panko, W. B.: Experimental hydronephrosis: A summary of research in progress I. Trans. Amer. Assoc. Genitourin. Surg., *64*:128, 1972.

Gottschalik, C. W., and Mylle, M.: Micropuncture study of pressures in proximal tubule and peritubular capillaries of the rat's kidney and their relation to ureteral and renal venous pressures. Am. J. Physiol., *185*:430, 1956.

Higgins, C. C.: Ureteral injuries during surgery: A review of 87 cases. J.A.M.A., *199*:82, 1967.

Jaffe, B. M., Bricker, E. M., and Butcher, H. R., Jr.,: Surgical complications of ileal segment urinary diversion. Ann. Surg., *167*:367, 1968.

Johnston, J. H.: Temporary cutaneous ureterostomy in the management of advanced congenital urinary obstruction. Arch. Dis. Child., *38*:161, 1963.

Kretschmer, H. L., and Kanter, A. E.: Effect of certain gynecologic lesions on the upper urinary tract: A pyelographic study. J.A.M.A., *109*:1087, 1937.

Krohn, A. G., Ogden, D. A., and Holmes, S. H.: Renal function in 29 healthy adults before and after nephrectomy. J.A.M.A., *196*:110, 1966.

Lapides, J.: Physiology of the intact human ureter. J. Urol., *59*:501, 1948.

Lapides, J., Koyanagi, T., and Diokno, A.: Ten year survey cutaneous vesicostomy. J. Urol., *105*:76, 1971.

Lapides, J., Diokno, A. C., Silber, S. J., and Lowe, B. S.: Clean intermittent self-catheterization in the treatment of urinary tract disease. J. Urol., 107:458, 1972.

Malt, R. A.: Compensatory growth of the kidney. N. Engl. J. Med., 280:1446, 1969.

Mogg, R. A.: The treatment of neurogenic urinary incontinence using the colonic conduit. Br. J. Urol., 37:681, 1965.

Mogg, R. A.: Urinary diversion using the colonic conduit. Br. J. Urol., 39:687, 1967.

Murnaghan, G. F.: The dynamics of the renal pelvis and ureter with reference to congenital hydronephrosis. Br. J. Urol., 30:321, 1958.

Ockerblad, N. F.: Reimplantation of the ureter into the bladder by a flap method. J. Urol., 57:845, 1947.

Perlmutter, A. D., and Tank, E. S.: Loop cutaneous ureterostomy in infancy. J. Urol., 99:559, 1968.

Rao, N. R., and Heptinstall, R. H.: Experimental hydronephrosis. A microangiographic study. Invest. Urol., 6:183, 1968.

Rose, J. G., and Gillenwater, J. Y.: The effect of chronic ureteral obstruction and infection upon ureteral function. Invest. Urol., *11*:471, 1974.

Sober, I.: Pelvioureterostomy-en-Y. J. Urol., *107*:473, 1972.

Vaughn, E. D., Surenson, E. J., and Gillenwater, J. Y.: The renal hemodynamic response to chronic unilateral complete ureteral occlusion. Invest. Urol., 8:78, 1970.

Witherington, R.: Experimental study on role of intravesical ureter in vesicoureteral regurgitation. J. Urol., 89:176, 1963.

Zimskind, P. D., Davis, D. M. D., Lewis, P. L., Decarstecker, J., and Berwind, R. T.: Complete obstruction of the ureter; immediate and long term effects on the renal pelvic pressure in dogs. Surg. Forum, *19*:538, 1968.

Chapter Twelve

OBSTRUCTIVE UROPATHY— PROSTATISM

A. Richard Kendall and Lester Karafin

PROSTATE GLAND

The anatomy and embryology of the entire genitourinary system have been well described in Chapters One and Two. In brief, the prostate is a fibromuscular glandular organ, arising during the twelfth week of embryonic life as outgrowths of the prostatic urethra (mesonephric duct). These outgrowths proceed in an orderly fashion and by the fourth month of fetal life are organized into five groups of glands that correspond to the lobes of the adult prostate (anterior, median, posterior, and two lateral) and which completely encircle the urethra. By the last trimester, lobulation is completed by the development of fibromuscular septa, and the entire gland is encased by a dense fibrous capsule.

Thus formed, the prostate completely surrounds the prostatic urethra, with its base at the neck of the bladder and its apex resting against the urogenital diaphragm. The posterior aspect lies against the anterior wall of the rectum and is separated by Denonvilliers' fascia, and the anterior portion of the gland is attached to the undersurface of the pubis by the puboprostatic ligaments. The ejaculatory ducts course obliquely through the prostate to empty into the posterior urethra on the verumontanum just lateral to the utricle.

Blood supply to the prostate arises mainly via branches of the inferior vesical artery, which is a branch of the internal iliac artery. As initially described by Flocks, these vessels at the base of the prostate branch into urethral and capsular arteries. The former penetrate the prostate at the vesicoprostatic junction to supply the vesical neck and periurethral portions of the gland. The capsular branches supply the periphery of the gland and the periurethral apical tissue. With prostatic hyperplasia, the urethral vessels assume more importance in supplying most of the adenomatous tissue.

317

The actual size of the prostate gland should only be of importance to the urologic surgeon. Symptomatic prostatism may be the result of only minimal enlargement as discerned by palpation, and conversely, marked enlargement may produce little symptomatology if the prostatic urethra is not obstructed. Although the average adult prostate weighs between 15 and 20 grams, the student is often confused by house staff nomenclature, such as the grading categories of +1, +2, +3, +4. It appears obvious that this form of estimation of prostatic size should be discarded, and the size of the prostate should be described in uniform terms, preferably by approximate dimensions in centimeters (normal size is 3 cm by 4 cm).

More important than the determination of size, the student must learn just how to perform rectal palpation of the prostate. He must recognize the normal landmarks (base, apex, median, and lateral sulci). Only through repeated examinations can one appreciate the normal consistency of the prostate and compare a firm gland (carcinoma, granulomatous inflammation, calculi, or infarction) with the normal or even the congested soft prostate described by some as indicative of prostatitis. Ideal prostatic palpation is best achieved either with the patient in the lateral decubitus position, facing the examiner with hips flexed, or while standing with knees slightly flexed and elbows resting on the table. The well lubricated index finger easily palpates the prostate and its normal landmarks immediately after gentle entrance through the anal sphincter. Rectal examination should always include an estimation of the tone of the external anal sphincter, should rule out any intraluminal lesions, and should be completed with testing of the bulbocavernosus reflex (see neurogenic bladder disease).

The prostate gland has no essential function except to produce a fluid which acts as a conveyance and nutrient for spermatozoa. Normal prostatic fluid is rich in acid phosphatase, which is excreted through the ductal system. Elevation of the serum acid phosphatase (especially the prostatic fraction) is usually indicative of prostatic carcinoma with local ductal obstruction or distant metastases. One should not expect elevations of prostatic acid phosphatase into the neoplastic range following simple prostatic examination.

Prostatism is a clinical term utilized to designate obstruction to urinary flow that is of prostatic origin. Although the symptoms may be similar, the obstruction may be due to fibromuscular hyperplasia (BPH), carcinoma, vesical neck contracture, or occasionally reversible inflammatory disease.

BENIGN PROSTATIC HYPERPLASIA

Benign prostatic hyperplasia (BPH) represents by far the most common cause of vesical neck obstruction. The term *hypertrophy* is a misnomer and should be discarded since the enlargement is the result of new growth of the periurethral glands and is not simple hypertrophy.

Most commonly, the two lateral lobes and the median lobe undergo hyperplasia that gives rise to the commonly employed term of *trilobar hyperplasia*. The anterior lobe usually remains rudimentary while the posterior lobe is the site of neoplastic change. True vesical neck contracture is quite uncommon, usually occurring in the younger male and possibly representing a fibrous response to infection. Temporary obstructive symptoms can occur with inflammatory lesions of the prostate, e.g., bacterial, nonspecific, or allergic (see Chapter Eight). Although prostatitis is a much overdiagnosed entity, its existence cannot be denied, and medical treatment may prevent an unnecessary operation. Conversely, urinary tract infection secondary to prostatic obstruction should never be diagnosed as chronic prostatitis and a definitive, curative operation be withheld while the patient is subjected to numerous antimicrobial agents and long term prostatic massage.

Currently, the cause of benign prostatic hyperplasia is completely unknown. Despite the lack of specific evidence, most researchers believe that some imbalance in sex hormones is directly responsible. It has been attributed both to sexual overindulgence and to celibacy as well as to chronic infection. Normal amounts of male hormones are necessary for the development and maintenance of the prostate gland, and hyperplasia is never seen in eunuchs. (For a more complete discussion of the various theories and investigations that pertain to origin, the reader is referred to the summation of Mostofi.)

Signs and Symptoms

Although "silent prostatism" is a definite entity in which the patient, denying symptoms, first appears with a distended bladder and azotemia, it must be realized that prostatic obstruction progresses slowly, and the disease is not truly silent. The patient lives with and adjusts to the symptoms so gradually that he believes that they are normal and have always been present. Significant symptoms attributable to benign hyperplasia rarely occur before fifty years of age.

IRRITATIVE SYMPTOMS

1. Urinary frequency.
2. Urinary urgency.
3. Nocturia or nocturnal incontinence.
4. Dysuria (usually secondary to infection).

Although the exact reason for these symptoms is poorly understood, it may be due to trigonal irritability by the enlarging prostate. In the presence of significant residual urine, the effective bladder capacity may be reduced, thus producing urinary frequency. It must be noted that irritative symptoms may be due to other (nonprostatic) problems, and injudicious operations may result in a more uncomfortable patient. Thus, neurogenic bladder disease, diabetes mellitus, fluid retention, or even psychosomatic problems may mimic the irritative symptoms of prostatism.

OBSTRUCTIVE SYMPTOMS

1. Difficulty or delayed initiation of micturition (hesitancy).
2. Straining to void.
3. Decrease in size and force of the urinary stream.
4. Interruption of the urinary stream.
5. Sensation of incomplete bladder evacuation.
6. Increased postmicturitional dribbling.
7. Previous bout of urinary retention.
8. Vesical or rectal tenesmus.
9. Complete urinary retention.

All of the above are evidences of obstruction, but in the differential diagnosis one must include neurogenic bladder disease (Chapter Six), urethral stricture, and "prostatitis." Following alcohol consumption, ulcer or asthmatic therapy, during cold weather, or after a prolonged delay in voiding, the patient with obstructive symptoms should be suspected of *underlying* prostatism. Rectal tenesmus may be due to an unsuspected distended bladder pressing on the rectum.

DIAGNOSIS

Office Physical Examination

Weight loss and pallor may be due to unsuspected renal insufficiency with accompanying anemia. Although advanced or silent prostatism may result in hydronephrosis (see Chapter Eleven), the enlarged kidneys are most often not palpable. A mass in the midline of the lower abdomen that is dull to percussion most likely represents a distended bladder. However, on rare occasions a severe fecal impaction can appear similar and produce secondary bladder symptoms. An asymmetric mass in the lower abdomen may represent a large vesical diverticulum.

The presence of a hernia may represent the gradual weakening of the abdominal wall from straining to void. Acute or chronic epididymitis may result from bacteria ascending along or through the lumen of the vas deferens. As described previously, rectal examination is most important to estimate the size of the prostate and to rule out neoplasm. Occasionally, a distended bladder is misinterpreted as a markedly enlarged prostate gland, and thus the prostate should be reevaluated approximately 24 to 48 hours following decompression, which allows subsidence of edema and permits a more normal palpation of the prostate. Prolapsed external hemorrhoids may result from increased intrapelvic pressure that is due to the distended bladder or straining to void. Bimanual examination permits the identification of a distended bladder previously unsuspected and is an excellent aid in determining significant quantities of residual urine.

Office Laboratory Examination

URINALYSIS

The patient should always void in the presence of the examiner so as to afford observation of the urinary stream. Despite more sophisticated methods, such as the uroflowmeter or stop watch, this is by far the best manner in which to evaluate potential urinary obstruction. What appears to be a satisfactory stream to the patient, owing to the gradual onset of symptomatology, may be quite markedly decreased to the observing physician. Voiding is observed to determine the presence or absence of hesitation, any decrease in force and flow of the stream, or an interruption. Routinely, a midstream specimen is analyzed, although if one suspects infection, the initial portion, midstream, and prostatic fluid can all be evaluated and the infection thus localized. Microscopic examination of the centrifuged sediment detects the presence of white blood cells, red blood cells, or casts. Staining (methylene blue or gram staining) is usually necessary to detect bacteruria. A properly performed stained sediment is almost as reliable as a culture in detecting infection and at no additional cost to the patient. Conversely, rather advanced prostatism may produce no changes whatsoever in the urine.

PROSTATIC FLUID

Much controversy still exists as to the significance of white blood cells in prostatic fluid. Although 20 per cent of normal males may have an increased number of white blood cells in prostatic secretions, the presence of irritative symptoms plus the "pus cells" makes one suspicious of possible inflammation. Bacteria are notoriously difficult to demonstrate.

Examination Follow-Up

Following this preliminary evaluation of the individual as an outpatient, the physician must then decide whether further investigation is indeed warranted. If the symptoms are mild, i.e., the patient is observed to void with a good stream, there is no evidence of a distended bladder, and urinalysis is negative, then only reassurance and supportive therapy may be necessary. An intelligent patient can be instructed to return every six months or sooner if symptomatology progresses. *Routine* catheterization to simply determine residual urine is to be condemned as a possible means of introducing infection.

UROLOGIC COMPLICATIONS OF PROSTATISM

URINARY TRACT INFECTION

Although a few patients with "prostatitis" develop transient obstructive symptoms that resolve on treatment of the inflammatory process, more frequently, underlying prostatism may result in recurrent or relapsing urinary tract infections that resist cure by medical means. The source of bacterial contamination is somewhat controversial, with the ascending urethral theory being more plausible in the female. In the male, bacterial dissemination from the gastrointestinal tract via the lymphatic system has received strong support. Lapides has more recently popularized the concept of a hematogenous origin. He postulates that prolonged elevations of intravesical pressure result in a decreased blood flow in the vesical tissues, thus reducing host resistance and permitting hematogenously disseminated bacteria to seed out and proliferate. Certainly, injudicious instrumentation may infect a mildly obstructed lower urinary tract.

Epididymitis. This condition is usually a result of ascending infection from the bladder and prostate. Prostatic hyperplasia may cause a reflux of urine and bacteria through the lumen of the ejaculatory ducts.

Cystitis. The introduction of bacteria into an obstructed urinary tract accentuates all irritative bladder symptoms and produces significant dysuria. Infection in the presence of residual urine resists antimicrobial eradication.

Pyelonephritis. Once one segment of the urinary tract is infected, the remaining portions are at risk.

Septicemia. This condition is usually due to gram-negative organisms and may occur spontaneously or more often, following instrumentation, especially in the male who has significant residual urine. "Septic shock" is an extremely grave complication with a significant mortality rate despite newer, sophisticated antibacterial therapy.

CHANGES IN THE VESICAL WALL

As the bladder attempts to evacuate against increased intraurethral resistance, progressive trabeculation (hypertrophy of muscle bundles) occurs (Fig. 12–1). Increased muscular hypertrophy produces cellules or small mucosal saccules between the muscle bundles. Further progression may result in vesical diverticula that are single or multiple, small or large (Fig. 12–2). A diverticulum thus represents herniation of vesical mucosa through a defect in the musculature, and on occasion the diverticulum is larger than the bladder itself. A narrow mouth diverticulum may drain quite poorly and may be the cause of persistent infections. Increased incidence of carcinoma has been reported in diverticula.

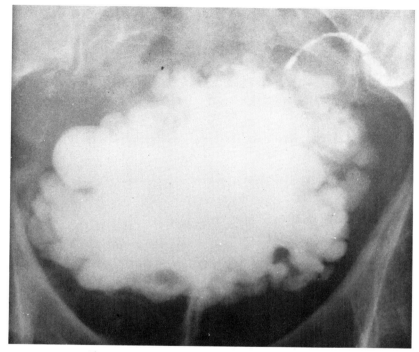

Figure 12-1 Diffuse, extensive vesical trabeculation.

Residual Urine

Residual urine is a result of detrusor decompensation, at which time the bladder is no longer able to be completely emptied. While the normal bladder is quite resistant to infection, the presence of significant residual urine may be associated with reduced host resistance. Thus, in the patient with suspected residual urine, unnecessary catheterization is to be condemned as a portal of infection. With progressive vesical decompensation, the patient may continue to void with little

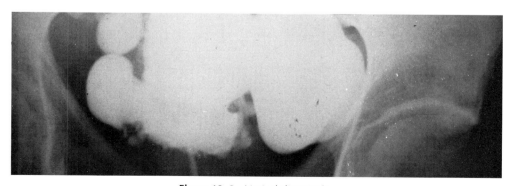

Figure 12-2 Vesical diverticula.

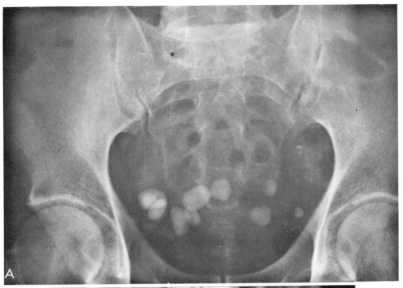

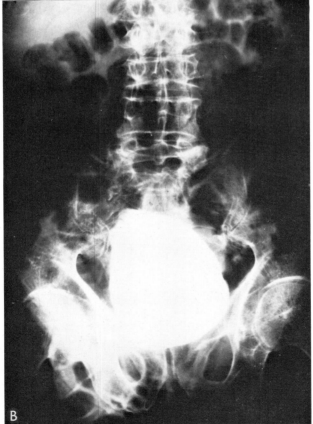

Figure 12–3   *A,* Multiple small vesical calculi. *B,* Giant vesical calculus.

subjective difficulty and yet carry over 1000 ml of residual urine and eventually develop azotemia. Acute urinary retention may occur early with high grade obstruction, while "chronic retention" with a large capacity bladder is indicative of a lower grade, long-term obstruction. Overflow incontinence, which is often nocturnal, is more frequent in "chronic retention."

VESICAL CALCULI

Any individual with a vesical calculus should be investigated for obstruction, and more specifically any male over 50 with such a calculus should be suspected of having prostatism (Figs. 12–3, A and 12–3, B). Residual urine predisposes to this complication, especially with secondary infection.

Prostatic calculi (Fig. 12–4) are usually of no real significance and may occur in normal males and those with prostatic hyperplasia or carcinoma. Usually the calculi are less than 0.5 cm in size, but occasionally they can replace the entire gland. When associated with benign hyperplasia, they often develop in the region of the surgical capsule. Their greatest significance lies in the fact that they are sometimes mistaken for carcinoma on rectal examination and occasionally may be a nidus for resistant infection.

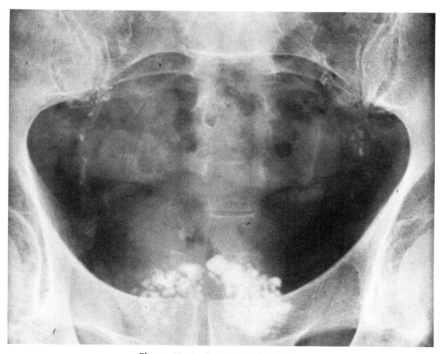

Figure 12–4 Prostatic calcification.

RENAL INSUFFICIENCY

Increasing intravesical pressure is eventually transmitted to the ureter, with pressures above 25 cm H_2O decreasing ureteric efflux while pressures between 40 and 50 cm H_2O may temporarily halt ureteric transport.

In response to increased intravesical pressure, there is a resultant increase in ureteric peristaltic activity and a subsequent early ureteric muscular hypertrophy. Varying degrees of regression of ureteric hypertrophy are apparent after relief of obstruction, but with prolonged elevations of intravesical pressure that are associated with long continued peristaltic hyperactivity, increasing dilatation, decompensation, and atony of the ureter, pelvis, and calyces can result. Thus, either mild or advanced hydroureteronephrosis may develop in elderly males who may already have some degree of nephrosclerosis (Figs. 12–5,A and 12–5,B). Acute or chronic pyelonephritis may further contribute to renal insufficiency. Any male over 45 with renal insufficiency should be evaluated for possible prostatism. Subtle symptoms of azotemia in the elderly male include anorexia, weight loss, drowsiness, and gastrointestinal complaints.

HEMATURIA

Often unrecognized is the fact that significant hematuria can occur as the result of the friability of telangiectatic veins in the prostatic mucosa. The sudden onset may be quite alarming to the patient, but in most cases hematuria ceases spontaneously or responds to catheter drainage. On only two occasions has semiemergent prostatectomy for severe bleeding been necessary in the authors' experience.

With the above information in hand relative to the potential course and complications of prostatism, the investigation and care of each patient must be individualized. If his symptoms are moderate or findings suggest significant residual urine, further urologic evaluation is indicated.

Excretory Urography

A great wealth of knowledge concerning the presence or absence of significant obstruction may be obtained by this rather safe, rapid x-ray study. If the upper tracts are normal, if there is only minimal to mild vesical trabeculation, and if the bladder empties fairly well after voiding (postvoiding film), then instrumentation may be deferred in the patient with mild symptomatology and an uninfected urine. Conversely, any or all of the following conditions demonstrated on urographic analysis may indicate the need for endoscopic examination or eventual prostatectomy:

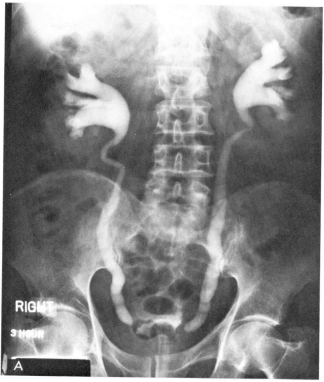

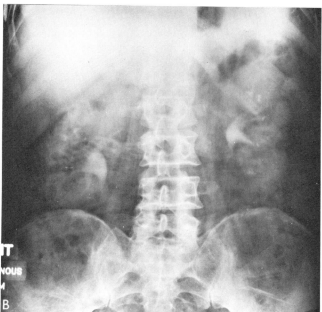

Figure 12–5 *A,* Hydroureter-onephrosis secondary to prostatic obstruction. *B,* Normal, unobstructed upper tract after prostatectomy.

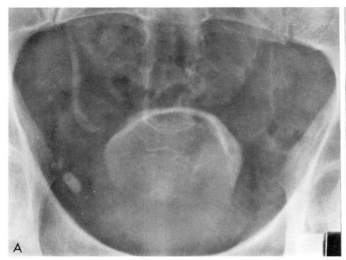
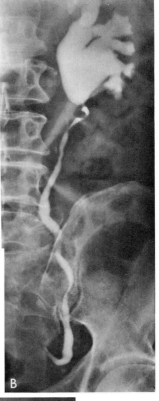

Figure 12–6 *A,* "Fish-hooking" of the lower ureters secondary to a large intravesical prostatic enlargement. *B,* "Fish-hooking" of lower ureter.

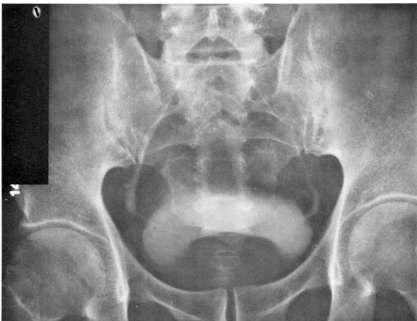

Figure 12–7 Filling defect in bladder caused by symmetrical intravesical protrusion of the prostate.

1. Hydroureteronephrosis.

2. "Fish-hooking" of lower ureters that is due to intravesical enlargement and upward displacement of the trigone (Figs. 12–6,A and 12–6,B).

3. Vesical calculi which are usually opaque but occasionally are lucent and appear as filling defects.

4. Significant vesical trabeculation or diverticula formation. The latter should be studied after voiding to determine the degree of emptying.

5. Significant residual urine. One must be careful in this determination for too often the patient may not have the urge to void or the surroundings may not be conducive to normal micturition. The absence of residual urine is indeed significant, but its presence may be "artifactual."

6. The presence of a large intravesical prostatic filling defect often supports the diagnosis of prostatism, *but* this can be noted in asymptomatic individuals and must be interpreted cautiously (Fig. 12–7).

7. The bladder may be elevated well above the pubic symphysis secondary to a large, long prostate gland (Figs. 12–8,A and 12–8,B).

Retrograde Cystography

With the improvement and sophistication of excretory urography, retrograde cystography (the injection of contrast material directly into the bladder via a catheter) is less often employed and has the hazard of urinary tract instrumentation which can introduce infection. Double contrast studies described in Chapter Three may provide information as to the status of the bladder and the size of the prostate when desirable, but cystoscopy is even more informative.

Pandendoscopic and Cystoscopic Examination

Many patients do not require further confirmation of prostatism after a complete evaluation as described previously, and these procedures usually are performed in conjunction with a contemplated prostatectomy. In those patients in whom the diagnosis cannot be completed, endoscopy is desirable. Although many major centers continue to employ general or regional anesthesia, approximately 90 per cent of the authors' diagnostic endoscopic examinations in the male are performed with only local anesthesia, frequently on an outpatient basis. At the time of endoscopy, one can determine:

1. The existence of residual urine.

2. The size and degree of visual obstruction by the prostate; the latter factor is quite unreliable, and frequently patients with little symptomatology appear to have significant visual obstruction while those with marked symptomatology may have an open or unobstructed-appearing outlet.

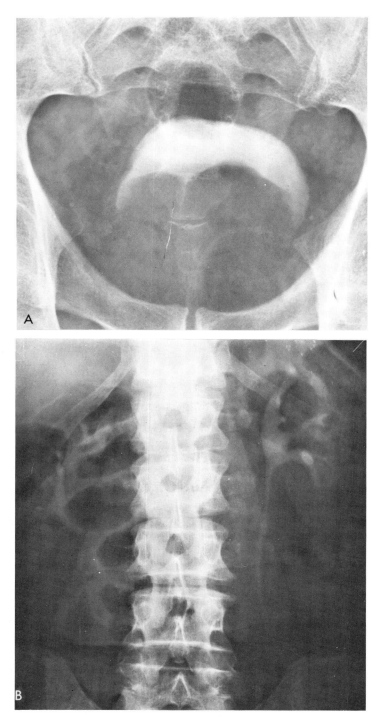

Figure 12–8   *A*, Elevation of the bladder above the pubic symphysis by a large prostate gland. *B*, Unobstructed upper tracts despite huge prostate.

3. The degree of vesical trabeculation and the presence of diverticula or calculi.

4. Any coincidental findings such as vesical neoplasm.

Whenever the possibility of a neurogenic bladder exists, cystometric studies are mandatory.

TREATMENT OF PROSTATISM

Irritative Symptoms. When very little evidence of obstruction exists, these symptoms are followed conservatively, with reassurance and possibly symptomatic therapy. Thus, mild frequency and nocturia may respond to low doses of anticholinergic medication (high doses may produce obstructive symptoms), sitz baths, and the avoidance of alcohol or any foods that appear to increase symptomatology.

Obstructive Symptoms. Patients having complete urinary retention require prompt drainage via a small (18 French) aseptically introduced urethral catheter. Patients with only several ounces of residual uninfected urine are best handled without a catheter prior to definitive operation, although those with vesical decompensation or complicating azotemia require a period of stabilization by bladder drainage prior to the operation.

Although there is the belief by some physicians that rapid decompression of a distended bladder can result in hypotension, there is no substantial evidence to support this myth. However, following decompression of a chronically obstructed bladder, it is not unusual to note the presence of hematuria. This is due to a rupture of blood vessels and hyperemia of the vesical wall, which has previously been under a great deal of pressure and is relatively ischemic. If catheter drainage is warranted but an inlying urethral catheter is contraindicated, suprapubic cystostomy may be necessary in cases of persistent sepsis, epididymitis, and the inability to pass a urethral catheter. If prolonged preoperative vesical drainage is necessary, some clinicians still prefer routine cystostomy, but most patients tolerate quite well a properly cared for urethral catheter. Recently, clean intermittent self-catheterization has been found quite useful.

Preoperative Evaluation

Modern methods of preoperative and postoperative care as well as refinements in techniques have reduced the overall mortality in prostatectomy to less than 2 per cent. All cardiovascular and general medical problems must be well controlled preoperatively. Ideally, elective prostatectomy should be deferred until approximately three to four months following significant cardiovascular insult (myocardial infarction or cerebral vascular accident). In azotemic patients it is important that renal function be stabilized prior to definitive operation. Although it is true that most patients who can ambulate survive an uncomplicated transurethral resection of the prostate, the mortality increases in the chronically ill; continued catheter drainage may be judicious. At a later date, improvement in the patient's overall condition will make an operation less hazardous.

Although infected urine cannot be effectively sterilized in patients with an indwelling catheter, an operation should certainly be deferred until symptomatic clinical infections, such as sepsis and epididymitis, are controlled. In recent years some institutions have routinely utilized antimicrobial agents preoperatively, while others do not use the drugs at all or have restricted their use to patients with a positive urine culture or indwelling catheter. A preoperative urine culture and sensitivity study should always be available to enable treatment of a significant postoperative sepsis. Baseline electrolytes and renal function studies are mandatory.

Choice of Operation

Although four clinical operations are available, i.e., transurethral resection, suprapubic prostatectomy, retropubic prostatectomy, and perineal prostatectomy, most often the choice is between transurethral resection of the prostate and any of the open procedures; and generally, regional anesthesia (spinal) is preferred.

Transurethral Resection

During the past 25 years approximately 85 to 90 per cent of all prostatectomies performed at our institution* have been done transurethrally. The goal of any prostatectomy is to remove all obstructing tissue with minimal risk to the patient. If performed properly all of the aforementioned procedures remove all obstructing prostatic tissue down to the surgical capsule (the true capsule plus a compressed portion of adenoma). Contrary to the protestations of some clinicians, it has been well documented that open operations with enucleation do not remove more tissue than a well executed transurethral resection. The advantages of transurethral resection are as follows:

1. Shorter period of postoperative catheter drainage (two to three days as contrasted to five to nine days with enucleative procedures).

2. No abdominal incision with pain to delay ambulation or to increase pulmonary, venous, or wound complications.

3. Superior hemostasis with less need for blood replacement.

4. Shorter hospitalization, with the patient usually being discharged on the fifth or sixth postoperative day.

Thus, the authors feel that transurethral resection is the operation of choice whenever feasible.

---

*Temple University School of Medicine.

Potential Contraindications to Transurethral Resection
1. Inability to satisfactorily position the patient (rare).
2. Severe urethral stricture. This problem may be obviated by urethral dilatation, internal urethrotomy, or preferably perineal urethrotomy.
3. Vesical calculi. If these are less than 2 cm in diameter and not too hard, they can be crushed and removed at the time of prostatectomy (litholapaxy). If the calculi are extremely large or too hard to crush, an open enucleative procedure may be combined with the removal of the calculi.
4. Large, poorly emptying vesical diverticulum. If diverticulectomy is necessary, this can be combined with a suprapubic prostatectomy, or performed after transurethral resection.
5. Small bladder capacity can render transurethral resection quite difficult, especially with a large prostate gland inasmuch as the constant need to empty the bladder prolongs the operation and poor visualization secondary to bleeding may be a problem.
6. An extremely large prostate gland. The definition of a large gland is relative; to an accomplished, skillful resectionist this might mean 150 grams, while to others, 25 grams might be a challenge. Most textbooks advocate a resection to take one hour and although this can in many cases be successfully extended, there are sound reasons for this limitation. It must be realized that the time required to perform a transurethral resection is directly proportional to the size of the gland as the tissue is essentially removed "piece by piece." Thus, the larger the gland, the more cuts necessary and the longer the operating time. Conversely, once the prostate is exposed, open enucleation of a large gland takes little more additional time than that of a smaller one. The rationale for avoiding transurethral resection in an extremely large prostate gland is described under the complication of water intoxication.

OPEN ENUCLEATIVE OPERATION

Retropubic Prostatectomy. Through a suprapubic incision the anterior surgical capsule of the prostate is incised, the plane between the capsule and adenoma developed, and the hyperplastic gland enucleated. The major advantages include:
1. Avoidance of an incision in the bladder and thus possibly less postoperative vesical spasm than that encountered in the classical suprapubic prostatectomy.
2. Excellent hemostasis as the entire prostatic fossa is readily visualized.
3. A shorter period of catheter drainage than in the suprapubic operation and the avoidance of a suprapubic catheter.
Suprapubic Prostatectomy. The bladder is approached suprapubically and opened just above the vesicoprostatic junction. A finger inserted through the vesical neck into the prostatic urethra breaks through the prostatic adenoma into the cleavage plane between the

adenoma and surgical capsule with subsequent enucleation. The major advantages are that the bladder can be well inspected, and secondary problems such as calculi and diverticula can be corrected. This operation can be performed more rapidly and demands somewhat less skill than the other forms of prostatectomy. In many institutions this procedure has been replaced by the retropubic approach because of the superior hemostasis, decreased bladder irritability, and shorter hospitalization.

Perineal Prostatectomy. The prostate is approached through an incision just above the anal margin. Although this is the oldest of the four modern approaches to prostatectomy, it is in general the least used and in most centers is performed only occasionally for benign prostatic hyperplasia. It is more likely to be utilized for total prostatectomy when one is attempting a cure in the patient with carcinoma. The disadvantages of this procedure include:

1. The exaggerated lithotomy position which may not be well tolerated by the elderly.

2. Possible rectal injury.

3. Possible increased incidence of impotence which has been refuted by some researchers.

4. Lack of experience with this approach by many younger urologists.

CRYOSURGERY

No discussion of various operations for prostatic obstruction would be complete without mention of this recent technique. Although introduced almost a decade ago, it still must be considered in its infancy and has few if any present indications in the treatment of benign prostatism.

Utilizing liquid nitrogen through a transurethrally placed probe the prostate gland is frozen, usually within 8 to 10 minutes. The probe is cooled to $-180°C$, and temperatures may reach $-30°C$ in the periphery of the gland. Following freezing, the probe is removed and a urethral catheter inserted. Tissue sloughing begins in about two days and can continue for many weeks.

Disadvantages of this inexact technique include:

1. Incomplete removal of adenoma.

2. Prolonged catheter drainage.

3. Inability to evacuate large necrotic fragments.

4. Rectal and surrounding tissue injury secondary to freezing.

Despite the advantages of rapidity and decreased blood loss, the disadvantages of this procedure limit its conventional utilization at least at the present time.

In summary most modern urologists prefer the transurethral approach but if an "open" operation is indicated, the expertise of the individual surgeon determines the procedure.

COMPLICATIONS OF PROSTATECTOMY

Besides those problems often encountered in any elderly male undergoing any form of operation, certain complications specifically related to the various procedures must be understood.

IMMEDIATE COMPLICATIONS

1. Excessive blood loss is usually due to inadequate hemostasis by the surgeon. Only rarely are significant problems such as fibrinolysis and disseminated intravascular coagulopathy encountered.

2. Extravasation of urine either by vesical or prostatic capsule perforation at the time of transurethral resection. When clinically detected, the operation should be terminated, and suprapubic cystostomy and drainage instituted.

3. Hypervolemia, hyponatremia, water intoxication (transurethral resection only).

As one resects the prostate, venous sinusoids in the capsule may be opened. If the resection is too prolonged especially in a large vascular gland, excessive irrigation fluid may enter the systemic circulation. For many years distilled water was utilized for irrigation but produced some degree of hemolysis when it entered the vascular system, either through the venous sinusoids or when reabsorbed from a clinically undetected perforation. At the present time most centers utilize a non-electrolyte, isotonic solution (with respect to the red blood cell) such as Glycine or Cytal to prevent this potential hazard. However, when these solutions dilute the vascular compartment, hyponatremia and hypervolemia occur. Subsequently, there is a shift of fluid into the cells by osmosis, resulting in water intoxication. The anesthesiologist may note a sudden increase in blood pressure, confusion, or bradycardia with eventual hypotension. This potential complication is the major reason why large prostate glands (over 80 grams) that require prolonged resection time are often removed by an open procedure. When water intoxication is encountered, the operation is terminated immediately. Serum electrolyte determinations should be obtained for confirmation, and fluid is limited until diuresis occurs. In severe situations hypertonic saline may be required to correct osmolality. During the past ten years, refinement in technique and the routine utilization of 25 grams of mannitol begun at the time of anesthesia have reduced this problem to a minimum. The osmotic diuresis produced by mannitol has also limited the need for routine postoperative bladder irrigations.

4. Sepsis. Although this is usually a more delayed complication, bladder and prostatic infections may be disseminated through the venous sinusoids. Thus, one can understand the rationale for the routine use of antimicrobials in patients with a preoperatively infected urine.

5. Electrical explosion at the time of transurethral resection (extremely rare).

EARLY POSTOPERATIVE COMPLICATIONS

1. Prolonged bleeding necessitating frequent bladder irrigations and occasionally a return to the operating room for secondary hemostasis.
2. Sepsis.
3. Any "nonurologic" complication, including thromboembolic and cardiovascular problems.

LATER POSTOPERATIVE COMPLICATIONS

1. Delayed hemorrhage.
2. Epididymitis. The incidence of this potentially morbid problem is about 4 per cent when a prophylactic vasectomy is not performed and 1 to 2 per cent following vasectomy. Vasectomy is less effective if performed after the urinary tract is already infected or if the patient has been maintained on urethral catheter drainage.
3. Urethritis. Secondary to the catheter or urethral manipulation. (See Urethral Stricture.)
4. Wound infection.
5. Thromboembolic problems.

LATE POSTOPERATIVE COMPLICATIONS

Urethral Stricture. Although this is the most common complication following prostatectomy (10 per cent), many could be avoided by improved care on the part of the surgeon. Meatotomy, the use of a smaller resectoscope sheath, internal urethrotomy, adequate urethral lubrication, perineal urethrotomy, early catheter removal, and meatal care all can reduce the incidence of stricture.

Impotence. There is no rational explanation for impotence except *possibly* as a result of nerve injury at the time of perineal exposure. Quite often elderly males complaining of postoperative impotence have performed sexually infrequently or inadequately prior to the operation.

Urinary Tract Infection. Frequently, patients develop a urinary tract infection prior to evaluation, following instrumentation, or postoperatively with the use of an indwelling urethral catheter. It is important to note that following all types of prostatectomy the entire prostatic urethra as well as the prostate itself is removed, leaving only the "raw" surgical capsule. Transitional epithelium from the area of the trigone and vesical neck slowly reepithelializes the prostatic capsule over the next 8 to 12 weeks. During this period of healing, overactivity or a voluntary delay in voiding may break loose a formed clot, producing hematuria that usually ceases spontaneously.

One should not expect sterilization of infected urine until complete reepithelialization occurs, and even without detectable bacteria, pyuria is to be expected until this process is completed. Postoperatively, antimicrobials should be utilized only in the symptomatic, infected patient but otherwise withheld until they can be successfully employed following complete healing of the prostatic fossa. Quite frequently, the spontaneous disappearance of infection or pyuria occurs with reepithelialization.

Incontinence. Postoperatively some degree of urge incontinence may be present for a short period of time. Occasionally, a short period of stress incontinence may follow relief of marked obstruction with a decrease in intraurethral resistance in the presence of a high intravesical pressure. Only rarely does stress incontinence persist, and it may be due to injury to the remaining portion of the internal sphincter (see Chapter Six). Rough enucleation or resection too far distally may account for this very serious complication. No patient should be considered truly incontinent until *at least* six months postoperative after which time improvement is less frequent. Many operations have been promoted for the correction of incontinence, but the ideal procedure has yet to be developed.

Ureteric Obstruction. This is an extremely rare occurrence that is due to resection and fulguration of the ureteric orifice *or* to misplaced hemostatic sutures in open operations.

Recurrent Obstruction. The inability to void satisfactorily upon removal of the catheter may be due to vesical atony (when severely decompensated), postoperative edema, residual tissue not removed, or a previously undiagnosed neurogenic bladder. Voiding problems at a later date may result from residual tissue, recurrent adenoma, vesical neck contracture, or urethral stricture. Following properly performed prostatectomy, less than 8 per cent of patients should require future reoperation. Unfortunately, carcinoma can develop following enucleation or transurethral resection for benign prostatic hyperplasia as prostatic tissue always remains in the surgical capsule.

VESICAL NECK CONTRACTURE

Congenital obstruction of the vesical neck is a rare entity, while about 10 per cent of adults with "prostatism" may develop the acquired form. This lesion develops earlier in life than glandular hyperplasia and is truly a fibrous contracture, possibly secondary to inflammatory changes. Symptoms and complications are similar to those described for benign hyperplasia, and although transurethral resection is usually successful therapy, plastic revision of the vesical neck is occasionally necessary. The latter is frequently employed when vesical neck contracture occurs as a complication following prostatectomy.

SUMMARY

The significant increase in longevity that has developed during the past fifty years has greatly increased the number of men who live into the prostatic age. Despite somewhat enthusiastic reports by a few physicians with regard to the medical treatment of benign prostatic hyperplasia utilizing cyproterone acetate and candicidin, at the present time prostatectomy is still the only proven modality in the treatment of prostatism. Thus, a thorough understanding of this condition, which may become symptomatic in 20 to 30 per cent of men over sixty, is imperative.

SELECTED REFERENCES

Flocks, R. H., and Scott, W. W. (eds.): The prostate. Urol. Clin. North Am., 2:1, 1975.
A current review of various aspects of prostatism, including inflammatory, obstructive, and neoplastic processes.

Mostofi, F. K.: Benign prostatic hyperplasia. *In* Campbell, M. F., and Harrison, J. H. (eds.): Urology. Philadelphia, W. B. Saunders Company, 1970.
A rather complete and informative discussion of the origin and pathophysiology of prostatic hyperplasia.

Weyrauch, H. W.: Surgery of the Prostate. Philadelphia, W. B. Saunders Company, 1959.
A classic work on prostatic surgery.

REFERENCES

Brendler, H.: Surgery for benign disease of the prostate and seminal vesicles. *In* Glenn, J. F., and Boyce, W. H. (eds.): Urologic Surgery. New York, Harper & Row, Publishers, 1969.
Gonder, M. J., Soanes, W. A., and Schulman, S.: Cryosurgical treatment of the prostate. Invest. Urol., 3:373, 1966.
Marshall, A., Brown, A. K., Jones, W. W., and Lindsay, R. M.: An assessment of cryosurgery in the treatment of prostatic obstruction. J. Urol., 109:1026, 1973.
Melchior, J., Valk, W. L., Foret, J. D., and Mebust, W. K.: Transurethral prostatectomy. Computerized analysis of 2223 conservative cases. J. Urol., 112:634, 1974.
Melchior, J., Valk, W. L., Foret, J. D., and Mebust, W. K.: Transurethral prostatectomy in the azotemic patient. J. Urol., 112:643, 1974.
Melchior, J., Valk, W. L., Foret, J. D., and Mebust, W. K.: Transurethral prostatectomy and epididymitis. J. Urol., 112:647, 1974.
Millin, T., and Macalister, C. L. O.: Retropubic prostatectomy. *In* Campbell, M. F., and Harrison, J. H. (eds.): Urology. Philadelphia, W. B. Saunders Company, 1970.
Mostofi, F. K.: Benign prostatic hyperplasia. *In* Campbell, M. F., and Harrison, J. H. (eds.): Urology. Philadelphia, W. B. Saunders Company, 1970.
Nesbit, R. M.: Transurethral prostatic resection. *In* Campbell, M. F., and Harrison, J. H. (eds.): Urology. Philadelphia, W. B. Saunders Company, 1970.
Thompson, I. M.: Transurethral surgery. *In* Glenn, J. F. (ed.): Urologic Surgery. New York, Harper & Row, Publishers, 1975.
Wear, J. B., Jr., and Haley, P.: Transurethral prostatectomy without antibiotics. J. Urol., 110:436, 1973.
Weyrauch, H. W.: Surgery of the Prostate. Philadelphia, W. B. Saunders Company, 1959.
Weyrauch, H. W., and Rous, S. N.: Benign lesions of the prostate and vesical neck. *In* Karafin, L., and Kendall, A. R. (eds.): Urology. New York, Harper & Row, Publishers, vol. 2, 1975.

Chapter Thirteen

TRAUMATIC LESIONS OF THE UROGENITAL TRACT

Russell Scott, Jr. and C. E. Carlton, Jr.

KIDNEY

Injuries of the kidney are becoming increasingly common because of the large number of industrial and automobile accidents and the increase in crimes of violence.

Etiology

Traumatic wounds of the kidney are ordinarily caused by forces delivered to the organ in four different ways.

Laceration of the Kidney or Its Pedicle by Penetrating Wounds. Injuries of this type are ordinarily accompanied by intraperitoneal injuries in 85 per cent of the cases, with rupture of the intestine, stomach, liver, spleen, or major vessels.

Crushing Injuries. These occur when the patient is run over by an automobile or crushed between two external forces. In this type of injury there is considerable trauma to surrounding structures (e.g., the lower thorax and the abdominal viscera). The kidney lesion is coincidental to and part of the picture of a generalized injury that involves several organs or parts of the body, and thus the kidney cannot be treated independently.

Injuries that Result from a Direct Blow over the Kidney. In this type of injury, the force is transmitted to the kidney without penetrating the overlying structures or without injuring them. In this situation, the force is transmitted to the organ in such a way as to cause an injury either to its vessels or to the parenchyma itself. One of the commonest injuries of this type is that which occurs during football and other body contact sports. Such injuries may cause rupture of the kidney without any sign of external injury to the overlying structures.

339

Inertial Injuries.   The fourth type of injury occurs when the victim is traveling at a high rate of speed and is suddenly stopped, as in an auto accident or a fall. In this injury the renal arteries are stretched and the intima tears. A subintimal dissection develops, which results in a renal artery thrombosis.

Pathology

The simplest traumatic lesion of the kidney is a renal contusion with ecchymosis or a small hematoma within the substance of the kidney but with no actual tear of the capsule or lining of the renal pelvis. This injury manifests by soreness in the flank, with or without microscopic hematuria or minimal gross hematuria.

More extensive lesions may vary from the laceration of a vessel in the perirenal fat with hematoma formation, to rupture of the true capsule of the kidney with a minimal laceration of the parenchyma, to rupture of the parenchyma, capsule, and lining of the pelvis. In the latter cases extravasation of blood will extend into the pelvis as well as to the perirenal space. More extensive injuries of the kidney may produce stellate or multiple lacerations of the renal parenchyma, with separation of one or more fragments of parenchyma from the kidney. In this type of injury the rapidly forming hematoma may not be confined within Gerota's fascia.

The renal pedicle may be torn with or without laceration of the parenchyma of the kidney. In such a circumstance, a hematoma develops rapidly about the kidney, but there is apt to be no hematuria. As mentioned previously, the intima of the renal artery may split, resulting in a subintimal dissection with thrombosis of the renal artery.

SECONDARY PATHOLOGY

The perirenal hematoma and the traumatized kidney constitute particularly favorable soil for bacterial invasion and growth, so it is not uncommon for acute suppuration to occur in the kidney and perirenal hematoma following trauma that is inadequately treated. A perinephric abscess may develop with great rapidity (see Perinephric Abscess, p. 284). Other secondary complications of renal trauma consist of continued bleeding or secondary hemorrhage that occurs several days later and may be a threat to life. Perirenal fibrosis may develop, resulting in a Goldblatt kidney with secondary hypertension. Ischemic fragments of kidney may also result in hypertension. Arteriovenous aneurysms may result from injury to renal vessels, and on rare occasions urinomas may develop and persist as pseudocysts of the kidney.

Symptoms and Signs of Renal Trauma

Shock.   The trauma that is responsible for injury to the kidney frequently results in immediate shock, probably because most blows that produce kidney injury occur in the region of the so-called "solar plexus." Thus, a college athlete who is suddenly struck over his kidney by a well-placed body block or who blocks a punt and receives the ball directly over his kidney anteriorly may lose consciousness immediately after the impact and may have to be carried from the football field. The immediate shock is of short duration, however, and if it lasts for more than a few minutes, one should suspect that intra-abdominal hemorrhage resulting from rupture of some intraperitoneal viscus has occurred or that there is some other cause for prolonged shock. After recovery from the immediate shock, the patient is in fairly good condition, and any subsequent relapse should be considered a sign of severe hemorrhage that occurs as a complication of the injury. It is important to recognize and differentiate between these two types of shock: immediate and delayed shock, both of which frequently accompany kidney injuries.

Pain. There is almost always pain in the flank, and this may result from the direct trauma to soft parts, or it may in some instances result from fracture of the ribs. Moreover, the injured kidney itself is painful. Soreness and muscle spasm on the side of the injury are common.

Mass. The examining physician should pay particular attention to the development of a mass in the flank in case of suspected injury to the kidney. One should make every effort to decide at an early stage whether or not the hematoma is localized. Extensive hematoma in the retroperitoneal space is usually indicative of widespread kidney injury and may demand emergency surgical intervention.

Hematuria. About 80 per cent of all injuries to the kidney are accompanied by hematuria of some degree (gross or microscopic). The patient may lose large quantities of blood in the urine if bleeding into the renal pelvis continues. It should be remembered, however, that even extensive injuries to the kidney or the pedicle vessels can occur without any hematuria, even microscopic. For this reason the diagnosis of traumatic injury to the kidney should never be overlooked because the urinary appearance is normal.

X-ray Appearance. Even with significant renal injury, approximately 25 per cent of the patients will have a "normal" intravenous pyelogram. A plain film of the abdomen following rupture of the kidney may show absence of the psoas on the affected side and lateral curvature of the spine with concavity on the side of the injury, thus presenting an x-ray picture identical with that seen in perinephric abscess. Intravenous pyelograms will generally reveal an enlarged kidney shadow that results from the hematoma and the irregularity of the pyelogram due to the extravasation of contrast material at the point of rupture through the pelvic mucosa; but traumatic suppression of renal function may prevent excretion of the contrast media and thus hinder successful pyelographic analysis of the injured kidney.

The primary usefulness of the conventional intravenous pyelogram is to establish the functional capacity of the uninjured kidney should nephrectomy of the injured kidney be required. The intravenous pyelogram is of limited value in determining the extent of renal injury. Where significant renal injury is suspected, a selective renal arteriogram is the single most useful test in determining the location and extent of injury. If it is impossible to obtain this study, a drip intravenous pyelogram with tomographic cuts may provide valuable information concerning the location and extent of renal injury. Rarely will it be necessary to resort to a retrograde pyelogram. The origin and clinical course of the patient (expanding flank mass, amount of blood replacement therapy and so on) are also important in judging the extent of injury.

Treatment

Penetrating Injury. In patients with penetrating renal injury, exploration is mandatory if for no other reason than to rule out or repair associated injuries to intraperitoneal viscera, which occur in 80 per cent of such patients. The principles of surgical repair of the injured kidney are similar to the repair of the kidney injured by blunt trauma, which are discussed in that section,

Blunt Trauma. The first step in deciding the treatment of blunt renal trauma is to ascertain the presence of injury to other viscera and the extent of renal damage, e.g., a simple contusion, a small laceration, a large laceration, a macerated kidney, or a thrombosis of the renal artery. It takes judgment and experience coupled with adequate objective data to reach a sound decision about the extent of injury. Information, such as the origin of the injury, the presence or absence of a mass, the amount of blood required, and the appearance of the intravenous pyelogram, tomogram, or arteriogram, is often necessary in order to select appropriate therapy.

Conservative Treatment

Such treatment consists of absolute bedrest for about 10 days, with review of serial urines, vital signs, and hematocrits. If a hematoma is present, prophylactic antibiotics should be administered in an attempt to prevent an abscess from developing in the perinephric hematoma. After the patient has recovered, the blood pressure should be followed for two years to be certain that hypertension does not develop. An intravenous pyelogram should be obtained at three and twelve months following injury to detect a correctable anatomical derangement of the kidney that might result in stone formation or progressive hydronephrosis.

Surgical Treatment

If, in the judgment of the surgeon, the extent of the injury is extensive enough so that significant life-threatening bleeding is occurring or so that delayed hemorrhage, abscess formation, renal parenchymal slough, or a urinoma is likely to develop, then exploration is probably wise. In past years only hemorrhage that was a threat to the patient's life was an indication for surgery, becuase as Gerota's fascia is opened and the tamponade released, there is usually a frightful outpouring of blood, and a hasty nephrectomy for the control of hemorrhage may be required. However, now when the anterior approach is used, the renal artery and vein may be isolated and brought under control before Gerota's fascia is opened, thus avoiding nephrectomy for the purpose of controlling hemorrhage. Therefore, the indications for exploration have been liberalized, and a number of the late complications of significant renal trauma can be avoided by early exploration in well-selected cases.

Once exploration is attempted, the abdomen is explored through an anterior, transperitoneal incision. Careful intra-abdominal exploration is carried out. If there is a large tense hematoma over the kidney, the renal artery and vein should be isolated at their junction with the aorta and vena cava before Gerota's fascia is opened. Bulldog clamps can then be applied to the renal vessels. The colon is reflected and Gerota's fascia opened, the hematoma evacuated, and the kidney inspected (Fig. 13–1).

Obviously, devitalized renal parenchyma should be debrided to prevent a late slough of tissue with secondary hemorrhage. If open, the collecting system should be closed. If possible, the renal parenchyma should be closed with superficial mattress sutures. If the parenchyma cannot be closed, a pedicle of live fat can be laid in the defect to eliminate dead space and minimize postoperative ooze. The flank should be drained in an extraperitoneal fashion in the case of subsequent develop-

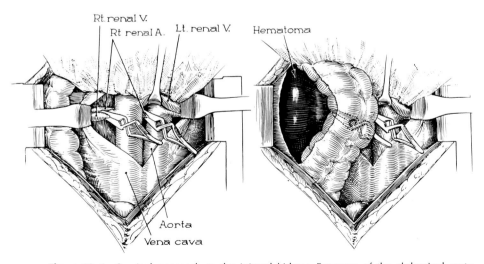

Figure 13–1 Surgical approach to the injured kidney. Exposure of the abdominal aorta and left renal vein through an incision in the posterior parietal peritoneum. Application of noncrushing vascular clamps to the appropriate renal artery and vein. Mobilization of the injured kidney and release of the perirenal tamponade only after vascular control.

ment of abscess or urinary leak. The follow-up management is as out-lined under conservative management. It should be emphasized that not all patients with significant injury from blunt trauma are operated upon. Those patients who in the judgment of an experienced surgeon have an injury of such location and extent that late complications may necessitate nephrectomy are prime candidates for early exploration, the purpose of which is to control hemorrhage, repair the injured parenchyma, and establish drainage in the hope of preventing late complications.

URETER

Etiology

Traumatic lesions of the ureter may occur as a result of injury inflicted by the surgeon or by blunt or penetrating injury. Injury may occur as a result of intraureteric manipulation with stiff catheters or metal instruments that are employed during attempts to manipulate or dislodge ureteric calculi. Under these circumstances the ureter is often friable because of the stone or infection, and the stiff instruments used to manipulate the calculus may easily penetrate the ureteric wall.

Other ureteric injuries that result from surgical trauma can occur from one of three causes. First, ligation of the ureter can be caused by deeply placed sutures. This type of injury occurs most frequently as a complication of operations upon the uterus and its adnexa. The second type of operative injury occurs as a result of clamping the ureter with a hemostat. This can occur when the surgeon is working deep in the pelvis, particularly in operations upon the uterus and its adnexa. Third, the ureter may be transected during operations performed in the pelvis. As mentioned previously, the ureter may be injured by a gunshot wound or stab wound. On rare occasions, the ureter may be torn by blunt trauma.

Symptoms, Signs, and Treatment of Ureteric Injury

Ureteric Injury from Intraureteric Manipulation. When ureteric injury from manipulation is complicated by extravasation of urine, the patient complains of pain in the lower abdomen that radiates upward toward the kidney; sepsis develops if infection is present, and there is usually reflex ileus. Severe pain, with or without sepsis or ileus, that occurs after ureteric manipulation for calculus should lead one to sus-pect traumatic rupture of the ureter. An excretory urogram should be obtained immediately, and if this does not satisfactorily visualize the entire ureter on the affected side, a retrograde pyeloureterogram should be made.

Treatment consists of immediate incision and drainage of the periureteric space, especially if there is significant extravasation. It is usually advisable first to establish ureteric catheter drainage via cystoscopy and then to provide open drainage of the periureteric area by operation if there is significant extravasation. If there is only minimal extravasation, ureteric catheter drainage alone may suffice. If there is significant injury to the lower ureter, ureteric reimplantation should be considered. One of the late sequelae of ureteric injury is ureteric stricture, which may necessitate ureteroplasty or reimplantation into the bladder.

The ligation of one or both ureters is suggested by the following symptoms and signs.

1. Total anuria is present following pelvic operation (if both are ligated).

2. There may be gradually developing pain with tenderness over the kidney, with or without sepsis, depending upon coexisting infection in the kidney.

3. Unexplained ileus may be the only clue to ureteric ligation in the heavily sedated postoperative patient.

4. Symptoms may be lacking if but one ureter is ligated, and the kidney is uninfected.

When ureteric ligation is suspected, an intravenous pyelogram should be obtained immediately. If there is hydronephrosis or nonvisualization, cystoscopic examination with ureteric catheterization should be performed for the purpose of demonstrating whether one or both ureters have been ligated and the approximate level of the ligature. If either of these catastrophes has occurred, immediate exploration of the site of ligation is recommended, provided the patient's general condition permits and the site of ligation is considered "operable." From 7 to 10 days following ligation and *in the absence of abscess,* excision of the entire injured portion of the ureter with reanastomosis or ureteroneocystostomy is usually possible. There is a tendency for the surgeon to want to "deligate" and splint the ureter in the hope that it will heal without stricture. This procedure usually fails, and in almost all cases it is safer to excise the area of ischemic ureter and anastomose healthy ureter to healthy ureter. If the site of ureteric injury is surrounded by more than mild periureteric reaction and edema, a nephrostomy should be done and the ureter repaired at a later time.

Transection of the Ureter. This is usually discovered at the time of operation, although it occasionally is not discovered until postoperatively when urine appears in the wound. If discovered at the time of surgery, immediate end to end anastomosis of the ureter should be effected, and satisfactory healing should take place, usually without stricture. However, several fundamental principles must be observed in carrying out a repair of this type (Fig. 13–2).

The first principle is to adequately debride the injured ureteric ends. This may involve removing several centimeters of ureter. Both ends are then spatulated. The ureter should be freed in both directions for a sufficient distance so that the ends meet without tension. Number

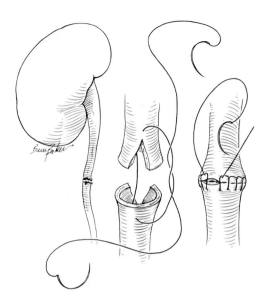

Figure 13–2. Technique of repair of injured ureter. Spatulation of opposing surfaces of the ureter after debridement of injured tissue. Meticulous watertight closure of the ureter employing 5–0 chromic catgut.

0000 or 00000 chromic sutures are placed to avoid ureteric stenosis and, it is hoped, to provide a watertight closure of the ureter. In most instances, proximal diversion of the urine in the form of a pyelostomy or linear ureterostomy at least 4 cm above the site of repair avoids urine from being forced through the site of repair. In selected cases, some surgeons prefer not to divert the urine. If the surgeon is unsure of his debridement, viability of the ureter, or the degree of tension, one of two procedures should be done: (1) the bladder should be opened and a tube passed up through the ureter to provide better diversion and also to act as a stent or (2) a nephrostomy can be done and a stenting catheter passed down into the bladder (Fig. 13–3). In any event, the area of repair should always be drained to avoid a collection of urine and the formation of abscesses.

BLADDER

The distended bladder may be ruptured by an exceedingly light blow, while the empty organ is rarely injured, except by crushing or penetrating wounds, which occur most frequently as a complication of a fractured pelvis or stab or gunshot wounds. The bladder may also be ruptured during the passage of catheters, sounds, and cystoscopes or during a transurethral resection of the prostate or a bladder tumor.

The signs and symptoms of a ruptured bladder depend on the location as well as the extent of the laceration. If extraperitoneal, there is usually moderate pain low in the pelvis, with spasm of the lower rectus muscles and gradual ascending dullness to percussion over the suprapubic areas up to the level of the umbilicus; the clinical picture is of pelvic cellulitis. If the rupture is intraperitoneal, the patient has severe

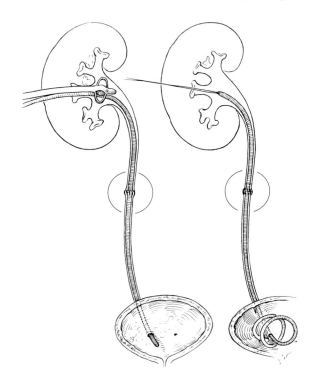

Figure 13–3 Alternate techniques of placing splinting ureteric catheters where urethral tension, infection, or other factors might result in failure of primary healing.

pain and boardlike rigidity of the entire abdomen and may develop shock; the clinical picture is of peritonitis. Patients have micturitional disturbance with either type of injury. They may urinate with difficulty and pass only small amounts of bloody urine, or else they may be unable to urinate at all. The inability to urinate may result from reflex spasm of the urinary sphincters, or it may derive from an empty bladder.

Diagnosis of a ruptured bladder is dependent upon x-ray demonstration of extravesical contrast material, which has previously been introduced into the bladder by catheter, or by cystoscopic examination. *Since omentum or clots may plug the laceration, it is necessary to fill the bladder to capacity and then force in an additional 50 to 100 ml of contrast material with an Asepto syringe.* It is also imperative to drain the contrast media from the bladder and to obtain a "postdrainage film" inasmuch as the bladder that is distended with contrast material may obscure small areas of extravasation in front of or behind the bladder.

Treatment

The treatment consists of suprapubic cystotomy with debridement and approximation of the edges of the tear in the bladder wall, followed by suprapubic and adequate extravesical drainage. Very little harm is done as a result of a ruptured bladder, provided the laceration is closed and adequate drainage of the bladder and extravesical space is maintained following the repair. Clear urine in the peritoneal cavity does little harm if the source of extravasation is closed.

ANTERIOR URETHRA

Injuries to the urethra are considered in two categories: (1) anterior urethral injury and (2) injuries to the prostatomembranous urethra.

Etiology

Traumatic injuries of the urethra may occur as the result of a straddle injury (falling astride a fixed object) or from traumatic instrumentation, either iatrogenic or self-inflicted. Injuries secondary to instrumentation usually are of limited extent, involve the mucosa, and are not accompanied by perineal hematoma. They will almost invariably heal with short-term urethral catheter drainage.

When the urethra is crushed against the pubic rami as in a straddle injury, the extent of damage may range from minor contusion of the urethra and corporeal bodies to complete rupture of the corpus spongiosum and urethra.

Symptoms of Anterior Urethral Injury

Pain. Trauma to the urethra usually causes pain localized to the site of injury.

Bleeding. There is usually rather brisk bleeding from the urethral meatus; however, there may be only a few drops of blood. If the urethra is lacerated or severed, there is hematoma formation in the perineum. If Buck's fascia is intact, the hematoma is confined to the periurethral area (Fig. 13–4). If Buck's fascia has been ruptured, blood extravasates into the subcutaneous tissue of the penis, scrotum, and perineum (Fig. 13–5).

Diagnosis of Anterior Urethral Injury

The history and physical findings readily suggest the presence of anterior urethral injury, but proper treatment of the lesion requires precise delineation of the location and extent of the injury. This precise delineation requires retrograde urethrography and in rare instances, urethroscopy.

In any patient in whom the slightest suspicion of urethral injury exists, retrograde urethrography should be performed as the first diag-

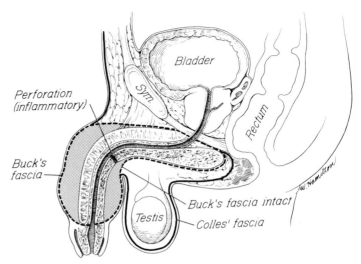

Figure 13–4 Penis only inflammatory perforation. Extravasation beneath intact Buck's fascia.

nostic study. All too often, a significant urethral laceration is overlooked by the hasty insertion of an indwelling Foley catheter, and, therefore, the diagnosis is not made. The retrograde urethrogram is performed by placing the patient in the oblique position on the x-ray table and gently and slowly inserting into the urethral meatus 30 ml of viscous contrast medium (Fig. 13–6). Regular intravenous pyelography medium alone or mixed with an equal amount of water-soluble surgical lubricant serves this purpose well.

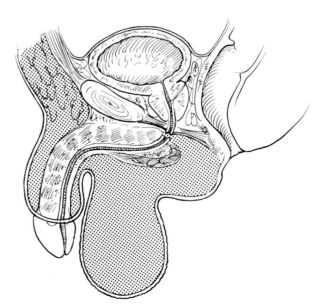

Figure 13–5 Typical route of urinary extravasation and blood collection with injury to the urethra distal to the urogenital diaphragm.

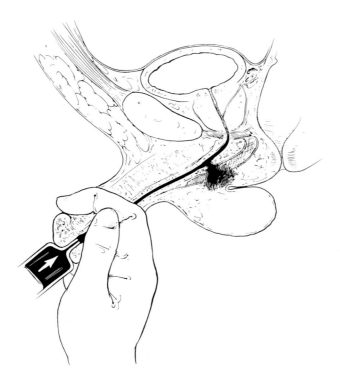

Figure 13–6. The technique of retrograde urethrography. The tip of a large syringe is impacted into the urethral meatus, and viscous contrast medium is injected in a retrograde manner.

Treatment

SURGICAL TREATMENT OF ANTERIOR URETHRAL INJURIES

Treatment of urethral injuries is based on the extent and severity of the injury and the presence and extent of hematoma or urinary extravasation. All but the most minor puncture wounds of the urethra should be treated by surgical exploration, with excision of injured tissue and primary repair. If crushed tissues surrounded by undrained infected hematoma are allowed to heal secondarily, the inevitable sequelae are dense fibrosis and stricture. Principles of primary surgical treatment include:

1. Surgical exploration and evacuation of hematoma.

2. Precise delineation of the location and extent of injury by urethrography and urethroscopy.

3. Wide mobilization of the urethra from the cavernous bodies, allowing debridement and reanastomosis under no tension (Fig. 13–7).

4. Spatulated watertight reanastomosis.

5. Adequate periurethral space drainage.

6. Proximal urinary diversion (suprapubic cystotomy) only if primary healing is not expected or watertight anastomosis is not obtained. If watertight anastomosis is obtained and primary healing is anticipated, a Foley catheter is employed for 24 to 48 hours.

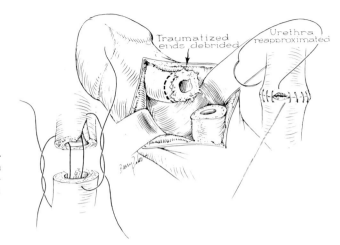

Figure 13–7 The injured urethra is mobilized from the corpora cavernosa. The injured ends debrided, spatulated, and closed in a watertight fashion.

NONSURGICAL TREATMENT OF THE URETHRA

If there is only contusion of the urethra that is confirmed by urethroscopy, the patient requires no treatment. If there is only a minor puncture wound of the urethra with minimal hematoma, the patient should receive antibiotics and should be placed on indwelling catheter drainage for 7 to 10 days.

PROSTATOMEMBRANOUS URETHRA

Etiology

Almost invariably, this injury is caused by a shearing effect at the rigid attachment of the apex of the prostate to the fixed urogenital diaphragm in association with fracture of the bony pelvis (Fig. 13–8). On

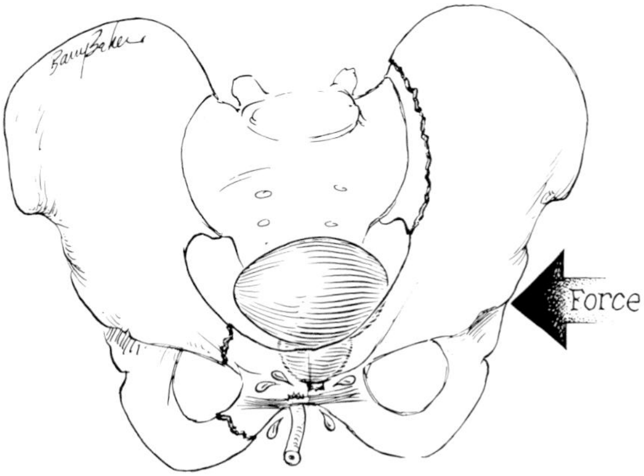

Figure 13–8 Typical mechanism of injury to the urethra at the junction of the prostatic apex and the membranous urethra. Note the shearing force applied to the urethra as the pelvic girdle is fractured.

rare occasions, this portion of the urethra may be damaged by a severe straddle injury associated with laceration of the urogenital diaphragm.

Diagnosis of Injury to the Prostatomembranous Urethra

Since these injuries usually occur in association with a fractured pelvis, the patient exhibits the usual findings of a fractured pelvis (severe pelvic and lower abdominal pain, hypotension, and rigidity of the abdomen). In addition, he complains of the inability to urinate or is able to urinate only small amounts of bloody urine.

Rectal examination reveals fluctuance in the area of the prostate, and if there is complete severance of the posterior urethra, the prostate cannot be palpated (Fig. 13–9). The diagnosis is confirmed by retrograde urethrography.

Treatment of Injury to the Prostatomembranous Urethra

Urinary diversion by suprapubic cystostomy should be done in all patients with injury to the posterior urethra. The hematoma should be left undisturbed and no attempt made to suture or approximate the laceration. After 21 days an antegrade cystourethrogram is performed. If the laceration has healed without stricture, the cystostomy catheter is removed. If stricture has occurred, approximate primary repair is accomplished. Treatment by Foley catheter alone should be avoided be-

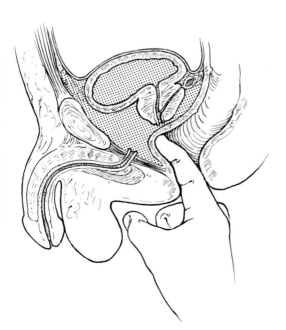

Figure 13–9 Rectal-digital findings with complete laceration of the prostatic urethra. There is a striking absence of the prostate to palpation and the balloonlike consistency of the pelvic hematoma.

cause of the likelihood of developing urethritis with long term catheter drainage.

The cogent argument for this form of therapy is that attempted initial repair of posterior urethral injuries yields an extremely high incidence of strictures and impotence and that if the area of injury is left undisturbed initially, the subsequent urethroplasty can be much more easily done.

URETHRAL STRICTURES

Any discussion of urethral trauma would be incomplete without detailed consideration of one of its sequelae, namely, stricture.

Etiology

Circumferential scarring of the urethra may occur with any type of injury to the urethral tissue. This tissue damage may be inflicted by internal or external forces applied to the urethra as previously discussed or may be due to bacterial, chemical, thermal, or pressure injury. In the past, most urethral strictures resulted from untreated gonorrheal urethritis or the various traumatic treatments of gonorrhea, e.g., intraurethral instillation of strong chemicals. With the advent of easily available antibiotic treatment of gonorrhea, this etiologic basis for stricture has been largely eliminated. The majority of urethral strictures now are due to direct trauma or urethritis secondary to indwelling urethral catheter.

Symptoms of Urethral Stricture

Obstruction to Urination. As the urethral lumen is reduced below about 16 Fr., progressive reduction of the caliber of the urinary stream occurs, and the patient develops hesitancy, frequency, intermittency, and nocturia, as in prostatic obstruction. Failure to seek treatment may result in urinary retention.

Bleeding from the Urethra. This may occur consequent to congestion or ulceration of the urethral mucosa at the site of the stricture.

Infection. Urethritis, prostatitis, and cystitis may occur as a result of obstruction to urinary flow. Not uncommonly, the prostatic infection spreads in a retrograde fashion down the vas deferens to cause epididymitis. Any patient with recurrent or bilateral epididymitis should be suspected of having a urethral stricture. Urethritis associated with the increased intraluminal pressure proximal to the stricture may result in extension of the infection outside the urethra, resulting in periurethral abscess.

Diagnosis of Urethral Stricture

Diagnosis is suggested by the history of urinary obstructive symptoms, particulary when the patient has pyuria and terminal dribbling. The diagnosis is confirmed by urethral instrumentation; "gripping" of the urethral sound or bougie by the stricture is a pathognomonic sign of stricture. Urethrocystograms made by injecting the urethra with opaque media and followed by x-ray exposures with the patient in the oblique position are another means of confirming the diagnosis.

Direct instrumental examination serves to determine the location, number, and caliber of the stricture. Prerequisites for instrumentation of the urethra are meticulous asepsis and gentleness in technique. Clean hands, sterile instruments, and an abundance of sterile water-soluble lubricants are essential. The genitalia are prepared as for minor surgery, and a topical anesthetic agent is gently introduced into the urethral lumen. The instruments required are steel sounds 20 Fr. or larger, since a steel sound of smaller size should never be introduced into the urethra because of the danger of its sharp point creating a false passage. The only exception to this rule is the use of LaForte sounds which are screw-tipped and are safely guided into the urethra by a filiform bougie to which they are securely attached. Filiform bougies may have straight or curved tips. A screw tip allows attachment to flexible bougies (Phillips bougie) or LaForte sounds. To determine an abnormal narrowing, a well-lubricated sound of size 24 or 26 Fr. is gently introduced into the urethra, almost of its own weight; it should follow the roof of the canal until its progress is arrested by an obstruction. If the meatus is too small for the passage of instruments, meatotomy should be performed. If the sound fails to "engage," smaller instruments are passed in succession until the lumen of the stricture is finally calibrated.

The distance from the meatus to the area of constriction is then measured on the shaft of the instrument. Metal sounds may be used above 20 Fr.; filiforms with a bougie down to the size of about 10 Fr. are used for calibration of smaller strictures. Unlimited patience and the utmost gentleness are essential to the passage of instruments through a stricture, particularly when the stricture is of small caliber. The distorted crooked canal may give rise to considerable difficulty, and if the filiform fails to pass the obstruction, it is gently manipulated by advancing, withdrawing, and rotating. It may be necessary to bend the tip of the filiform at an angle, producing a gentle curve toward its tip. Straight as well as screw-tip or "pigtail" filiforms may have to be employed in order finally to penetrate the channel. If instrumentation fails to establish the location and the caliber of the stricture, then urethrocystograms may be of great value in obtaining this information.

Treatment

The treatment of urethral stricture consists of enlarging the urethral lumen at the site of stricture either by instrumental dilation or by various surgical techniques. The treatment of a specific type of urethral stricture varies with the character and position of the stricture.

DILATIONS

A stricture is a scar, and it is well to remember that, with few 'exceptions, scar tissue continues to contract indefinitely and that periodic dilations may always be necessary. The key to treatment of urethral dilation is *gentleness,* so as not to inflict further urethral trauma and thus pain that would discourage the patient from further treatment. As a general rule, the stricture should not be dilated more than 4 Fr. at any one visit.

Large Caliber (20 Fr. or over).   Steel sounds are used and dilations carried out at progressively increasing intervals of time with the hope of eventually obtaining the objective of having dilatations every six months. Most strictures require dilatations at about that interval in order to maintain the full caliber of the urethra.

Strictures of Small Caliber.   Strictures of small caliber are invariably treated by bougies. The main objective in the treatment of either filiform or small stricture is to convert it to a stricture of large caliber, the treatment of which has been outlined above. Strictures of small caliber may be treated according to two methods.

INTERMITTENT DILATATION.   In this method, the patient is ambulatory and comes into the clinic or physician's office every four to seven days initially for dilatation as described above. This interval is increased as the stricture begins to soften and stay open between visits.

CONTINUOUS DILATATION.   In many cases it is desirable to convert a stricture of small caliber to one of large caliber with a minimum expenditure of time in order to return the patient to his occupation or to his home. In the latter instance, it is a particularly valuable procedure when patients come to a large medical center for diagnosis and treatment. Thus, the patient coming to University Hospital with a filiform or small caliber stricture is frequently treated in this manner. He is hospitalized for a few days so that his stricture may be converted to one of large caliber; thus, he can be returned to his home and to the care of his local physician who is then able to carry out intermittent dilatations by the use of steel sounds.

Upon calibration of the urethra, a filiform bougie is left indwelling and tied in place, and the patient is admitted to the hospital and given chemotherapy as a prophylaxis against sepsis. He is able to urinate around the filiform without difficulty. If the patient has a stricture which will admit a No. 14 or No. 16 bougie, then a 12 or 14 soft rubber catheter is introduced and left indwelling. Twenty-four hours later the filiform or the catheter is removed, the urethra is gently dilated and a larger catheter is introduced and left indwelling. It generally takes about 48 to 72 hours to convert a filiform stricture to one of large caliber by this method. Those which require a longer period of treatment by this method generally fall into the category of intractable stricture and require operation.

Treatment of Stricture with Urinary Retention. It is well to remember that retention may occur with a relatively large caliber stricture. For that reason, any patient having a stricture with urinary retention should have an attempt made at passage of a steel sound, size No. 24 or 26 Fr., and if this instrument fails to pass easily, then bougies of diminishing size are used in an effort to bypass the obstruction. Under no circumstance should much force be applied to these instruments.

If the stricture proves to be impassable and the patient's condition is satisfactory, he should be given morphine and put into a tub of hot water; frequently, the relaxation which is afforded by these two therapeutic measures will allow him to urinate. If this procedure fails, then surgery is necessary. Operative treatment of impassable stricture with urinary retention consists of suprapubic drainage. After a few days of such drainage the acute congestion in the urethra generally subsides and allows the passage of urethral instruments.

Intractable Stricture. This is one form of stricture that does not dilate by either intermittent or continuous dilatation; it also may be one which dilates with some difficulty and whose caliber cannot be maintained by intermittent dilatation. Intractable strictures inevitably require operative treatment.

Finally, a specimen of all urethral strictures should be taken for biopsy when the stricture is first diagnosed to rule out carcinoma of the urethra, which can mimic exactly the symptoms and findings of urethral stricture. For the same reason, a stricture which suddenly changes its behavior, i.e., requires more frequent dilation or becomes harder to dilate should be examined to rule out carcinoma. Most carcinomas of the male urethra have been treated for varying periods of time as urethral strictures.

SURGICAL TREATMENT

Operative treatment of urethral stricture is reserved for those patients with intractable strictures and for those young patients in whom a lifetime of urethral dilations would impose considerable disability. The surgical techniques employed are (1) internal urethrotomy, (2) primary excision of the stricture, and (3) urethroplasty.

Internal Urethrotomy. This is a technique by which a urethrotome containing a concealed knife is introduced into the urethra to a point above the stricture; then after bringing the knife to the surface of the instrument, the knife is withdrawn making a longitudinal cut through the entire thickness of the stricture. In order to prevent reapposition of the cut edges of the stricture, a Foley catheter must be left indwelling for several weeks or a large caliber sound passed at weekly intervals for four to six weeks.

Primary Excision of the Urethral Stricture. This may be performed in selected cases when the stricture is short (2.5 cm or less) and located far enough distal to the membranous urethra to allow adequate mobilization of the proximal urethra for closure without tension. The surgical technique includes primary watertight reanastomosis of the urethra as described under treatment of trauma of the anterior urethra (see Fig. 13–7).

Urethroplasty. This procedure should be performed in patients with strictures that are intractable to urethral dilation or internal urethrotomy and who are not candidates for primary excision because of the extent of the stricture or its location in the proximal bulbous or prostatomembranous urethra. This procedure is done in two stages. The first stage of the operation is performed by surgically exposing the strictured portion of the urethra, making an incision in the ventral surface of the urethra extending through the length of the stricture and into normal urethra for at least 2 cm proximal to and distal to the stricture. Depending on the location of the stricture, penile or scrotal skin is sutured to the cut urethral margins, marsupializing that portion of the urethra. This skin is used in the second stage of the operation for reconstructing the urethra. In strictures distal to the midbulbous urethra, the technique of Denis-Browne is favored. In strictures proximal to the midbulbous urethra, the technique described by Turner-Warwick is used.

Complications of Urethral Stricture

The most common complications of old and neglected stricture are those that result from obstruction and chronic infection. Chronic cystitis occurs frequently, and it is not at all uncommon in neglected cases of stricture for the bladder to decompensate and carry residual urine.

Likewise, ascending urinary infection with chronic pyelonephritis is a frequent accompaniment of chronic stricture. All degrees of pathologic change within the bladder, the ureters, and the kidney are thus to be seen in neglected stricture.

A less common but more urgent complication is periurethral infection with its many manifestations. In considering the pathogenesis and pathology of periurethral infection occurring as a complication of urethral stricture, it should be borne in mind that all strictures of the urethra produce some degree of obstruction, and that practically all strictures are accompanied by chronic inflammatory changes in the urethra proximal to the stricture itself. In this area of chronic urethritis, there occasionally occurs ulceration which, in turn, may eventually allow extravasation of small quantities of infected urine beyond the submucosa of the urethra. Likewise, small periurethral abscesses can form as the result of suppurative infections in the urethral glands above the site of stricture. In either circumstance the tendency to extravasation at this point is enhanced since there exists hydrostatic pressure above this point of the stricture, exerted by the patient in his effort to force urine beyond the obstructive lesion. The pathologic sequence of events may follow either one of two courses.

Periurethral Abscess. If the extravasation occurs gradually and the infecting organisms are of low virulence, there develops a well-defined abscess wall to protect surrounding structures from rapid extravasation. Thus, a localized periurethral abscess points into the perineum; there is a hot, red, tender swelling which eventually fluctuates and, if it is not drained by surgical incision, eventually ruptures spontaneously in the perineum. The perineal opening drains pus and urine, and the fistula persists unless the stricture is adequately dilated. A patient who develops one periurethral abscess with resulting urinary fistula and who continues to neglect his stricture not infrequently develops subsequent periurethral abscesses which likewise rupture in the perineum to form additional urinary fistulae. In far advanced cases of this type it is not unusual to see patients who void all of their urine through multiple perineal fistulae. Such cases have been very appropriately described as having "water-pot perineum."

The treatment of acute periurethral abscess involves two procedures: (1) drainage of the abscess and (2) proximal diversion of the urine by suprapubic cystostomy. The stricture itself is best left untreated until the acute inflammatory reaction has subsided.

Treatment of urinary fistula or "water-pot perineum" requires proximal urinary diversion to allow subsidence of acute inflammatory reaction. If the fistulae do not close with urinary diversion, antibiotics, and dilation of the stricture, they must be excised, usually in conjunction with a first stage urethroplasty.

Periurethral Extravasation. When periurethral suppuration occurs as described above and a rapid extension of infection takes place, owing to the presence of anaerobic virulent organisms accompanied by a relatively high intraurethral hydrostatic pressure, the infection does not become walled-off in the form of an abscess but rather takes the form of a diffuse urinary phlegmon; it spreads, rapidly involving the entire genital tract. The scrotum becomes edematous, then inflamed, and finally gangrenous. After involvement of the scrotum and perineum the subcutaneous structures of the penis become involved, and then extravasation follows along the subcutaneous planes and extends upward involving the abdominal wall. Deep involvement of the pelvis does not occur because of the protective barriers afforded by the pelvic fascia. The disease runs a rapidly progressive course and, if early surgical drainage is not afforded, the patient dies of sepsis.

Diagnosis never offers any difficulty, although too frequently the attending physician fails to recognize the underlying stricture in the management of the case.

Treatment of periurethral extravasation (urinary phlegmon) consists of incision and drainage with debridement and removal of all necrotic tissue. Likewise, the underlying urethral strictures should be adequately treated, and urinary diversion by cystostomy accomplished.

Under no circumstances should the testes be removed, even in the most extensive cases of gangrene. The testes derive their vascular supply by way of the inguinal cord, and this structure is not involved by periurethral extravasation. In extreme cases it is occasionally necessary to remove the entire scrotum and drain as high as the 12th rib in performing adequate and complete debridement. When this is necessary, the testes may be left entirely exposed since they suffer very little from this exposure. Rapid regeneration of epithelium sufficient to cover the testes eventually takes place after granulation and healing has occurred. It is not necessary to sacrifice the gonads in this type of case, and skin grafting is rarely necessary for covering the testes.

GENITAL INJURIES

Penis

Amputation. If the amputated segment is in good condition, reanastomosis should be attempted in the first few hours after injury. The rich vascularity of the corporeal bodies will allow survival of some such autografts.

If reanastomosis is not feasible because of elapsed time or crush injury of the amputated segment, the stump of the penis should be debrided and closed (Fig. 13–10). Spatulation of the urethra with the insertion of a skin flap into the spatulation is important in preventing stricture of the new urethral meatus.

Fracture or Laceration of the Corpus Cavernosum. When the corpus cavernosum is fractured by a crush injury or lacerated by penetrating wounds, there is marked hematoma formation along the shaft of the penis that extends into the scrotum and lower abdomen. Careful palpation will reveal a defect in the firm tunica albuginea.

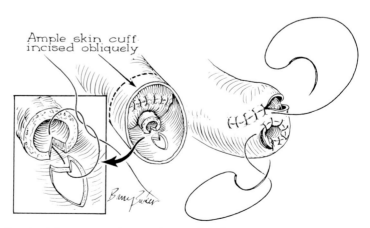

Figure 13–10 Repair of the amputated penis. Corporeal bodies are oversewn with horizontal mattress sutures. A new spatulated urethral meatus is created as demonstrated.

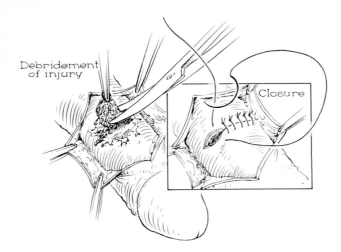

Figure 13–11 Debridement and repair of laceration of the corpus cavernosum.

This injury should be treated by prompt surgical exploration, evacuation of hematoma, and repair of the tunica albuginea (Fig. 13–11). This will markedly decrease the possibility of secondary infection and deforming cicatrization of these erectile bodies.

Avulsion of the Penile and Scrotal Skin. In the past these injuries were usually the result of the genitals being caught in farm or factory machinery, and their incidence was declining due to increasing safety precautions. However, these injuries are presently on the rise again because of the proliferation of motorbikes and motorcycles. Hundreds of young men in the United States annually leave parts or all of their genital skin on the handlebars of these machines. The diagnosis of these injuries is obvious.

TREATMENT

Initial. There should be minimal debridement of skin in order to leave all possible tissue; this is particularly true with scrotal skin, which has a unique ability to regenerate.

Definitive Care

PENIS.   All remaining distal penile skin should be excised and the penis covered by a split thickness skin graft.

SCROTUM.   When any remnant of scrotal skin remains, scrotal regeneration will occur, and during this period of time, simple topical care of the granulating surface should be carried out. If all scrotal skin has been avulsed, the testes should be implanted into the medial aspects of the thighs (Fig. 13–12). Skin grafts over the testes are unsatisfactory because of their tendency to painfully constrict and immobilize the testes.

Testicular Injury

Because of their extreme mobility, the testes are seldom injured. Such injuries, however, do occur secondary to straddle injury or oc-

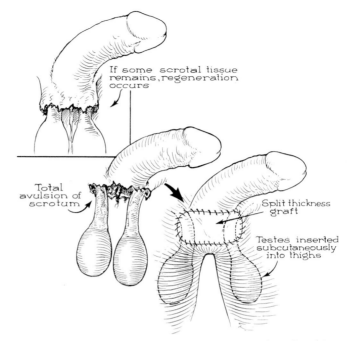

If some scrotal tissue remains, regeneration occurs

Total avulsion of scrotum

Split thickness graft

Testes inserted subcutaneously into thighs

Figure 13–12 Expectant treatment where remnant of scrotum remains. With total avulsion of the scrotum, the testes are implanted into the medial aspect of the thigh.

casionally, gunshot wounds. If the testis is simply contused, with no palpable defect in the tunica albuginea, the patient should be treated with bedrest, ice packs, and scrotal elevation until the pain subsides. Adequate palpation of the testis for laceration of the tunica albuginea is greatly enhanced by infiltration of the spermatic cord with xylocaine at the level of the pubic tubercle. If there is scrotal hematoma or a defect in the tunica albuginea, primary surgical repair is indicated. Evacuation of hematoma, debridement, and primary repair obviate secondary hemorrhage, infection, and necrosis. Any viable part of the testis should be preserved for possible hormone production. The tunica vaginalis should be excised to prevent hydrocele.

SELECTED REFERENCES

Carlton, C. E., Jr., Scott, R., Jr., and Guthrie, A. G.: Surgical correction of ureteral injury. J. Trauma, 9:457, 1969.
A detailed article on the rationale and technique of repair of the injured ureter.

Glenn, J. F., and Boyce, W. A.: Urological Surgery. 2nd ed. New York, Harper & Row Pubs., Inc., 1974.
The second edition, now in press, has several chapters which deal in detail with surgical techniques of the repair of injury to the kidney, ureter, and bladder.

Scott, R., Jr., and Carlton, C. E., Jr.: Genitourinary tract. In American College of Surgeons, Committee on Trauma: Early Care of the Injured Patient. Philadelphia, W. B. Saunders Company, 1972, pp. 160–181.
An excellent summary of the diagnosis and initial management of genitourinary injuries.

Scott, R., Jr., Gordon, H. L., Carlton, C. E., Jr., Scott, B. F., and Beach, P. D.: Current Controversies in Urologic Management. Philadelphia, W. B. Saunders Company, 1972.

This book discusses in detail the controversial aspects of management of injuries to the kidney, membranous urethra, and ureter. For the reader interested in more than one approach to the problem, this is an excellent book.

REFERENCES

Anderson, H. V., Hodges, C. V., Benham, A. M., and Ocker, J. M.: Transuretero-ureterostomy (contralateral uretero-ureterostomy): Experimental and clinical experiences. J. Urol., 83:593, 1960.

Badenoch, A. W.: Injuries of the ureter. Proc. R. Soc. Med., 52:101, 1959.

Baird, H. H., and Justis, H. R.: Surgical injuries of the ureter and bladder. J.A.M.A., 162:1357, 1956.

Braasch, W. F., and Strom, G. W.: Renal trauma and its relation to hypertension. J. Urol., 50:543, 1943.

Carlton, C. E., Jr., Scott, R. Jr., and Guthrie, A. G.: The initial management of ureteral injuries: A report of 78 cases. Trans. Am. Assoc. Genitourin. Surg., 62:114, 1970.

Glenn, J. F., and Harvard, B. M.: The injured kidney. J.A.M.A., 173:1189, 1960.

Hamm, F. C., and Weinberg, S. R.: Management of the severed ureter. Trans. Am. Assoc. Genitourin. Surg., 48:130, 1956.

Hamm, F. C., and Weinberg, S. R.: Experimental studies of regeneration of ureter without intubation. J. Urol., 75:43, 1956.

Hamm, F. C., Weinberg, S. R., and Waterhouse, R. K.: Repair of the injured ureter: A new technique for end-to-end anastomosis. Surgery, 45:575, 1959.

Hinman, F., Jr.: Ureteral repair and the splint. J. Urol., 78:376, 1957.

Hinman, F., Jr.: Experimental evidence of ureteral reconstitution. In Bergman, H. (ed.): The Ureter. New York, Hoeber Medical Division, Harper & Row Pubs., Inc., 1967, pp. 67–80.

Lapides, J., and Caffery, E. L.: Observations on the healing of ureteral muscle: Relationship to intubated ureterotomy. J. Urol., 73:47, 1955.

Mahoney, S. A., and Persky, L.: Intravenous drip nephrotomography as an adjunct in the evaluation of renal injury. J. Urol., 99:513, 1968.

Massumi, R. A., Andrade, A., and Kramer, N.: Arterial hypertension in traumatic subcapsular perineal hematoma (Page kidney). Am. J. Med., 46:635, 1969.

Morse, T. S., Smith, J. P., Howard, W. H. R., and Rowe, M. I.: Kidney injuries in children. J. Urol., 98:539, 1967.

O'Connor, V. J.: Immediate management of injured ureter. J.A.M.A., 162:1201, 1956.

Scott, R., Jr., Carlton, C. E., Jr., Ashmore, A. J., and Duke, H. H.: Initial management of non-penetrating renal injuries. Clinical review of 111 cases. J. Urol., 90:535, 1963.

Spence, H. M., and Boone, T.: Surgical injuries to the ureter. J.A.M.A., 176:1070, 1961.

Staubitz, W. J., Macoss, I. V., Lent, M. H., Sigman, E. M., and Oberkirscher, O.: Management of ureteral injuries. J.A.M.A., 171:1296, 1959.

Turner-Warwick, R. T.: A technique for posterior urethroplasty. J. Urol., 83:416, 1960.

Chapter Fourteen

RENAL CALCULUS DISEASE

Robert D. Johnson

Renal calculus disease is surprisingly common. It is reported that about 200,000 Americans are hospitalized each year for this problem, but this is an underestimation of its magnitude. Not included in this number are the many instances of spontaneous passage of small calculi and of single visits to emergency rooms for renal colic. Another study reports that 1 of every 150 hospitalized patients in North America has a diagnosis of renal calculus disease, although that was not necessarily the reason for hospital admission. In one large autopsy series, renal calculi were found in slightly more than 1 per 100 (1.12 per cent).

Urinary tract stones have plagued man from antiquity, and history has left several tantalizing clues that point to possible etiologic factors. Urinary tract stones are exceedingly rare in children in the United States today, although bladder calculi were quite common here a half century ago. Today, however, they have virtually disappeared in this age group. This problem remains endemic, though, in some areas of the Mid and Far East, particularly in those regions noted for their poor nutrition. The reduction in the frequency of stones seems best related to an improved economic status of the people and a shift from a diet primarily of grain to that which includes meat, milk, and milk products. Among other things, this shift very likely has resulted in an increase in urinary orthophosphate and pyrophosphate concentrations. Vesical stones virtually disappeared in children in Norfolk, eastern England, between 1910 and 1930, coincident with an improved standard of living in that region. Curiously, these stones were found almost exclusively in boys, as continues to be the case in the endemic stone areas of the world today, perhaps because of the slower flow rate of urine leaving the bladder and progressing through the much longer and narrower male urethra. The marked reduction in bladder stones, however, has unfortunately been associated with a simultaneous increase in renal calculus disease. "Stone waves" were well documented following World Wars I and II in Europe but involved noncombatant as well as warring nations. "Waves" were also noted in the Scandinavian countries, Switzerland, and Japan but strangely were not apparent in the British Isles. The involved countries were relatively free of renal stones for seven or eight years following World War I, during which time there were severe caloric, protein, and calcium restrictions, but later during the postwar period of improved economic status the stones began to reappear. The exact cause for this occurrence is indeed an enigma.

On the other hand, renal calculi are relatively *rare* among the native populations of South Africa, particularly in the Bantu tribe, and also on the islands of the West Indies. It is interesting to note that the Bantu have a rather high urinary sodium concentration and that the inhabitants of the islands of the West Indies drink mostly distilled ocean water. In spite of these and other intriguing associations, the useful application and an understanding of their roles in the production of renal calculus disease remains meager.

The dramatic and severe pain of renal colic is not the least of the complications from renal calculi, but of much greater significance are obstruction and recurrent urinary tract infection, which can lead to irreversible renal damage. Renal complications require the removal of one kidney from almost one third of patients who have calculus disease. Prompt surgical relief of obstruction is an extremely important part of the management of renal calculus disease. This section, however, deals with medical aspects of stone disease: the pathophysiology, diagnosis, treatment, and prevention.

PATHOPHYSIOLOGY

It was natural for early students of calculi to seek to learn the composition of each in the hope that the cause could be better understood and a rational treatment developed. Calcium is the most common component of renal calculi, making up a major part of more than 90 per cent of them, and oxalate, found in 65 to 75 per cent of such stones, is the second. In one large series of stones investigated, it was found that calcium in association with *mixed* phosphate and oxalate occurred in 51 per cent, phosphate in 20 per cent, oxalate alone in 13 per cent, and mixed phosphate and uric acid in 8 per cent. In addition, 6 per cent were pure uric acid stones, and less than 1 per cent were cystine, cystine and phosphate, uric acid, and other rare stones such as xanthine, silicate, and matrix calculi.

With the finding of calcium as the major component of almost all urinary calculi, it was reasonable to deduce that the urine of such patients should contain greater amounts of calcium than that found in urine from normal subjects and that this difference would probably be due to an elevation in blood calcium. This hypothesis was true in some instances but not in most. In fact, *hypercalcemia* is found relatively infrequently in the population of stone formers, only 4 per cent of whom are found to have hyperparathyroidism and another 1 or 2 per cent who develop stones from less common causes of hypercalcemia, such as Vitamin D intoxication, immobilization, Paget's disease, sarcoidosis, berylliosis, and milk alkali syndrome. *Hypercalciuria*, without obvious hypercalcemia, is more common in stone formers and suggests either an *intermittent* hypercalcemia, as is seen in some patients with primary hyperparathyroidism, or an abnormal renal tubular handling of the filtered load of calcium, as in renal tubular acidosis, Type I, or in idiopathic hypercalciuria, which is discussed more fully on pages 367 and 382. Since in almost all oxalate stone formers urinary oxalate concentrations fall within the range of normal and since urinary calcium concentrations in some calcium stone formers are normal, the cause of the stone disease is not obvious on the simple basis of the concentration of those ions in urine. Many documented instances of patients with marked hypercalciuria who do *not* form renal calculi further emphasize this fact.

Presence of "Precipitators" in Urine

What information is there that might be useful to better understand the cause or pathophysiology of renal calculus production? Is this a single or is it a multifactoral disorder? See Table 14-1. Urine is a metastable supersaturated solution of crystalloids and other substances. Precipitation of crystalloids from such a solution can be encouraged upon the introduction of an appropriate nidus. The presence of specific substances found in the "core" of every stone, even those that are essentially pure cystine or pure uric acid, suggests a common denominator for stone formation. This central matrix is a mixture of serum proteins and mucoproteins found in the urine and extractable from the kidneys of patients with chronic stone disease. These proteins may be absent in the case of the incidental or occasional stone former and are usually absent from the urine of normal persons. They have been identified, however, in the urine of patients who have *not* formed stones but who do have urinary tract infections. The implication is that the stones were generated in response to tissue injury.

Matrix Hypothesis.   Recently, a calcium binding protein, somewhat similar to Matrix substance A of Boyce, has been reported found in normal chick intestinal mucosa and kidney that has some immunologic similarities. As attractive as the matrix hypothesis is, it has neither been wholly accepted nor entirely rejected by investigators in this field. If the metabolism of the matrix proteins were better understood and manipulation of them were possible, research would be further stimulated in this area. Boyce and his colleagues, who have done perhaps the most outstanding research on the role of the organic matrix in renal stone formation, offer it as a possible explanation for the development of renal calculi but hesitate to assign it a primary role in calculus formation because "(1) this [hypothesis] has not been proved;

TABLE 14–1   Possible Etiologic Factors in Renal Calculus Formation

PRESENCE OF "PRECIPITATORS" IN URINE
   Mucoproteins (Boyce)
   Bacteria
SOLUTE CONCENTRATION
   Dehydration
   Increased solute load
     Hypercalciuria
      Idiopathic
      Hyperparathyroidism
      Sarcoidosis
      Vitamin D excess
      Cushing's disease
     Hyperuricemia and hyperuricuria
      Gout
      Lymphoma; leukemia
      Cancer therapies
      Probenecid
     Cystinuria
     Xanthinuria
     Hyperoxaluria
ABNORMAL pH CONTROL
   Renal tubular acidosis — Type I
   Use of carbonic anhydrase inhibitors
   Infection with urea-splitting bacteria
   Chronic diarrhea (including ileostomy)
   Henneman's renal tubular dysfunction
DEFICIENCIES OF "SOLUBILIZERS" IN URINE
   Citrate
   Pyrophosphate
   Magnesium, zinc, manganese
   Sodium
   Glucuronides
   Organic acids
   Amino acids
   Colloids
   Unknowns
PRESENCE OF "ANTISOLUBILIZERS" IN URINE
   Aluminum
   Ferric iron
   Silicon
MISCELLANEOUS
   Stasis
   Randall's plaque
   Inducement from medications

(2) every crystalline component of native calculi can be induced to homogeneous nucleation and growth from metastable or supersaturated solutions without the presence of organic molecules; and (3) the very diversity of clinical situations in which concretions are formed of the most concentrated and precipitable components of urine (oxaluria, cystinuria, etc.) argues against the assumption of a 'special' macromolecule essential to concrement formation." In spite of these objections, the role of the matrix substance as a possible initiator of stone formation remains an open question.

Bacteria or cellular elements of inflammation, in the case of urinary tract infections, may be additional precipitators or initiators of stone formation.

Solute Concentration

Whether the matrix mucoprotein of Boyce or a critical concentration of Brushite (calcium phosphate monohydrate) acts as an initiator for stone formation, the fact remains that the specific crystalloids found in the stone *do* precipitate and can be encouraged to do so by one or more of several means (Table 14-1). The concentration of the crystalloids is increased under conditions of dehydration or increased solute load presented to the urine. Changes in urinary pH diminish the solubility of specific solutes. Reduction in the concentration of substances naturally found in urine that act as "solubilizers," the presence of substances that antagonize the action of such "solubilizers," and finally mechanical factors such as stasis, Randall plaque formation, or foreign bodies also may be important factors in stone production.

The increased incidence of renal calculus disease in troops moved under battle conditions to a hot, dry climate may be related to dehydration. Under these circumstances the composition of the stones is most often uric acid or calcium oxalate. Whether, in addition to the dehydration, the rise in urinary uric acid seen with acute stress and adrenal cortical stimulation is a factor in the production of the uric acid stones or whether a critical increase in oxalate concentration from dehydration encourages calcium oxalate stone formation is conjectural.

HYPERCALCIURIA

Idiopathic Hypercalciuria. The most common cause of hypercalciuria, idiopathic hypercalciuria has been a poorly understood entity until recently. It is seen mostly in young to middle-aged males, may be familial, and appears in one of two ways. One form is associated with gastrointestinal hyperabsorption of calcium. Serum calcium remains normal, however. Reduction in oral calcium intake or the administration of cellulose phosphate, which reduces gastrointestinal calcium absorption, abolishes the hypercalciuria. A second form is related to an abnormality in renal tubular rather than gastrointestinal handling of this ion, which results in hypercalciuria. It has been demonstrated that in this form parathyroid hormone concentration in the blood is elevated and that the secondary hyperparathyroidism can be abolished by reducing renal losses of calcium with the use of chlorothiazide. Recently, it has been suggested that the gastrointestinal and renal forms of idiopathic hypercalciuria may be variants of the same process and related to the unexplained hypophosphatemia common in this condition. Hypophosphatemia *per se* causes hypercalciuria and also is one factor which stimulates 1,25-dihydroxycholecalciferol production by the kidney. The latter would independently stimulate gastrointestinal absorption of calcium. Thus, the hypothesis can be tested.

Primary Hyperparathyroidism. When renal function is otherwise normal, the hypercalciuria associated with primary hyperparathyroidism is not proportional to the degree of hypercalcemia and the filtered load of calcium. Since parathyroid hormone increases renal tubular reabsorption of calcium, its excessive activity reduces the percentage of calcium in the filtered load that appears in the urine. Hypercalciuria usually does occur, however, because of the increased filtration of calcium secondary to the hypercalcemia, but when the serum calcium is elevated to 11.5 mg/100 ml, the urinary calcium may be little more than 150 to 160 mg per 24 hours, with the patient on a 140 mg calcium diet. Obviously, in the presence of excessive circulating parathyroid hormone there can occur a minimal degree of serum calcium elevation, which allows a filtered load that is just able to balance the increased rate of calcium reabsorption. In this case there is no hypercalciuria. It is noteworthy that the phosphaturic effect of parathyroid hormone added to the hypercalciuria results in an increase in the product of urinary calcium and phosphate that would be expected to encourage stone formation. In spite of this effect, it is interesting to note the relative infrequency with which patients with primary hyperparathyroidism continue to form stones. It is not uncommon to obtain a history of the passage of a stone 20 years earlier; yet, at the time of examination there may be no evidence of renal calculus disease. This lack of calculi could be due to increased fluid intake from the thirst often seen with hypercalcemia and to the reduced renal tubular concentrating power secondary to chronic hypercalcemia, which results in a dilute urine.

Vitamin D Excess. Though it does not appear to effect directly the renal clearance of calcium in man, vitamin D excess in the otherwise healthy individual does have a direct renal phosphaturic action. Hypercalciuria observed with an excess of this vitamin is most likely due to several secondary effects of its action. It increases bone resorption and gastrointestinal absorption of calcium, both of which tend to elevate serum calcium and increase the renal filtered load of calcium. Suppression of parathyroid hormone secretion follows. This, in turn, reduces renal tubular reabsorption of calcium, adding further to the hypercalciuria. Finally, from the action of excessive vitamin D, bone resorption releases buffer into the circulation, producing a mild alkalosis and reducing the urinary concentration of hydrogen ion. This activity would be expected to encourage the precipitation of calcium phosphate stones.

HYPERURICURIA

Hyperuricuria is an important factor in the production of uric acid calculi, which are seen in one quarter of the patients with primary gout and one third to one half of patients with secondary hyperuricemia. Hyperuricuria results from the rapid turnover of nucleoproteins, e.g., during the course of leukemia, lymphoma, and cancer chemotherapy. Some researchers have suggested that calcium oxalate crystal growth may be encouraged by the presence of urates and uric acid because of shared physical-chemical properties. Recent reports have emphasized the frequency of hyperuricuria in *calcium* stone formers and their effective management by correction of the hyperuricuria with the use of allopurinol.

CYSTINURIA

The maximal solubility of *cystine* in a 24 hour urine specimen is about 300 mg, within a pH range of 4.5 to 7.0. The degree of cystinuria associated with liver disease and most other aminoacidurias is ordinarily below that level, and renal calculi are rarely seen. The exception is found in cystinuria, a familial disorder inherited as an autosomal recessive in which homozygotes excrete between 500 and 1300 mg per day. Heterozygotes, on the other hand, though excreting more than normal individuals, rarely exceed 300 mg output per day and rarely develop calculi. The condition is called "cystinuria" because of the clinical implications of that particular amino acid, but it is also a disorder of renal tubular handling, and in some subgroups also of gastrointestinal handling, of four dibasic amino acids (cystine, lysine, arginine, and ornithine). It is the relative insolubility of cystine at the usual range of urinary pH, in contradistinction to the other amino acids, that creates the problem. A further complication may arise from obstruction and a secondary urinary tract infection which, when added to the therapeutic program of alkalinization of the urine, may result in mixed stones containing also calcium, oxalate, or phosphate.

XANTHINURIA

Xanthine, another relatively insoluble substance in urine, has been found to be the main constituent of renal calculi in about 25 per cent of patients with hereditary xanthinuria, a rare condition that is due to an inherited reduction in xanthine oxidase activity in various tissues of the body. This enzyme plays a key role in the metabolism of xanthine to uric acid; thus its deficiency results in low concentrations of uric acid in the blood and urine but high concentrations of xanthine and hypoxanthine. *Hypoxanthine* stones, however, have not been reported, probably because hypoxanthine is 10 to 30 times more soluble in urine than xanthine. The solubility of xanthine in urine at pH 5 is 5 mg/100 ml and at pH 7 is 13 mg/100 ml. The concentration of xanthine in five of nineteen reported patients with hereditary xanthinuria and renal calculus disease ranged between about 160 and 725 mg per 24 hour urine. An expected appearance of xanthine stones in patients placed on allopurinol, a xanthine oxidase inhibitor, has not materialized, with a rare exception, probably because suppression of the enzyme activity by it is incomplete, and urinary concentrations of xanthine do not ordinarily exceed the solubility.

Hyperoxaluria

Oxalate is relatively insoluble in urine, and its solubility is only slightly influenced by changes in pH. Although oxalate is a major constituent of two thirds to three quarters of all renal calculi, past observations have indicated that urinary oxalate concentration is within the normal limits in almost all oxalate stone formers, with the exception of those with primary hyperoxaluria, a rare inherited enzyme deficiency that results in high concentrations of oxalate in the urine, blood, and tissues. Recently, however, the case of the ordinary oxalate stone former has been reexamined, and there is some evidence to suggest that minor, but perhaps significant, elevations in urinary oxalate are found. Also, the frequent finding of hypercalciuria in this group of patients may be important and together with even minor constant or intermittent elevations in urinary oxalate may be critical in this type of stone formation.

Dietary Factors in Calcium Oxalate Stone Formation. As regards dietary factors which may be active in the production of calcium oxalate stones, it has been reported in a group of such patients that an increase in carbohydrate in the diet induces more calciuria and is associated with a greater antidiuresis in the stone formers than in the control group members. Vitamin B_6 (pyridoxine) deficiency has been shown to result in nephrocalcinosis and hyperoxaluria in the cat, though as yet a deficiency of Vitamin B_6 or an abnormality in its metabolism has not been shown in humans who form renal calcium oxalate stones. A renewed interest has been directed to a possible role of dietary oxalate in the oxalate stone former since *small* increments in urinary oxalate may be important. In addition, a state of hyperabsorption of oxalate has been found in chronic small bowel disease, usually in association with steatorrhea. Methoxy flurane anesthesia and also the chronic use of very large doses of ascorbic acid are potential causes for significant hyperoxaluria and possible stone formation. Dietary purines may be responsible for the frequent finding of hyperuricuria in calcium stone formers, which may induce epitaxic growth of calcium oxalate crystals.

Abnormal pH Control

Normally, urinary pH fluctuates throughout the day from 4.5 or 5.0 to 6.5 or 7.0 with the "alkaline tide" appearing in the postprandial period. Renal calculi are seen in patients who have distal *renal tubular acidosis (Type I)*, a condition in which the distal renal tubules are unable to maintain the normal gradient for hydrogen ion, thus resulting in a urine which rarely has a pH below 6.0. A similar situation pertains to patients taking carbonic anhydrase inhibitors, such as acetazolamide for glaucoma. This persistent "alkaline" pH encourages the precipitation of calcium phosphate and stone formation. A relatively persistent "alkaline" urine is also found in patients with urinary tracts infected by urea-splitting organisms such as Proteus. On the other hand, very acid urines persistently encourage the formation of uric acid calculi because of the relative insolubility of uric acid at a low pH. Examples of this condition can be found in states of severe chronic diarrhea (including that from ileostomies), with the loss of bicarbonate, dehydration and a fixed "acid" urine, and a renal tubular dysfunction most commonly seen in peoples of Mediterranean origin in whom there is a defect in the renal tubular secretion of ammonium. The urine pH in these patients is usually 5.5 or lower throughout the entire 24 hour period, and undoubtedly this low pH is a factor in the high frequency of uric acid stones they produce.

Deficiencies of "Solubilizers" in Urine

CITRATE

About 35 to 58 per cent of urinary calcium is un-ionized, and most of the remainder is bound to citrate in a freely diffusible form. Although groups of renal stone formers have been shown to have urinary citrate to calcium ratios below those of controls, it has been difficult to demonstrate a urinary citrate deficiency common to stone formers. Hypercalciuria explains the low ratio best. Urinary citrate is low, however, in cases of urinary tract infection with urea-splitters or during the prolonged use of acetazolamide as in the treatment of glaucoma. Since citrate complexes with magnesium, it is reduced with the administration of magnesium in the form of sulfate, oxide, or trisilicate.

PYROPHOSPHATES

Pyrophosphates have been known for a long time in industry where they are used as "crystal poisons" to prevent the development of boiler scale and scale within the cooling systems of automobiles. Pyrophosphate is another solubilizer which appears in human urine in small amounts, probably as a metabolite of orthophosphate, because its oral ingestion results in a very little increase in urinary pyrophosphate. The ingestion of large amounts of orthophosphate, however, does increase urinary concentrations of pyrophosphate to some degree. Pyrophosphate is reduced in the urine when dietary phosphate is limited or when aluminum hydroxide, which binds orthophosphate in the gut, is administered, apparently by reducing the orthophosphate substrate for the production of the pyrophosphate. Males normally excrete more pyrophosphate than young females, but both may show an increase above those levels normally found in urine after the administration of oral or parenteral orthophosphate. The pyrophosphates have little effect on preventing uric acid or magnesium ammonium phosphate stone formation.

MAGNESIUM

Magnesium has been reported to increase the solubility of hydroxy apatite and of calcium oxalate and has been only occasionally found in smaller than normal amounts in the urine of stone formers. Many stone formers, however, have a high urinary calcium/magnesium ratio. It is observed that chlorothiazides increase the urinary content of magnesium. *Zinc* and *manganese* also inhibit mineralization in vitro in low concentrations, but no deficiency of either of these has been reported found in the urine of stone formers. It is interesting to note that the soil is low in magnesium in the southeastern part of the United States where the highest incidence of renal calculus disease exists.

SODIUM

Urinary sodium concentration is dependent upon sodium intake unless there is significant renal insufficiency or secondary aldosteronism. There is no evidence for low urinary sodium concentration in stone formers, but a high calcium to sodium osmolar ratio has been reported in a group of them, sodium being one of the most significant elements of that osmolality. Under these conditions, urine supersaturated with calcium oxalate or phosphate is transformed from a metastable to a highly unstable state. Other researchers have suggested that a high sodium to calcium ratio such as is seen in the African Bantu, who has a low incidence of renal stone, is due to the fact that sodium competes with calcium in the formation of hydroxy apatite crystals and is more soluble.

OTHER SUBSTANCES

In addition, other substances found in urine, such as glucuronides, organic acids, amino acids, and colloids, further increase the solubility of crystalloids by their mere presence but make up in only a small part the total solubilizing activity of human urine. One group of investigators no longer believes that there are small peptides in urine which are potent solubilizers, but their most recent studies with simple synthetic urines, containing 12 chemical components commonly found in normal urine, have shown that most, if not all, of the "calcification inhibiting activity" in the urine is apparently due to interactions among a few known components, essentially eliminating the need for another unknown. Of the twelve components, four (magnesium, citrate, calcium, and inorganic phosphate) are the most important in modifying the calcification inhibiting capacity of the urine. In particular, the activity attributable to citrate is enhanced by inorganic phosphate in the presence of calcium and magnesium ions. Further enhancement occurs with acidification followed by neutralization. This new line of investigation may open up understanding to other differences between normal and stone-forming urine.

Presence of "Antisolubilizers" in Urine

Aluminum and *trivalent iron* block the solubilizing activity of pyrophosphate, and *silicon*, though not affecting pyrophosphate, blocks the other inhibitors in urine. Drinking water is the most common source of silicon, but the medication magnesium trisilicate is another.

Obstruction within the Urinary Tract and Randall's Plaque Formation

These may be factors in renal stone formation in special circumstances.

Stones Induced by Medications

Patients with glaucoma treated with *acetazolamide* may form calcium phosphate or oxalate stones. Stone formation may cease with discontinuation of the drug, but if it is important to continue it, successful management may be accomplished by the addition of urinary dilution and the use of oral orthophosphate. Peptic ulcer patients taking large doses of *magnesium trisilicate* occasionally form silicate stones. These patients may respond favorably by switching to an antacid containing a combination of aluminum hydroxide and magnesium oxide. *Absorbable alkali,* such as calcium carbonate and sodium bicarbonate, may produce nephrocalcinosis or calcium phosphate or oxalate stones. Discontinuation of the absorbable alkali and the use of a nonabsorbable antacid is therapeutic. Patients who have a propensity to form calcium stones may have an exacerbation of their problem upon the administration of large doses of *aluminum hydroxide* for prolonged periods of time. This use results in a decrease in urinary pyrophosphate concentration (a natural solubilizer) and an increase in urinary aluminum, which has an antisolubilizing action. Massive oral doses of *vitamin C*, currently popular, in doses greater than two grams a day may increase urinary oxalate concentration significantly and encourage oxalate stone formation in some patients. *Oral* orthophosphate given to a calcium ammonium magnesium phosphate stone former may induce further stone formation. *Allopurinol* has been reported to produce xanthine stones in situations in which there is a very high uric acid production, such as in the Lesch-Nyhan syndrome. This problem is best approached by dilution of urine, alkalinization, and reduction of the allopurinol to the minimal effective dose.

DIAGNOSIS

Frequently, the diagnosis of renal calculus disease is made at the time of the stone's ureteric migration when the patient develops the typical excruciating pain of renal colic. This pain often begins deep in the lumbar region and progresses with radiation around the side into the groin, the testicle or the penis in the male, or the labia in the female. Pain may come in waves and be only partially relieved by narcotics. Occasionally, however, stones are passed in a relatively painless way, associated with only a dull ache and may be brought to the attention when the patient notes a momentary interruption of the urinary stream or actually hears the "clink" of the stone against the toilet bowl. Asymptomatic stones are often uncovered at the finding of silent microscopic hematuria, azotemia, hypertension, a positive family history for renal stone disease, or by the discovery of opaque calculi at the time of routine roentgenologic studies.

Roentgenograms, in particular, are a fruitful source since over 90 per cent of renal calculi contain calcium. Pure cystine stones, contrary to some reports, are also radiopaque (Fig. 14–1). In addition, although pure uric acid stones, as well as the very rare xanthine calculi, are radiolucent, such stones can occasionally be identified radiologically,

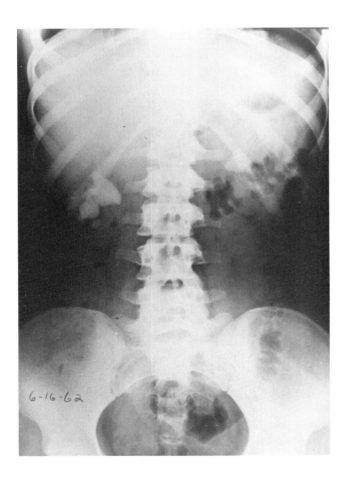

Figure 14–1   Bilateral opaque cystine calculi shown in plain film over the abdomen.

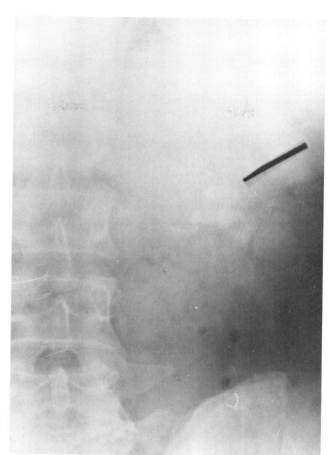

Figure 14–2 *A,* X-ray over abdomen showing a mixed uric acid and calcium stone. Note a very large nonopaque uric acid stone from a patient with urinary tract infection. Urea-splitting organisms have produced concretions of calcium ammonium magnesium phosphate on the stone's surface which makes it faintly visible.

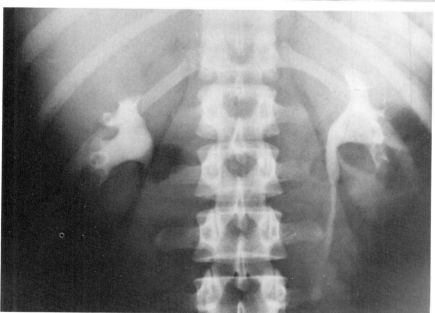

Figure 14–2 *B,* Nonopaque uric acid stone made visible as a negative shadow or filling defect on x-ray during intravenous pyelography.

even without the use of contrast medium because they frequently are mixed with calcium that is the result of urinary tract infection (Fig. 14–2,A). The uric acid stones which contain no calcium usually can be identified as a negative shadow by intravenous pyelography (Fig. 14–2,B). Other characteristics of the stone's composition may sometimes be suspected from the radiologic appearance. For example, staghorn or branched calculi that fill one or more calyces or even the entire pelvis of the kidney are almost invariably composed of calcium magnesium ammonium phosphate, secondary to urinary tract infection. Cystine stones are usually bilateral and usually appear in childhood. Calcium phosphate stones may appear radiologically as rather smooth stones that often show concentric rings of varying density. Oxalate stones are more likely to show irregularities of the surface, which at times are described as "stellate" or "mulberry" in form.

SILENT RENAL STONE DISEASE

Historical and physical findings may lead one to suspect the possibility of silent renal stone disease. For example, hypercalcemia can cause one or more of the following symptoms: weakness, anorexia, weight loss, change in psyche, pruritus, bone pain or fractures, symptoms of peptic ulcer, nocturia and polyuria, and signs such as calcification in the cornea near the limbus (band keratopathy) or within the conjunctivae or on the tympanic membranes. When stone disease is found in children, it is usually secondary to cystinuria, urinary tract infection, inflammatory intestinal disease, or the rare condition, primary hyperoxaluria. The possibility of renal calculi in adults should be considered with chronic inflammatory bowel disease and chronic diarrhea as well as in those with arthritis who may have atypical gout. Patients with myeloproliferative disorders, those undergoing cancer chemotherapy, and patients with glaucoma who are being treated with acetazolamide also are potential candidates for stone formation.

The Stone

Every effort should be made to recover a stone a patient has passed because of its value in determining probable etiologic factors in its formation and to suggest a more rational approach to treatment. Not all stones passed during an acute episode are brought to the physician, but inquiry by him can often discover one tucked away at home "in the dresser drawer." The gross appearance of the stone may also suggest its composition (Fig. 14–3). Calcium phosphate stones are usually white, cream colored, or a very light tan, are composed of lamellar concretions, and may be rather soft and easily flaked off with a knife blade. This is most often the case with apatite calculi, whereas the calcium hydrogen phosphate (Brushite) stones have a more nodular appearance to their surface; the calcium magnesium ammonium phosphate (Stru-

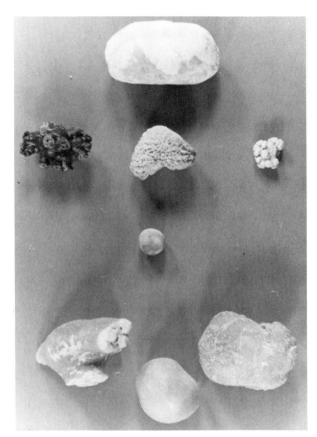

Figure 14–3 Physical characteristics of several types of stones. *Top,* Calcium phosphate stone with concretions of calcium magnesium ammonium phosphate on its surface. *Second row (left to right),* Calcium oxalate monohydrate (Jack stone) type, calcium oxalate dihydrate calculus, calcium oxalate dihydrate calculus. *Third row,* Uric acid calculus. *Fourth row,* Three cystine calculi. The first is part of a staghorn calculus (waxy, honey colored stones).

vite) stones, secondary to urinary tract infection, tend to have a more crystalline inner surface with a somewhat columnar structure in the inner zones. Calcium oxalate stones usually occur in one of two forms, the monohydrate with one molecule of water of hydration or the dihydrate with two. The oxalate monohydrate (Whewellite) occasionally has a rather smooth surface (Hempseed type), but much more commonly the surface is rough, convoluted, and often sharply contoured. The surface of the calculus usually has a metallic sheen or varnished appearance with a reddish brown or even black color (Fig. 14–4,*A*). The dihydrate oxalate (Weddellite) stone is lighter in color, and its surface is usually studded with sharp-edged, sometimes knife-bladelike crystals (Fig. 14–4,*B*). Oxalate stones are much harder than the phosphate stones and more difficult to break or cut.

Stone Screen and "Workup"

Although the majority of renal stone problems are idiopathic, it is well to first uncover any possible contributing factor (Table 14–2).

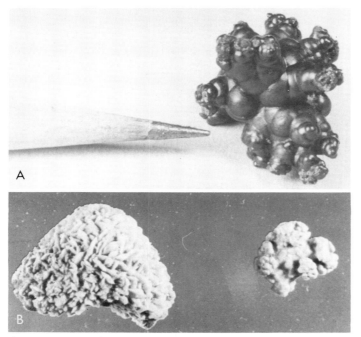

Figure 14–4 *A,* Calcium oxalate monohydrate calculus (jet black in color). *B,* Calcium oxalate dihydrate calculi.

First, the patient should be questioned about the chronic use of medications such as acetazolamide (Diamox), uricosuric drugs (probenecid), vitamin D, allopurinol, magnesium trisilicate, aluminum hydroxide, and vitamin C in large doses. In addition, an estimate is obtained concerning the daily intake of milk and any use of absorbable alkali, such as sodium bicarbonate or antacids containing carbonate.

If a stone is available, it should be submitted for analysis, preferably by x-ray diffraction. The stone's nucleus or central area should be assayed separately from its outer zones because the initial cause of its production may be suggested by the nuclear analysis, whereas the outer zones may show evidence of mixing of constituents as is seen, for example, in infected urine where the outer zone of a uric acid stone may contain calcium magnesium ammonium phosphate. The latter finding in either a pure or a mixed stone is pathognomonic of urinary tract infection with urea-splitting bacteria such as Proteus. Not infrequently an analysis report will return indicating that a stone contains calcium phosphate and uric acid. When not expressed quantitatively, the uric acid may be due to blood adhering to the stone at the time of its analysis and usually is not at all related to the problem of its genesis. If cystine is reported in the stone analysis, the diagnosis of cystinuria is almost certain. So-called matrix calculi are somewhat soft but may have gritty concretions imbedded within them. X-ray diffraction studies are particularly helpful in identifying stones such as xanthine or silicate.

TABLE 14–2 Laboratory Assessment

ANALYSIS	SPECIFIC TESTS
Of Stone	Calcium, phosphorus, oxalate, ammonium, magnesium, uric acid, and cystine
Of Blood	Calcium, phosphorus, alkaline phosphatase, creatinine, sodium, potassium, chloride, CO_2 content, pH, uric acid, and protein electrophoresis
Of Urine	Complete urinalysis, including evaluation for infection and crystals Check pH of every fresh voided specimen for 48 hours (Nitrazine paper: range 4 to 8) Calcium, phosphorus, creatinine, cystine and, if available, oxalate (24 hour urine acidified for cystine and oxalate) Uric acid (24 hour urine)
Radiologic	KUB (plain abdominal x-ray over kidneys, ureters, and bladder) Excretory urogram Hands Chest

URINALYSIS

Although the routine urinalysis is of limited value, it is important for the physician to examine it himself to be sure that cystine crystalluria is not overlooked since it is very easily missed. The best conditions for finding these crystals are in a first voided morning specimen that is acidified and chilled in the refrigerator for a short time. Typical hexagonal crystals (Fig. 14–5) may be present in abundance but can be missed if they are sought for under the usual intensity of light because they are very transparent and extremely thin. They look very much like tiny hexagons of clear plastic film floating in the urine and can be very nicely seen when the light is reduced, preferably when it is somewhat obliquely cast through the slide. Crystals of oxalate, magnesium, ammonium phosphate, and uric acid are commonly found in the urine of patients without renal calculi and have little clinical significance. If a *fresh* voided specimen has a pH of over 7.0, one may suspect an infection with urea-splitting organisms. Pyuria and bacteriuria indicate infection in urine properly collected. Culture and antibiotic sensitivity studies are necessary for proper therapy.

A biochemical screening test for cystinuria is also available in most hospitals (Fig. 14–6). It is best determined on a first voided specimen in the morning. Pure uric acid, xanthine and cystine stones can be ignited, leaving almost no ash and giving off the odor of burning flesh, or in the case of cystine, of burning hair owing to the sulfur content of the latter.

Hypercalcemia

As concerns an increased solute load in the production of renal calculus disease, hypercalcemia and hypercalciuria are first to be con-

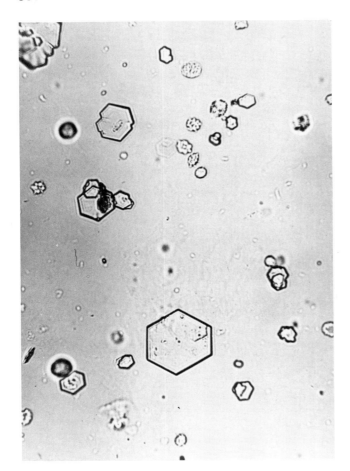

Figure 14–5 Cystine crystals in urine.

sidered. Hypercalcemia may not be a persistent finding even in primary hyperparathyroidism. Serum calcium concentrations may fluctuate between the upper limits of normal and clearly elevated levels from day to day or week to week. Therefore, hypercalcemia cannot be excluded with the finding of a single normal serum calcium concentration. It is best to have three, and ideally five, specimens spaced over

---

To about 5 ml of urine add a few drops of concentrated ammonium hydroxide.

Add 2 ml of a freshly prepared 5 per cent sodium cyanide solution and mix.

Wait for five to ten minutes, then add, by drops, a freshly prepared solution of 5 per cent sodium nitroprusside.

A deep purplish color is a positive result.

Figure 14–6 Screening test for cystine.

several days or several weeks. It is critical to know the normal range for calcium in the specific laboratory. In general the reported normal ranges have been too high. In most laboratories the upper limit has been reduced from 11.0 mg/100 ml to 10.5 mg/100 ml but even this may be too high, particularly in young women where anything above 10.2 mg/100 ml may be a significant elevation above normal.

Hypercalcemia and renal stone disease can be seen together in sarcoidosis, vitamin D excess, and milk-alkali syndrome in addition to primary hyperparathyroidism. The hypercalcemia seen with malignancy and in some cases of hyperthyroidism is usually not of long enough duration to result in renal calculus disease.

PRIMARY HYPERPARATHYROIDISM

A diagnosis of primary hyperparathyroidism is established by documenting hypercalcemia, though it may be intermittent or borderline, and subperiosteal bone resorption, which is best seen with x-rays of the hands. The latter must be found in the absence of significant renal insufficiency, vitamin D deficiency, or chronic intestinal malabsorption, all of which produce secondary hyperparathyroidism. Unfortunately, subperiosteal resorption is found in only about 15 per cent of patients having primary hyperparathyroidism. In its absence, the diagnosis can be established by exclusion after ruling out the other causes of hypercalcemia. The current availability of measurements of parathyroid hormone (PTH) concentrations in serum allows some refinement in the diagnosis of uncertain cases and in those with borderline or intermittent hypercalcemia. When parathyroid hormone and calcium concentrations are measured simultaneously in serum, a simple discriminate analysis of these may uncover an *inappropriately* high concentration of parathyroid hormone for the level of serum calcium. Since normally these concentrations are inversely related, parathyroid hormone may be found inappropriately high while still within the upper limits of the "normal range" if the serum calcium concentration is also within the upper limits of normal. Measurement of the hormone elevation is, however, not specific for *primary* hyperparathyroidism, but the causes of secondary hyperparathyroidism are not usually difficult to rule out. Sampling from the right and left venous drainage areas of the thyroid may help in localizing primary hyperparathyroidism and circumventing uncertainties as to whether the elevated peripheral concentrations of the hormone are due to secretion from a primary parathyroid adenoma or to an ectopic nonparathyroid neoplasm that produces a parathyroidlike hormonal substance.

One other condition in which serum PTH is secondarily elevated is idiopathic hypercalciuria (renal type) with normal serum calcium concentration. It should be possible to differentiate this from the so-called normocalcemic primary hyperparathyroidism by the use of hydrochlorothiazide for several weeks to eliminate the hypercalciuria. Serum calcium concentration should be carefully monitored during this time because, in the case of primary hyperparathyroidism, hypercalcemia usually appears and elevation of the PTH level persists, while in idiopathic hypercalciuria with secondary hyperparathyroidism, the serum calcium remains normal and the PTH level is suppressed to normal.

SARCOIDOSIS

When hypercalcemia is found *in association with renal stone*, the most likely diagnosis other than primary hyperparathyroidism is sarcoidosis. The diagnosis of sarcoidosis, however, is not always easy to confirm. It is suspected by finding the large, usually bilateral hilar lymph nodes that occur with or without evidence of parenchymal disease, iritis or uveitis, erythema nodosum, allergy to delayed sensitivity skin tests such as old tuberculin and mumps antigen, and leukopenia and serum protein electrophoresis abnormality, with elevations of alpha-2 or gamma globulin. There is a difference of opinion about the value of the Kveim test, but the biopsy and pathologic examination of paratracheal lymph nodes or of sarcoid skin lesions (not erythema nodosum) may be more definitive. Of help is the fact that hypercalcemia is seen in less than 5 per cent of patients with sarcoidosis and then only in those with evidence of disseminated disease, usually with pulmonary parenchymal involvement. The incidence of *hypercalciuria*, however, is very high and occurs in the majority of patients. Sarcoidosis is associated with increased sensitivity to vitamin D and the gastrointestinal hyperabsorption of calcium. Even in the absence of hypercalcemia, hypercalciuria is usually marked in sarcoidosis and may range from 300 to 1000 mg per 24 hours. This excess of calcium undoubtedly is due to both the hyperabsorption and to a suppression of parathyroid hormone secretion that results in decreased renal tubular reabsorption of calcium. Contrastingly, in an individual with primary hyperparathyroidism the amount of calcium, though above that found in the normal person, is surprisingly less than that expected to be found when considering the filtered load.

Hypercalciuria

IDIOPATHIC HYPERCALCIURIA

The most common type of hypercalciuria is the *idiopathic* form. It is a diagnosis made by the exclusion of hyperparathyroidism, sarcoidosis, vitamin D excess, and Cushing's disease. It may be somewhat difficult to separate from so-called normocalcemic hyperparathyroidism and that form which has intermittent hypercalcemia. As mentioned above, however, the degree of hypercalciuria in primary hyperparathyroidism is relatively small when considering the filtered load of calcium, but in idiopathic hypercalciuria, urinary calcium excretion is high in the absence of hypercalcemia. Idiopathic hypercalciuria is seen four times as commonly in males and may present in one of two forms: (1) the gastrointestinal (hyperabsorption of calcium) or (2) the renal ("calcium-leak").

Although serum calcium is within the normal range, parathyroid hormone (PTH) concentration is reported elevated in the renal type. This elevation can be suppressed to normal by reducing the renal loss of calcium with the administration of chlorothiazide. Placing the patient on a low calcium intake further increases plasma PTH concentration and does not greatly reduce the hypercalciuria. On the other hand in the gastrointestinal type, reduction in calcium absorption from the gut, by low calcium intake or the use of oral phytate or cellulose phosphate, results in the reduction of urinary calcium to normal. Administration of chlorothiazide, however, may result in elevation of the serum calcium in normocalcemia primary hyperparathyroidism and perhaps, at least transiently, in the gastrointestinal type of idiopathic hypercalciuria.

Screening for the presence or absence of hypercalciuria can best be accomplished by allowing the patient to maintain a normal diet which usually includes 500 to 1000 mg of calcium per day and which results in a normal urinary excretion of calcium of less than 300 mg per day in males and 250 mg per day in females (see Table 14–3).

CUSHING'S DISEASE

The increased resorption and diminished formation rate of bone in Cushing's disease often results in hypercalciuria without hypercalcemia. The diagnosis is made by finding typical physical features of Cushing's syndrome and an elevation of 17-hydroxycorticosteroids in the urine not suppressible below 2.5 mg (Porter-Silber chromogens) per 24 hours on the second day of two days by the administration of 0.5 mg of dexamethasone every 6 hours.

TABLE 14–3   Concentrations of Urinary Crystalloids per 24 Hours

	NORMAL (MG)	CONSIDERED ABNORMAL (MG)	DIETARY CONDITIONS
Calcium	100 to 200	300 (male) 250 (female)	General
Oxalate	20 to 55	65	No deficiency of folic acid; low glycine intake
Phosphate	300 to 1000	1000	Normal protein and milk intake
Uric acid	250 to 550	750	Low purine; low protein
Cystine	10 to 20	100	Normal
Xanthine	5 to 20	20	Normal

Hyperuricemia and Hyperuricuria

Hyperuricemia occurs in both primary and secondary forms. It may also appear after the use of chlorothiazides and a moderate elevation of serum uric acid is found in a number of patients with primary hyperparathyroidism. In fact, mixed calcium stones with a uric acid component may occur in this condition. A diagnosis of primary gout can be established by finding hyperuricemia and hyperuricuria in the absence of myeloproliferative disease, cancer therapies, chlorothiazides, hyperparathyroidism, and gouty arthritis, though not always with classic podagra. Joint fluid aspirates show the birefringent crystals of uric acid within the cells of the polymorphonuclear leukocytes. It should be remembered that probenecid, salicylates, and glucocorticoids can cause a moderate degree of hyperuricuria. Hyperuricuria is also seen in some calcium oxalate stone formers.

Cystinuria

Homozygotic cystinurics excrete greater than 300 mg of cystine in the urine each day as well as large amounts of three other dibasic amino acids, lysine, arginine, and ornithine, all of which can be demonstrated by chromatography. Ordinarily this technique is not necessary to establish the diagnosis if, however, urinary cystine crystals can be demonstrated in a patient with renal calculus disease, which is usually bilateral and appears in childhood. The stones are opaque and may become staghorn. A qualitative screening test is indicated in Figure 14–6.

Xanthinuria

Small amounts of xanthine are found in normal urines, but excessive amounts that result in renal calculus disease appear only in the rare genetic disorder xanthinuria, in which there is a low or absent xanthine oxidase enzyme activity in tissues. Only a few of these rare cases have actually produced stones. Since xanthine is a precursor in the metabolism of purines to uric acid, it is not surprising to find extremely low levels of uric acid in both serum and urine in this condition. Xanthinuria has also been described in association with hemochromatosis and during the use of allopurinol (Zyloprim), but under these circumstances recognizable xanthine stone production has not yet resulted. An exception is a case of Lesch-Nyhan syndrome (a hereditary disorder of purine metabolism with excessive production of purines) that was treated with this drug.

Oxaluria

Hyperoxaluria may be caused by (1) one of the two types of *primary hyperoxaluria*, (2) inflammatory bowel disease, in which increased conversion of the bile acid glycine to oxalate by bacterial action occurs and results in increased absorption of oxalate, (3) vitamin B_6 (pyridoxine) deficiency, (4) ingestion of large amounts of oxalate, glycolate, ethylene glycol, or glyoxalate, (5) a high carbohydrate ingestion in idiopathic oxalate stone formers, and (6) a low dietary calcium intake.

The clinical picture for primary hyperoxaluria is identical for both types. The condition usually manifests itself in childhood with the appearance of renal calculi or renal failure. There are a number of milder cases, however, which make their clinical appearance in adulthood. In the absence of pyridoxine deficiency, the diagnosis is made by finding greater than 120 mg oxalate excretion in the urine during 24 hours. Slight elevations of urinary oxalate, 50 to 150 mg per 24 hours, have also been reported in patients with Klinefelter's syndrome, cirrhosis, renal tubular acidosis, and sarcoidosis. Type I is due to a deficiency of the enzyme α-ketoglutarate-glyoxalate carboligase that is measurable from a biopsy of liver, kidney, or spleen and also is diagnosed by demonstrating an excessive (greater than 60 mg per 24 hours) urinary excretion of glycolic acid. Type II is due to a diminished activity of D-glyceric dehydrogenase, assayable in leukocytes. In this type there is an increased excretion (greater than 225 mg per 24 hours) or urinary L-glyceric acid. Although the administration of Vitamin B_6 (pyridoxine) may result in a reduction of urinary oxalate in most forms of hyperoxaluria, the hyperoxaluria is not abolished as it is in an individual deficient of pyridoxine. In the case of hyperoxaluria in association with inflammatory bowel disease, if the latter is the cause, the hyperoxaluria may be diminished or removed by the oral administration of cholestyramine or taurine.

Abnormal pH Control

Normally, following a meal there is an alkaline tide in the urine. Urinary pH ordinarily varies between 4.5 and 6.5 to 7.0. Patients can be taught to read accurately a Nitrazine paper (range pH 4 to 8) and to record the pH of each voided specimen over a 48 hour period so that the diurnal variations can be assessed. Patients with renal tubular acidosis (Type I), those with infection of the urinary tract with urea-splitting bacteria, and those using carbonic anhydrase inhibitors (e.g., Diamox) find that the pH of all urines is above 5.5, while those patients with chronic diarrhea, including some ileostomies, and those with the renal tubular dysfunction of Henneman remain at a pH below 5.5 throughout the 24 hour period. Those with pH persistently below 5.5 tend to form uric acid stones, while patients with diarrhea, oxalate stones. Those with pH persistently higher than 5.5 or 6.0 are more likely to form phosphate or calcium oxalate stones.

Renal Tubular Acidosis

Patients with renal tubular acidosis, Type I (distal form), develop nephrocalcinosis and sometimes renal calculi, but those with Type II (proximal form) have been free of this complication to date. Renal tubular acidosis may manifest itself in muscular weakness and bone pain, particularly in the pelvic region, producing what has been described as a "waddling" gait. There is a metabolic acidosis with hyperchloremia and hypokalemia. Measurement of urinary pH after a 12 hour fast offers a screening test. Those with this disorder maintain a urinary pH above 5.5. If the screening test is positive, an ammonium chloride challenge may help to confirm the diagnosis. Ammonium chloride solution, 100 mg/kg over 24 hours in four divided oral doses at a concentration of 500 mg/5 ml is given, and the pH and bicarbonate content of plasma in urine are measured at intervals. If the urine pH has not fallen below 5.5 when the plasma bicarbonate reaches 20 mEq per liter, the diagnosis is confirmed provided that urinary bicarbonate is not high (suggesting a proximal leak) and the urine is not infected with urea-splitting bacteria.

Urea-Splitting Bacterial Infection

Identification of an infection caused by urea-splitting organisms, such as Proteus, is accomplished by finding the organism in significant numbers on two consecutive urine cultures. It can be suspected, however, by a simple office procedure. A small volume of freshly voided urine from the patient is placed in a sterile test tube at room temperature alongside a known uninfected urine specimen, also freshly voided, and allowed to stand overnight. The following morning a urine specimen infected with urea-splitting organisms will be much more alkaline than the control when tested with Nitrazine paper. Of course, if the initial freshly voided urine specimen has a pH of 7.0, the likelihood of infection with a urea-splitting organism is great, just on this evidence alone.

TREATMENT AND PREVENTION

General Measures

There is general agreement that the maintenance of a dilute urine is a very important adjunct to any and all of the other therapeutic and preventative measures. Too often, however, the patient is merely told to "drink a lot of water." This action may improve urinary output and increase dilution during the day, but considerable urinary concentration may continue to occur during the night. It is also more important to emphasize output than intake to the patient since, with a fixed intake, the output can vary considerably depending on extrarenal losses of fluid from the skin and gastrointestinal tract. For example, in order to maintain an optimal output, it is necessary to drink more in the hot summer months. The patient is encouraged to develop the habit of drinking a large glass of water at least every two hours during the day and two glasses at bedtime. This should produce nocturia at about 2 or 3 a.m. at which time another glass or two should be taken. Stone formers adapt surprisingly well to this once nightly nocturia. The second general measure is to correct obstructive lesions and to remove obstructive or infected stones. Successful treatment of patients with infected stones requires prolonged antibiotic therapy after stone removal. The third measure is the vigorous treatment of any urinary tract infection that appears after the removal of or the spontaneous passage of a renal stone.

Calcium Stone Therapy

STONE FORMATION IN HYPERCALCEMIA

Hyperparathyroidism. Hypercalcemia, in association with renal calculi, is seen with hyperparathyroidism, vitamin D excess, sarcoidosis, Paget's disease, milk alkali syndrome, and from significant immobilization as with some forms of poliomyelitis. Although renal calculi are seen in frequent association with hyperparathyroidism, many observers have noted that more often these appear at long intervals, and evidence may be found of only one stone over a 20 to 30 year history. One group of researchers have documented the fact that only 11 per cent of their patients with proven hyperparathyroidism have had a "metabolically active" status regarding stone formation. Such a status is defined as evidence of a new stone formation, or stone growth, or the documented passage of gravel within the past year. In patients considered "active" producers or whenever obstruction occurs that requires surgical intervention, a parathyroidectomy almost always restores the patient to a "metabolically inactive" state. When parathyroid surgery is not possible or the parathyroid tumor is unable to be located surgically, the oral administration of orthophosphate (1 to 2 grams of inorganic phosphorus per day as K-Phos or Neutraphos) may prevent further stone formation.

Vitamin D Excess. Since stone formation with vitamin D excess is a self-limited problem, one needs only treat the temporary hypercalcemia and hypercalciuria. It should be remembered, however, that vitamin D is stored in body fat, and the excess may not disappear for many weeks. During this time, of course, vitamin D should be stopped, including sources from fortified foods, and the patient should be placed on a low calcium diet. Fluid intake should be high around the clock, and during hypercalcemia, hydrocortisone or an analogue can be used temporarily to block the increased gastrointestinal absorption of calcium.

Sarcoidosis. Since patients with sarcoidosis are extremely sensitive to small doses of vitamin D and since the condition is often more chronic, the protracted use of a low calcium diet, intermittent three week courses of hydrocortisone or its analogue and the oral ingestion of orthophosphate may be useful in reducing stone formation.

Milk Alkali Syndrome. This is treated by removing milk and milk products from the diet as well as the absorbable alkali. Fluids are forced around the clock.

Paget's Disease. This can be treated with a low calcium diet, mobilization, and if the hypercalciuria persists, by the use of orthophosphate or hydrochlorothiazide, the latter in doses of 25 to 50 mg twice daily.

Immobilization. In the case of hypercalcemia with immobilization from poliomyelitis, the foremost factors in therapy are a reduction in the intake of vitamin D and calcium, urinary dilution by forcing fluids, the use of a rocking bed, and finally the vigorous treatment of urinary tract infections that almost invariably follow the use of a catheter.

STONE FORMATION IN HYPERCALCIURIA

Idiopathic Hypercalciuria. Hypercalciuria and renal calculi are most often found together in the conditions of idiopathic hypercalciuria, hyperparathyroidism, sarcoidosis, vitamin D excess, and Cushing's syndrome. Idiopathic hypercalciuria of the renal type may be treated successfully with the use of hydrochlorothiazide, which may reduce urinary calcium by 50 per cent. The gastrointestinal (hyperabsorptive) type responds with a reduction of urinary calcium by placing the patient on a low calcium diet with the addition of oral orthophosphate. Cellulose phosphate (an experimental drug, see p. 392) may soon become the single drug of choice for this condition. In addition, it has been recognized that hyperuricuria is commonly associated with the syndrome of idiopathic hypercalciuria and the production of *calcium* stones. These may be prevented by the use of allopurinol.

The management of hyperparathyroidism, sarcoidosis, and vitamin D excess were previously discussed.

Cushing's Syndrome. The hypercalciuria of Cushing's syndrome is secondary to increased resorption and an associated decreased accretion of bone, together with an increased glomerular filtration rate. If renal calculi become a problem, administration of oral phosphate may be helpful. Direct treatment of Cushing's syndrome is the most effective therapeutic measure, however.

Other Stone Therapy

CALCIUM AMMONIUM MAGNESIUM PHOSPHATE STONES

Calcium ammonium magnesium phosphate stones are the indicators of *urinary tract infection*, which is usually caused by urea-splitting bacteria such as Proteus. The presence of infected stones is a great deterrent to successful treatment, and the progressive growth and recurrence of stones is likely to occur unless infected calculi are completely removed under antibiotic coverage continued for many weeks thereafter. In addition, acidification of the urine to a pH of 5.5 or less for several months with the use of ammonium chloride or cranberry juice is a helpful adjunct. Oral orthophosphate therapy is definitely contraindicated in dealing with this type of stone.

CALCIUM OXALATE STONES

Calcium oxalate stones are usually idiopathic. They are among the most common of all stones and often the most difficult to treat, but in the past few years some definite gains have been made in their management. If they are found in association with hypercalciuria, hydrochlorothiazide is the drug of choice, unless the hypercalciuria disappears with calcium restriction, in which case a low calcium diet or cellulose phosphate is preferable. Allopurinol is indicated in the calcium oxalate stone former if there is hyperuricuria, with or without hypercalciuria. If *both* hypercalciuria and hyperuricuria are found, hydrochlorothiazide can be given in combination with small doses (150 to 200 mg per day) of allopurinol.

Factors Stimulating Increases in Urinary Oxalate Concentration. Since the recognition that very minor increases in urinary oxalate concentration may be important in the production of calculi in some patients, factors which may have such minor influence are being reevaluated. It should be kept in mind that the increased gastrointestinal absorption of oxalate occurs with a low calcium diet, with inflammatory bowel disease, with large intakes of dietary oxalate, such as are found in rhubarb, beets, tea, coffee, spinach, and chocolate, as well as in the very rare patient with intestinal sucrase-isomaltase deficiency, in which case there is an increased formation of soluble oxalates in the bowel by the fermentation of sugars. A high carbohydrate diet in patients without this enzyme deficiency may also produce some elevation in urinary oxalate concentration. One other dietary source for increased urinary oxalate is massive doses of vitamin C (greater than 2 grams per day), which is currently a popular item for self-medication. The increase in urinary oxalate seen with inflammatory bowel disease can be treated successfully with cholestyramine or taurine. In the case of renal tubular acidosis (Type I), one should treat the acidosis and replace the deficits of sodium, potassium, and bicarbonate. After this therapy, urinary citrate rises and urinary calcium declines. Stones usually cease to form, but if they continue to do so, treatment with oral orthophosphate may be helpful. The use of magnesium oxide has been popular in the past because it increases urinary magnesium, a solubilizer, and decreases urinary oxalate. Gastrointestinal tolerance to it is limited, however, and other methods of treatment are currently more favored.

URIC ACID STONES

Uric acid stones are usually very successfully treated by the measures of urinary alkalinization and dilution. Special attention should be paid to the nighttime urine concentration by maintaining an adequate fluid volume through liquids taken at bedtime and in the early morning hours. The urine pH should be kept at about 6.5 by the use of alkali, but higher pH levels should be avoided since calcium stones may form. It is not difficult to keep the urine alkaline to that pH by the administration of sodium bicarbonate or citrate (Polycitra syrup). In cases of significant hyperuricemia, allopurinol may not only prevent but also assist in the dissolution of uric acid stones. It is particularly useful during cancer chemotherapy when serum uric acid is rising. In chronic diarrhea that includes a hyperactive ileostomy and in the case of the renal tubular inability to secrete normal concentrations of ammonium, alkalinization of the urine and the forcing of fluids is often adequate, but when recurrent uric acid stone formation is persistent, the addition of allopurinol may be decisive.

CYSTINE STONES

Cystine stones may respond to careful and consistent dilution by forcing fluids and alkalinization with sodium citrate and potassium citrate (Polycitra syrup), persistently keeping the urine pH at 7.5. A very low methionine diet is not practical and cannot be tolerated for long by most patients, but dietary protein excess should be avoided and kept near the minimum requirement. D-penicillamine or N-acetyl-D-penicillamine is usually not required except when anticipating that calculi can be dissolved medically. Following this dissolution, penicillamine should be discontinued because of the high incidence and seriousness of the side effects.

XANTHINE STONES

Xanthine stones are best treated by 24 hour urinary dilution and alkalinization with sodium bicarbonate or citrate (Polycitra syrup).

Medications Used in the Therapy of Renal Calculus Disease

ORTHOPHOSPHATES

Orthophosphates are given orally in divided doses that provide 1 to 2 grams of inorganic phosphorus per day. Forcing the dose much beyond this may produce some diarrhea, though most patients have some gastrointestinal tolerance to the drug. It can be provided as potassium acid phosphate (K-Phos) or as a neutral sodium and potassium phosphate (Neutra-Phos). Its method of action is unclear, but it has been suggested that it increases urinary orthophosphate, which competes with pyrophosphate for renal tubular reabsorption, thereby raising the concentration of the urinary pyrophosphate, a somewhat potent solubilizer. Extraskeletal calcification has been reported with oral phosphate, but the doses of elemental phosphorus given per day exceed by two to six times those recommended.

HYDROCHLOROTHIAZIDE

Hydrochlorothiazide, apparently by a direct renal tubular effect, lowers urinary calcium concentrations by 30 to 50 per cent. In addition, urinary magnesium increases, and there is a slight increase in pyrophosphate, both favorable changes in the case of recurrent calcium stone formation. Hydrochlorothiazide is especially useful in treating recurrent calcium stone formers who have idiopathic hypercalciuria, particularly the "renal type." Some side effects of the drug are a tendency for hypokalemia, hyperuricemia, hyperglycemia, and sometimes the feeling of fatigue. These effects are minimal in most patients. The smallest effective dose is recommended, 25 to 50 mg twice daily. It is said that there is somewhat less renal loss of bicarbonate and potassium with hydrochlorothiazide than with chlorothiazide. Occasionally hypercalcemia develops during hydrochlorothiazide administration. Should this occur, one should suspect a concomitant diagnosis of primary hyperparathyroidism, sarcoidosis, or vitamin D excess.

MAGNESIUM OXIDE

Use of magnesium oxide is limited by gastrointestinal intolerance but has been used successfully by some urologists for the treatment of idiopathic calcium oxalate stone formation. It causes a decrease in urinary oxalate as well as an increase in urinary magnesium concentration. It is given as the oxide, 100 mg orally three times a day and usually in association with pyridoxine (vitamin B_6), 100 mg a day, which in some patients may also further reduce the urinary oxalate concentration.

ALLOPURINOL

Allopurinol (Zyloprim) is especially useful in the treatment of patients with hyperuricemia secondary to cancer chemotherapy or to myeloproliferative disorders. It is also a helpful agent to use in dissolving uric acid calculi. Following their dissolution, however, it is usually possible to rely on alkalinization and dilution alone to prevent further stone formation. Sometimes it can be used in patients with severe stone problems secondary to ileostomy. The dose ranges from 200 to 800 mg a day. In addition, it is useful in patients with recurrent *calcium* stone formation and hyperuricuria, with or without hypercalciuria. In the latter case it can be used in combination with hydrochlorthiazide.

ALKALINIZING AGENTS

Sodium bicarbonate, though inexpensive, is not usually a favorite with patients because of the abdominal distention it causes. A better tolerated preparation is sodium and potassium citrate (Polycitra syrup). Each ml contains 1 millimol each of sodium, potassium, and citrate, and 15 to 20 ml after each meal and at 2 a.m. is enough to maintain a urinary pH usually between 7.4 and 7.6. This preparation is especially useful in patients with cystinuria but also helps those with persistently acid urine and uric stone formation, though smaller doses normally are used to maintain a pH at about 6.5. The solubility of uric acid is about doubled at that pH.

D-PENICILLAMINE

D-Penicillamine is used to dissolve nonobstructing cystine calculi and must be given 30 minutes before meals, 250 mg three to four times a day. It must be used with caution, however, since side effects include nephrotic syndrome, serum sickness, neutropenia, dermatitis, gastrointestinal disturbances, and iron deficiency.

Experimental Drugs of Potential Usefulness

CELLULOSE PHOSPHATE

Cellulose phosphate is not yet commercially available in this country but has promise in the treatment of recurrent calcium stones. In cases of absorptive hypercalciuria and nephrolithiasis, urinary calcium was reduced to less than 200 mg a day by the oral administration of 5 grams of cellulose phosphate two to three times a day. The state of saturation of urinary Brushite decreased, and stone formation practically ceased. Since the material also binds magnesium, a magnesium chloride supplement of about 150 mg is given at bedtime. During the administration of this substance, there was no change in serum iron, calcium, or zinc, and parathyroid hormone concentrations remained normal throughout the study. There was no escape from the effects of the treatment over a nearly five year period of constant administration in some patients. Extraskeletal calcification would not be expected to occur with the use of this poorly absorbed drug.

DISODIUM ETIDRONATE

Disodium Etidronate (Diphosphonate) inhibits calcium deposition in bone and perhaps will inhibit renal calculus formation in vivo. The most likely mechanism of action is a strong chemisorption on hydroxy apatite crystals that blocks further crystal formation. Its chronic use in man, however, has resulted in osteomalacia, which may limit its usefulness.

METHYLENE BLUE

Methylene blue is a cationic dye which inhibits calcification of rachitic rat's cartilage and is said often to keep indwelling catheters free of crystallization. Its mode of action is perhaps that of competing with calcium ions at binding sites in matrix. Its experimental use has caused some stones to vanish over a two-year period of treatment, and it has the rather remarkable property of being active even in the presence of infection, perhaps with the exception of Pseudomonas.

ISOCARBOXAZID

Isocarboxazid (Marplan) is a monoamine oxidase inhibitor that blocks the metabolism of ethanolamine to oxalate and could be useful in treatment of oxalate stone formers who are resistant to other therapies.

RENACIDIN

A 10 per cent solution of Renacidin at pH 4 of the anhydrides, lactones, and acid salts of gluconic and citric acid has been successfully used for the irrigation and dissolution of stones by retrograde catheterization. Some deaths have occurred with its use, however, probably secondary to hypermagnesemia.

PYROPHOSPHATASE INHIBITORS

Pyrophosphatase inhibitors are being investigated as possible means of increasing urinary pyrophosphate above normal in order to take advantage of its solubilizing activity.

CALCIUM CARBINIDE

Calcium carbinide has been used with some success in the treatment of congenital hyperoxaluria.

DISTILLED WATER

Finally, with resistant problems and in selected cases, the adjunctive use of distilled water exclusively may result in control of stone formation. Its action may be to remove dietary silicon, which is found in significant concentrations in drinking water in many areas and which may be an important inducer of stone formation in some patients.

SELECTED REFERENCES

Howard, J. E.: Etiology, treatment and prevention of kidney stones. Med. Times, 98:107, 1970.
> *This is an overview by a well-known investigator and clinician interested for many years in the medical management of urinary stone disease.*

Smith, L. H., Jr., and Williams, H. E.: Kidney stones. *In* Strauss, M. B., and Welt, L. G. (eds.): Diseases of the Kidney. 2nd ed. vol. II. Boston, Little, Brown & Company, 1971, pp. 973–996.
> *The chapter deals with historical, etiologic, biochemical and physical aspects of the stone problem. Illustrations are excellent. There are 100 appended references.*

Smith, L. H., Jr.: Symposium on Stones. Am. J. Med., 45:649, 1968.
> *The symposium is composed of ten papers given by recognized experts concerning the genesis, composition, and pathophysiology of urinary calculi. References are extensive.*

Williams, H. E.: Nephrolithiasis: N. Engl. J. Med., 290:33, 1974.
> *This is a recent concise review of physiologic considerations in the formation and treatment of urinary stones.*

Yendt, E. R.: Renal calculi. Can. Med. Assoc. J., 102:479, 1970.
> *This paper was presented as the Osler oration at the 102nd Annual Meeting of the Canadian Medical Society June 11, 1969. It is a survey of the renal stone problem that reports the author's investigation of 439 patients with renal calculi and particularly the use of thiazides in their management. It is philosophical and entertaining as well. There are 61 references.*

REFERENCES

Barker, L. M., Pallante, S. L., Eisenberg, H., Joule, J. A., Becker, G. L., and Howard, J. E.: Simple synthetic and natural urines have equivalent anticalcifying properties. Invest. Urol., 12:79, 1974.

Bernstein, D. S., and Newton, R.: The effect of oral sodium phosphate on the formation of renal calculi and on idiopathic hypercalciuria. Lancet, 2:1105, 1966.

Bourke, E.: Recent advances in the pathogenesis of renal calculi. J. Ir. Med. Assoc., 66:14, 1973.

Boyce, W. H.: Organic matrix of human concretions. Symposium on Stones. Am. J. Med., 45:673, 1968.

Coe, F. L., Canterbury, J. M., Firpo, J. J., and Reiss, E.: Evidence for secondary hyperparathyroidism in idiopathic hypercalciuria. J. Clin. Invest., 52:134, 1973.

Chadwick, V. S., Modha, K., and Dowling, R. H.: Mechanism for hyperoxaluria in patients with ileal dysfunction: N. Engl. J. Med., 289:172, 1973.

Ehrig, U., Harrison, J. E., and Wilson, D. R.: Effect of long-term thiazide therapy on intestinal calcium absorption in patients with recurrent renal calculi. Metabolism, 23:139, 1974.

Ettinger, B., and Kolb, F. O.: Inorganic phosphate treatment of nephrolithiasis. Am. J. Med., 55:32, 1973.

Gordon, E. E., and Sheps, S. G.: Effect of acetazolamide on citrate excretion and formation of renal calculi. N. Engl. J. Med., 256:1215, 1957.

Greene, M. L., Fujimoto, W. Y., and Seegmiller, J. E.: Urinary xanthine stones: A rare complication of allopurinol therapy. N. Engl. J. Med., 280:426, 1969.

Joekes, A. M., Rose, G. A., and Sutor, J.: Multiple renal silica calculi. Br. Med. J., 1:146, 1973.

King, J. S., Jr.: Currents in renal stone research. Clin. Chem., 17:971, 1971.

Lemann, J. L., Jr., Piering, W. F., and Lennon, E. J.: Possible role of carbohydrate: Induced calciuria in calcium oxalate kidney-stone formation. N. Engl. J. Med., 280:232, 1969.

Pak, C. Y. C.: Hydrochlorothiazide therapy in nephrolithiasis. Effect on the urinary activity product and formation product of brushite. Clin. Pharmacol. Ther., 14:209, 1973.

Pak, C. Y. C., Delea, C. S., and Bartter, F. C.: Successful treatment of recurrent nephrolithiasis (calcium stones) with cellulose phosphate. N. Engl. J. Med., 290:175, 1974.

Pak, C. Y. C., East, D. A., Sangenbacher, L. J., Delea, C. S., and Bartter, F. C.: Gastrointestinal calcium absorption in nephrolithiasis. J. Clin. Endocrinol. Metab., 35:261, 1972.

Pak, C. Y. C., Ohata, M., Lawrence, E. C., and Snyder, W.: The hypercalciurias: Causes, parathyroid functions and diagnostic criteria. J. Clin. Invest., 54:387, 1974.

Shaw, D. G., and Sutor, J.: Cystine stone dissolution. Br. J. Radiol., 45:664, 1972.

Yendt, E. R., Guay, G. F., and Garcia, D. A.: The Use of thiazides in the prevention of renal calculi. Can. Med. Assoc. J., 102:614, 1970.

Chapter Fifteen

NEOPLASMS OF THE GENITOURINARY SYSTEM

Marvin W. Woodruff,
William S. Oberheim,
and Harold E. Marden, Jr.

The development and application of antibiotic and immunization techniques during the twentieth century have resulted in a marked diminution of mortality from infectious and contagious diseases. During this same period, the incidence of cancer has steadily increased both in absolute frequency and in relation to incidence figures of other disease occurrence, and this generalization has also been noted in the great majority of genitourinary tumors.

The state of perfection of investigative techniques such as urography, endoscopy, biopsy, cytology, angiography, enzymatic and isotope study presently available to the urologist makes the genitourinary system highly accessible for an early and accurate diagnosis of neoplastic disease.

A high index of suspicion on the part of the examining physician concerning any patient with an unexplained genitourinary system mass, hematuria (gross or microscopic), persistent pyuria, fever, weight loss, or edema, as representing neoplasm until proven otherwise, is certainly the most important key to an early diagnosis of urologic malignancy. The earlier the diagnosis, the greater the likelihood the tumor can be localized and cured by surgical extirpation, while diagnostic procrastination may result in discovery only after metastasis has taken place.

MALIGNANT TUMORS OF THE KIDNEY

Renal malignancy occurs most frequently in the first and sixth decades of life. There are three principal types of primary renal neoplasms:

(1) Wilms' tumor (adenosarcoma) of early childhood, (2) adult parenchymal tumors (adenocarcinoma), and (3) tumors of the collecting system (transitional, or squamous cell carcinoma, or very rarely adenocarcinoma).

Wilms' Tumor

Although Wilms' tumor is occasionally reported in adults, the vast majority occur in children below the age of three. First reported by Wilms in 1899, other names used to describe this tumor include adenosarcoma, embryoma, and nephroblastoma.

PATHOLOGY

Grossly, as seen in Figure 15–1, the tumor characteristically is well-encapsulated, smooth, and globular. The rapid growth feature of

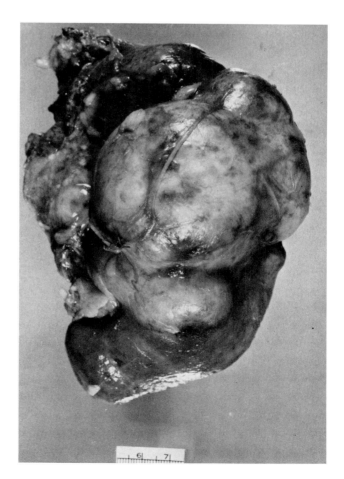

Figure 15–1 Gross appearance of Wilms' tumor. Note the smooth, well encapsulated globular appearance.

this malignancy, coupled with its occurrence in an age group where verbalization of symptoms is not possible, frequently is responsible for the large size of the tumor at the time of discovery. These tumors have attained weights of 5 kg and larger and often represent a significant percentage of the child's total body weight.

Histologically, one sees abortive epithelial tubules of varying maturity embodied in mesenchymal and muscular stroma with rhabdomyosarcomal elements frequently noted. Calcification is uncommon and is more characteristic of neuroblastoma than of Wilms' tumor.

Metastasis

Sixty per cent of children with Wilms' tumor present with metastasis. The vigorous growth potential of this tumor coupled with frequently noted early hematogenous dissemination to the lungs should preclude any procrastination on the part of the clinician in proceeding with definitive diagnosis and treatment. In addition to the hematogenous dissemination to the lungs and liver, lymphatic spread to para-aortic and mediastinal nodes and local extension to the adrenal gland are frequently seen. Unlike the adult adenocarcinoma or the childhood neuroblastoma, bony metastasis is rare.

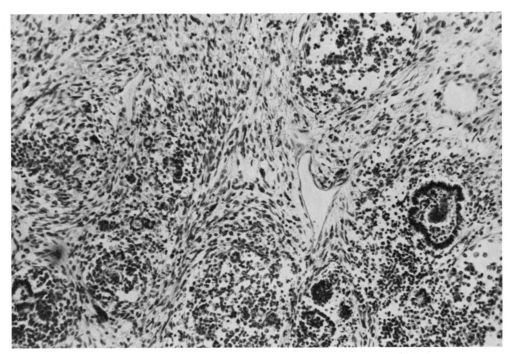

Figure 15-2 Histologic appearance of Wilms' tumor showing characteristic of abortive tubules embodied in malignant muscular stroma.

SIGNS AND SYMPTOMS

The commonest presenting sign is an abdominal mass. Pain is frequently noted, while hematuria, gastrointestinal symptoms, fever, malaise, abdominal vein distention, and hypertension are occasionally seen.

DIAGNOSIS

Differentiation from other causes of abdominal mass, such as enlarged spleen, renal cyst, and hydronephrosis, is made by pyelography. Where urographic visualization is not feasible because of obstruction, laminagraphy and angiography may be required. Additional information can sometimes be obtained by perirenal CO_2 insufflation and radioisotope renal scanning techniques. The preoperative differentiation between Wilms' tumor and neuroblastoma is difficult and on occasion is made only at the time the tumor is exposed at surgery.

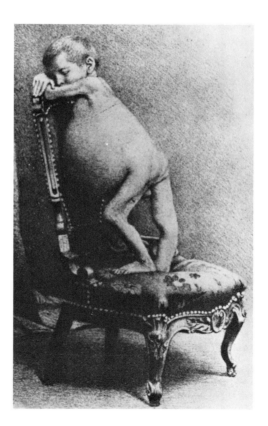

Figure 15–3 Early plight of children with Wilms' tumor prior to nephrectomy era. (From Huber and Boström: Deutsches Arch. Klin. Med., 1879.).

TREATMENT

Since the tumor is extremely radiosensitive and responds to chemotherapy, present day therapy consists of combination transabdominal nephrectomy, irradiation, and chemotherapy. Historically, four sequential eras of therapeutic approach to Wilms' tumor have evolved.

1. The presurgical era, when all children with this tumor died of disease.

2. Surgery alone with a 20 per cent cure.

3. Surgery and irradiation therapy, further increasing the cure rate to 40 per cent.

4. Combined surgery, irradiation, and chemotherapy, presently employed, that results in a cure rate of over 60 per cent, and when the child is below the age of one year, approaches 90 per cent.

Metastatic disease is a mixed discipline problem, and combination chemotherapy (actinomycin D or vincristine) or radiation is employed. Occasional successes from surgical excision of solitary metastatic lesions have been reported, as well as successful renal transplantation following the removal of bilateral Wilms' tumors.

The risk formula proposed by Collins is of great help in Wilms' tumor prognosis. It states that if the child survives a period equal to his age at the time of tumor removal plus nine months, without evidence of recurrence, there is greater than a 90 per cent chance of cure.

Adenocarcinoma of the Kidney

Adenocarcinoma of the kidney has also been referred to as hypernephroma, renal cell carcinoma, Grawitz's tumors, and clear cell carcinoma. It makes up 80 per cent of all malignant renal tumors and occurs primarily in the later decades of life. Adenocarcinoma is found twice as frequently in males as in females.

This malignancy exhibits several extraordinary properties. Unusual latency in growth of the primary tumor as well as indolent appearance of metastasis is frequently noted. Another peculiarity of the tumor, the occasional spontaneous regression of the untreated primary lesion, and disappearance of pulmonary metastasis following nephrectomy, strongly suggests that the tumor on occasion may lack autonomy. The kidney also functions as a target organ for hormones from the pituitary and adrenal glands and is capable of producing hormones of its own, including renin and erythropoietin. The production of a parathyroidlike hormone has also been observed by several investigators. The experimental induction of renal tumors in the hamster with estrogen, combined with the series of responses of pulmonary metastases in humans with Provera or testosterone, further suggests an extrarenal hormonal influence on the behavior of this tumor.

PATHOLOGY

Grossly, these tumors appear nodular, well-encapsulated, and characteristically have a yellowish appearance. Associated areas of hemorrhagic necrosis can be seen on cut section and neighboring vascularity is frequently greatly increased.

Histologically, the tumor usually consists of large clear cells with abundant foamy cytoplasm, although one may also see smaller cells with dense, granular eosinophilic-staining cytoplasm that more closely resemble renal tubular cells. Attempts to prognosticate based on whether the tumor is clear cell or granular cell in histologic type is presently under study. Frequently, if multiple sections are made, both histologic types are found within the same tumor.

STAGING

The urologist can stage kidney tumors on the basis of his operative findings and gross examination as follows:

Stage I: Tumor confined to the kidney.
        A. Within tumor capsule.
        B. Within renal capsule.
Stage II: Extrarenal tumor.
        A. Direct extension.
        B. Renal vein.
        C. Lymphatic.
Stage III: Distant metastasis.

METASTASIS

Metastasis from hypernephroma can be hematogenous, lymphatic, or by direct extension. The lungs, para-aortic nodes, renal vein, bone, brain, and skin are common sites of local or distant metastasis.

SIGNS AND SYMPTOMS

The classic triad of a flank mass, hematuria, and flank pain may be present. A left varicocele is occasionally noted secondary to obstruction of the spermatic vein where it enters into the left renal vein. Fever, malaise, hypertension, weight loss, and anemia may also be present. Occasionally, the patient can present with symptoms secondary to pulmonary or bony metastasis rather than those related to the primary tumor in the kidney. Erythropoietin-induced erythrocytosis occurs relatively frequently but is not specific for malignancy and has been observed in a variety of renal diseases. Rarely, tumor elaboration of a parathyroidlike hormone may induce symptoms of hyperparathyroidism.

DIAGNOSIS

The presence of a renal malignancy is suspected when one notes a tumor deformity (stretching or splaying of the collecting system) on pyelographic analysis. Renal angiography is of paramount importance in differentiating renal cysts from malignancy, with a characteristic puddling of contrast media noted within the malignant tumor as compared to only vascular displacement seen with renal cysts. Adrenalin injection during selective angiography causes the renal vessels related to benign lesions and normal kidney to contract while those vessels related to renal malignancy are autonomous and remain unaffected. Nephrotomography and radioisotope scanning techniques may also provide adjuvant diagnostic information. Cytologic examination rarely is positive with parenchymal renal tumors and is of greater diagnostic value in tumors of the collecting system, ureter, and bladder. Needle aspiration of suspected cysts combined with contrast media injection and cytologic studies of aspirated fluid may be of considerable help in differentiating cyst from solid tumor in selected cases.

TREATMENT

The treatment of adenocarcinoma of the kidney is nephrectomy. Any unexplained lesion that manifests a tumor deformity on a pyelo-

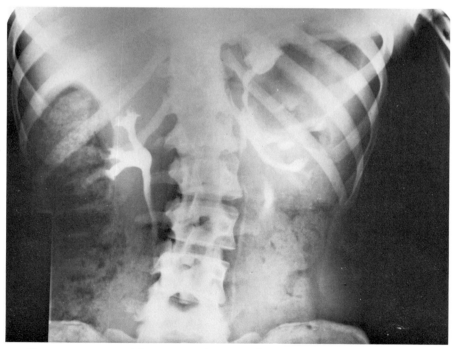

Figure 15-4 Tumor deformity secondary to renal carcinoma. Note stretching and splaying of the infundibula.

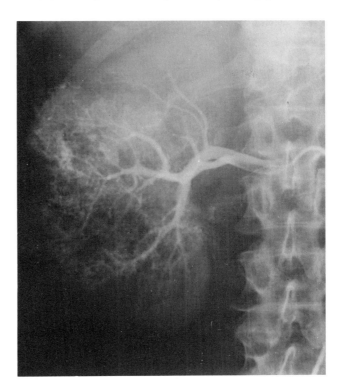

Figure 15–5 Selective renal angiography showing a large renal carcinoma characterized by marked neovascularity.

gram should be surgically explored. The renal pedicle is approached through a flank, transabdominal, or thoracoabdominal incision, and the renal vessels are ligated promptly. The tumor, kidney, perirenal fascia, and proximal ureter are removed with as little trauma as possible to the tumor mass. Since lymph node metastasis carries with it a worse prognosis than renal vein extension, more urologic surgeons are adding a local para-aortic lymph node dissection to nephrectomy in the treatment of this tumor.

Postoperative radiation therapy appears to significantly improve the prognosis. Preoperative radiation has been reported to shrink and delineate the tumor, making nephrectomy easier, and its effect on the ultimate prognosis is presently under study by a large cooperative study group of urologists and radiotherapists.

Solitary metastasis may be treated with local excision or radiotherapy. The most impressive results in the chemotherapy of pulmonary metastasis from renal adenocarcinoma have been reported using the hormonal agents Provera and testosterone. Recognition that the kidney can function both as an endocrine organ, as well as a target organ for extrarenal hormones, adds plausibility to the results of these hormonally treated patients.

One must remember that because of the indolent growth properties of this tumor, the survival figures cannot be limited to five years. Several long-term studies indicate that significant numbers of patients surgically treated for adenocarcinoma of the kidney continue to die of the disease during the five to ten year period postoperatively.

Sarcoma of the Kidney

Sarcoma of the kidney is an extremely rare neoplasm. Although the exact origin is obscure, sarcoma probably arises from the connective tissue of the parenchyma or capsule. Many are of mixed variety and sometimes are histologically difficult to distinguish from Wilms' tumor. Metastasis occurs early by hematogenous dissemination, and the prognosis is generally poor. The surgical treatment, nephrectomy, is similar to that for parenchymal renal tumors.

MALIGNANT TUMORS OF THE RENAL PELVIS

Carcinoma of the renal pelvis is a relatively uncommon tumor and constitutes about 7 per cent of all malignancies of the kidney. These tumors are primarily urothelial in origin and are of three main histologic types: transitional cell carcinoma, squamous cell carcinoma, and adenocarcinoma.

Transitional cell carcinoma is more common, (80 per cent of all collecting system tumors), usually papillary in type, and carries with it a better prognosis than the more sessile squamous cell type. Squamous cell carcinoma frequently is associated with pre-existing chronic renal irritation, such as calculous disease.

Hematuria is the most common presenting symptom, and hydronephrosis-induced renal colic secondary to obstruction from tumor or blood clot is not uncommon.

Retrograde pyeloureterography is the primary diagnostic technique employed. Because these tumors are frequently multicentric in origin, a thorough urographic and endoscopic evaluation of the entire urinary tract is performed. Characteristically, one sees a filling defect in the renal pelvis, and the pyelographic appearance is sometimes difficult to distinguish from that of a nonopaque stone or blood clot. If the ureteropelvic junction is obstructed, hydronephrosis may ensue, while if only an infundibulum is occluded, caliectasia is noted. Cytologic examination of the urine obtained from the ureteric catheter at the time of retrograde pyelography is frequently positive and is a useful diagnostic adjuvant. Renal arteriography may be misleading and is frequently normal unless parenchymal invasion has taken place. These tumors may be multicentric, with a 30 per cent ipsilateral ureteric and 20 per cent bladder involvement reported.

The surgical treatment of malignant tumors of the renal pelvis is nephroureterectomy that includes a cuff of adjacent bladder. The prognosis depends upon a histologic examination and the stage of the disease. The five-year survival rate of transitional cell carcinoma is 50

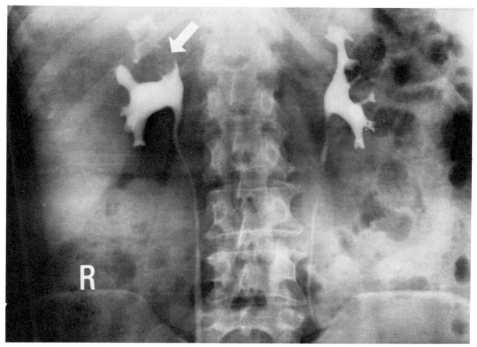

Figure 15–6 Retrograde pyelogram showing filling defect of right upper infundibulum caused by transitional cell carcinoma of collecting system.

per cent with the survival of individual cases, as with bladder carcinoma, related to the stage of disease at the time of surgery. Squamous cell carcinoma has a more ominous prognosis, and as noted with squamous cell tumors of the bladder and ureter, it has a five-year survival rate of less than 10 per cent.

Because of the multicentric nature of these tumors and their propensity to recur, these patients are followed carefully postnephroureterectomy and partial cystectomy in the same fashion as those treated for carcinoma of the urinary bladder. Observation cystoscopy and pyelography are performed every three months for two years, every six months for the following two years, and yearly thereafter.

CARCINOMA OF THE URETER

Ureteric tumors have a marked resemblance to those of the renal collecting system in having similar presenting signs, symptoms, histologic types, staging, grading, treatment, and prognosis. Primary ureteric tumors are very rare and present most frequently in the sixth and seventh decades of life and occur twice as commonly in males as in females. The lower third of the ureter is the most common site of tumor involvement.

The two most common histologic ureteric tumors are transitional cell carcinoma and squamous cell carcinoma. On gross examination, the more common type, transitional cell carcinoma, is papillary and consists of a pedunculated fibrovascular pedicle covered by transitional cells of varying grades of malignancy. The rarer squamous cell carcinoma is sessile and more scirrhous in its infiltration.

Due to the relatively thin wall and abundant lymphatic drainage of the ureter, metastasis by direct extension and to the regional lymph nodes occurs frequently and early in the course of the disease.

Painless hematuria is the most common symptom. Renal colic presents in 50 per cent of the patients and may be due to the passage of clots down the ureter or to mechanical obstruction by tumor. Occasionally, a ureteric tumor can be palpated on vaginal or rectal examination.

Carcinoma of the ureter is diagnosed preoperatively in about 50 per cent of patients. Intravenous pyelography may reveal a nonfunctioning kidney, hydronephrosis or hydroureter, or a filling defect. The differential diagnosis of such filling defects include nonopaque calculus, blood clot, ureteritis cystica, and secondary compression. A cystoscopic investigation to determine the concomitant presence of a bladder tumor and a retrograde ureterogram to delineate the ureteric filling defect are essential. Ureteric tumors are characterized by a helmet-shaped filling defect with proximal dilatation of the ureter.

Nephroureterectomy with excision of the adjacent cuff of bladder is the treatment for ureteric carcinoma. Bilateral ureteric tumors are rare, and their treatment requires a modification of the usual procedure, with most being treated with a segmental excision or ureteric replacement with ileum. Adjunctive radiotherapy is frequently employed. The postoperative management includes periodic intravenous pyelography and cystoscopy. The prognosis for transitional cell carcinoma of the ureter is related to the stage of the disease at the time of diagnosis and treatment. Squamous cell carcinoma of the ureter, similar to that of the collecting system and bladder, has a dismal prognosis.

MALIGNANT TUMORS OF THE URINARY BLADDER

Except for the carcinogenic effect of aniline dye derivatives and those associated with chronic intravesical irritative disease such as stones and parasites, the cause of bladder cancer is unknown. If one were to review the information published on the subject of carcinoma of the urinary bladder during the past half century, he would immediately realize that much confusion exists concerning the appraisal of the numerous methods used in treating patients with this disease. It would also be apparent that the major difficulty lies with the large number of important variables encountered in the analysis of results of various therapeutic approaches to bladder cancer.

The significant variables encountered in carcinoma of the urinary bladder are noted in Table 15–1.

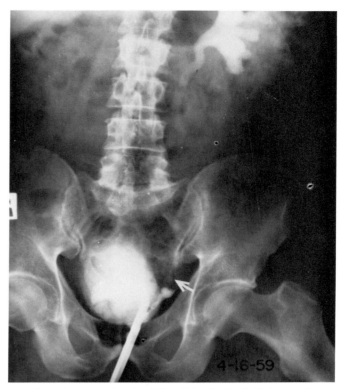

Figure 15–7 Left retrograde ureterogram showing filling defect in distal third secondary to transitional cell carcinoma.

HISTOLOGY

Four major histologic types of bladder cancer are recognized: transitional cell, squamous cell, adenocarcinoma, and rhabdomyosarcoma.

Transitional cell carcinoma is the most common histologic type of bladder cancer in the United States and ranks as the seventh most frequent cause of death of all male patients who die of malignant tumor. All papillomatoid tumors of the bladder are malignant or at least potentially malignant. Grossly, the majority are located in the region of the vesical neck and trigone and are characteristically papillary, although the less differentiated tumor has a more sessile appearance. Histologically, one sees a basic core of loose connective tissue covered with transitional epithelium, which, depending on the grade of tumor, displays varying degrees of differentiation and numbers of mitotic figures.

Squamous cell carcinoma is encountered less commonly and has a poorer prognosis than the transitional cell type; the five-year survival rate ranges between 5 and 10 per cent. It is often associated with concomitant disease that causes chronic irritation and infection in the

TABLE 15–1   Variables Encountered in Carcinoma of the Urinary Bladder

HISTOLOGIC TYPE	Transitional cell Squamous Adenocarcinoma Rhabdomyosarcoma
JEWETT STAGE OF DISEASE	O Mucosa A Lamina propria B_1 Inner muscle B_2 Outer muscle C Serosa D_1 Local extension D_2 Distant metastasis
TUMOR GRADE	I Well-differentiated II Median-differentiated III Poorly differentiated IV Anaplastic
SIZE OF TUMOR	Small Medium Large
LOCATION	Floor Lateral wall Trigone Dome Vesical neck
NUMBER OF TUMORS	Single Multiple
LENGTH OF SYMPTOMS	Less than 1 year Greater than 1 year

THERAPY	Biopsy and fulguration
	Transurethral resection
	Segmental resection
	Total or radical cystectomy with urinary diversion
	   Ileal loop
	   Ureterosigmoidostomy
	   Cutaneous ureterostomy
	   Nephrostomy
	Radiation therapy
	Chemotherapy

urinary tract, such as prolonged calculous disease. Histologically, the tumor consists of large squamoid-type cells with intercellular bridges. Keratinization and pearl formation are frequently noted.

Adenocarcinoma is a rare form of vesical cancer and can originate from urachal remnants in the dome of the bladder or from glandular elements located in the subtrigonal area. It also may arise by glandular metaplasia and the type of malignant degeneration noted in exstrophy of the bladder. Microscopically, the tumor consists of glandular structures of varying degrees of anaplasia, which may or may not secrete mucus.

Rhabdomyosarcoma, or sarcoma botryoides, is primarily a malignant tumor of infancy. Only a handful of five-year survivors of this disease may be found in the literature. All patients reported surviving this disease were treated by radical surgical procedures consisting of supravesical diversion and total cystectomy.

STAGING

Jewett and Strong's establishment in 1946 of a sound method of clinical staging of vesical cancer according to the depth of penetration is greatly responsible for the strides made during the past two decades, both toward better understanding the potential curability of this disease and toward improving the evaluation of the therapeutic results obtained. The correlation of Jewett's staging, Broders' grading, and the International Staging System are combined in Figure 15–8.

Stage O.   This stage refers to vesical papillomas involving the mucosa alone. They are low-grade malignant tumors and are considered much the same as carcinoma in situ of the cervix. It has been observed that 20 per cent of Stage O bladder tumor patients will develop deeper forms of bladder carcinoma within five years after discovery. Unless frequent recurrence is noted, more radical forms of surgical extirpation are avoided in this early stage since the five-year survival rate closely follows the actuarial life expectancy.

Stage A.   This stage describes those bladder tumors which penetrate through the mucosa into the suburothelial layer of the lamina propria.

Stage B.   The bladder detrusor is made up of a meshwork of muscle. In transitional cell carcinoma, metastasis is primarily by lymphatic and direct extension. Thus, the location of the lymphatics, which become prominent in the outer half of the vesical muscle layers, is important. This is borne out by studies that compare curability with depth of penetration. Most patients whose tumors were confined within the superficial one half of the bladder muscle layer, Stage B_1, survived five years regardless of surgical approaches. Once the tumor invaded the outer half of the muscle layer, Stage B_2, lymph node metastasis was often present and the majority, more than 80 per cent, died of disease

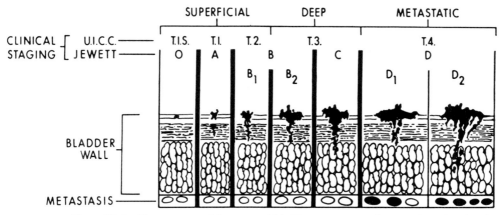

Figure 15–8   The seven possible stages of bladder carcinoma indicating clinical and pathologic equivalents of the Jewett and Strong and International Union against cancer symptoms.

within five years no matter how radical the surgical procedure employed.

Stage C. This stage refers to bladder tumor penetrating all layers of the bladder including the serosa, but not involving regional lymph nodes or adjacent organs.

Stage D₁. This stage denotes local extension within the confines of the pelvis to the internal iliac lymph nodes, rectum, prostate, vagina, or bony pelvis. Reported surgical cures for this stage of disease are almost nil, except for an occasional patient in which only one or two pelvic lymph nodes are involved. Most of the D_1 patients are dead within 18 months, and five-year survivals approach zero.

Stage D₂. This stage signifies distant metastasis. These patients are invariably dead of disease within one year. Metastasis outside the confines of the pelvis from primary bladder cancer frequently are noted in the lung, liver, intra-abdominal lymph nodes, bone, and brain.

HISTOLOGIC GRADING

Bladder tumor grading based on histologic differentiation and mitotic activity was first proposed by Broders in 1922. It is considered an important feature of the disease because it essentially correlates with the growth potential of the tumor.

Grading varies from one to four depending on the degree of differentiation and the percentage of tumor cells showing mitotic figures.

LOCATION

The location of the tumor within the bladder is important in that it often dictates the type of surgical approach to be used. Areas high on the dome or on the superior portion of the posterior wall may be poorly accessible for transurethral resection. Similarly, tumors ordinarily managed elsewhere in the bladder by segmental resection may not be amenable to this procedure and require total cystectomy when they are located in the vicinity of the vesical neck or trigone where the bladder is relatively fixed.

SIZE AND NUMBER OF TUMORS

The size and number of tumors also play a significant role in determining the therapeutic approach to bladder cancer. Patients with a few small superficial papillary growths may be easily treated by transurethral resection. However, in multiple bladder papillomatosis the growths, although equally superficial, may number in the hundreds, with total cystectomy being the only possible treatment. Similarly, a low-stage bladder tumor, 1 to 2 cm in diameter, may be adequately excised transurethrally, whereas a tumor five times as large with the same stage and grade requires a more extensive surgical procedure, such as segmental resection or total cystectomy because of its large size.

SIGNS AND SYMPTOMS

The majority of patients with bladder neoplasm will present with hematuria. The physician should consider any unexplained bleeding from the urinary tract as neoplastic in origin until proven otherwise. Irritative symptoms such as frequency, dysuria, and urgency may be present. Depending on the size and location of the bladder lesion, symptoms secondary to obstructive uropathy may ensue, including diminution of the force and caliber of the urinary stream. Ureteric orifice obstruction may cause flank pain secondary to hydronephrosis. Disseminated metastasis may result in weight loss, debilitation, gastrointestinal disturbance, and bone pain. Since the length of symptomatology is related to eventual prognosis, procrastination should be avoided if bladder neoplasm is suspected.

DIAGNOSIS

Definitive diagnosis is made by cystoscopic examination and biopsy performed under general anesthesia. At the conclusion of the endoscopic procedure, a muscle relaxant may be given so that adequate bimanual examination can be made to accurately assess the stage of disease.

An accurate evaluation is made of the upper urinary tract by pyelographic and renal function studies, while a thorough search for metastatic disease is accomplished by appropriate roentgenographic and laboratory studies.

URINE CYTOLOGY

The most satisfactory urologic application of cytology is in the study of bladder carcinoma. By cytologic examination alone, however, it is not possible to locate the anatomic source of the cancer cells. False positive and false negative reports are common. Therefore, unless ample confirmatory evidence exists, either clinical or histologic, no treatment should be instituted on the basis of a positive cytologic report alone.

TREATMENT

In the foregoing discussion, it is apparent that it does not necessarily follow that the more extensive the bladder cancer, the more radical the surgical procedure. Location, size, and number of the tumors, frequency of recurrence, and the patient's age and general physical condition are the primary factors that determine the type of extirpative surgical procedure required. Some of the therapeutic modalities for treatment for bladder cancer are as follows: biopsy and fulguration, transurethral resection, segmental resection, total or radical cystectomy, radiation therapy, and chemotherapy.

Transurethral Resection. These endoscopic methods are utilized when the tumors are relatively small and superficial and in an accessible location in the bladder. During these procedures, care should should be taken to obtain a piece of tumor tissue for histologic study. If doubt exists as to the possibility of neoplasm remaining in the base of the tumor during transurethral resection, cuts from the depth and margins of the tumor should be submitted as separate specimens for biopsy.

Segmental Resection. The indications for segmental resection are similar to total cystectomy with the exception of location. Tumors anatomically located in a mobile portion of the bladder which may be sacrificed can be treated by this method. Most patients with medium-sized bladder tumors located away from the trigone or vesical neck may be treated in this fashion. Adequate tumor-free margins without extravesical tumor contamination are essential for the success of this procedure.

Total Cystectomy. This operation entails a complete removal of the bladder, prostate, and seminal vesicles in the male, and the bladder and urethra in the female. It is employed when adequate surgical extirpation of an operable neoplasm cannot be effected by less radical means.

Radical cystectomy combines total cystectomy with pelvic lymph node dissection. It does not result in any significant improvement of the five-year survival rate of any stage of bladder cancer. It does allow, however, for a more accurate assessment of the stage of disease because of the additional lymph node information obtained.

Supravesical Diversion. Several methods of supravesical urinary diversion have been used following total cystectomy that include ureteroileostomy, ureterosigmoidostomy, cutaneous ureterostomy, and nephrostomy. As seen in Figures 15–9 and 15–10, when part of the intestine is used for bladder substitution, it may function as a conduit or reservoir.

URETEROILEOSTOMY. The diversion of the urinary stream by means of ureteroileostomy is the most widely used intestinal conduit method for supravesical urinary diversion. This procedure minimizes back pressure, pyelonephritis, reflux, and electrolyte disturbance inherent in many of the other types of urinary diversion.

URETEROSIGMOIDOSTOMY. Although this method is appealing because no external apparatus is required for the collection of urine, two serious complications are involved in ureterosigmoidostomy: hyperchloremic acidosis and chronic pyelonephritis. Hyperchloremic acidosis is caused by the absorption of chloride from the urine in the intestine. A normal kidney can excrete this excess chloride load with-

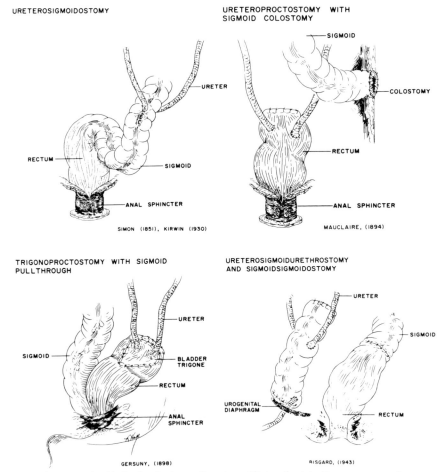

URETEROSIGMOIDOSTOMY

URETEROPROCTOSTOMY WITH
SIGMOID COLOSTOMY

SIMON (1851), KIRWIN (1930)

MAUCLAIRE, (1894)

TRIGONOPROCTOSTOMY WITH SIGMOID
PULLTHROUGH

URETEROSIGMOIDURETHROSTOMY
AND SIGMOIDSIGMOIDOSTOMY

GERSUNY, (1898)

RISGARD, (1943)

Figure 15–9   Methods of urinary diversion utilizing the intestine as a reservoir.

out difficulty. As reported by Lapides, once chronic pyelonephritis occurs secondary to the reflux of bacteria from the fecal stream, there is a deterioration of tubular function, and the excess chloride load cannot be entirely excreted, resulting in systemic acidosis. This procedure should never be attempted in patients with dilated ureters or chronic renal insufficiency.

CUTANEOUS URETEROSTOMY.   This procedure does not require bowel anastomosis following cystectomy, thereby reducing the operative time and morbidity. The major problem is the frequent occurrence of circumferential cicatrical stenosis of the cutaneous ureteric stoma. In attempting to obviate the stricture of the cutaneous ureteric stoma, several procedures have been offered in remedy, including the use of Z-plasty, skin flaps, grafts, and tubes. None of these techniques, however, has uniformly prevented circumferential cicatrical stenosis when normally calibered ureters were used.

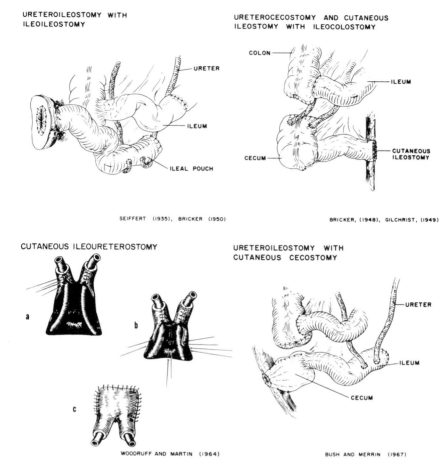

Figure 15–10   Methods of urinary diversion using the intestine as a conduit.

NEPHROSTOMY.   In this poor method of diversion, the presence of an indwelling catheter invariably results in chronic infection with pyelonephritis and sometimes with calculous disease. It defeats the basic purposes of urinary diversion, i.e., the protection and conservation of renal function. Nephrostomy is primarily a temporary rather than a definitive means for urinary diversion.

Radiation Therapy.   This has been frequently shown to eradicate local transitional cell carcinoma in the bladder. However, it is of little value in the control of disseminated disease. It appears that radiation therapy is more effective with the less differentiated transitional tumor, an observation that can be theoretically explained by the more actively dividing cells being more prone to radiation injury.

Chemotherapy.   This has been used locally and systemically. The local intravesical use of thiotepa and the use of systemic 5-fluorouracil in combination with radiation therapy in advanced disease has been described extensively. More recently, bleomycin has been utilized in squamous cell carcinoma of the bladder with a few regressions noted.

Since bladder cancers frequently recur, periodic endoscopic followup is of extreme importance in control of the disease. Quarterly cystoscopy for two years, then every six months for two more years, and yearly examination thereafter is the ideal method of follow-up.

MALIGNANCY OF THE PROSTATE

Carcinoma of the prostate is the second most frequent cause of cancer deaths in men. About 20 per cent of men past the age of sixty have prostatic carcinoma, and the incidence increases with each subsequent decade of life. The disease frequently presents as an insidious process with few or no symptoms related to the local lesion and unfortunately, often is discovered only after widespread dissemination has occurred. The necessity for early diagnosis is reflected in the high cure rate by radical extirpation when the tumor is confined to the gland. The hormonal responsiveness of prostate carcinoma was described by Huggins in 1941, and this historic contribution is the keystone to the present day hormonal therapeutic approach of the disseminated form of the disease.

PATHOLOGY

Carcinoma of the prostate most frequently arises in the posterior lobe of the gland. Grossly, the tissue exhibits marked increased consistency, and on cut section, yellowish nodules, which may be solitary or confluent, are evident.

On histologic examination, the neoplasm, which originates primarily from the epithelium of the acini, may display varying degrees of differentiation. The more differentiated tumors present a distinct glandular pattern of small back-to-back acini, loss of the normal two cell lining, and small cells with nuclear pleomorphism. The less differentiated tumors may show abortive or no glandular pattern at all and are composed of small cells having variable amounts of cytoplasm with pleomorphic hyperchromatic nuclei. Perineural invasion is a common histologic feature of this tumor.

Prostatic carcinoma may be staged clinically as follows:

Stage A: Incidental microscopic focus.
Stage B: Localized nodule confined within the prostate gland.
Stage C: Local extension to adjacent structures.
Stage D: Distant metastasis.

The tumor may be graded on its histologic pattern and cytologic features as follows:

Grade 1:   Well-differentiated
Grade 2:   Moderately differentiated.
Grade 3:   Poorly differentiated.
Grade 4:   Totally anaplastic.

METASTASIS

Adenocarcinoma of the prostate can spread by direct extension to involve adjacent structures such as the posterior urethra, bladder, and seminal vesicles. Lymphatic metastasis is common, with the initial site being the pelvic nodes along the internal iliac vessels. Hematogenous spread through Batson's veins is responsible for the early dissemination to bone.

SYMPTOMS

Posterior urethral invasion frequently results in obstructive uropathy and symptoms of bladder neck obstruction. Bone and neuritic pain are commonly present secondary to bone metastasis and nerve compression. The patient may present with anemia of a myelophthisic type from marrow replacement by neoplasm. Clinically, advanced carcinoma of the prostate gland mimics premature aging. It is not uncommon for the patient to take to bed with weakness and bone pain, become progressively immobile, anorexic, cachectic, and finally succumb to an intercurrent episode of bronchopneumonia.

DIAGNOSIS

The diagnosis of prostatic carcinoma is suspected by rectal examination and acid phosphatase studies and confirmed by prostatic biopsy. On digital palpation the gland has a stony consistency. Since chronic prostatitis and prostatic calculi can simulate the feel of carcinoma on rectal examination, differentiation can be definitely made by prostatic biopsy. Tissue diagnosis can be made by excisional and needle perineal biopsy, transrectal needle biopsy, or by transurethral resection. The reported diagnostic accuracy with prostatic biopsy ranges from 70 to 95 per cent.

Acid phosphatase determination is an important adjunct to definitive diagnosis. Although an elevated serum acid phosphatase is not specific for prostatic disease, determination of the prostatic fraction greatly increases its diagnostic specificity. An elevated serum prostatic acid phosphatase denotes systemic dissemination with abnormal levels reported in 30 per cent of Stage C and 75 per cent of Stage D carcinoma of the prostate gland. More recently, bone marrow acid phosphatase has been reported to be an early reliable index of prostate carcinoma dissemination.

Skeletal survey is an essential part of the evaluation since 50 to 55 per cent of patients with prostatic carcinoma present with osteoblastic metastasis when first seen by the urologist. Additional studies that may be of assistance in the evaluation of bony metastasis include serum alkaline phosphatase and a bone marrow smear. A radioisotope bone scan may demonstrate skeletal metastasis prior to being noted on routine skeletal x-ray studies.

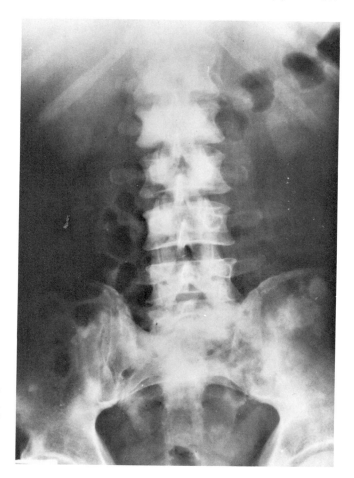

Figure 15–11 Carcinoma of the prostate: characteristic osteoblastic metastasis in the bony pelvis and lumbar spine.

TREATMENT

The therapeutic management of adenocarcinoma of the prostate is determined by the stage of the disease, age of the patient, and presenting symptoms. For those carcinomas that are discovered incidentally on subtotal prostatectomy, some urologists recommend a radical prostatectomy, while others would pursue a more conservative, watchful course. Many would agree, however, that a radical prostatectomy, either by the perineal or retropubic approach, is the treatment of choice for carcinoma confined to the prostate gland, provided the patient fulfills the criteria of being a good surgical candidate with a 15 year life expectancy and has normal serum acid phosphatase and no evidence of metastasis on skeletal survey. Although radical surgery has been performed by some investigators for prostatic carcinoma with extracapsular extension into contiguous structures, more commonly a transurethral resection to alleviate obstructive symptomatology, combined with or-

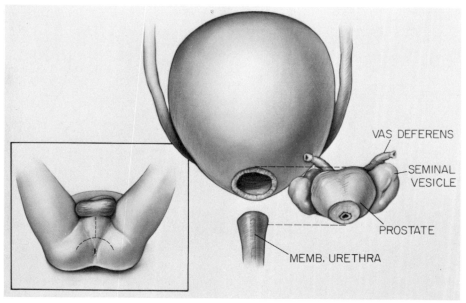

VAS DEFERENS

SEMINAL VESICLE

PROSTATE

MEMB. URETHRA

Figure 15–12 Diagrammatic representation of radical perineal prostatectomy procedure for carcinoma prostate.

chiectomy and estrogen therapy to suppress the tumor growth, has been utilized. A similar therapeutic regimen is employed in the patient with distant metastasis. The cooperative Veterans Administration Study described the potential cardiovascular complications from estrogen therapy. One milligram of stilbestrol daily appears to minimize cardiovascular complications, while providing significant antiandrogenic effect.

Radiation therapy is presently under evaluation as the definitive treatment of prostatic carcinoma and has been successfully employed for the palliative treatment of bony metastasis. Evanescent relief of pain in advanced prostatic carcinoma has been occasionally achieved with adrenalectomy or hypophysectomy, but the beneficial results are difficult to interpret, since prolonged survival is infrequent in those reported treated by these modalities.

PROGNOSIS

In general, the lower the stage of the tumor, the better the prognosis. Furthermore, the more differentiated the tumor the greater its propensity for hormonal suppression. Radical extirpation for Stage A and B tumors with or without adjuvant endocrine therapy provides the best chance for cure, with ten-year survival rates approaching 50 per cent being reported in several large series. With high-stage, high-grade malignancy, the survival rate markedly diminishes. The serum acid phosphatase has been valuable in prognostication, with a return to normal correlating well with remission, while a subsequent elevation is frequently associated with relapse.

TUMORS OF THE TESTES

Primary testicular tumors constitute 2 per cent of all malignant neoplasms in males and account for 10 per cent of all genitourinary tumors. The majority occur in the younger age group, with 70 per cent noted between the ages of 20 and 40. Excluding tumors of the hematopoietic and lymphoid systems, testicular tumors are the most common malignancy in young adult men. Bilateral testicular tumors are extremely rare and usually occur sequentially rather than simultaneously.

The cryptorchid testis is more prone to develop malignancy than the normally descended one, and orchiopexy does not appear to significantly reduce this malignant propensity.

There are two general categories of primary testicular tumors based on cell origin: germinal and nongerminal. The germinal tumors compose 97 per cent and are highly malignant. Nongerminal tumors, in contradistinction, account for only 3 per cent, commonly are benign, and take their origin from the Sertoli or Leydig cells.

The germ cell origin and interrelationship of testicular tumors is shown in the following diagram. The development from germ cell origin by seminoma, embryonal carcinoma, teratoma, and choriocarcinoma readily explain the frequently noted testicular tumors of mixed types.

Classification of germ cell tumors of the testis according to the histologic element with the greatest malignant potential:

Group I: Pure seminoma.
Group II: Embryonal carcinoma with or without seminoma.
Group III: Teratocarcinoma with or without seminoma.
Group IV: Choriocarcinoma, pure or with seminoma, embryonal carcinoma, or teratocarcinoma.

Tumors of Germ Cell Origin

PATHOLOGY

Seminoma is the most common and the least malignant of the germinal testicular tumors. It is extremely radiosensitive and tends to metastasize less frequently and later. Primary extragonadal seminoma has been reported in the retroperitoneum, mediastinum, and pineal body. Grossly, the tumor is firm, well-encapsulated, and covered by a smooth, glistening tunica. The cut surface appears gray-white in color with occasional foci of hemorrhagic necrosis seen. Seminoma attains the largest size of the malignant testicular tumors and demonstrates the least amount of hemorrhage. Histologically, one sees a monotonous pattern consisting of large, round or polyhedral cells that have distinct cell borders and clear cytoplasm, with large central hyperchromatic nuclei with conspicuous nucleoli. The presence of lymphoid stroma, as seen in Figure 15–14, has been correlated with improved prognosis and may represent an immunologic resistance of the host to his tumor.

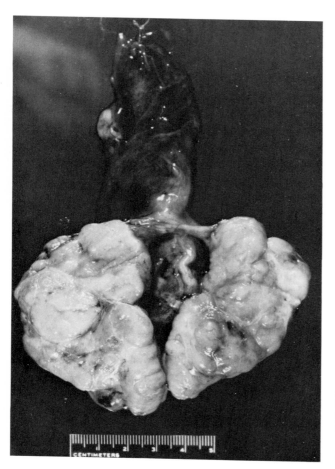

Figure 15–13 Gross appearance of testicular seminoma. Note the homogenous gray-white appearance with very little hemorrhagic necrosis.

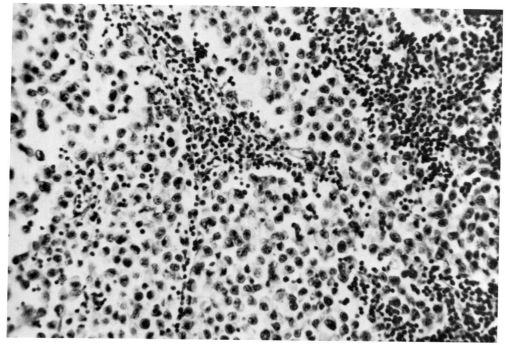

Figure 15–14   Monotonous histologic appearance of seminoma with lymphoid stroma.

Embryonal carcinoma is second in frequency to seminoma. It is more malignant than seminoma, relatively radioresistant, and metastasizes early by way of lymphatic channels. On gross examination the tumor is firm and nodular with frequent areas of hemorrhage seen. Microscopically, the tumor is composed of large anaplastic cells that have homogenous eosinophilic cytoplasm with indistinct cell borders containing pleomorphic nuclei with prominent nucleoli. Frequently, one sees a glandular or organoid pattern and papillary or acinar differentiation. Embryoid bodies resembling a one to two-week-old embryo are occasionally observed.

Teratocarcinoma occurs less frequently than embryonal carcinoma. Histologically, it consists of a combination of embryonal carcinoma with somatic elements of variable differentiation and malignancy. Grossly, the tumor has a variegated nodular appearance with cystic spaces filled with gelatinous material. A gritty sensation on sectioning is due to the presence of cartilage and bone. Microscopically, one sees a chaotic array of ectodermal, endodermal, and mesodermal derivatives of varying degrees of somatic differentiation, along with areas typical of embryonal carcinoma. Teratoid elements frequently found include smooth muscle, connective tissues, cartilage, bone, gastrointestinal and respiratory epithelium, nervous tissue, and cutaneous structures.

The morbid prognosis of pure choriocarcinoma is well-recognized, and it ranks as the most malignant tumor found in man. Fortunately, it is the rarest of the testicular tumors. Because of its hematogenous mode of dissemination, it characteristically metastasizes early and diffusely. Widespread metastasis in the face of a primary tumor measuring less than 1 cm in diameter has been frequently observed. Of all the testicular tumors, it is associated with the most hemorrhagic necrosis owing to the rapidity with which it outgrows its blood supply. Microscopically, a villouslike formation is noted which is composed of two elements: cytotrophoblasts and syncytiotrophoblasts. The cytotrophoblastic components consist of uniform closely packed cells with clear cytoplasm and distinct cell borders. The syncytiotrophoblastic element consists of large cells containing multiple smudgy-appearing hyperchromatic nuclei. In addition to the similarity of the histologic pattern of choriocarcinoma to the human placenta, these testicular tumors secrete high levels of chorionic gonadotropin as well.

The staging of testicular tumors is as follows:

Stage I: Tumor limited to testis.
Stage II: Tumor in regional para-aortic lymph nodes.
Stage III: Disseminated metastasis beyond the para-aortic nodes.

Metastasis

Testicular tumors are spread primarily by lymphatics, which follow the spermatic vessels to the para-aortic nodes in the region of the renal hilum. Once para-aortic lymph node involvement takes place, subsequent spread is to the mediastinum, left supraclavicular nodes, and lungs. With pulmonary metastasis, tumor may then spread systemically to involve the brain, liver, soft tissues, and bone. Direct extension along the spermatic cord and to the scrotum commonly occurs. Choriocarcinoma differs from the other germinal testicular tumors in that its metastasis is primarily hematogenous.

Signs and Symptoms

The presenting signs and symptoms of testicular neoplasm may be related to its location in the scrotum, to distant metastasis, or to target organ responsiveness to circulating hormone produced by the tumor. The most common symptom is pain in the scrotum, while testicular mass is the most common presenting sign. Trauma to the testis has not been implicated in the cause of testicular tumor; however, because of its increased size, the testicular tumor is more prone to injury, and frequently minor trauma first focuses the patient's attention to a previously existing tumor. Hydrocele is commonly co-associated with testicular tumor and may obscure the diagnosis. Whenever both are suspected, aspiration of the testis may be performed.

Metastatic spread of a testicular tumor may occasionally give rise to palpable left supraclavicular lymph nodes or to dyspnea secondary to

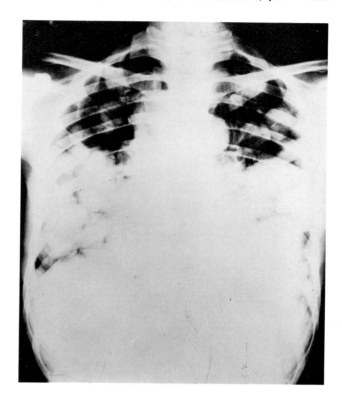

Figure 15–15 Multiple cannonball metastases characteristic of malignant germ cell tumors.

the multiple "cannonball" metastases in the lungs. Elaboration of high titers of human chorionic gonadotropin by choriocarcinoma may cause gynecomastia.

DIAGNOSIS

The initial evaluation of a patient suspected of having a testicular tumor should include a chest x-ray for pulmonary metastasis, an intravenous pyelogram for para-aortic lymph node involvement with secondary lateral displacement of the proximal ureters, and a chorionic gonadotropin titer. Lymphangiography has also been employed for the preoperative evaluation of para-aortic node involvement. The completeness of a retroperitoneal lymph node dissection can be determined by a postoperative x-ray of the abdomen when lymphangiography has been performed preoperatively.

Definitive diagnosis must be based on the microscopic examination of serial sections of the testis after radical orchiectomy. Simple biopsy of a tumor of the testis is to be condemned since it may result in tumor dissemination.

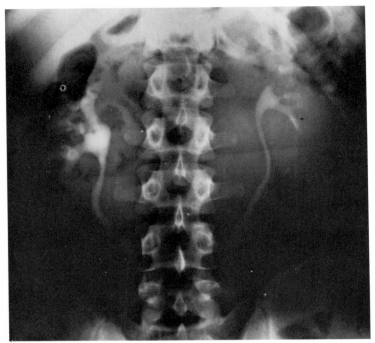

Figure 15–16   Lateral displacement of proximal ureters secondary to para-aortic lymph node metastasis from embryonal carcinoma.

TREATMENT

The initial treatment of all testicular tumors is radical orchiectomy through an inguinal incision with a high ligation of the spermatic cord at the level of the internal ring. If the testicular tumor is pure seminoma and there is no clinical evidence of metastasis, radiation therapy in a total dose of 3000 rad is delivered to the para-aortic and ipsilateral iliac lymph nodes. Radiation therapy is also utilized to treat seminoma metastasis. A recurrence of seminoma in a site previously radiated is rare.

With embryonal carcinoma, teratocarcinoma, or choriocarcinoma, a bilateral para-aortic retroperitoneal lymph node dissection is performed. The dissection removes en bloc all the lymphatic and areolar tissue between the ureters, including that surrounding the great vessels from the level of the renal vessels to the bifurcation of the iliac vessels. Although adjuvant postoperative radiation therapy is recommended to the para-aortic bed if excised nodes are reported positive, some investigators recommend its routine use regardless of whether the nodes are involved.

Several chemotherapeutic agents have been evaluated in testicular tumors. Actinomycin D has been beneficial in the treatment of germinal tumors other than seminoma. Mithromycin is specifically effective in the treatment of embryonal carcinoma. Interestingly, the agent used successfully in the treatment of choriocarcinoma in the female, methotrexate, is absolutely of no benefit in the male. Although many evanescent regressions of pulmonary metastasis in testicular tumors treated with chemotherapy occur, long-term survival with this stage of the disease is essentially nonexistent.

PROGNOSIS

The prognosis of testicular tumors is determined by several variables. The histologic type, stage, and degree of anaplasia are all significant. In general, pure seminoma has the best survival statistics with five-year cures approaching 90 per cent when no evidence of distant spread is present at the time of orchiectomy and radiation therapy. The five-year survival rate in embryonal carcinoma and teratocarcinoma treated with radical orchiectomy and retroperitoneal node dissection with or without chemotherapy approaches 50 per cent. Pure choriocarcinoma, as previously noted, has almost 100 per cent mortality; however, the mixed choriocarcinoma, especially if teratoma is present, has a much better prognosis than the pure type.

TUMORS OF THE PENIS

Benign Tumors of the Penis

CYSTS

Penile cysts may be congenital or acquired. Congenital cysts arise in the area of the penoscrotal raphe as a result of incomplete closure. Histologically, congenital cysts may be dermoid or, more rarely, mucoid. Retention cysts, usually sebaceous in type, can occur secondary to acquired retention of secretions from cutaneous glands. Epithelial cysts that result from previous trauma or circumcision may occur in the area of cutaneous infolding.

Cysts of the penis usually require no treatment unless they become symptomatic or interfere with organ function, and then simple excision may be performed.

NEVI

Moles of the penis are seen frequently; they resemble nevi found elsewhere in the skin. They may be pigmented or nonpigmented and histologically may be junctional, intradermal, or compound in type. It is important to distinguish penile nevi from melanoma. When there is doubt, excisional biopsy is recommended.

HEMANGIOMAS

Penile hemangiomas may be superficial or deep. The superficial type, punctate or macular in appearance, causes little concern. Because of surface size or depth of penetration, the larger hemangioma may require surgical excision. Local radiation therapy has also been used in the treatment of penile hemangiomas.

PAPILLOMATOID LESIONS — ACUMINATE CONDYLOMAS

These exophytic growths may be single or multiple and, although usually small, may occasionally become very large. The origin of condyloma acuminatum has been ascribed by most investigators to a filterable virus. There is a predilection for the mucocutaneous junction of both the male and female genitalia, and venereal transmission has frequently been observed. Histologically, condyloma acuminatum may be distinguished from verrucous carcinoma, even though the epithelium in both shows marked proliferation and frequent mitosis, by the absence of anaplastic characteristics and infiltration.

Condylomas are most frequently treated by local excision with adjunctive fulguration of the base. Local application of 25 per cent podophyllin is also effective.

SUPPORTING TISSUE TUMORS

Keloids occur secondary to trauma and most frequently are observed in the operative site following circumcision. Other supporting tissue tumors, e.g., fibromas and myomas, are extremely rare. Lipomas of the penis are also rare, perhaps as the result of the paucity of adipose tissue in the penis as compared to the subcutaneous fat deposition elsewhere in the body.

Precancerous Tumors of the Penis

QUEYRAT'S ERYTHROPLASIA

Erythroplasia of Queyrat is included as a premalignant penile tumor because of its high frequency of malignant transformation. Classically, erythroplasia of Queyrat appears as a raised, red, velvet-appearing plaque that is usually located on the dorsal aspect of the glans of the penis. Histologically, the lesion shows acanthosis, with frequent mitotic figures seen in all layers of the epithelium accompanied by subepithelial infiltration of lymphocytes, polymorphonuclear leukocytes, and plasma cells with associated proliferation of capillaries.

The treatment of this lesion is local excision, although once it attains large size, partial amputation may be required.

Balanitis Xerotica Obliterans

This lesion is included in the precancerous category more because of tradition than scientific fact. It may appear as a pale sclerotic plaque and frequently involves the urethral meatus. It is a disease of collagen, and histologically one sees an atrophic epidermis with a loss of rete pegs and a homogenization of collagen, with an underlying dense zone of lymphocytes. Balanitis xerotica obliterans is thought to represent the penile form of lichen sclerosis, a nonmalignant dermatologic disease seen elsewhere in the skin. Treatment by local excision usually suffices, although a careful periodic follow-up is indicated.

Leukoplakia

Leukoplakia appears as a raised, white, plaquelike lesion usually limited to the glans of the penis. It frequently results from chronic irritation by the prepuce. Circumcision is the initial treatment. Histologically, the two basic features observed are marked hyperkeratosis and elongation of the rete pegs. Local excision is recommended for leukoplakia, although, as in the other premalignant penile lesions, one cannot predict with any degree of accuracy the frequency of malignant transformation.

Malignant Tumors of the Penis

Epidermoid Carcinoma

Squamous cell carcinoma of the penis is a rare malignancy, accounting for only 2 to 3 per cent of tumors in various series reported in the United States. It is a disease found in uncircumcised males. Chronic irritation from phimosis or poor hygiene is frequently a factor. Smegma has been indicted by some as the precancerous agent.

Signs and Symptoms. In an organ handled several times daily, it is difficult to understand how a growth would not be noted immediately and brought promptly to the attention of a physician. However, several authors have noted an attitude of neglectfulness in many patients with this disease, with unexplainable delays of months and even years between the onset of symptoms and presentation for treatment.

The presenting symptoms are those of a local ulcer or mass that is frequently associated with hemorrhage and pain. Preputial inflammation, which may cause progressive phimosis, is almost always present. With urethral invasion, urinary obstruction may occur.

Inguinal lymphadenopathy secondary to lymphatic metastasis or inflammatory origin may also be present. It has been reported that palpable inguinal adenopathy correlates poorly with this histologic finding of the excised nodes. Of 60 patients in whom lymph node structure was studied, 43 patients had significant palpable adenopathy; only 23 (53.5 per cent) of these patients had lymph node metastasis, while 12 per cent of patients with no adenopathy had metastasis. From this study, it appears that the determination of the need for lymphadenectomy on the basis of clinical suspicion alone is highly inaccurate.

Pathology. Grossly, one sees a papillary lesion with varying degrees of inflammatory ulceration and superimposed infection. Microscopically, the tumor shows the typical characteristics of an epidermoid carcinoma with keratinization, pearl formation, and intercellular bridges.

Metastasis. Early metastasis is primarily via the lymphatics to the deep and superficial inguinal nodes. Iliac node metastasis may occur secondary to advanced disease or urethral invasion, and cure by iliac lymphadenectomy at this stage is rare.

Treatment. The surgical approach to carcinoma of the penis consists of subtotal or total penectomy combined with bilateral inguinal lymphadenectomy. The surgical technique of inguinal lymphadenectomy is performed as described by Baronofsky in 1948. It can be performed even in the presence of advanced inguinal node metastasis and should be considered in such cases, since inguinal lymphadenectomy may prevent secondary hemorrhage from tumor erosion into the femoral vessels and may aid in the control of sloughing and infection of the ulcerated groin metastasis. Also, because of the poor correlation be-

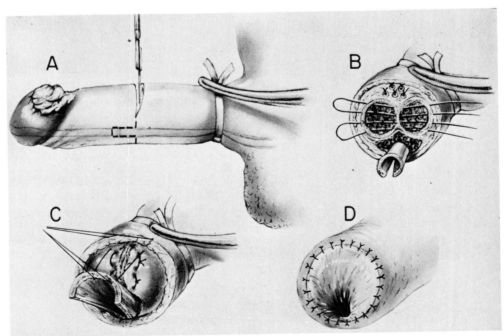

Figure 15–17 Segmental resection of penis for carcinoma. Note spatulation technique to prevent meatal stricture.

tween palpable adenopathy and groin metastasis, lymph node excision helps in disease prognostication and the direction of future therapy.

Squamous cell carcinoma of the penis is sensitive to radiation therapy, and this mode of therapy is advocated by some in small early tumors.

For the most part, primary malignant disease of the penis is synonymous with epidermoid carcinoma. However, there is a small group of malignant tumors that arise from the supportive tissue elements of the penis. Included in this group are fibrosarcoma, myosarcoma, undifferentiated sarcoma, endothelioma, and Kaposi's sarcoma. Also to be distinguished from the epithelial penile tumors are the malignant melanomas, which rarely arise from the skin of the penis.

FIBROSARCOMA

The fibrosarcomas are thought to arise from the fibrous sheaths and septums of the erectile tissue and from fibrous elements within the subcutaneous tissue. Usually, the fibrosarcomas are of a lesser order of malignancy than the other penile sarcomas; only about 10 per cent develop distant metastasis. Treatment consists of wide local excision; however, local recurrence is the rule rather than the exception.

MYOSARCOMA

The myosarcomas (leiomyosarcoma and rhabdomyosarcoma) develop from muscular elements of the penis. They are the least common of the mesenchymal penile tumors; only nine leiomyosarcomas and five rhabdomyosarcomas have been reported. The lesions are characterized by interlacing bundles of spindle-shaped cells that contain frequent mitotic figures. The rhabdomyosarcomas are differentiated from the leiomyosarcomas by the presence of striated muscle cells. Generally, the rhabdomyosarcomas are more malignant than the leiomyosarcomas and are less responsive to radiation therapy. Accordingly, a more radical surgical approach is applied in the treatment of rhabdomyosarcomas, whereas local excision or partial amputation may suffice in the treatment of penile leiomyosarcoma.

HEMANGIOENDOTHELIOMA

Hemangioendothelioma is also known as angiofibrosarcoma, hemangioblastoma, hemangioendothelioblastoma, and hemangioendotheliosarcoma. Two criteria for histologic diagnosis are (1) the formation of vascular tubes with a delicate framework of reticulum fibers and (2) the formation of atypical endothelial cells in greater numbers than normally line the vessels.

Radical surgical excision is essential in the treatment of this tumor since it is particularly resistant to radiation. Hemangioendothelioma has a great tendency to recur following surgery, and the prognosis is guarded in all cases.

KAPOSI'S SARCOMA

Kaposi's sarcoma is a generalized malignant disease which only rarely develops with an initial lesion of the penis. The disease usually presents with a reddish-blue macule on the lower extremity; later, lesions appear elsewhere on the skin and then in the gastrointestinal tract, lymph nodes, and heart.

Histologically, the primary macule is composed of dilated venules within the dermis that are surrounded by a zone of inflammatory cells. The disease progresses through several stages; these include a granulomatous phase with endothelial proliferation and the formation of abnormal vascular sinuses, and a final sarcomatous phase. In this final phase, Kaposi's sarcoma retains its relationship to the vascular elements, and one often sees vascular channels interspersed with bundles of spindle-shaped cells.

MALIGNANT MELANOMA

Malignant melanoma, like Kaposi's sarcoma, is a disease which may originate in the skin in any area of the body and only rarely begins in the skin of the penis. The initial lesion is usually red to black in color and may appear as a macule, papule, or ulcer. Histologically, there is evidence of malignant change within junctional nevus cells in the dermis and epidermis associated with an inflammatory cell infiltrate. The lesions do not necessarily contain melanin.

The results of treatment of malignant melanoma of the penis (as well as malignant melanomas in other areas) are poor. In the penis, metastases occur early by direct extension into the corpora cavernosa, by lymphatic spread to the inguinal nodes, and by hematogenous spread to the liver, lungs, and adrenal gland. Partial or complete amputation of the penis, together with bilateral groin dissections, is recommended for tumors of the shaft or prepuce.

CARCINOMA OF THE SCROTUM

Carcinoma of the scrotum was observed by Pott in 1775 to be occupationally related in chimney sweeps; however, the disease has become extremely rare today, and carcinogens other than coal derivatives have been implicated, including paraffin and arsenic. A latency period of from 10 to 70 years between exposure to the carcinogen and development of scrotal carcinoma has been reported.

Grossly, this tumor appears as a papillary or nodular lesion in the scrotal skin and is frequently associated with areas of ulceration. The ulcer displays elevated, rolled indurated edges and is indolent in its development. Microscopically, one sees squamous carcinoma composed of typical large polyhedral cells, intercellular bridges, and keratin deposition. The tumor can be confined to the scrotum for long periods of time. Metastatic spread is through the lymphatics to the superficial and deep inguinal lymph nodes. Distant metastasis from hematogenous dissemination is uncommon.

Definitive diagnosis is established by biopsy of the scrotal lesion. Although clinical experience with this tumor is scant, the treatment recommended is local excision of the scrotal skin with a bilateral inguinal lymph node dissection. When inguinal lymph nodes are negative, the five-year prognosis exceeds 50 per cent.

TUMORS OF THE MALE URETHRA

Benign Tumors of the Male Urethra

The only benign tumors of the male urethra that occur with any frequency are condylomas; these are most often associated with similar lesions of the penile skin. Other benign tumors of the penis are uncommon.

The major symptoms of these tumors are urethral bleeding and obstruction. If the growth is in the posterior urethra, hematuria is likely, whereas anterior urethral tumors are more apt to cause a bloody discharge between voidings.

Small lesions near the external meatus can be readily excised and fulgurated through the meatus, although a meatotomy may be needed. Single or multiple growths located more proximal in the urethra are more difficult to approach. These may be excised and fulgurated with the rectoscope if they are small. With the larger lesions, an external urethrotomy or partial urethrectomy may be necessary for complete removal.

Squamous cell carcinoma may develop as a complication of condyloma acuminatum, especially if neglected for a long period of time. Instillation of triethylenethiophosphoramide (thiotepa) has been used by some with apparent good results. Podophyllin, which can be used in treating external lesions, must be applied with care in the urethra since it is equally injurious to normal mucosa.

Malignant Carcinoma of the Male Urethra

Carcinoma of the urethra is relatively uncommon and occurs less frequently in the male than in the female, if carcinoma of prostatic origin is excluded. The neoplasms may arise in any portion of the urethra, the histologic type varying according to the epithelium of the area involved. The lining of the prostatic urethra is transitional cell, that of the bulbomembranous urethra is transitional cell with islands of squamous cell epithelium, while the very distal portion of the urethra is lined with squamous cells. The glands of Littre in the fossa navicularis and Cowper's glands opening into the bulbous urethra all have a glandular type of epithelium.

Squamous cell carcinoma is the most common malignant urethral tumor, composing about 65 per cent of reported cases; 25 per cent are anaplastic carcinoma, and the remainder are transitional cell or adenocarcinoma.

The urethra has a very ample lymphatic and blood supply. The anterior urethra drains primarily to the inguinal lymph nodes and the remainder of the urethra to the iliac nodes. In spite of the vascular corporal structures, hematogenous metastases are relatively rare.

The bulbomembranous urethra is the most common site of carcinoma, with 57 per cent of these tumors found there; 36 per cent arise more anteriorly in the urethra, and 7 per cent occur in the prostatic urethra. The prognosis is poorest with the bulbomembranous lesions.

Chronic inflammation appears to be an etiologic factor in the male and perhaps would account for the preponderance of disease in the bulbomembranous urethra where strictures are common.

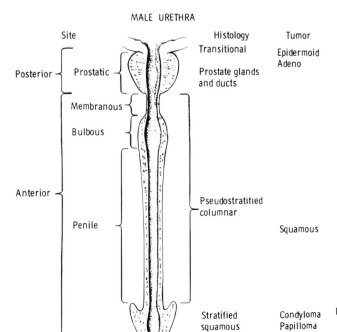

Figure 15-18 Histologic components of the male urethra.

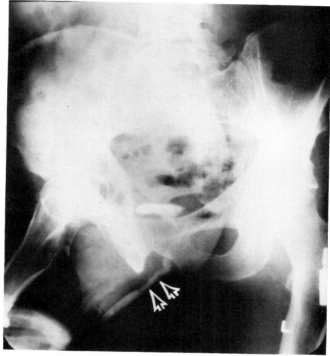

Figure 15–19 Urethrogram study showing irregularity in bulbomembranous urethra caused by squamous cell carcinoma.

TREATMENT

The location and extent of urethral involvement, as well as the presence or absence of local soft tissue spread, is most important in choosing the form of treatment. There is little agreement as to the relative merits of surgery or x-ray therapy in the management of this disease. The number of comparable cases reported with various forms of therapy do not warrant any final conclusions. If surgery is decided upon, the exact procedure depends on the location and extent of the tumor, its degree of anaplasia, and whether metastases to lymph nodes or distant organs are present.

Partial penectomy or partial urethrectomy with urethral reanastomosis may be possible with small lesions of the anterior urethra. More extensive tumors necessitate removal of the entire anterior urethra and penis with perineal urethrostomy.

Some authors feel that the treatment of choice in carcinoma of the anterior urethra or bulbomembranous urethra is radiation. The prognosis for untreated patients is very poor, and few survive for one year.

The question of whether prophylactic or therapeutic iliac and inguinal lymph node dissection should be performed in urethral carcinomas is not settled. The true incidence of lymph node involvement

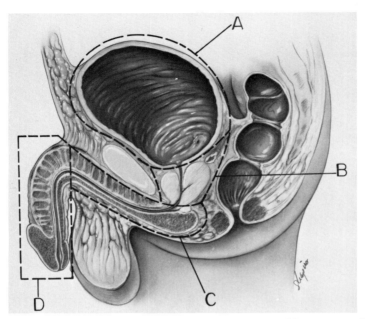

Figure 15–20 Sagittal section of male pelvis showing different zones of lower genitourinary tract requiring excision, depending upon urethral tumor location.

is unknown, and the survival chances with lymph node invasions would require a series of patients treated with lymphadenectomy that could be evaluated statistically. Certainly, at the present time, no other method of treatment offers much hope for this group of patients.

TUMORS OF THE FEMALE URETHRA

Benign Tumors of the Female Urethra

The most common benign lesions are caruncles; these occur near or at the external meatus and can be readily removed by local excision. Caruncles are probably not true tumors but are rather the result of a chronically inflamed edematous portion of prolapsed urethral mucosa.

Other benign lesions such as condyloma acuminatum and fibrous polyp also can be removed by local excision if they are adjacent to the meatus.

Lesions which can be mistaken for urethral tumors are diverticula of the urethra or large prolapsing ureteroceles. Both can be differentiated by appropriate endoscopic and urographic evaluation.

Malignant Tumors of the Female Urethra

Malignancy of the urethra is reported to be twice as common in the female as in the male; the incidence is greatest during the fifth and sixth decades.

In the female, unlike in the male, no correlation has been established between malignant tumors and other urethral diseases that cause acute or chronic irritation. Urethral stricture, chronic infection, cystocele, and pregnancy have not been shown to have an etiologic association. Urethral caruncle and malignancy are often confused in the early stages, but apparently caruncle is not a premalignant disease.

For purposes of treatment and prognosis, urethral tumors in the female are usually divided into three groups: (1) lesions of the proximal urethra, (2) lesions of the distal urethra, and (3) lesions of the entire urethra. Tumors may also arise in a urethral diverticulum although these are relatively rare.

Approximately 65 per cent of the malignancies of the female urethra are squamous cell carcinoma, 35 per cent are transitional cell, and the remainder are adenocarcinoma, melanoma, and sarcoma. Most female urethral adenocarcinomas arise from the periurethral glands.

DIAGNOSIS

The most common presenting sign in malignancy of the female urethra is hematuria or bloody urethral discharge with dysuria and frequency. Urethral mass, perineal pain, dyspareunia, urinary incontinence, and urethrovaginal fistula are also frequent manifestations. The most common differential diagnostic conditions are urethral caruncle, prolapse, urethral diverticulum, and carcinoma of the vagina. Since women are often uncertain as to the exact source of vaginal bleeding, the urethra must be considered as one of the possible points of origin in evaluating this presenting symptom.

Careful inspection and palpation of the urethra should be included whenever a pelvic examination is done. Most urethral tumors can be either seen or palpated or both. Lesions of the distal urethra or meatus may be biopsied directly or endoscopically. Tumors of the proximal urethra may be biopsied endoscopically. If vaginal extension has occurred, this may be biopsied transvaginally. Cystourethrography helps to determine the size and extent of the tumor and also aids in the differential diagnosis of urethral diverticulum. A voiding cystourethrogram is particularly helpful if a diverticulum is suspected. The status of

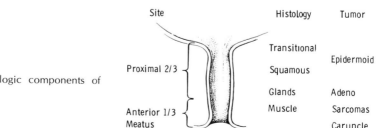

Figure 15–21   Histologic components of female urethra.

FEMALE URETHRA

Site	Histology	Tumor
	Transitional	Epidermoid
Proximal 2/3	Squamous	
	Glands	Adeno
Anterior 1/3	Muscle	Sarcomas
Meatus		Caruncle

the upper urinary tracts should be evaluated by intravenous pyelography, since retroperitoneal lymph node involvement may cause lateral displacement of the ureters.

The proximal portion of the urethra drains directly to the iliac lymph nodes, while the distal portion and meatus drain first to the inguinal nodes so that careful palpation must be performed.

Some researchers believe that distant spread is uncommon and report, in one instance, that only 14 per cent of 79 patients had extralymphatic metastases.

TREATMENT

Surgery alone, radiation alone, and surgery plus radiation have been used in different centers. No clear-cut advantage has been demonstrated with any mode of treatment. The results with lesions over 3 cm in diameter or with involvement of the entire urethra have been uniformly poor with any form of therapy.

Tumors of the proximal or entire urethra require total urethrectomy and cystectomy with supravesical urinary diversion. Anterior exenteration is recommended by some, especially if there is local extension to the vagina.

There is no agreement on the advisability of prophylactic or therapeutic lymph node dissection. Antoniades found lymph node metastases already present in 25 per cent of patients when first seen. The type of lymphadenectomy performed depends on the location of the tumor: inguinal lymph node dissection for distal urethral lesions and iliac dissection for proximal urethral lesions. However, the prognosis with positive nodes when lymphadenectomy is performed appears uniformly poor.

External or interstitial radiation has been widely used, the usual dose being about 5500 rads. Those who use radiation as the primary form of treatment in urethral carcinoma advocate radical surgery for recurrence or for patients with urinary obstruction.

PRIMARY TUMORS OF THE EPIDIDYMIS

Primary epididymal tumors are quite rare when compared with the frequency of involvement of this organ by inflammatory processes. A review of the literature indicates a total of 218 cases.

Benign Mesoblastic Tumors of the Epididymis

ADENOMATOID TUMOR

The adenomatoid tumor, which composes nearly 60 per cent of the total number reported, is the most commonly encountered primary epididymal tumor.

The typical patient with an adenomatoid tumor of the epididymis presents with a painless intrascrotal mass which may be of long standing. Rarely do patients present with pain as the initial symptom, and the tumor frequently is an incidental finding on physical examination. The tumor is noted as a firm, usually nontender, discrete nodule, well-localized in the epididymis. It does not transilluminate light. While the size of the tumor may vary, it is most often less than 2.5 cm in diameter and occurs twice as commonly on the left side as on the right.

Grossly, the lesion is well-circumscribed and encapsulated. The cut surface resembles that of a uterine fibroid with whorled masses of homogenous tissue. Microscopically, there are glandlike structures within an abundant connective tissue stroma that characteristically include smooth muscle fibers. Histologic variation ranges from areas which appear as solid cords of cuboidal and low columnar cells to greatly dilated spaces lined by markedly flattened cells. Many of the lining cells are vacuolated, giving a signet ring appearance because of the peripherally displaced nuclei.

The cellular origin of the adenomatoid tumor is still uncertain, but several theories have been discussed in the literature. The most widely accepted ones suggest that they are either of mesothelial origin or that they arise as hamartomas of the mesonephros or from müllerian vestiges in the epididymis. One bit of circumstantial evidence supporting mesonephric origin is the location of such tumors. They have been found associated with epididymis, tunica vaginalis, and spermatic cord in males, as well as along the course of the ovaries, fallopian tubes, and posterior uterus in females. No other sites for adenomatoid tumors have been described, and it is precisely in these areas that the definitive embryologic kidney develops. Furthermore, the mesonephros and its collecting system contain all the elements known to occur in adenomatoid tumors, including smooth muscle.

Leiomyoma

After the adenomatoid tumors, the leiomyomas are the most frequently encountered benign tumors of the epididymis.

Histologically, leiomyoma of the epididymis is identical to leiomyoma of any other organ, and one sees whorling bundles of uniform-appearing, smooth muscle cells that contain oval nuclei and long slender, bipolar cytoplasmic processes.

Fibroma

Fibromas of epididymal origin are extremely rare and usually present as small solid tumors. However, fibromas of quite large proportions have been reported; one measured 20 by 25 cm at the time of surgery. Histologically, the fibroma is composed of interlacing bundles of normal-appearing fibrocytes and fibroblasts interspaced with a variable amount of collagen.

CYSTADENOMA

This is another rare benign tumor of the epididymis, and is thought to develop within the efferent ductules of the epididymis and to arise embryologically from either the mesonephros or mesonephric duct. Grossly, the lesions are multicystic, while microscopically one sees cystic spaces containing a colloidlike material lined by a single row of cuboidal or columnar cells. Characteristically, there are areas which contain papillary projections of uniform cells with clear cytoplasm.

Four of the reported cases of clear cell cystadenoma were found as part of the complex of von Hippel-Lindau disease, an association of cerebellar hemangioblastoma with tumors of various organs (frequently included are the retina, spinal cord, pancreas, liver, kidney, and epididymis). Clear cell cystadenomas may also be associated with renal neoplasms.

Other benign neoplasms of the epididymis which have been reported are angiomas, lipomas, and cholesteatomas. They are rare, and all are treated by local excision.

Malignant Tumors of the Epididymis

Malignant lesions are more uncommon than benign tumors of the epididymis. The statistics on the incidence of malignant epididymal tumors are subject to debate since case reports prior to the 1940's include in the malignant category some lesions which would today be classified as benign adenomatoid tumors. The assignment of malignancy or benignancy to an epididymal tumor depends on its morphology. Histologically, the diagnosis of malignancy depends on finding cellular atypia, mitotic figures, invasion, destruction of surrounding structures, and vascular involvement.

In spite of the relative rarity of malignant epididymal lesions, this diagnosis must be considered in any patient who presents with an intrascrotal, extratesticular mass. Malignant tumors of the epididymis are often more difficult to differentiate from inflammatory conditions than are the benign lesions. Age and mode of onset, duration, rate of growth, type of pain, and associated diseases must all be considered. Does the lesion transilluminate? Is it tender, solid, or cystic? If the differentiation between benign and malignant conditions cannot be made, exploration is mandatory. The differentiation between neoplastic and nonneoplastic disease has been found most difficult when dealing with cystic dilatation of the epididymal ducts, spermatoceles less than 2 cm in diameter, and chronic nonspecific epididymitis. Torsion of the appendix epididymis, tuberculous epididymitis, and granulomatous lesions of various types should also be considered in the differential diagnosis.

Mesoblastic Origin

The sarcomas are malignant lesions of mesoblastic origin and are more prevalent than the carcinomatous lesions of epithelial origin. As of 1968, 34 sarcomas had been found in the literature. Most of the sarcomas were untyped, but leiomyosarcoma, fibrosarcoma, and rhabdomyosarcoma have all been reported.

Epithelial Origin

In 1968 a total of twenty cases of primary carcinoma of the epididymis was reported. Patients with these tumors are more apt to present with pain and tenderness than are those with benign solid neoplasms; thus, differentiation from inflammatory conditions is difficult, and most of these patients die within two years of their diagnosed epididymal carcinoma.

Treatment of Benign and Malignant Lesions of the Epididymis

The treatment for benign lesions of the epididymis is simple excision or epididymectomy. Rarely is orchiectomy required. The treatment of malignant epididymal lesions requires radical orchiectomy and epididymectomy with resection of the spermatic cord to the internal ring. Some authors also recommend radiation therapy to the para-aortic lymph nodes in spite of the fact that these tumors often metastasize primarily hematogenously.

TUMORS OF SEMINAL VESICLES

Benign Tumors of the Seminal Vesicles

Benign tumors of the seminal vesicles are very rare. If they are small, the lesions are usually asymptomatic but must be differentiated from malignant lesions. They usually are discovered incidentally on rectal examination. The best exploratory approach is through the perineum unless the tumor is very large, in which case a transabdominal route is more suitable.

Cysts of the seminal vesicles are of two types: müllerian and retention. They are distinguished by their location and content. Müllerian duct cysts lie in the midline and do not contain spermatozoa, whereas retention cysts are more lateral and do contain spermatozoa. The definitive diagnosis of seminal vesical cysts is made on exploration. If it is not possible to remove the entire cyst, partial excision and drainage can be performed.

Malignant Tumors of the Seminal Vesicles

Primary malignancy of the seminal vesicles is rare, whereas metastatic lesions in this area are relatively common. Primary carcinoma and sarcoma do occur, but it is difficult to determine their true incidence because the primary site is often uncertain. Some lesions classified as primary prostatic carcinoma may quite possibly be of seminal vesical origin. The usual criteria for considering a lesion in the seminal vesicles to be primary are that it is an anaplastic or papillary adenocarcinoma and that it occupies solely or mainly the seminal vesicles. A total of 44 cases has been reported in the literature.

The symptoms of malignancy of the seminal vesicles usually present later after extension has already occurred to adjacent organs. It has only rarely been possible to attempt a curative procedure. Routine periodic rectal examinations might detect the malignancy at an earlier, potentially curable stage.

When practicable, excision of the seminal vesicles, bladder, and prostate, with supravesical urinary diversion, is the operation of choice. In the event one is dealing with a small low-grade tumor, perhaps removal of the seminal vesicles alone might be sufficient, although this would certainly be a rare circumstance. There is insufficient information available to evaluate the cure rates or the advisability of lymph node dissection or radiation therapy as a surgical adjunct. In most patients, only palliative treatment is possible, consisting mainly of urinary diversion if ureteric obstruction has taken place.

SELECTED REFERENCES

Abeshouse, B. S.: Primary benign and malignant tumors of the ureter. Am. J. Surg., 91:237, 1956.
Extensive review of ureteric carcinoma comprising the clinical, histopathologic, and therapeutic features. Excellent bibliography is included.

Collins, V. P.: The treatment of Wilms' tumor. Cancer, 11:89, 1958.
Describes the appropriate length of the postoperative period for evaluating cure in Wilms' tumor surgery.

Cox, C. E., Cass, A. S., and Boyce, W. H.: Bladder cancer: A 26 year review. Trans. Am. Assoc. Genitourin. Surg., 60:22, 1968.
Long-term follow-up of bladder carcinoma which reveals that regardless of the modality of treatment, low-grade, low-stage tumors have a favorable prognosis whereas high-grade, high-stage tumors have a poorer prognosis.

Flocks, R. H.: Clinical cancer of the prostate: A study of 4000 cases. J.A.M.A., 193:559, 1955.
An excellent introduction to all aspects of carcinoma of the prostate. The use of interstitial radiation as an adjunctive modality is emphasized.

Grabstald, H.: Tumors of the urethra in men and women. Cancer, 32:1236, 1973.
Thorough presentation of urethral carcinoma. Correlates anatomical location and tumor staging with survival. The surgical approaches to the tumor depending on portion of urethra involved are discussed.

Hardner, G. J., and Woodruff, M. W.: Operative management of carcinoma of the penis. J. Urol., 98:487, 1967.
Review of carcinoma of the penis with emphasis on penectomy and bilateral inguinal node dissection as the definitive mode of therapy. The surgical technique of penectomy and groin dissection is vividly illustrated.

Huggins, C. B. et al.: Studies on prostatic cancer. J. Urol., 46:997, 1941.
  A classic paper on the endocrine control of prostatic carcinoma.
Lucke, B., and Schlumberger, H.: Tumors of the kidney, renal pelvis and ureter. *In* Atlas of Tumor Pathology. Washington, D.C., Armed Forces Institute of Pathology, 1957.
  Although dated, still a sound monograph with extensive illustrations of parenchymal and urothelial tumors of the kidney and ureter.
Mostofi, F. K., and Price, E. B.: Tumors of the male genital system. *In* Atlas of Tumor Pathology. Washington, D.C., Armed Forces Institute of Pathology, 1973.
  Contains extensive data on the largest available series of testicular tumors. Well-illustrated and documented.
Skinner, D. G., Colvin, R. B. et al.: Diagnosis and management of renal cell carcinoma. Cancer, 28:1165, 1971.
  An excellent concise paper which correlates clinical, laboratory, and pathologic material related to renal malignancy.
Woodruff, M. W., Wagle, D. et al.: Current status of chemotherapy of advanced renal carcinoma. *In* King, J. S. (ed.): Urological Neoplasia, Boston, Little Brown & Co., 1967, pp. 573–592.
  Comprehensive review and evaluation of chemotherapeutic modalities utilized in the management of renal carcinoma.

REFERENCES

KIDNEY

Bloom, H. J. G., Roe, D. M., and Mitchley, B. C. V.: Sex hormones and renal neoplasia. Cancer, 20:2118, 1967.
Damon, A., Holub, D. A., Melicow, M. M., and Uson, A. C.: Polycythemia and renal carcinoma. Am. J. Med., 25:182, 1958.
D'Angio, C. J., Farber, S., and Maddock, C. L.: Potentiation of x-ray effects by actinomycin D. Radiology, 73:175, 1959.
DeLorimier, A. A., Belzer, F. O., Kountz, S. L., and Kushner, J. H.: Simultaneous bilateral nephrectomy and renal allotransplantation for bilateral Wilms' tumor. Surgery, 64:850, 1968.
Farber, S., D'Angio, G., Evans, A., and Mitus, A.: Clinical studies of actinomycin D with special reference to Wilms' tumor in children. Ann. N. Y. Acad. Sci., 89:421, 1960.
Farrow, G. M., Harrison, E. G. et al.: Sarcomas and saracomatoid and mixed malignant tumors of the kidney in adults — Part I. Cancer, 22:545, 1968.
Glenn, J. F., and Rhame, R. C.: Wilms' tumor: Epidemiological experience. J. Urol., 85:911, 1961.
Jenkins, R. H.: Embryonal adenomyosarcoma of the kidney in adults. N. Engl. J. Med., 205:479, 1931.
Lacy, S. S., Cox, C. E., and Blade, C.: Preoperative radiotherapy of renal cell carcinoma: A feasibility study. Am. Surg., 33:943, 1967.
McDonald, J. R., and Priestley, J. T.: Carcinoma of renal pelvis: Histopathologic study of 75 cases with special reference to prognosis. J. Urol., 51:245, 1944.
Miller, H. C., Woodruff, M. W. et al.: Spontaneous regression of pulmonary metastasis from hypernephroma. Ann. Surg., 156:852, 1962.
Rubin, P.: Cancer of the urogenital tract: Kidney. J.A.M.A., 204:219, 1968.
Wagenvoort, C. A., Morrow, G. W., Jr., and Ten Cate, W. H.: Squamous cell carcinoma of the renal pelvis with muco-epidermoid metastasis. J. Urol., 85:727, 1961.
Woodruff, M. W., Kibler, R. S. et al.: The Neohydrin HG-203 renal scan as an adjuvant to diagnosis of renal disease. J. Urol., 89:746, 1963.
Woodruff, M. W., Wagle, D. et al.: The current status of chemotherapy for advanced renal carcinoma. J. Urol., 97:611, 1969.

URETER

Brady, L. W. et al.: Radiation therapy: A valuable adjunct in the management of carcinoma of the ureter. J.A.M.A., 206:2871, 1968.
Scott, W. W.: Review of primary carcinoma of the ureter presenting two cases. J. Urol., 50:45, 1943.
Senger, F. L., and Furey, C. A., Jr.: Primary ureteral tumor with a review of the literature since 1943. J. Urol., 69:243, 1953.

BLADDER

Bricker, E. M.: Substitution for the urinary bladder by the use of isolated ileal segments. Surg. Clin. North Am., 36:1117, 1956.

Broders, A. C.: Carcinoma: Grading and practical application. Arch. Pathol., 2:376, 1926.

Damon, J. E., and Woodruff, M. W.: Care and management of the ureteroileostomy patient. N.Y. State J. Med., 62:3244, 1962.

Flocks, R. H.: Treatment of patients with carcinoma of the bladder. J.A.M.A., 145:295, 1951.

Friedman, M.: Supervoltage (2-mvp) rotation irradiation of cancer of the bladder. Radiology, 73:191, 1959.

Jewett, H. J., and Strong, G. H.: Infiltrating carcinoma of the bladder: Relation of depth of penetration of the bladder wall to incidence of local extension and metastases. J. Urol., 55:366, 1946.

Jewett, H. J.: The surgical treatment of carcinoma of the bladder. J. Urol., 79:87, 1968.

Jewett, H. J.: Infiltrating carcinoma of the bladder; Relation of early diagnosis to five year survival rate after complete extirpation. J.A.M.A., 148:187, 1952.

Lapides, J.: Mechanism of electrolyte imbalance following ureterosigmoid transplantation. Surg. Gynecol. Obstet., 93:691, 1951.

Lapides, J.: Butterfly cutaneous ureterostomy. J. Urol., 88:735, 1962.

Marshall, V. F.: Current clinical problems regarding bladder tumors. Cancer, 9:543, 1956.

Rubin, P., and Buran, R.: Supervoltage irradiation in bladder carcinoma. Radiology, 73:209, 1959.

Thompson, I. M., and Coppridge, A. J.: The management of bladder tumors in children: A study of sarcoma botryoides. J. Urol., 82:590, 1959.

Thompson, I. M., and Ross, G.: Single stoma skin flap interposition cutaneous ureterostomy. Surg. Gynecol. Obstet., 115:363, 1962.

Whitmore, W. F. et al.: Preoperative irradiation with cystectomy in the management of bladder cancer. Am. J. Roentgenol. Radium Ther. Nucl. Med., 102:570, 1968.

Whitmore, W. F., and Marshall, V. F.: Radical total cystectomy for cancer of the bladder: 230 consecutive cases 5 years later. J. Urol., 87:853, 1962.

Woodburne, R. T.: Essentials of Human Anatomy. New York, Oxford University Press, 1973.

Woodruff, M. W., Hodson, J. M., and Murphy, W. T.: Further observations on the use of combination 5-fluorouracil and supervoltage irradiation therapy in the treatment of advanced carcinoma of the bladder. J. Urol., 90:747, 1963.

Woodruff, M. W., Hardner, G. H. et al.: Advanced carcinoma of the urinary bladder. Cancer Bulletin, 19:29, 1967.

Woodruff, M. W., and Graham, R. M.: Cytologic methods. In Glenn, J. F.: Diagnostic Urology. New York, Hoeber Medical Div., Harper & Row, Publishers, pp. 330–354, 1964.

PROSTATE

Batson, O. U.: The function of the vertebral veins and their role in the spread of metastases. Ann. Surg., 112:138, 1940.

Faber, D. D. et al.: An evaluation of the strontium 85 scan for the detection and localization of bone metastases from prostatic carcinoma: A preliminary report of 93 cases. J. Urol., 97:526, 1967.

Flocks, R. H. et al.: Treatment of carcinoma of the prostate by interstitial radiation with radioactive gold (Au 198): A preliminary report. J. Urol., 68:510, 1952.

Huggins, C., and Scott, W. W.: Bilateral adrenalectomy in prostate cancer: Clinical features and urinary excretion of 17-ketosteroids and estrogens. Ann. Surg., 122:1031, 1945.

Jewett, H. J. et al.: The palpable nodule of prostatic cancer: Results 15 years after radical excision. J.A.M.A., 203:403, 1968.

Nesbit, R. M., and Baum, W. C.: Endocrine control of prostatic carcinoma: Clinical and statistical survey of 1818 cases. J.A.M.A., 143:1317, 1950.

Rubin, P.: Cancer of the urogenital tract: Prostate cancer: Introduction. J.A.M.A., 209:1695, 1969.

Scott, W. W.: An evaluation of endocrine control therapy plus radical perineal prostatectomy in the treatment of selected cases of advanced carcinoma of the prostate followed five or more years. J. Urol., 77:521, 1957.

Scott, W. W., and Boyd, H. L.: Combined hormone control therapy and radical prostatectomy in the treatment of selected cases of advanced carcinoma of the prostate: A retrospective study based upon 25 years experience. J. Urol., *101*:86, 1969.

Veterans Administration Co-operative Urological Research Group: Treatment and survival of patients with cancer of the prostate. Surg. Gynecol. Obstet., *124*:1011, 1967.

TESTIS

Dixon, F. J., and Moore, R. A.: Tumors of the male sex organs. *In* Dixon, F. J., and Moore, R. A. (eds.): Armed Forces Institute Atlas Of Tumor Pathology. Washington, D. C., Armed Forces Institute of Pathology, 1952.

Friedman, M.: Treatment of trophocarcinoma of the testis. Radiology, *80*:550, 1963.

Kennedy, B. J.: Mithramycin therapy in advanced testicular neoplasms. Cancer, *26*:755, 1970.

Kurohara, S. S., Badib, A. O. et al.: Prognostic factors in the common testis tumors. Am. J. Roentgenol. Radium Ther. Nucl. Med., *103*:827, 1968.

Kurohara, S. S., Webster, J. H. et al.: Clinical features of common testicular tumors. J. Urol., *101*:587, 1969.

Lewis, L. G.: Testis tumors: Report of 250 cases. J. Urol., *59*:763, 1948.

Li, M. C., Whitmore, W. F. et al.: Effects of combined drug therapy on metastatic cancer of the testis. J.A.M.A., *174*:1291, 1960.

Mackenzie, A. R.: Chemotherapy of metastatic testis cancer. Cancer, *19*:1369, 1966.

Martin, L. S. J., Woodruff, M. W., and Pickren, J.: Testicular seminoma: A review of 179 patients treated over a 50-year period. Arch. Surg., *90*:306, 1965.

Mostofi, F. K., Theiss, E. A., Ashley, D. J. B.: Tumors of specialized gonadal stroma. Cancer, *12*:944, 1959.

Nesbit, R. M., and Lynn, J.: Malignant testicular neoplasms. Surgery, *20*:273, 1946.

Patton, J. F., and Mallis, N.: Tumors of the testis. J. Urol., *81*:457, 1959.

Skinner, D. G., and Leadbetter, W. F.: The surgical management of testis tumors. J. Urol., *106*:84, 1971.

Staubitz, W. J., and Magoss, I. V. et al.: Surgical management of testis tumors. J. Urol., *101*:350, 1969.

Woodruff, M. W., and Phalakornkule, S.: Extragonadal retroperitoneal seminoma. J. Urol., *91*:579, 1964.

PENIS

Baronofsky, I. D.: Techniques of inguinal node dissection. Surgery, *24*:555, 1948.

Lapides, J.: Partial amputation of the penis without postoperative stricture. Mich. Med., *64*:24, 1965.

Schrek, R., and Lenowitz, H.: Etiologic factors in carcinoma of the penis. Cancer Res., *7*:180, 1947.

Woodruff, M. W., and Mecanas, H.: Hemangioendothelioma of the male genitalia. J. Urol., *87*:560, 1962.

SCROTUM

Graves, R. C., and Flo, S.: Carcinoma of the scrotum. J. Urol., *43*:309, 1940.

Henry, S. A.: Cancer of the scrotum in relation to occupation. London, Oxford University Press, 1946.

Pott, P.: Chirurgical Observations. London, 1775.

URETHRA

Grabstald, H., Hilaris, B., and Henschke, U.: Cancer of the female urethra. J.A.M.A., *197*:835, 1966.

Kaplan, G. W., Buckley, G. J., and Grayhack, J. T.: Carcinoma of the male urethra. J. Urol., *98*:365, 1967.

McCrea, L. E.: Malignancy of the female urethra. Urol. Survey, *2*:85, 1952.

McCrea, L. E., and Furlong, J. H., Jr.: Primary carcinoma of the male urethra. Urol. Survey, *1*:1, 1951.

Mandler, J. I., and Pool, T. L.: Primary carcinoma of the male urethra. J. Urol., 96:67, 1966.

Marshall, V. F.: Radical excision of locally extensive carcinoma of the deep male urethra. J. Urol., 78:252, 1957.

Wishard, W. N., Jr., Nourse, M. H., and Mertz, J. H.: Diverticulum of the female urethra with special reference to diverticular carcinoma. Southern Med. J., 52:890, 1959.

Accessory Organs

Broth, G., Bullock, W. K., and Morrow, J.: Epididymal tumors: I. Report of fifteen new cases including a review of the literature; II. Histochemical study of the so-called adenomatoid tumor. J. Urol., 100:530, 1968.

Gray, G., Biorn, C. L., and Drinken, H. R.: Tumors of the epididymis. J. Urol., 86:620, 1961.

Smith, B. A., Jr., Webb, E. A., and Price, W. E.: Carcinoma of the seminal vesicle. J. Urol., 97:743, 1967.

Woodruff, M. W., Marden, H. E., Jr., and Schoenfeld, L. V.: Benign and malignant tumors of penis, urethra, epididymis and seminal vesicles. In Medical Department Loose Leaf Reference Services: Practice of Surgery: Karafin, L., and Kendall, A. R.: Urology. Vols. I and II, Hagerstown, Maryland, Harper and Row, Pubs., Inc., 1974.

Chapter Sixteen

ADRENAL GLAND

Karl R. Herwig

The adrenals, located above and medial to each kidney, are actually two glands in one, the adrenal cortex and the adrenal medulla (Fig. 16–1). The cortex secretes steroid hormones which are essential for normal body function. It develops from mesodermal cells that arise near the cranial end of the mesonephros. The medulla secretes catecholamines which play a role in the acute reaction to stress but are not essential to the individual. It arises from neuroectoderm along the aorta and becomes surrounded by the mesodermal cells that form the cortex. Primary diseases of the adrenal cortex and medulla are rare, but their manifestations of distinct clinical characteristics are of great interest.

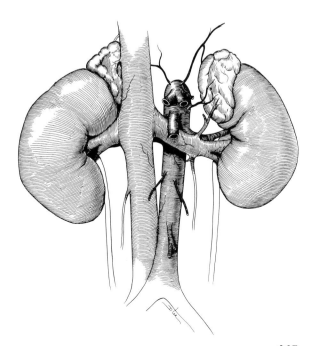

Figure 16–1 Line drawing showing the relationship of the adrenal glands to the kidneys. Also shown are the multiple arterial supply and the single central vein.

ADRENAL CORTEX

Early in fetal life the cortex begins synthesizing steroids from cholesterol and secreting them. Three types of steroids are produced, depending on their main physiologic effect: the glucocorticoids represented by cortisol, the mineral corticoids represented by aldosterone, and the androgenic steroids represented quantitatively by dehydroepiandrosterone (Fig. 16–2). The conversion of cholesterol to one of the steroids involves many enzymatic transformations and occurs in response to various stimuli from outside the adrenal cortex. Knowledge of some of these enzymatic transformations is important for the understanding of abnormalities of steroid synthesis such as occur in the congenital adrenogenital syndrome. The external stimuli and their mechanism of action are also important to the understanding of adrenal physiology and pathophysiology.

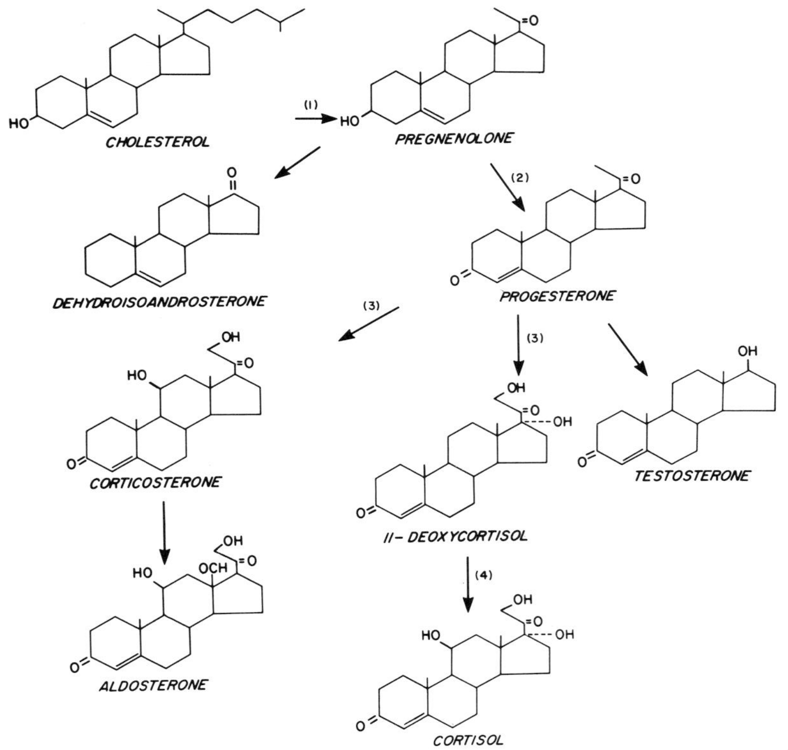

Figure 16–2   Major steps of steroid synthesis from cholesterol. Important enzymatically controlled steps are identified: *1*, ACTH; *2*, 3β-Hydroxysteroid dehydrogenase; *3*, 21-Hydroxylase; *4*, 11β-Hydroxylase. More complete schematics of steroid synthesis are included in the selected readings.

GLUCOCORTICOIDS

The primary stimulus for glucocorticoid synthesis is adrenocortico-tropic stimulating hormone (ACTH), which is produced by the anterior pituitary and mediated by cyclic AMP. ACTH causes the adrenal cortex to accumulate cholesterol, activates the conversion of cholesterol to pregnenolone, and maintains the enzymes active in converting preg-nenolone to hormone steroids. ACTH is produced in response to cortico-tropic release factor (CRF), which is produced and released from the hypothalamus. CRF is produced in response to various stresses such as trauma, fever, anxiety, and hypoglycemia. The hypothalamus also has a basic rhythm, depending on the sleep-wake pattern of an individual, and it releases CRF in response to this rhythm. Cortisol also regulates CRF and ACTH production by depressing their secretion when it is present. This activity is known as a negative feedback mechanism of hormone production, and it is inherent in everyone with normal gluco-corticoid function (Fig. 16–3).

Glucocorticoids function in organic metabolism by stimulating spe-cific enzymes as a permissive hormone, i.e., by enabling other hor-mones to exert their effects. Glucocorticoids also act on the nucleus of a cell to change its metabolism. Steroids are lipid soluble and diffuse freely through cell membranes. In the cytoplasm they attach to a recep-tor protein and migrate into the nucleus where they cause new RNA to be formed. Glucocorticoids affect all cells and thus all systems, al-though this effect is unequal depending on the affinity of the target cell to steroid hormones.

Glucocorticoids stimulate the breakdown of protein and its conver-sion to glucose in the liver. This is gluconeogenesis, and it leads to increased liver glycogen, a rise in blood sugar, and a negative nitrogen balance. The effects upon lipid metabolism under basal conditions are unclear. Overproduction of glucocorticoids induces the centripetal dis-tribution of fat.

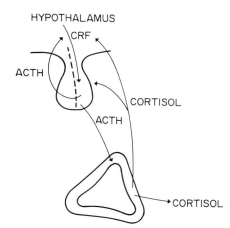

Figure 16–3 Schematic representation of stimulus for cortisol production from the hypothalamus and pituitary. The negative loop feedback regulation of cortisol is shown. (From Siegel, J. R., and Chodoff, P. D. (eds.): Surgical Management of the Aged and High Risk Patient. New York, Grune & Stratton, 1976.)

Other effects of glucocorticoids include: immunosuppression by impairing humoral antibody production; inhibiting the proliferation of lymphoid tissue and inhibiting phagocytosis, their anti-inflammatory effect; blood pressure alteration through their ability to potentiate or permit the vasoconstrictive action of epinephrine; and normal central nervous system functional activity. They also stimulate hematopoiesis, appetite, and uric acid excretion, and they effect calcium metabolism and blood coagulation. As one soon appreciates, cortisol affects every cell, tissue, and system of the body.

MINERAL CORTICOIDS

Renin release from the juxtaglomerular cells of the kidney is the primary stimulus for the production of mineral corticoids. This release seems to depend on sodium concentration of the distal portion of Henle's loop and effective circulating blood volume. Renin causes the conversion of angiotensin I to angiotensin II, a potent vasoconstricting substance. Angiotensin II stimulates the glomeruli of the adrenal cortex to produce the mineral corticoid, aldosterone (Fig. 16–4). Other stimuli of aldosterone production that act directly on the adrenal cortex are ACTH, potassium, and sodium; however, these are not as strong a stimulus as the renin-angiotensin system.

Aldosterone promotes the retention of sodium and the excretion of potassium in the distal convoluted tubule of the kidney. It is important in maintaining sodium balance in fluid volume, especially extracellular fluid volume. Aldosterone has a negative feedback effect on the renin-angiotensin system, since reconstitution of extracellular volume or elevated sodium concentration in the distal loop of Henle depresses the production of renin by the juxtaglomerular cells.

ANDROGENIC STEROIDS

The physiologic significance of the adrenal androgens in the normal individual is unclear. However, it is known that overproduction leads to virilization in the female or precocious puberty in the male.

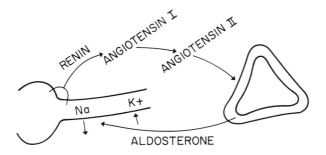

Figure 16–4 Schematic representation of the renin-angiotensin-aldosterone system. Aldosterone has a negative feedback regulation in this system. (From Siegel, J. R., and Chudoff, P. D. (eds.): Surgical Management of the Aged and High Risk Patient. New York, Grune & Stratton, 1976.)

Measurement and Metabolism of Adrenal Steroids

Cortisol. After cortisol is secreted, it becomes associated with transcortin, a plasma glycoprotein. In normal conditions, 75 per cent of the plasma cortisol is bound to transcortin, 15 per cent is bound to albumin, and 10 per cent is unbound. Cortisol can be measured in the blood and urine colorimetrically, fluorometrically, and isotopically. Measurements of secretory rates by isotope dilution are an important index of cortisol production in normal and abnormal situations. The major pathway of steroid inactivation occurs in the liver and involves the enzymatic reduction of the 4–5 double bond to form a dihydrosteroid derivative that is quickly converted to a tetrahydro derivative. This is conjugated with glucuronic acid, forming a water-soluble product that is excreted by the kidney. Measurement of this excreted product colorimetrically by the Porter-Silber method results in the 17-hydroxysteroid and is a useful index of cortisol secretion (Table 16–1).

Aldosterone. Aldosterone is secreted in much smaller quantities and is difficult to measure. Recent development of radioimmunoassays has resulted in sensitive measurements of this important hormone (see Table 16–1). Dehydroepiandrosterone, the principal androgenic steroid, is conjugated with sulfuric acid and is the principal precursor of urinary 17-ketosteroids in the urine. The biochemical evaluation of adrenal cortical function usually includes plasma and urinary cortisol levels and 24 hour measurement of urinary 17-hydroxysteroids and 17-ketosteroids (see Table 16–1). Because of the biologic rhythm of the hypothalamus, ACTH and cortisol are not evenly produced but show a diurnal variation with higher levels in the morning and lower levels in the evening. This phenomenon represents one of the basic principles of determining the status of pituitary adrenal function. Variations from normal suggest certain disease processes.

Adrenal Insufficiency

Inadequate amounts of steroid production result in adrenal insufficiency that can develop into a life-threatening situation. Primary failure

TABLE 16–1   Normal Blood and Urine Levels of Steroid Hormones and Their Metabolites

STEROID	DETERMINED FROM	LEVEL
Cortisol	Serum	11 to 30 μg/100 ml (Higher in a.m. than in p.m.)
17-Hydroxysteroids	Urine	5 to 10 mg/24 hr
17-Ketosteroids	Urine	6 to 20 mg/24 hr (male) 4 to 14 mg/24 hr (female)
Aldosterone	Urine	2 to 17 μg/24 hr

of the adrenal cortex is termed *Addison's disease*, after Thomas Addison, who described the clinical setting in 1855. When seen acutely it is often associated with meningococcemia with adrenal hemorrhage (Waterhouse-Friderichsen syndrome). It has a poor prognosis because of late recognition. Tuberculosis was the most common cause of Addison's disease in the past, but today other factors, such as idiopathic atrophy, fungal diseases, and bilateral adrenalectomy, are more common causes.

The symptoms and signs are due to both aldosterone and cortisol deficiency. A lack of aldosterone results in impaired ability to conserve sodium and excrete potassium and hydrogen. A lack of cortisol results in impaired gluconeogenesis, hypoglycemia, the wasting of fat deposits, and elevated ACTH and MSH (melanocyte stimulating hormone) levels (Table 16–2). The patient complains of easy fatigability, muscular weakness, weight loss, nausea, vomiting, and anorexia. Examination usually reveals mucosal pigmentation, hypotension, lethargy, and often prerenal azotemia and hypoglycemia. The plasma and urinary cortisol concentrations are low, and the urinary 17-hydroxysteroid and 17-ketosteroid excretions are depressed.

Secondary Adrenal Insufficiency. Hypopituitarism results in secondary adrenal insufficiency. The manifestations are the same as primary adrenal insufficiency except for the lack of hyperpigmentation owing to the absence of MSH. The distinction between primary and secondary adrenal insufficiency is therapeutically important. In primary adrenal insufficiency, both mineral corticoid and glucocorticoid are deficient, but in the secondary form, only glucocorticoid is deficient. Thus, therapy in secondary adrenal insufficiency does not require a mineral corticoid substitute. In addition, secondary adrenal insufficiency is often accompanied by other endocrine deficiencies that require replacement, such as hypothyroidism.

Treatment of Adrenal Insufficiency. Treatment consists of replacing the specific hormones that are lacking. When there is acute crisis, large doses of glucocorticoids, rapid restitution of the extracellular volume with saline solutions, and treatment of the underlying cause are necessary. Mineral corticoids are unnecessary in acute situations. Chronic primary insufficiency maintenance steroids include hydrocortisone 30 mg per day (20 mg in morning, 10 mg in evening) and fluorohydrocortisone 0.1 mg per day for mineral corticoid replacement. The patient should carry identification at all times concerning the presence of adrenal insuf-

TABLE 16–2   Symptoms and Signs of Addison's Disease

Easy fatigability
Weight loss
Nausea and vomiting
Muscular weakness
Anorexia
Hyperpigmentation
Hypotension

ficiency. In secondary adrenal insufficiency, fluorohydrocortisone is not needed because the patient can produce adequate amounts of aldosterone. The amount of steroids should be increased during stress, such as during illness or surgical operations (Table 16–3).

STEROID-PREP

Anyone who has received steroid medication for any reason in the recent past or who faces the possible total loss of adrenal function from operation requires preoperative glucocorticoid preparation, a steroid-prep. A satisfactory loading of glucocorticoids preoperatively is obtained by giving hydrocortisone (50 mg) the night before the operation and hydrocortisone (100 mg) when the patient is taken to the operating room. During the operation, hydrocortisone infuses at a rate of 10 mg per hour. If no complications from the operation occur, the steroids are rapidly tapered to a maintenance level or discontinued if the adrenal glands are functioning. Tapering is carried out by giving hydrocortisone (200 mg) on the day of the operation and on the first postoperative day in divided doses, 150 mg on the second, 100 mg on the third, 75 mg on the fourth, 50 mg on the fifth and so forth. If both adrenal glands are removed, then fluorohydrocortisone 0.1 mg is added for salt balance when the hydrocortisone is reduced below 75 mg per day. The dosage is not rigid but is modified according to each patient's needs. After surgery one can usually reach maintenance levels or complete withdrawal within a week. Often after removal of an adrenal tumor, the remaining adrenal tissue does not begin functioning immediately, and,

TABLE 16–3 **Preparation and Tapering Doses of Hydrocortisone Used in Adrenal Surgery**

STEROID ADMINISTRATION	TIME OF ADMINISTRATION	DOSE OF HYDROCORTISONE
Preoperatively	12 midnight	50 mg I.M.
	6 a.m. or on call to operating room	100 mg I.M.
	In operating room	10 mg I.V. per hr
Postoperatively	Day of operation	50 mg every 6 hr
	Post-op day #1	50 mg every 6 hr
	#2	50 mg every 8 hr
	#3	25 mg every 6 hr
	* #4	25 mg every 8 hr
	#5	15 mg every 8 hr
	** #6	15 mg a.m.
		10 mg noon
		5 mg p.m.
	#7	10 mg twice daily
	#8	none

*If patient has had bilateral total adrenalectomy, add 0.1 mg fluorohydrocortisone for salt balance.

**Maintenance level for patient requiring replacement steroids.

in these instances, replacement with exogenous steroids may be required for a few months or ACTH used to stimulate the adrenal cortex.

Hyperfunction of the Adrenal Cortex

Overproduction of cortisol leads to the development of Cushing's syndrome, which is characterized by truncal obesity, hypertension, fatigability and weakness, amenorrhea or impotence, hirsutism, osteoporosis, emotional instability, and increased susceptibility to infection. The negative nitrogen balance from protein loss and gluconeogenesis results in muscle wasting and weakness. Osteoporosis also occurs because of the protein catabolism, which may result in hypercalcemia and the formation of renal calculi. Abdominal striae occur because of the decrease of elastic tissue and collagen secondary to protein catabolism. The skin thins and blood vessels become close to the surface, giving the patient a plethoric appearance without the presence of erythrocytosis (Fig. 16–5).

In large amounts, cortisol depresses the production of lymphocytes and interferes in the normal inflammatory reaction, causing the patient with Cushing's syndrome to be more vulnerable to infection. Glucone-

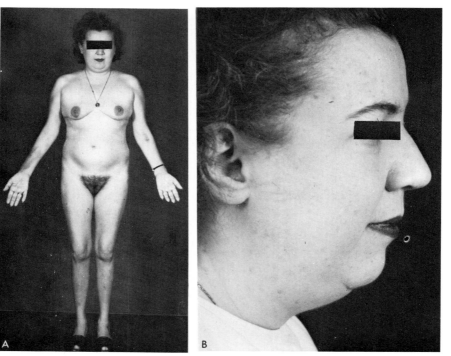

Figure 16–5   *A*, The appearance of a patient with Cushing's syndrome. One should particularly notice the thin extremities in relation to the truncal obesity. In *B* note the facial acne and fullness of the face ("moon shaped").

ogenesis raises insulin requirements and may lead to the exhaustion of pancreatic beta cells and the development of overt diabetes mellitus. Sodium retention, a result of excessive amounts of cortisol, may lead to hypertension. The redistribution of fat in a centripetal fashion gives rise to the buffalo hump, moon facies, and truncal obesity. The thin extremities that are due to muscle wasting exaggerate this effect (see Fig. 16–5). Emotional instability with rapid mood swings occurs owing to the effect of cortisol upon the central nervous system.

Etiology of Cushing's Syndrome. The causes of Cushing's syndrome vary, and differentiation of the causes is necessary for proper therapy. Primary causes can be divided into three groups: (1) excessive production of ACTH by the pituitary due to primary pituitary disease or excessive CRF production from the hypothalamus, (2) production of ACTH or an ACTH-like substance from a malignant neoplasm such as oat cell carcinoma of the lung, and (3) primary tumor of the adrenal cortex that is either benign or malignant. Increased ACTH results in bilateral hyperplasia of the adrenal cortex and is the cause of Cushing's syndrome in over 70 per cent of the affected patients. Primary tumors are found in approximately 20 per cent of the affected patients. A secondary cause of Cushing's syndrome is exogenous steroid, an all too common finding at present.

Cushing's syndrome occurs more frequently in females. Its highest incidence of occurrence is between the ages of 20 and 40 years. If it is found in children, it is more likely due to a malignant tumor of the adrenal gland and has a poor prognosis.

Diagnosis of Cushing's Syndrome. Diagnosis is not simple, and the signs and symptoms are important (Table 16–4). Finding an elevated plasma cortisol level with the loss of diurnal variation along with elevated levels of urinary 17-hydroxysteroids and 17-ketosteroids suggests the diagnosis. At times an obese patient or febrile patient may demonstrate these findings. Photographs of the patient prior to the onset of his symptoms with comparison to his present appearance may be helpful in documenting the physical change. However, the diagnosis remains biochemical. To differentiate the Cushingoid patient without Cushing's syndrome from the patient with true Cushing's syndrome, one can manipulate the pituitary-adrenal axis. Low doses of

TABLE 16–4   Common Symptoms, Signs, and Findings of Cushing's Syndrome

Muscular fatigue or weakness
Menstrual cycle disturbance
Moon facies
Hirsutism
Plethora
Hypertension ($> 150/90$)
Truncal obesity
Acne
Psychiatric disorder
Increased tendency to ecchymosis

dexamethasone 0.5 mg every 6 hours depress the production of ACTH in the obese or febrile patient but not in the patient with Cushing's syndrome. The plasma cortisol and urinary 17-hydroxy-steroids and 17-ketosteroids measure this response. Once Cushing's syndrome is suspected, the cause of the problem, whether excess ACTH or primary tumor, should be determined because therapy varies with the cause. Biochemical means can usually differentiate adrenal hyperplasia from adrenal tumors (Fig. 16–6).

Since most adrenal tumors are independent of pituitary function, attempting to suppress the pituitary with large amounts of dexametha-sone does not result in decreased plasma cortisol and urinary 17-hydroxysteroids and 17-ketosteroids as it does in the patient with hyperplasia. Two milligrams of dexamethasone every 6 hours for three days is utilized to suppress activity of the pituitary gland. Metyrapone stimulates ACTH production and is also used to differentiate hyperpla-sia from tumor; the patient with hyperplasia demonstrates increased urinary 17-hydroxysteroid and 17-ketosteroid excretion when compared to baseline, while the patient with a tumor shows no response. Usually, the patient with ectopic production of ACTH is discovered during the evaluation of a primary malignancy.

Radiologic means of diagnosing adrenal cortical tumors also exist. The intravenous pyelogram offers little help unless a large tumor

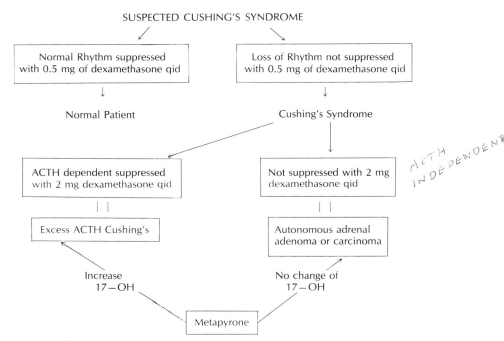

Figure 16–6 Schematic representation of the biochemical differentiation of suspected Cushing's syndrome. (Adapted from Little, G. W.: The adrenal cortex. *In* Williams, R. H. (ed.): Textbook of Endocrinology, 5th ed. Philadelphia, W. B. Saunders Company, 1974.)

displacing the kidney is present (Fig. 16–7). Retroperitoneal CO_2 insufflation has been used, but the technique is difficult and causes some morbidity. Because of the multiple arterial supply to the adrenal gland, adrenal arteriography is usually useless. However, adrenal venography, by catheterizing the central adrenal vein, often discloses the tumor deformity when one is present (Fig. 16–8,A). The use of [131]I-19-iodocholesterol adrenal scanning can differentiate hyperplasia from tumor, since the isotope is evident only in the active tumor while both glands are visualized with hyperplasia (Fig. 16–8,B). At the present time, the scan appears to be the most useful radiographic method for diagnosing adrenal cortical tumors that produce Cushing's syndrome and for localizing their position.

Treatment of Cushing's Syndrome. The treatment of bilateral adrenal hyperplasia due to ACTH excess rests on nonoperative techniques with the reservation of bilateral adrenalectomy for patients who do not respond to therapy. Nonoperative techniques include radiation of the pituitary gland and small doses of o,p'DDD, a suppressor of

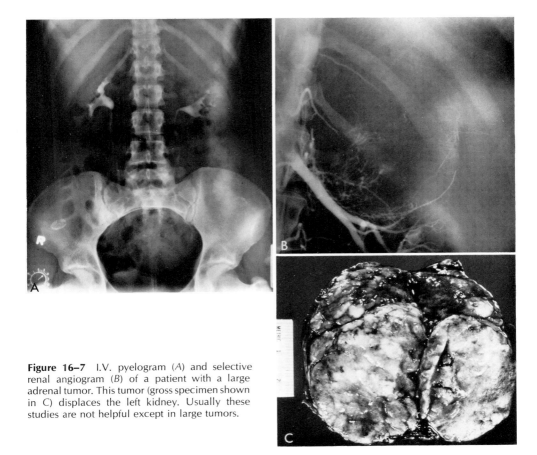

Figure 16–7 I.V. pyelogram (*A*) and selective renal angiogram (*B*) of a patient with a large adrenal tumor. This tumor (gross specimen shown in *C*) displaces the left kidney. Usually these studies are not helpful except in large tumors.

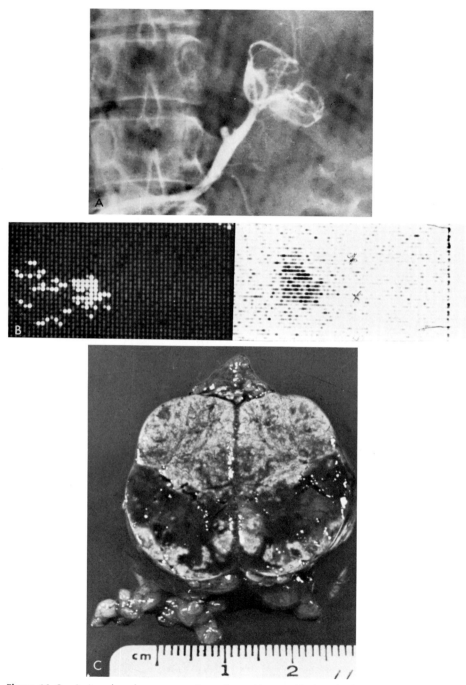

Figure 16–8   *A*, An adrenal venogram of a patient with a small adrenal adenoma causing Cushing's disease. *B*, The iodocholesterol scan demonstrates activity only in the tumor. *C*, The gross specimen is a typical adrenal adenoma found in these patients. (From Herwig, K. R. et al.: Localization of adrenal tumors by photoscanning. J. Urol., *109*:2, 1973. © 1973 The Williams & Wilkins Company, Baltimore.)

steroid synthesis. If total adrenalectomy is undertaken, all cortical tissue should be removed because of the risk of Cushing's syndrome recurring from remnants. Primary adrenal tumors should be removed operatively (Fig. 16–8,C). Therapy for ectopic ACTH production is directed toward the primary malignancy. In patients with functioning adrenal cortical carcinoma o,p'DDD may be used as an adjunct to operative removal. It has been found useful in suppressing the hormonal effects of the tumor when the entire tumor cannot be removed.

Prognosis of Cushing's Syndrome. If Cushing's syndrome persists, 50 per cent of the patients with it will die within five years. In addition, there may be a significant morbidity from cerebral vascular accidents that are due to hypertension. The overwhelming majority of these patients can be cured or controlled with therapy, but even the treated patients have an increased morbidity, since the disease is often replaced by a dependence on exogenous sources for the necessary steroids. This therapy is not without risk, especially if the patient faces stress.

Hyperfunction of Mineral Corticoid Production

Overproduction of mineral corticoid is known as *aldosteronism.* When due to disease in the adrenal cortex, it is known as primary aldosteronism, or Conn's syndrome. If it is related to increased renin states, it is known as secondary aldosteronism. Secondary aldosteronism occurs with congestive heart failure, renal vascular hypertension, and other states when there is decreased effective circulating blood volume. Treatment of secondary aldosteronism is directed toward the causes of the decreased circulating blood volume rather than toward the increased aldosterone production.

Primary Aldosteronism. Primary aldosteronism represents the cause of hypertension in approximately 1 to 5 per cent of all patients with essential hypertension. Its true incidence is unknown because of the difficulty in diagnosis. Symptoms and signs of primary aldosteronism include muscle weakness, headache, easy fatigability, polyuria, polydipsia, and hypertension (Table 16–5). The hypertension of primary aldosteronism is not high, and severe eyeground changes are uncommon. The exact cause of the hypertension is unclear, although it appears to be related to sodium retention and increased circulating blood volume. The potassium loss is both extracellular and intracellular and

TABLE 16–5   Common Symptoms and Signs of Primary Aldosteronism

Muscle weakness
Polyuria, nocturia
Headache
Polydipsia
Visual disturbance
Tetany
Fatigue
Muscle discomfort

**TABLE 16–6 Laboratory Studies Necessary to
Confirm the Diagnosis of Primary Aldosteronism**

Elevated blood and urine aldosterone with high salt diet
Suppressed peripheral plasma renin activity on low salt diet and upright position
Normal glucocorticoids
Hypokalemia (not necessary)

gives rise to muscular weakness, easy fatigability and muscle cramps. Hypokalemic nephropathy impairs renal concentrating ability, which leads to polyuria and polydipsia. Approximately 50 per cent of the patients have an abnormal glucose tolerance curve owing to the effects of hypokalemia on the pancreatic islet cells.

DIAGNOSIS. One suspects the presence of primary aldosteronism in patients with benign hypertension and hypokalemia, in patients with benign hypertension who rapidly develop hypokalemia after receiving thiazide diuretics, and in hypertensive patients who develop hypokalemia after a salt load. The diagnosis is made by finding normal glucocorticoid production, increased aldosterone production, and depressed plasma renin activity (Table 16–6). The aldosterone is measured in 24 hour urine collections, with the patient on a high sodium diet which normally should depress aldosterone production. The renin measurements are made with peripheral plasma after the patient has received a low sodium diet. This diet as well as the upright position should normally stimulate renin production. The normal feedback mechanism of the renin-angiotensin-aldosterone system is inoperative in primary aldosteronism because the tumor is independent of this mechanism (see Fig. 16–4). The presence of hypokalemia is unnecessary for the diagnosis but is usually present.

After entertaining the diagnosis and confirming it biochemically, it is helpful to determine whether the primary aldosteronism results from an adenoma of the adrenal cortex or bilateral nodular hyperplasia. Bilateral hyperplasia occurs in approximately 16 per cent of patients with primary aldosteronism. In the majority of patients, the differentiation can be accomplished by adrenal venography, [131]I-19-iodocholesterol scan, and adrenal vein blood aldosterone measurements (Fig. 16–9).

TREATMENT. No steroid preparation is required. The hypokalemia can be corrected with spironolactone or potassium chloride administered orally preoperatively. The treatment of bilateral nodular hyperplasia is unsettled at the present time; some urologists advocate bilateral adrenalectomy while others prefer to control symptoms with spironolactone. Adenomas are excised, usually leaving the uninvolved adrenal tissue. If primary aldosteronism remains untreated, irreversible hypertensive changes can occur.

Hyperfunction of Adrenal Androgens

The synthesis of cortisol and aldosterone from cholesterol involves many enzymatically regulated steps. Defects in the enzymes, which are

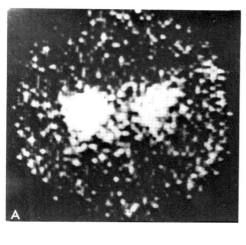
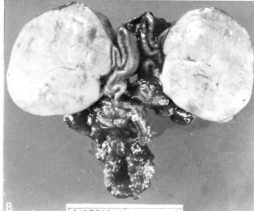
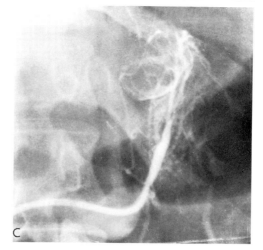

Figure 16-9 An iodocholesterol scan *(A)*, tumor *(B)*, and adrenal venogram *(C)* of a patient with primary aldosteronism due to an adrenal adenoma. (From Herwig, K. R., et al.: Localization of adrenal tumors by photoscanning. J. Urol., *109*:2, 1973.)

genetically determined, can cause accumulations of substances that are precursors of the regulated steps with diminished derivatives of the steps. The end result is diminution of cortisol production, which leads to increased secretion of ACTH. The increased secretion of ACTH results in hyperplasia of the adrenal cortex as it attempts to increase cortisol production. The result is known as congenital adrenal hyperplasia. Under normal conditions, the precursors of cortisol have little biologic activity, but as large amounts accumulate, their biologic effect becomes evident.

Congenital Adrenal Hyperplasia. This condition appears to be inherited through autosomal recessive genes and is often familial. It is a cause of female pseudohermaphroditism, the most common intersex problem in the female. In males, it can cause precocious puberty or infertility. In its mildest form, congenital adrenal hyperplasia presents as ambiguous genitalia, but it may also be associated with hypertension and hyponatremia and may threaten the life of the newborn. Its presentation depends on which enzymes are deficient and the completeness of the defect. The most common deficit is 21-hydroxylase deficiency (see Fig. 16-2). This causes accumulation of androgenic steroids with diminished cortisol and aldosterone. It usually presents as ambiguous genitalia accompanied by hypertension and some salt losing. Other enzyme deficits `include 11-hydroxylase and 3 β-dehydrogenase deficiency.

One suspects the presence of congenital adrenal hyperplasia in any newborn with ambiguous genitalia or severe failure to thrive in the newborn period. The diagnosis is confirmed by finding diminished derivatives and elevated precursors such as elevated levels of pregnanetriol and 17-ketosteroids in the urine. Therapy is directed toward the replacement of the deficient steroids. In addition, this replacement diminishes ACTH secretion and depresses accumulation of precursors. Often, some reconstruction of the ambiguous genitalia is needed.

ADRENAL MEDULLA

The adrenal medulla is the part of the sympathetic nervous system that prepares the individual for stress. Like other parts of the sympa-

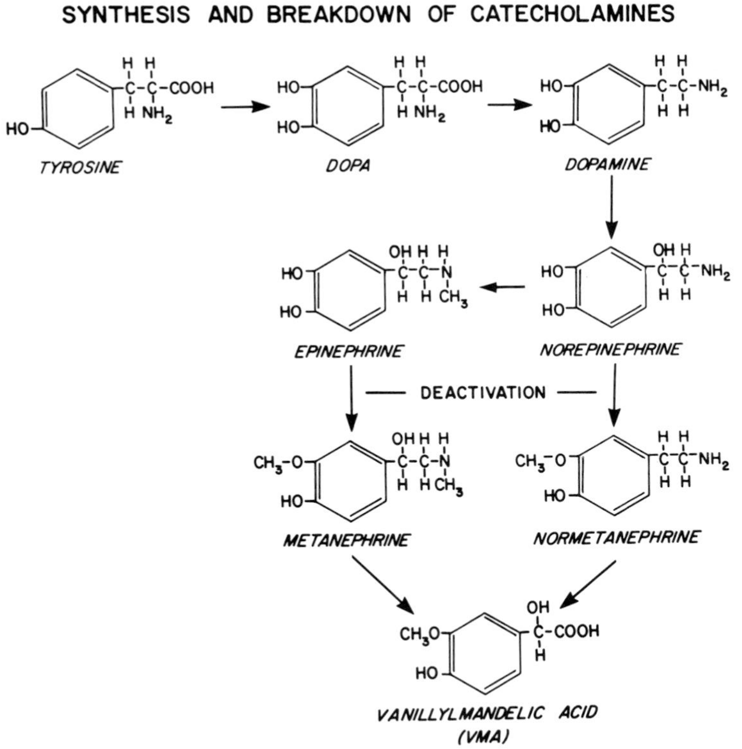

SYNTHESIS AND BREAKDOWN OF CATECHOLAMINES

Figure 16-10 Schematic representation of the synthesis and catabolism of epinephrine and norepinephrine.

tively limits the maximum capacity of the tubule to reabsorb bicarbonate, which appears in the urine. Serum bicarbonate levels decrease until the new threshold level is reached. At this point a steady state of metabolic acidosis exists. The proximal tubule can handle the decreased filtered load of bicarbonate and the distal tubule is not flooded with bicarbonate. Distal acidification and net acid excretion are possible.

However, decreased hydrogen ion secretion in the distal nephron impairs bicarbonate regeneration (table 2). Decreasing urinary ammonium and titratable acid limits net acid excretion. When net acid excretion decreases below the fixed acid production of the body (normally 1 mEq./kg. per 24 hours) progressive acidosis ensues.[6]

This brief discussion of the pathophysiology of renal tubular acidosis explains many of the clinical features that form the basis for diagnosis and classification of the disease (table 3). (Other forms of renal tubular acidosis have been described but they are beyond the scope of this report.) Although the diagnosis often is suggested by routine laboratory tests incomplete forms of distal renal tubular acidosis do not present with acidosis and require acid loading studies for diagnosis. Such investigations usually are prompted by a family history of renal tubular acidosis, history of nephrolithiasis or the presence of a condition known to be associated with secondary renal tubular acidosis. Table 4 lists some conditions associated with renal tubular acidosis likely to be seen by urologists.

Current concepts of stone formation in renal tubular acidosis relate to altered metabolism of calcium and citrate in systemic acidosis. Chronic acid retention titrates alkaline bone salts, leading to mobilization of calcium and hypercalciuria. Direct effects of acidosis on the renal tubule also may have a role in increasing urinary calcium.[7] Acidosis per se reduces urinary citrate, a well known inhibitor of crystallization. Alkaline urine decreases the solubility of...

TABLE 3. *Clinical features of renal tubular acidosis*

	Proximal	Distal
Serum chloride	High	High
Serum bicarbonate	>20 mEq./l.	<15 mEq./l.
Serum potassium	Normal to low	Normal to low
Anion gap	Normal	Normal
Urine pH (a.m.)	May be <6.0	>6.0
Urine pH (acid load)	<5.3	>5.3
Stones	Uncommon	Common
Fanconi's syndrome	Common	Rare
Bicarbonate requirement	High	Low

TABLE 4. *Secondary renal tubular acidosis*

Proximal	
Lowe's syndrome	Outdated tetracycline
Amyloidosis	Acetazolamide
Nephrotic syndrome	Mafenide
Renal transplantation	Heavy metals
Medullary cystic disease	

Distal	
Primary hyperparathyroidism	Renal transplantation
Idiopathic hypercalciuria	Amphotericin B
Medullary sponge kidney	Lithium carbonate
Pyelonephritis	Toluene
Obstructive uropathy	

require more medication. In secondary forms of renal tubular acidosis treatment of the underlying disease or removal of the toxin may ameliorate the tubular dysfunction, making bicarbonate therapy unnecessary. In these cases it is prudent to put the patient on the alkalizing agents until definite evidence for complete reversal of the defect is obtained.

The acute complication of hypokalemic paralysis in our case has been reported previously.[4] Impaired sodium-hydrogen ex-

have urolithiasis.

This pathogenetic scheme seems valid for patients with complete renal tubular acidosis but it does not explain why patients with incomplete renal tubular acidosis (not acidotic by definition) also tend to form stones. Also unexplained is the relative rarity of urolithiasis in proximal renal tubular acidosis. Thus, it seems likely that other metabolic abnormalities contribute to calculogenesis in this disease. In this regard recent evidence has suggested that some familial types of renal tubular acidosis are actually secondary to a primary disturbance of calcium metabolism.[8]

Treatment of renal tubular acidosis with sodium bicarbonate or other alkalizing medications can be expected to decrease the rate of stone formation. Alkali should be given in amounts sufficient to produce a normal serum bicarbonate. In general, patients with distal renal tubular acidosis are relatively sensitive to alkalization, while proximal renal tubular acidosis patients

management of these patients requires continuous monitoring of the electrocardiogram and frequent determinations of serum electrolytes while potassium chloride is being given. Administration of solutions containing bicarbonate or glucose will drive potassium into the intracellular compartment and exacerbate the hypokalemia. Therefore, no attempt is made to correct the acidosis until the serum potassium is at least 3.0 mEq./l. Respiratory insufficiency owing to ascending paralysis precipitated by bicarbonate administration in this setting has been reported.[9] A normal or elevated carbon dioxide pressure in the presence of metabolic acidosis may be an early clue to hypoventilation. While the high priority of potassium replacement deserves emphasis it also is important to indicate that rapid infusion of potassium to an acidotic patient can lead to dangerously high serum levels of potassium. Therefore, the proper approach depends on carefully titrating the patient with potassium and subsequently bicarbonate, and using the electrocardiogram and frequent determinations of serum electrolytes to monitor therapy.

REFERENCES

1. von Oettingen, W. F., Neal, P. A. and Donahue, D. D.: Toxicity and potential dangers of toluene; preliminary report. J.A.M.A., 118: 579, 1942.
2. Press, E. and Done, A. K.: Solvent sniffing. Physiologic effects and community control measures for intoxication of organic solvents. I. Pediatrics, 39: 451, 1967.
3. Press, E. and Done, A. K.: Solvent sniffing. Physiologic effects and community control measures for intoxication of organic solvents. II. Pediatrics, 39: 611, 1967.
4. Taher, S. M., Anderson, R. J., McCartney, R., Popovtzer, M. M. and Schrier, R. N.: Renal tubular acidosis associated with toluene "sniffing". New Engl. J. Med. 290: 765, 1974.
5. Wyse, D. G.: Deliberate inhalation of volatile hydrocarbons: a

TABLE 1. *Characteristics of bicarbonate reabsorption*

85-90% proximal tubule
10-15% distal tubule
1 hydrogen ion secreted for each bicarbonate reabsorbed
No net hydrogen ion excreted
Carbonic anhydrase required

TABLE 2. *Characteristics of bicarbonate regeneration*

Distal tubule and collecting duct
1 hydrogen ion excreted for each bicarbonate regenerated
Net hydrogen ion excretion does occur
Net acid excretion = urinary ammonium + titratable acid − bicarbonate
Carbonic anhydrase not required

thetic nervous system, it produces catecholamines, principally norepinephrine and epinephrine, which are synthesized from tyrosine (Fig. 16–10). The stimulus for their production includes physical, psychic, and environmental stress.

Epinephrine is one of the most potent vasopressors known; its principal pressor effect results from direct myocardial stimulation and increased cardiac output. Norepinephrine's pressor effect occurs by increasing peripheral vascular resistance. In addition, there are qualitative and quantitative differences in the action of these two catecholamines on the same receptor organ. These differences give rise to the concept of different receptor sites in the same organ for epinephrine and norepinephrine, the alpha and beta receptors. Both epinephrine and norepinephrine have alpha and beta receptor activity. This activity can be blocked by specific drugs such as phenoxybenzamine, an alpha blocker, and propranolol, a beta blocker. The catecholamines produce increased peripheral vascular resistance, cardiac excitation, increased cellular metabolism, and central nervous system excitability; they also cause relaxation of the vascular smooth muscle of the gut, bronchial tree, coronary arteries, and skeletal muscle in addition to relaxing the smooth muscle of the gut and bronchial tree.

Catecholamines are inactivated to normetanephrine, metanephrine, and vanillyl mandelic acid (VMA) peripherally by enzymatic action (see Fig. 16–10). These products of sympathetic activity can be measured in the urine (Table 16–7).

The physiologic function of the adrenal medulla is difficult to determine since absence of the medulla, such as occurs after bilateral adrenalectomy, alters the total catecholamines little. Tumors of chromaffin tissue occur, which produce distinct clinical symptoms and signs. The most important are neuroblastoma and pheochromocytoma.

NEUROBLASTOMA

Neuroblastomas arise from the neural crest tissue and are usually seen in children, especially infants. The adrenal medulla is a frequent site of neuroblastoma. The term *neuroblastoma* is a general term describing tumors of three histologic cell types: sympathogonioma, sympathoblastoma, and ganglioneuroma. The former two are more often malignant than the latter one. Neuroblastoma is suspected whenever an

TABLE 16–7   Normal Blood and Urine Levels for Catecholamines

PRODUCT	DETERMINED FROM	LEVEL
Epinephrine	Serum	0.1 to 0.5 μg/liter
Norepinephrine	Serum	2 to 6 μg/liter
Metanephrine	Urine	up to 130 μg/24 hr
Normetanephrine	Urine	up to 240 μg/24 hr
Vanillyl mandelic acid	Urine	2 to 6 mg/24 hr

abdominal mass is found in an infant. It is the most common abdominal tumor of infancy. It may be asymptomatic but usually is associated with fever, diarrhea, anemia, and lethargy. Metabolically, catecholamines can be produced by the tumor, leading to elevated VMA, meta-nephrine, and normetanephrine levels in the urine. These are helpful laboratory guides in the differential diagnosis of abdominal masses in infants. The plain film of the abdomen and intravenous pyelogram are also helpful with the differential diagnosis of infantile abdominal masses. In particular, it is necessary to differentiate between Wilms' tumor and neuroblastoma. Neuroblastomas are more often calcified, with a fine stippled calcification most characteristic; Wilms' tumor is rarely calcified. Neuroblastomas displace the kidney; Wilms' tumor dis-torts the collecting system of the kidney. Neuroblastomas invade the bone marrow and flat bones of the skull; Wilms' tumor more often spreads to the lungs.

Therapy of neuroblastoma includes operative removal, radiation therapy, and chemotherapy. Surgical removal, even incomplete remov-al, should be attempted because these tumors have been known to regress in size or mature to a more benign form after any operative procedure. The reason for this action is unknown. Various chemother-apeutic agents such as actinomycin D, vincristine, cyclophosphamide, and amethopterin have been tried with varying degrees of success. Combinations of these agents in association with radiation and opera-tion are being used by many investigative groups. In spite of vigorous therapy, the prognosis of neuroblastoma is poor, with less than 30 per cent of patients surviving five years.

PHEOCHROMOCYTOMA

The functioning cells of the adrenal medulla are the chromaffin cells. Tumors of these cells are known as pheochromocytomas and are rare. Because chromaffin cells lie along the aorta in addition to being in the adrenal medulla, 10 per cent of pheochromocytomas are outside the adrenal glands. Pheochromocytomas have occurred in the bladder, mediastinum, and brain. Ten per cent may be bilateral and multiple; this is especially true in children. They may also be associated with malignancies of other endocrine organs, such as the parathyroid and thyroid, and there appears to be a familial distribution for these tumors.

Pheochromocytomas cause hypertension. Classically, the hyperten-sion is episodic, occurring at intervals and associated with sweating, tachycardia, and flushing. However, this is present in less than one half of the patients with this tumor. Most patients have sustained hyperten-sion so that pheochromocytoma must be differentiated from other causes of hypertension since it represents a curable cause of hyperten-sion. Other symptoms include palpitation, excess of sweating, head-aches, and tremulousness. The patient is often underweight because of the increased metabolic rate caused by the catecholamines. No distinct clinical signs are usually seen. A palpable tumor is rare. Suggestive signs include fluctuation of the blood pressure taken over a period of time and orthostatic hypotension. An abnormal glucose tolerance curve is often found. If the diagnosis is suspected, the catecholamines metanephrine, normetanephrine, and VMA are measured in the urine. If the levels of all are elevated, the diagnosis is confirmed. All of these urinary products should be measured, since relying on one often can be misleading (see Table 16–7). Pharmacologic tests with histamine and phentolamine were used in the past, but because the results produced were often dangerous, unreliable, and inaccurate, they should not be used today.

Once the diagnosis is confirmed, attempts to control the symptoms with alpha and beta adrenergic blocking agents is an important preoperative adjunct. Many of the diagnostic studies utilized for localization of the tumor and the stress of operation can cause hypertensive crises or death if prior control of the pharmacologic effects of pheochromocytoma have not been obtained. Phenoxybenzamine blocks the alpha adrenergic effects of epinephrine and norepinephrine and allows replacement and re-expansion of the contracted extracellular fluid volume. A patient begins on 10 mg every 12 hours, and the dosage is increased until the cardiovascular manifestations are controlled. If cardiac arrhythmias are present, a beta adrenergic blocker, propranolol (10 to 40

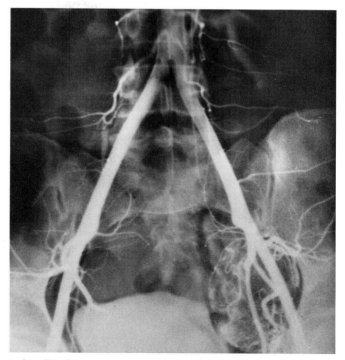

Figure 16–11 Angiogram of a pheochromocytoma involving the urinary bladder. This patient developed hypertension with micturition.

mg per day), is used also. With reasonable control of the pharmacologic effects of epinephrine and norepinephrine, one can undertake studies to determine the location of the pheochromocytoma. Since these tumors are not large, they usually do not displace contiguous organs, so that the intravenous pyelogram is often of little help. Abdominal aortography often demonstrates these highly vascular tumors (Fig. 16–11). However, care in performing the procedure is necessary to prevent a crisis. Sampling of venous blood from various levels of the inferior vena cava and analyzing the blood for catecholamines have also been successful in localizing pheochromocytoma.

Although pharmacologic agents can control the symptoms of pheochromocytoma, surgical removal remains the treatment of choice. Since these tumors may be ectopic, an anterior transperitoneal approach is preferred. The anesthesia must be carefully planned and performed. Certain anesthetic agents should be avoided such as cyclopropane and ether, which stimulate sympathetic activity. The patient's vital signs need careful monitoring, and drugs such as phentolamine should be available to control any pharmacologic effects that occur with manipulation of the tumor. The preoperative preparation with alpha and beta adrenergic blockers restores effective blood volume and aids in preventing intra- and postoperative fluctuations in cardiovascular dynamics. The therapy for pheochromocytoma is formidable and should be performed only by experienced personnel familiar with the nuances of the disease. In general the outcome is usually successful.

MISCELLANEOUS LESIONS

Nonfunctioning tumors of the adrenal gland and adrenal cysts occur. Usually, they are found as masses in the upper abdominal quadrants. They have no detectable function and usually are treated by operative removal. Some adrenal cortical carcinomas demonstrate no function. These have a poor prognosis because diagnosis is often late.

SELECTED REFERENCES

Glenn, J. F.: Surgery of the adrenal glands. *In* Glenn, J. F., and Boyce, W. H. (eds.): Urologic Surgery. New York, Hoeber Medical Division, Harper & Row, Pubs., Inc., 1969, pp. 1–36.
  This chapter presents current concepts of various surgical therapeutic approaches to adrenal disease as well as preoperative and postoperative care.
Jenkins, D., and Harrison, J. H.: The adrenals. *In* Campbell, M. F., and Harrison, J. H. (eds.): Urology. 3rd ed. Philadelphia, W. B. Saunders Company, 1970, pp. 2663–2762.
  This chapter in the standard urologic text offers a broad exposure to adrenal physiology, pathophysiology, manifestations, and therapy of adrenal diseases.
Thorn, G. W.: Symposium on the adrenal cortex. Am. J. Med., 53:529, 1972.
  This multiauthored symposium presents the current understanding of the physiology and pathophysiology of steroids and the adrenal cortex.
Williams, R. H. (ed.): Textbook of Endocrinology. 5th ed. Philadelphia, W. B. Saunders Company, 1974.

This multiauthored text is the standard reference in endocrinology. In addition to specific chapters about the adrenal gland, there are chapters concerning the pituitary gland and concepts of the organization and control of endocrine systems. An excellent list of references is appended to each chapter to assist the interested reader.

Wintrobe, M. M. et al. (eds.): Harrison's Principles of Internal Medicine. 7th ed. New York, McGraw Hill Book Company, 1974.
This reference text in internal medicine contains excellent chapters on endocrinology, especially the adrenal gland. It has excellent references at the end of each chapter.

REFERENCES

Beierwaltes, W. H. et al.: Visualization of human adrenal glands in vivo by scintillation scanning. J.A.M.A., *216*:275, 1971.

Bongiovanni, A. M., and Root, A. W.: The adreno-genital syndrome. N. Engl. J. Med., *268*:1283, 1342, 1391, 1963.

Conn, J. W., et al.: Preoperative diagnosis of primary aldosteronism. Arch. Intern. Med., *123*:113, 1969.

Egdahl, R. H.: Surgery of the adrenal glands. N. Engl. J. Med., *278*:939, 1968.

Engelman, H.: Principles in the diagnosis of pheochromocytoma. Bull. N. Y. Acad. Med., *45*:851, 1969.

Forsham, P. H.: Abnormalities of the adrenal cortex. Clin. Symp., *15*:315, 1963.

Gifford, R. W., Jr. et al.: Clinical features, diagnosis and treatment of pheochromocytoma: A review of 76 cases. Mayo Clin. Proc., *39*:281, 1964.

Glenn, F., and Mannix, H.: Diagnosis and prognosis of Cushing's syndrome. Surg. Gynecol. Obstet., *126*:762, 1971.

Harrison, T. S., Bartlett, J. D., Jr., and Seaton, J. F.: Current evaluation and management of pheochromocytoma. Ann. Surg., *168*:701, 1968.

Hutter, A. M., Jr., and Kayhoe, D. E.: Adrenal cortical carcinoma. Results of treatment with o,p'DDD in 138 patients. Am. J. Med., *41*:581, 1966.

Melby, J. C.: Assessment of adrenocortical function. N. Engl. J. Med., *285*:735, 1971.

O'Malley, B. W.: Mechanism of action of steroid hormones. N. Engl. J. Med., *284*:370, 1971.

Orth, D. N., and Liddle, G. W.: Results of treatment in 108 patients with Cushing's syndrome. N. Engl. J. Med., *285*:243, 1971.

Ross, E. J. et al.: Preoperative and operative management of patients with pheochromocytoma. Br. Med. J., *9*:191, 1967.

Wurtman, R. J.: Catecholamines. N. Engl. J. Med., *273*:637, 693, 746, 1965.

Chapter Seventeen

RENOVASCULAR HYPERTENSION

Ralph A. Straffon

The potential curability of hypertension secondary to unilateral renal disease has evoked widespread clinical interest since the classical experiments of Goldblatt in 1934. Renal lesions associated with hypertension may be parenchymal, perinephric, or vascular in type; they may be unilateral or bilateral and can occur singly or in combinations. These are the clinical counterparts of the experimental hypertension caused by cellophane perinephritis, nephrotoxic serum hepatitis, and renal artery narrowing produced by clamps or silver clips.

Since 1934 many efforts have been made to answer the fundamental question regarding participation of the kidney in systemic hypertension and the diagnosis of curable renal causes of hypertension in patients. Although a great deal of progress has been made in this area, a gap still exists in our knowledge. This discussion is limited to renovascular causes of hypertension, the clinical findings that suggest this disease, the diagnosis, evaluation, and selection of patients for operation, and the results that can be expected from appropriate therapy.

CAUSES

Experimental Renovascular Hypertension

Partial obstruction of the arterial supply to one or both kidneys by a silver clamp results in hypertension which begins in 24 to 72 hours and reaches its maximum level in about seven days. Unilateral constriction of the renal artery alone has rarely produced permanent hypertension in the dog unless combined with a contralateral nephrectomy. Removal of the constriction to the renal artery usually results in normotension, provided the hypertension has not been present more than six to eight weeks.

Cellophane wrapping of the whole kidney and partial infarction of the kidney by occlusion of a branch of the renal artery also produces hypertension in the experimental animal. Total infarction of the kidney is rarely associated with sustained hypertension as there must be some surviving tissue around the area of infarct, abnormal as it may be, to produce a pressor response.

In general, the severity of pathologic changes in the kidney distal to the point of arterial obstruction parallels the degree of obstruction and the severity of the hypertension. There are usually some atrophic but viable tubules or areas of definite infarction that are surrounded by areas of atrophic but viable tubular cells.

Renal Pressor System

In 1939 it was discovered that the pressor activity of the kidney was the result of a chemical reaction that culminated in the production of a polypeptide with potent vasoconstrictor properties that was called angiotensin. Through the efforts of a number of investigators in recent years, the interrelationship of the renin-angiotensin system has been elucidated.

Renin is a proteolytic enzyme secreted by the kidney. Evidence now suggests that renin is secreted by the juxtaglomerular apparatus. An abundance of granules in the juxtaglomerular apparatus closely parallels the secretion of renin, and the amount of renin available, if it is extracted from the kidney, is directly related to the number of granules in the cytoplasm of the juxtaglomerular cell (J.G. cells). In addition to this observation, it has been shown that fluorescein-labeled renin antibodies localize only in the cytoplasm of the juxtaglomerular cells.

Renin splits a plasm substrate, an alpha 2-globulin, to form a decapeptide called angiotensin I, a substance with virtually no pressor activity. Angiotensin I is converted to the octapeptide angiotensin II by the cleavage of the dipeptide histadyl-leucine. This conversion to angiotensin II, a potent vasopressor, takes place in the pulmonary circulation.

It is now well established that angiotensin II is the principal aldosterone stimulating hormone in man, although the potassium ion and ACTH also have a stimulatory effect.

The control of renin production by the kidney is not fully understood. Two theories are generally most widely accepted: (1) that the juxtaglomerular apparatus serves as a renal baroceptor sensitive to mean changes in arterial blood pressure and (2) that the sodium load to the macula densa is detected and that there is a reciprocal relation between sodium load and renin release (e.g., the less sodium presented to the macula densa the more renin released).

In renal artery stenosis renal blood flow is reduced, and the renal sensor, e.g., juxtaglomerular apparatus, interprets this reduction to represent an effective lowered blood volume. This stimulates release of renin that results in the production of increased amounts of angiotensin II. The increased angiotensin II stimulates peripheral vasoconstriction and aldosterone production. Aldosterone stimulates the kidney to increase its sodium and water reabsorption in an attempt to increase blood volume. The presence of renal artery stenosis continues to produce a decreased renal blood flow, interrupting the normal feedback mechanism that would normally decrease renin output; thus, renin production continues, resulting in hypertension.

Patients with untreated essential hypertension usually do not have elevated plasma renin activity. In malignant hypertension the renin production may be normal or elevated, and in renal artery stenosis renin production is usually increased.

In a functioning aldosteronoma, excess aldosterone excretion results in increased reabsorption of salt and water by the kidneys that produces an effective expanded blood volume. The renal sensor mechanism responds to this expanded volume by decreasing the renin production, but the interruption in the feedback loop here is due to the autonomously functioning adrenal tumor, which simply continues to produce aldosterone in spite of a decrease in the levels of renin and angiotensin II in the plasma. The low plasma renin levels found in a hypertensive patient with primary aldosteronism is an important diagnostic finding.

Very high renin levels are found in patients with cirrhosis, in Bartter's syndrome, in which high levels of renin and aldosterone are found in the absence of hypertension, and in renin-producing juxtaglomerular cell tumors. A working classification of reninism in patients with and without hypertension is presented in Table 17–1.

Although the renal pressor system has been the subject of a great

TABLE 17–1   Classification of Reninism °

WITH HYPERTENSION	WITHOUT HYPERTENSION
Primary Reninism	*Primary Reninism*
Juxtaglomerular cell tumor	Not yet described
Some Wilms' tumors	
Other neoplasms (not yet described)	
Secondary Reninism	*Secondary Reninism*
Accelerated (malignant) hypertension	Sodium and water depletion
Stenosis of renal artery	Dieting
(or one of its branches)	Sodium-losing nephropathy
	Chronic diarrhea states
	Adrenal cortical insufficiency
	Hepatic cirrhosis with ascites
	Nephrosis with edema
	Congestive cardiac failure
	Bartter's syndrome (diffuse juxtaglomerular
	cell hyperplasia)

°Adapted from Conn, J. W., et al.: The syndrome of hypertension, hyperreninemia and secondary aldosteronism associated with renal juxtaglomerular cell tumor (primary reninism). Trans. Am. Assoc. Genitourin. Surg., *64*:47, 1972.

deal of research, there is also evidence that the kidney may produce an antipressor substance and that hypertension may result when it is lacking. Arterial blood pressure tends to rise in bilateral nephrectomized patients and is returned to normal with a successful renal allograft.

CLINICAL FEATURES

Hypertension associated with renal artery disease has some clinical characteristics which help to sort out these patients from the large number of patients with hypertension. In order to determine the clinical features of renal hypertension, patients with known essential hypertension were compared with a group of patients with renovascular hypertension cured by surgery.

Age and Sex. Patients with renovascular hypertension are more often over 50 years of age than those with essential hypertension. Any patient less than 35 years of age with hypertension should be carefully evaluated to search for a correctable cause of the hypertension, such as renovascular disease, pheochromocytoma, or primary aldosteronoma.

There is little difference in the incidence of renovascular disease based on sex except that arteriosclerotic renal artery lesions are more prominent in the male and fibrous dysplasia of the renal artery occurs more frequently in the female. Renovascular hypertension appears to be less frequently encountered in black patients.

Duration of Hypertension. Hypertension of sudden onset suggests some definable cause such as a renovascular lesion. A history of long-standing elevated blood pressure is more often seen with essential hypertension but can also be present in renovascular hypertension.

Family History. A negative family history for hypertension in patients less than 35 years of age is as common in patients with essential hypertension as in those with renovascular hypertension. However, in patients over 35 there is more apt to be a family history of hypertension in patients with essential hypertension.

Change in the Severity of the Hypertension. A sudden increase in the severity of pre-existing hypertension is often seen in patients with renal hypertension. This is particularly true in older patients with arteriosclerosis of the renal artery.

Malignant Hypertension. Malignant hypertension may develop as frequently in patients with essential hypertension as in those patients with renovascular hypertension. The poor outlook for this group of patients with medical treatment makes it important to study these patients carefully to look for a correctable cause of the hypertension.

Retinopathy. Progressive retinopathy does not always accompany renovascular hypertension. Severe retinopathy (grade 3 or 4) is found more frequently in patients with arteriosclerotic renal artery disease than in those patients with fibrous renal artery lesions.

Abdominal Bruit. A most helpful physical finding in patients with renovascular lesions is a bruit heard best in the mid-epigastrium. The bruit may be transmitted to either side of the midline. The bruit is due to the turbulence of flow produced by the obstructive lesion in the renal artery.

DIAGNOSIS

UROGRAM

Intravenous pyelography should be performed on all hypertensive patients. The contrast material should be rapidly injected and films made at intervals of one, two, three, five, ten, fifteen, and thirty minutes. Laminagrams of just the renal area should be obtained at the time of the one, two, and three minute films to aid in definition of renal size and in the appearance time of the contrast material. The clinician should look carefully for one or more of the urographic abnormalities described below, which are found in patients with renovascular hypertension.

Disparity in Renal Size. Significant disparity in renal size should be considered when the left kidney is more than 1.5 cm shorter or 2.0 cm longer than the right kidney. Renal contour can be evaluated on the laminagrams to look for cortical scarring, which may be an indication of a segmental vascular lesion.

Disparity in Calyceal Appearance Time. A disparity of one minute or more in the calyceal appearance of the contrast material or an obvious increase in the amount of contrast material in one kidney as compared with the other on the early films of the urogram suggests a significant disparity in the renal handling of the contrast material.

Disparity in Concentration. A major physiologic consequence of renal artery stenosis is the increased renal tubular reabsorption of salt and water on the affected side. This results in an increased concentration of the contrast material during the urogram that is usually observed in the later films of the intravenous pyelogram. The entire collecting system may also be smaller due to the decreased volume of urine passing through the collecting system on the side of the vascular lesion.

Ureteric Notching. Small ureteric indentations due to collateral vessels may sometimes be seen, particularly in the area of the upper ureter.

In interpreting the findings of the properly performed intravenous pyelogram, the presence of one or more of the major findings listed above would be an indication for further evaluation to determine if a renovascular lesion is a factor in hypertension. Table 17–2 shows the incidence of abnormal urograms in various reported series of patients with essential hypertension as compared with patients with proven renovascular hypertension. This confirms the value of the urogram in screening hypertensive patients for renovascular hypertension.

TABLE 17-2   Comparison of Urographic Abnormalities in Various Reported Series

SERIES	ESSENTIAL HYPERTENSION		RENOVASCULAR HYPERTENSION	
	Number of Cases	*Per Cent Abnormal*	*Number of Cases*	*Per Cent Abnormal*
Cooperative Study	771	11.4	138	83
Maxwell et al. (1964)	121	17	42	93
Wilson et al. (1963)	127	8	128	72
Stewart et al. (1962)	105	25	22	86
Totals	1124		330	

RADIOISOTOPE RENOGRAM

The chief advantages of the renogram are its simplicity and safety and the fact that it can compare the renal handling of I 131-labeled orthoiodohippurate (Hippuran) by the two kidneys. The normal renogram has three basic phases: the initial rapid uptake by the kidney (vascular phase), the handling of the radioisotope material by the nephron (secretory phase), and the disappearance of the radioactive material from the kidney (excretory phase). In normal subjects the curves obtained simultaneously over the two kidneys should be similar.

There is no characteristic pattern of the renogram curve which serves to differentiate renal artery stenosis from renal parenchymal disease. The curve tends to be abnormal on the involved side in unilateral main renal artery disease but may be confusing in segmental and bilateral renal artery lesions. There is a high rate of false-positive curves (around 20 per cent) in the essential hypertension group and even more important are the false-negative curves that may be seen in the presence of a significant lesion of the renal artery.

The renogram should not be used as a screening test for patients with renovascular hypertension. Its main utility is that it is a reasonably good way to determine the function of the two kidneys preoperatively, and this result can be used as a control to compare with a postoperative renogram to be sure that the operative procedure to revascularize the involved kidney has been sucessful. There are now available more sophisticated ways of using radioactive materials to determine renal blood flow using the Anger camera and the computer. These techniques may prove to be more useful as screening tests for renovascular disease in hypertensive patients.

RENAL ANGIOGRAPHY

Renal angiography is the only available method for detecting the anatomic lesions that involve the renal arteries. Renal hypertension can be associated with lesions in the main renal artery, which includes the primary branches of the renal artery as well as segmental vessels. In addition, segmental or diffuse renal parenchymal disease (e.g., arteriolar nephrosclerosis) may produce hypertension of renal origin. The only technique of angiography that gives sufficient detail to identify the various lesions of the renal vasculature is selective renal angiography (percutaneous puncture of the femoral artery). Radiographs must be obtained initially in the aorta in the region of the renal arteries in order to visualize the takeoff of each renal artery and the number of renal arteries present on each side. Then, selective catheterization of each renal artery is carried out with radiographs made in both the anteroposterior and the oblique projections. This technique permits visualization of all segments of the blood supply to the kidney, eliminating the confusion produced by the simultaneous visualization of extrarenal arteries, such as the superior mesenteric artery and celiac axis, which overlie the renal blood supply.

Current indications for selective renal angiography in a patient with hypertension are listed in Table 17–3. Using this list of indications, one is unlikely to miss studying a hypertensive patient who may have an underlying renovascular lesion.

CLASSIFICATION OF RENAL ARTERY DISEASE

An updated classification of renal artery disease, based on the histologic examination of resected surgical specimens, is presented in Table 17–4. A correlation has been made between the angiographic findings and the histologic characteristics of the various renal artery lesions. It is now possible to predict with reasonable accuracy a pathologic lesion involving the renal artery from the selective renal angiogram. There are two basic disease processes that affect the renal vascular system, namely, atherosclerosis and the fibrous dysplasias.

Atherosclerosis

This is still the most frequent lesion involving the renal artery that produces hypertension and is the disease that causes renovascular hypertension in about 60 per cent of patients with renal hypertension. Two basic lesions are usually found; in about one third of the patients there is a circumferential plaque producing stenosis, and in the

TABLE 17–3 Indications for Selective Renal Angiography
in a Hypertensive Patient

Abnormal hypertensive urogram
Abrupt onset of hypertension in patient over 35 years of age
Malignant hypertension
Sudden acceleration of pre-existing hypertension
Hypertensive patient with diffuse arteriosclerosis
All hypertensive patients less than 35 years of age
Presence of an epigastric bruit

TABLE 17–4   Classification of Renal Artery Disease

Atherosclerosis
Fibrous Dysplasias
   Intimal
      Primary Intimal Fibroplasia
      Secondary Intimal Fibroplasia
   Medial
      Medial Hyperplasia
      Medial Fibroplasia with Aneurysms
      Perimedial Fibroplasia
      Medial Dissection
        Isolated
        With Intimal Fibroplasia
   Adventitial
      Periarterial Fibroplasia

remaining patients the plaque is eccentric. With both types of lesions, thrombosis or dissection into the media of the renal artery can complicate the disease process with a loss of function in the involved kidney.

Renal arteriography shows these lesions to occur primarily in the first 2 cm of the renal artery. Poststenotic dilatation is common, and the disease is often bilateral (Fig. 17–1). Since atherosclerosis is a systemic disease, the aorta and other extrarenal vessels (e.g., coronary and carotid arteries) may also be involved to a significant degree.

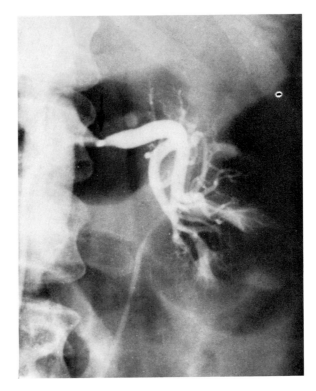

Figure 17–1 Angiographic appearance of an arteriosclerotic plaque involving the takeoff of the left renal artery.

Fibrous Dysplasia of the Renal Artery

This group of lesions accounts for about 40 per cent of the renal vascular lesions producing hypertension. They may be grouped into intimal, medial, and adventitial lesions.

INTIMAL LESIONS

Primary Intimal Fibroplasia. This accounts for about 10 per cent of the fibrous lesions that involve the renal arteries. The lesion consists of a circumferential mass of primitive collagen tissue within the internal elastic membrane, compromising the lumen of the vessel. Disruption and reduplication of the internal elastic membrane occurs more frequently in younger patients. This lesion may involve other arteries of the body as well. It is usually a lesion that progresses in severity, with dissection into the media a frequent complication.

Renal angiography reveals a smooth, tapering lesion, usually involving the midportion of the renal artery, and the disease may extend into the branches. The characteristic angiographic lesion is shown in Figure 17–2.

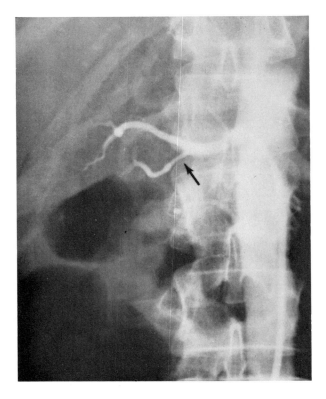

Figure 17–2 Angiographic appearance of primary intimal fibroplasia involving a major branch of the right renal artery.

Secondary Intimal Fibroplasia.   This occurs under a wide variety of circumstances. It can be produced by inflammatory reaction, and such intimal thickening is a prominent feature of rejection in renal transplantation. This lesion is prominent in certain patients with malignant hypertension.

MEDIAL LESIONS

Medial hyperplasia was initially called fibromuscular hyperplasia and is the only lesion seen producing renal artery stenosis where hypertrophy of muscle and fibrous tissue occurs in the media. This lesion was first seen in a young boy with bilateral renal artery stenosis, but it also occurs in young women. In some cases there may be a disruption of the internal elastic membrane with a resulting intramural hematoma.

Angiographically, this lesion usually appears as a small, tight stenosis of the main renal artery or its branches and may be difficult to distinguish from primary intimal fibroplasia. It is the least common of the lesions which cause renal hypertension, accounting for only 2 to 3 per cent of the fibrous lesions.

Medial Fibroplasia with Aneurysms.   This is one of the most common of the fibrous lesions (accounting for 75 to 80 per cent of these lesions) and occurs most often in young women. Microscopically, the lesion is best seen with the artery sectioned longitudinally, showing alternating areas of fibrous thickening and areas of destruction of the media. The internal elastic membrane is focally thinned and absent in the areas where medial destruction occurs, producing a series of microaneurysms lined only by the external elastic membrane. The lesion resists dissection and rupture and has not produced thrombosis of the renal artery.

On renal angiography the lesions produce a "string of beads" appearance, which many authors have termed fibromuscular hyperplasia (Fig. 17–3). It involves the distal portion of the renal artery and its branches and is frequently bilateral. The aneurysms themselves are greater in diameter than the normal renal artery proximal to the disease, and this is an important point in differentiating this disease angiographically from perimedial fibroplasia. Extensive collateral vessels are rarely seen. The areas of stenosis are often overshadowed by the contrast material in the aneurysms, making the degree of the actual stenosis difficult to assess. The disease tends to be progressive in patients less than 40 years of age but appears to be "burned out" and not progressive in older patients.

Perimedial Fibroplasia.   This lesion is a tightly stenotic one produced by a dense collar of collagen tissue deposited at the outer border of the media within the external elastic membrane. In some areas the fibrous tissue may completely replace the media. The lesion occurs predominantly in women between the ages of 15 and 30 and constitutes about 10 to 15 per cent of all the fibrous lesions.

The arteriogram often gives the appearance of "beading," but

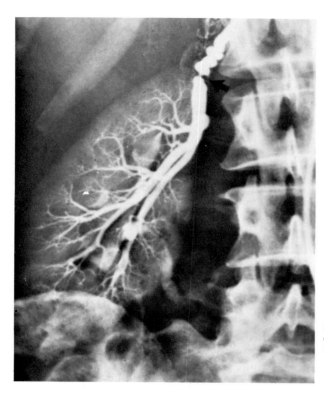

Figure 17–3   Selective renal angiogram of medial fibroplasia with aneurysms involving the right renal artery.

careful inspection shows that the areas of dilation do not exceed the diameter of the normal renal artery (Fig. 17–4). This finding plus the frequent occurrence of extensive collateral vessels helps differentiate this lesion from medial fibroplasia with aneurysms on renal angiography.

Medial Dissection.   This may occur independently of any underlying disease of the renal artery. It may result from a defect in the internal elastic membrane, which allows blood to escape into the medial, producing a hematoma. A clot may then be produced within the lumen of the artery with eventual organization by fibrous tissue or the dissection may re-enter the lumen of the renal artery at a more distal site, thus maintaining a blood supply to the affected kidney.

Dissection of this type can also be associated with primary intimal fibroplasia. The dissection in these patients occurs distal to the primary lesion and is produced by the jet stream of blood that results from the primary stenosis.

ADVENTITIAL LESIONS

Periarterial Fibroplasia.   This is a rare fibrous lesion of the renal artery that is produced by an inflammatory reaction in the adventitia

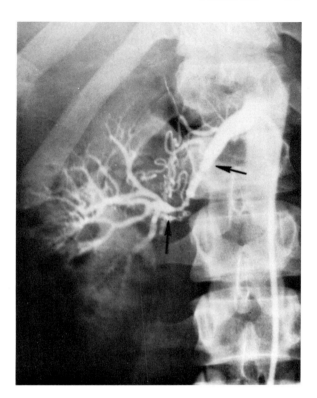

Figure 17–4 Perimedial fibroplasia as seen on an angiogram of the right renal artery. Note the extensive collateral circulation.

and is similar to that seen in retroperitoneal fibrosis. This lesion has not been encountered in the author's experience with the surgical treatment of renal hypertension.

DETERMINATION OF THE SIGNIFICANCE OF RENAL ARTERY LESIONS IN PRODUCING HYPERTENSION

It is well known that stenosis of the renal artery can be present without hypertension and that surgical repair of an existing renal artery stenosis in a hypertensive patient does not always result in a cure or improvement of the hypertension. One research group found that 53 per cent of 295 normotensive and hypertensive subjects studied at autopsy had a 25 per cent or greater narrowing of the lumen of the renal arteries as a result of atherosclerosis. Such lesions were found in 49 per cent of normotensive patients and in 77 per cent of hypertensive patients. It is thus essential that once a renal artery lesion is demonstrated in the hypertensive patient additional studies must be done to determine if repairing the lesion can cure or improve the hypertension. Tests that have been used to evaluate the significance of these lesions are shown in Table 17–5.

TABLE 17–5   Tests Used in Determining the Significance of Renal Artery Lesions in Hypertensive Patients

Excretory Function Tests
    Urogram
        Rapid sequence
    Renogram
    Split function tests
Pressor Substances
    Renin assays
        Peripheral
        Renal vein
    Juxtaglomerular cell counts
Pressure Gradients
    Phonorenogram
    Direct measurement
Status of the Renal Parenchyma
    Renal biopsy

Excretory Function Tests

UROGRAM

The rapid sequence intravenous pyelogram is used as a screening test for renal vascular disease in the hypertensive population. The major urographic abnormalities seen, i.e., decrease in renal size, delayed appearance time of the contrast material, and late hyperconcentration on the involved side, are all based on the physiologic changes produced in the kidney by renal artery stenosis. These include a decreased renal blood flow, a decreased glomerular filtration rate, an increased reabsorption of salt and water by the renal tubules, and a decreased transit time of contrast material through the kidney.

In the recent report of the cooperative study of renal hypertension, the use of these major urographic features had no significance in predicting preoperatively the group of patients who responded favorably and those who did not respond favorably to surgical treatment. Of those responding favorably to surgical treatment, 83 per cent had one or more urographic abnormalities, while 81 per cent of those failing to respond to surgical treatment also had one or more abnormalities. The urogram is therefore not a good prognosticator for the results that may be obtained in the surgical treatment of a renovascular lesion.

RENOGRAM

The renogram is usually abnormal in unilateral main renal artery lesions but is of little value in bilateral segmental disease. It has not been found useful in predicting the success of renovascular surgery.

INDIVIDUAL FUNCTION TESTS

In dogs, partial occlusion of one main renal artery produces a decreased urine volume, decreased urine sodium, and increased urine osmolarity from the affected side. However, if the number of functioning nephrons is decreased by complete occlusion of the renal artery or parenchymal renal disease, such as glomerulonephritis, a decreased urine volume and urine osmolarity results. These experiments suggest that differences in renal function would be found in hypertensive patients with occlusive renal artery disease, depending on whether the occlusion was in the main renal artery, in a branch of the renal artery, or in a small vessel in the parenchyma.

Various techniques have evolved for doing "split" renal function studies. The criteria for abnormalities with these techniques are shown in Table 17–6. Technically good "split" function tests are time-consuming and are frequently associated with morbidity. Some institutions[*] have not used this test for several years because, although the test is usually reliable in the majority of patients with unilateral main renal artery stenosis, it is of little value in branch lesions or bilateral renal artery lesions. In addition, a significant number of patients with unilateral main renal artery disease who had a negative (false-negative) split function study were cured by surgery; false-positive results have also been reported.

TABLE 17–6   Criteria for Abnormality of "Split" Function Test

STAMEY	HOWARD	RAPOPORT
Urine volume 50 per cent	Urine volume 50 per cent	T.R.F.R.[°°] =
PAH[°] concentration in urine: 100 per cent or more on side of renal artery lesion	Na$^+$ concentration in urine: 15 per cent or more on side of renal artery lesion	$\dfrac{\text{Left } U_{Na} \times \text{Right } U_{Cr}}{\text{Left } U_{Cr} \times \text{Right } U_{Na}}$ Normal: 0.6 to 1.5

[°]Para-aminohippuric acid.
[°°]Tubular reabsorption fraction ratio.

Renal Pressor Substance

If renal hypertension is caused by the release of renin from the involved kidney, measurement of the amount released and comparison with the contralateral side should be a good predictive test for the results that may be obtained with surgical repair of the renal artery lesions.

Peripheral Vein Renin Activity. The measurement of peripheral vein renin has not been a good prognosticator of the results that may be obtained in the treatment of renal hypertension. In a series[†] of 29 patients with proven renal hypertension treated surgically, the predictive accuracy of peripheral vein renin was only 46 per cent.

Bilateral Renal Vein Renins. Sampling of blood from each renal

[°]Specifically, the Cleveland Clinic.
[†]The author's.

vein and from the vena cava can be performed after selective renal angiography. The ratio of the renal vein renin on the involved side to the renal vein renin on the contralateral side is determined. A ratio of 1.5 or higher is believed to be significant. The output of renin from the involved kidney can be stimulated prior to renal vein sampling by use of a low sodium diet for two or three days or a diuretic (e.g., ethacrynic acid), plus having the patient in the upright position several hours prior to the study. When the renal vein renin was elevated above normal on the involved side and the ratio was greater than 1.5, the predictive value of this particular test varied from 71 per cent to as high as 100 per cent in various series reported in the literature. In the author's experience the best results were obtained when the ratio of the involved side to the contralateral side was greater than 1.5, and the peripheral vein renin was also elevated above the normal value. These renin determinations should not be used as an absolute guide in the selection of patients for surgical revascularization, since good results can be obtained in patients with a renal artery stenosis who do not have significant vein renin ratios.

Juxtaglomerular Cell Counts. These have been reported to have some predictive value but require a good-sized biopsy specimen of the kidney to do the study. Such cell counts are not widely employed in the preoperative evaluation of patients with renovascular hypertension.

Pressure Gradients across the Stenosis in the Renal Artery

Phonorenogram. The measurement of transmitted renal artery pulse pressure in the renal pelvis using a cardiac photocatheter has been done preoperatively in a number of patients. It is the only way to estimate the pressure gradient across a renal artery stenosis prior to the operative procedure. It has been abandoned as a useful study in renal hypertension.

Direct Measurement of Pressure Gradients. Measurement may be done at the operating table both before and after revascularization of the kidney. If the gradient is above 40 mm of mercury, it is probably significant stenosis. The greatest value of this procedure, however, has been to determine if the surgical repair has eliminated any pressure gradient.

Status of Renal Parenchyma

Although preoperative bilateral renal biopsies to determine the presence and severity of arteriolar nephrosclerosis have been advocated, they are seldom used clinically. In nearly all cases, the severity of arteriolar sclerosis is greater on the contralateral side, suggesting that the renal artery stenosis had a protective effect on the small vessels of the involved kidney.

TREATMENT

Increasing knowledge regarding the natural history of renal artery disease and its response to medical and surgical therapy makes it obvious that not all patients should have operative repair of renal arterial lesions. Renal hypertension usually responds to the same therapeutic regimens that are effective in the treatment of essential hypertension. There are a number of factors that must be considered in selecting a patient with a renal artery lesion for an operation.

Age of Patient.   In general, the older the patient the greater the indication for medical management. The renal artery lesion most frequently seen in patients over 50 years of age is atherosclerosis. This lesion is a part of a generalized vascular disease that affects the arteries of other vital organs, such as the heart and brain, markedly increasing the risk of any operative procedure.

Co-Existing Disease.   Irrespective of the age of the patient, coexisting diseases, such as cerebral coronary insufficiency and hepatic or pulmonary disease may increase the surgical risk to the point that the wisest choice of management would be medical treatment. Greater surgical risks must be accepted, however, when renal function is threatened by the renal artery lesion.

Personality.   Certain patients refuse any operative procedure, while other patients are so unreliable that they would be incapable of following a medical program. Each patient must be assessed individually.

Duration of the Hypertension.   Patients with hypertension of long duration (over three years) generally do not respond as well to surgical treatment, but this should not be held as a strict contraindication to revascularization, since good results have been obtained in patients with long-standing hypertension.

Significance of the Renal Artery Lesion.   Patients with renal artery lesions of doubtful significance should be carefully screened before there is any decision to repair the lesion surgically.

Natural History of the Arterial Lesions.   Since it is possible to predict fairly accurately the type of renal artery lesion on the basis of the angiographic appearance, it is important to know the natural history of the various lesions. This is probably one of the most important factors in determining whether to treat the patient medically or surgically. The author has had the opportunity to follow a group of 88 patients with known renal artery disease of various types for a period of from one to eight years in duration. This experience has given some insight into the natural history of the lesions and has helped develop a general philosophy regarding the management of these lesions.

ATHEROSCLEROSIS.   Thirty-six patients with arteriosclerotic plaques obstructing the renal arteries have been placed on a program of medical management and monitored. One third of these patients have shown progression of disease, but it has been impossible to predict which lesions will progress and which will remain unchanged. Currently, only good risk patients who have a recent onset of hypertension and in whom the diagnostic evaluation suggests a significant renal arterial lesion are operated on. Since this is a systemic disease, the status of the cerebral and coronary circulation must be evaluated, even to the point of cerebral or coronary angiograms if indicated. If technically feasible, surgical repair of either carotid or coronary artery occlusion should take precedence over the renal artery lesion repair. Those patients with long-standing hypertension, evidence of generalized arteriosclerosis, or renal artery lesions of questionable significance do much better with medical management. An operation is advised in this group only if the hypertension cannot be controlled medically or the vascular lesion progresses, producing renal insufficiency.

INTIMAL FIBROPLASIA. This disease progressed in all four patients followed by the author with conservative therapy. Because of the progressive nature of this disease and because it occurs in a younger age group that is generally a good surgical risk, early operative repair is advisable. Revascularization should be the procedure of choice, since the disease may later develop in the contralateral renal artery.

MEDIAL HYPERPLASIA. Radiographically, it is difficult to distinguish this disease from intimal fibroplasia. Two of three patients followed medically showed progression of the disease process, and it is believed that this disease should be managed the same way as intimal fibroplasia, namely, early revascularization.

MEDIAL FIBROPLASIA WITH ANEURYSM. In the author's experience, this lesion occurs most often in women between the ages of 25 and 50. The right renal artery was the only vessel involved in 34 per cent, the left in 6 per cent, and both renal arteries in 60 per cent. Of 41 patients followed two to eight years, progressive arterial lesions developed in only two patients, and both of these were less than 40 years of age. This disease appears to be self-limiting and becomes relatively stable and nonprogressive in the older age group. The lesion does not dissect, thrombose, or cause hemorrhage from rupture of the aneurysm, and the development of ischemic renal atrophy is unlikely to occur in this older age group.

If the hypertension is of recent onset in a good-risk patient with a unilateral renal artery lesion or if the diagnostic evaluation indicates a significant arterial lesion, surgical repair should be performed. In a young, good-risk patient with bilateral disease, the side producing the larger output of renin from the renal vein is repaired first. The contralateral side is later repaired only if the blood pressure cannot be controlled medically. In those patients with bilateral medial fibroplasia who were managed in this manner, the hypertension has either been cured or easily managed medically, and the opposite side has rarely had to be repaired. In the older age group with bilateral disease, especially when the hypertension is of long duration, medical management with antihypertensive drugs is the treatment of choice.

PERIMEDIAL FIBROPLASIA. This lesion occurs chiefly in women 15 to 30 years of age, predominantly involving the right renal artery.

This lesion always progresses and should be surgically repaired, not only to improve the renal hypertension but also to preserve renal function.

Surgical Treatment

Once a patient with renal hypertension has been selected for operative repair, attention must be given to the type of operation which is best suited for the patient. There are a variety of surgical procedures available as indicated in Table 17–7.

SURGICAL APPROACH TO THE KIDNEY

The kidney to be revascularized is approached through a subcostal incision, curving the medial end across the midline (Fig. 17–5, A). The right kidney is exposed by reflecting the hepatic flexure downward and medially, using the Kocher maneuver on the duodenum (Fig. 17–5, B). The left kidney can be exposed by reflecting the splenic flexure of the colon downward and medially (Fig. 17–5, C). The exposure that can be obtained is excellent and can be maintained with the use of the Smith ring retractor (Fig. 17–6).

Nephrectomy. Every attempt is made to salvage a kidney by revascularization procedures. In some cases, the kidney is simply too severely damaged to make salvage possible. In the author's experience, if the involved kidney is less than 9 cm in length and the ischemic process is diffuse rather than localized, nephrectomy is the operative procedure of choice.

Segmental Nephrectomy. This operative procedure is used chiefly in lesions of the branches of the renal artery that produce segmental areas of ischemia. The technique utilized is to identify the arterial branch going to the area to be removed (Fig. 17–7A). This branch is injected with methylene blue to color the area supplied by the branch, or one can simply ligate the branch and note the color change. The capsule is stripped off the area of the kidney to be removed, and the segmental nephrectomy is accomplished by blunt and sharp dissec-

---

TABLE 17–7   Operative Procedures Used in Treating Renal Hypertension

Total nephrectomy
Segmental nephrectomy
Renal revascularization
    Resection and reanastomosis
    Endarterectomy with or without patch graft angioplasty
    Aortorenal reimplantation
    Aortorenal bypass graft
    Sphenorenal arterial shunt
    Autotransplant of the kidney

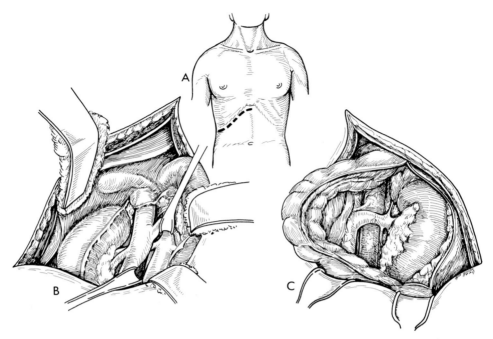

Figure 17–5   Surgical exposure of the kidney through the anterior transabdominal approach. *A*, Right subcostal incision. *B*, Exposure of the right renal artery and aorta by medial mobilization of the duodenum. *C*, Exposure of the left renal artery by mobilization downward of the splenic flexure of the colon.

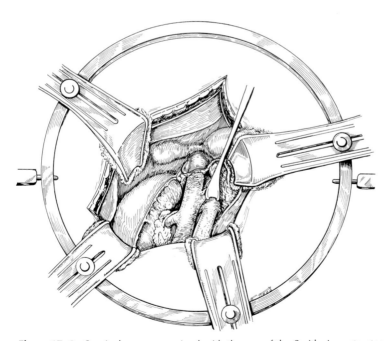

Figure 17–6   Surgical exposure gained with the use of the Smith ring retractor.

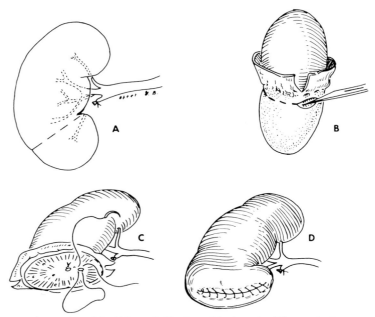

Figure 17–7   Segmental resection of the kidney. *A*, Ligation of the branch of the renal artery supplying the segment of the kidney to be removed. *B*, Stripping of the renal capsule and incision into the renal parenchyma. *C*, Suture ligation of the renal arteries and veins. The collecting system which is opened must also be identified and closed with sutures. *D*, Completed resection of the lower pole of the kidney.

tion (Fig. 17–7, *B*). The exposed collecting system is closed tightly, and bleeding vessels are suture-ligated to control bleeding (Fig. 17–7, *C*). The capsule is then closed over the area (Fig. 17–7, *D*).

RENAL REVASCULARIZATION

Resection and Reanastomosis.   This operative procedure is infrequently used in renal revascularization (Fig. 17–8). It can only be applied to those lesions that are focal in nature, as are sometimes seen in intimal fibroplasia or perimedial fibroplasia, and there the segment in-

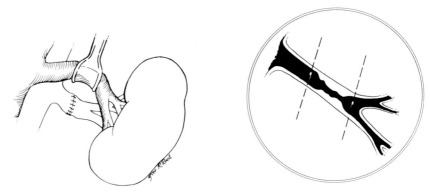

Figure 17–8   Surgical excision of a lesion in the renal artery with end to end reanastomosis.

volved is short enough to allow easy approximation of the renal artery after excision of the diseased segment. There is a tendency to remove as little renal artery as possible in order to facilitate the repair, and hence one is apt to leave some diseased vessel behind after the repair, thus causing a recurrence of stenosis postoperatively.

Endarterectomy with Patch Graft Angioplasty.   This used to be the operation of choice for arteriosclerotic plaque involving the renal artery, and it is still used in selected patients. A patch graft of saphenous vein is sutured into the incision in the renal artery to insure a wide lumen in the area of the endarterectomy (Fig. 17–9). Some surgeons prefer the transaortic approach, particularly when there is bilateral disease, cleaning out both renal arteries through their orifices within the aorta.

Aortorenal Reimplantation.   This operation can be applied only in a few selected cases. The lesion must involve only the take-off or first part of the renal artery, and the renal artery must be of sufficient length that it can be moved downward for reimplantation into the aorta (Fig. 17–10).

Aortorenal Bypass Graft.   The bypass graft is the operative procedure used most frequently by the author to revascularize the kidney and

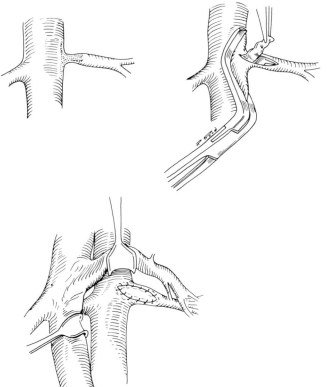

Figure 17–9 Surgical technique of endarterectomy and patch graft angioplasty used in removing an arteriosclerotic plaque in the renal artery.

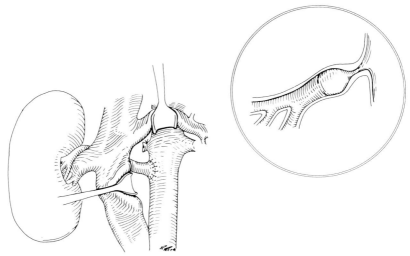

Figure 17–10   Surgical technique of ligation and aortorenal reimplantation of the renal artery.

is the most versatile of the revascularization procedures. Saphenous vein, internal iliac artery, or a synthetic graft may be used for the bypass. The aortic anastomosis is done first, and then the distal end of the graft is sutured to the renal artery distal to the renal artery lesion. This allows a very short ischemia time for the kidney, since the distal anastomosis is usually easy to perform and can be done in a matter of 8 to 10 minutes. The procedure also allows removal of as much of the main renal artery as the surgeon wishes, minimizing the chances of leaving the disease in place. If the disease extends into smaller branches, this problem can sometimes be bypassed with the graft, or if the disease extends into the branches to a degree which makes bypassing the lesions technically impossible, the bypass is sutured to the

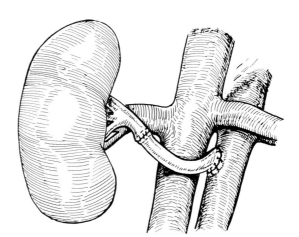

Figure 17–11   Saphenous vein bypass graft.

renal artery as far distally as possible. The distal lesions are then simply dilated by passing sounds of gradually increasing caliber into the vessels involved. This is particularly effective in patients with medial fibroplasia with aneurysms since the branch lesions are easily dilated by the passage of sounds. The bypass graft is usually brought in front of the vena cava, a procedure which facilitates revascularization (Fig. 17–11). The angiographic appearance that follows a saphenous vein bypass graft for the patient with medial fibroplasia with aneurysms (demonstrated in Fig. 17–3) is shown in Figure 17–12.

   Splenorenal Anastomosis.   If the splenic artery is not involved in the same disease process as the renal artery, a splenorenal bypass graft may be done to the left kidney. A segment of splenic artery may also be excised and used as a bypass graft on the right side as well. A splenectomy is usually not required since there is sufficient collateral circulation to keep the spleen viable.

RESULTS OF SURGERY

   The results which can be obtained in the surgical treatment of renal hypertension in various medical centers are summarized in Table

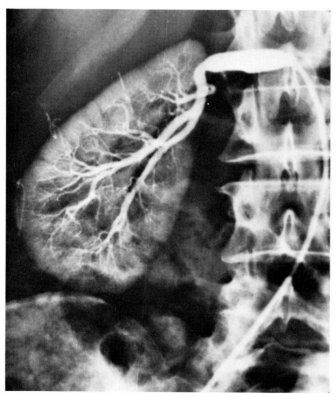

Figure 17–12   The postoperative angiographic appearance of a saphenous vein bypass graft.

TABLE 17–8   Results of Surgery in Renovascular Hypertension

RESEARCH SERIES[*]	NUMBER OF PATIENTS	PER CENT CURED	PER CENT IMPROVED	PER CENT FAILED	PER CENT EXPIRED
1	43	40	42	14	4
2	76	62	26	12	10
3	67	37	45	13	5
4	63	43	26	31	9
5	100	55	29	16	0
6	122	37	28	35	8
7	35	46	31	22	6
8	26	38	41	21	8
Total	532				
Average		50	26	18	6

[*] Listed by senior author:
1. Stewart (Arch. Surg., 85:617, 1962)
2. Dustan (Circulation, 27:1018, 1963)
3. Kaufman (J.A.M.A., 190:709, 1964)
4. Owen (Br. J. Urol., 36:7, 1964)
5. Hunt (Circ. Res., 21:211, 1967)
6. Perloff (Am. Heart J., 74:614, 1969)
7. Foster (Surgery, 60:240, 1966)
8. Baird (Can. Med. Assoc. J., 96:1299, 1967)

17–8. This is not a complete listing but the general averages, for well-selected patients, are as follows: 50 per cent cured, 26 per cent improved, 18 per cent sustained failure. The postoperative mortality was 6 per cent.

These results deal with renal vascular lesions of all types and do not sort out the results that can be obtained with the various types of renal artery lesions.

In a series of 80 patients with arteriosclerotic renal artery lesions, the results were excellent in 39 per cent, improved in 27 per cent and failed in the remaining patients. The operative mortality was 7 per cent, and seven patients died during the follow-up period, which averaged 30 months after treatment, including six patients whose hypertension was cured. Most of these deaths were due to systemic effects of atherosclerosis (e.g., myocardial infarct or cerebrovascular accident). These figures contrast markedly with the results which can be obtained in patients with fibrous dysplasias of the renal artery, since the operative mortality should be less than 1 per cent and a cure or marked improvement in the hypertension can be expected in nearly 90 per cent of well-selected patients treated with one of the surgical procedures.

SELECTED REFERENCES

Goldblatt, H., Lynch, J., Hanzel, R. F., and Summervile, W. W.: Studies in experimental hypertension: I. The production of persistent elevation of systolic blood pressure by means of renal ischemia. J. Exp. Med., 59:347, 1934.
Classical experiments by Goldblatt on the production of renal hypertension in dogs. The experimental counterpart for human renovascular hypertension.

Harrison, E. G., Jr., and McCormack, L. J.: Pathologic classification of renal artery disease in renovascular hypertension. Mayo Clin. Proc., 46:161, 1971.
Histologic description of the current classification of diseases of the renal artery. Emphasis is placed on the pathologic features.

McCormack, L. J., Poutasse, E. F., Meaney, T. F., Noto, T. J., and Dustan, H. P.: A pathologic-arteriographic correlation of renal artery disease. Am. Heart J., 72:188, 1966.
The description of the angiographic features of the various diseases of the renal artery is correlated with the pathologic findings. In most patients it is possible to identify preoperatively the disease process producing renovascular hypertension.

Meaney, T. F., and Dustan, H. P.: Selective renal angiography in the diagnosis of renal hypertension. Circulation, 23:1035, 1963.
An excellent description of the technique and findings on selective renal angiography in renovascular hypertension. Emphasis is placed on the radiographic appearance of the various lesions.

Page, I. H.: On the nature of the pressor action of renin. J. Exp. Med., 70:521, 1939.
The first description of the pressor activity of renin. A classic article in the field of renovascular hypertension.

Seldinger, S. I.: Catheter replacement of the needle percutaneous arteriography. Acta Radiol., 39:368, 1953.
The technique of selective renal angiography, an important advance in the diagnostic methods used for evaluating hypertension.

Stewart, B. H., Dustan, H. P., Kiser, W. S., Meaney, T. F., Straffon, R. A., and McCormack, L. J.: Correlation of angiography and natural history in evaluation of patients with renovascular hypertension. J. Urol., 104:231, 1970.
The knowledge of the natural history of the various diseases affecting the renal artery plays an important role in deciding the best method to use in treating the patient.

REFERENCES

Bookstein, J. J., Abrams, H., Buenger, R. E., et al.: Radiographic aspects of renovascular hypertension: Part I. Aims and methods of the radiology group study. J.A.M.A., 220:1218, 1972.

Bookstein, J. J., Abrams, H., Buenger, R. E., et al.: Radiologic aspects of renovascular hypertension: Part II. The role of urography in unilateral renovascular disease. J.A.M.A., 220:1225, 1972.

Hunt, J. C., Bernatz, P. E., and Harrison, E. G., Jr.: Factors determining diagnosis and choice of treatment of renovascular hypertension. Circ. Res., 21:Suppl. 2:211, 1967.

Hussain, R. A., Gifford, R. W., Jr., Stewart, B. H., et al.: Differential renal vein activity in the diagnosis of renovascular hypertension. Am. J. Cardiol., 32:707, 1973.

Page, I. H.: The production of persistent arterial hypertension by cellophane perinephritis. J. Exp. Med., 70:521, 1939.

Kiser, W. S., Guirguis, A. B., and Straffon, R. A.: Clinical evaluation of the phonorenogram for the diagnosis of occlusive renal artery disease. Trans. Am. Assoc. Genitourin. Surg., 60:150, 1968.

Maxwell, M. H., Gonick, H. C., Weilta, R., and Kaufman, J. J.: Use of rapid sequence intravenous pyelograms in the diagnosis of renovascular hypertension. N. Engl. J. Med., 270:213, 1964.

Simon, N., Franklin, S. S., Bliefer, K. H., and Maxwell, M. H.: Clinical characteristics of renovascular hypertension. J.A.M.A., 220:1209, 1972.

Stamey, T. A.: Renovascular hypertension. Baltimore, Williams & Wilkins Co., 1963.

Vander, A. J.: Control of renin release. Physiol. Rev., 47:359, 1967.

Vidt, D. G., Yutani, F. M., McCormack, L. J., et al.: Surgical treatment of renal vascular disease: Prognostic role of vascular changes in bilateral renal biopsies. Am. J. Cardiol., 30:827, 1972.

Wilson, L., Dustan, H. P., Page, I. H., and Poutasse, E. F.: Diagnosis of renal artery lesions. Arch. Intern. Med., 112:270, 1963.

Chapter Eighteen

MEDICAL MANAGEMENT OF THE HYPERTENSIVE PATIENT

Andrew J. Zweifler

Any discussion of hypertension must begin with a definition of that term. A preferred one states that hypertension is a disease characterized by the sustained elevation of diastolic blood pressure and progressive cardiovascular injury. As far as diastolic pressure is concerned, however, this definition leaves open the question of "how high is high?" This lack of any specific limit is necessary since it has been clearly established that the risk from hypertension is directly related to blood pressure and that this risk extends down into the "normotensive" range. This definition is not intended to imply that systolic hypertension is unimportant. In fact, systolic blood pressure is as reliable as diastolic blood pressure in predicting cardiovascular morbidity and mortality. However, it has not been established that treatment of systolic hypertension reduces morbidity and mortality if the diastolic blood pressure is normal. Similarly, borderline hypertension in young adults is clearly a major predictor of sustained hypertension, but currently there is no evidence to suggest that treatment of patients with this disorder has any significant effect on outcome.

Since there is no cut-off point between normal and high blood pressure, the decision about when to treat is an arbitrary one. It should be based on what is known about the efficacy of treatment of patients at various blood pressure levels and should be modified by considerations such as expected life span at the age of diagnosis. With these qualifications in mind, it is suggested that individuals less than 40 years of age be considered hypertensive if they have diastolic pressures consistently greater than 90 mm Hg and that those over the age of 40 with diastolic pressures greater than 95 mm Hg also be classified as hypertensive. All patients with hypertension should be treated and so should individuals with borderline readings, especially if they also have associated cardiovascular risk factors such as hyperlipidemia or diabetes. Blacks and individuals with a strong family history of hypertension also should be treated for borderline hypertension.

GOALS OF THERAPY

The immediate objective of antihypertensive therapy is the reduction of blood pressure to normal or near normal levels, but in individual cases medication is prescribed with the expectation of a variety of results. These goals of therapy include relief of symptoms, prevention of cardiovascular complications, prevention of acceleration of hypertension, and reversal of complications. Although most patients who are found to be hypertensive have no major complaints, some may be bothered by such symptoms as headaches and "dizzy spells." In such individuals relief of these complaints is an important therapeutic goal. The primary goal of therapy in the majority of individuals with high blood pressure, however, is the prevention of complications, with associated prolongation of useful life. Those conditions which have been shown to be partially preventable are the so-called pressure-related complications such as strokes, heart failure, and renal failure. To date, however, there is no evidence that the frequency of the major arteriosclerosis-related complication, myocardial infarction, is reduced by antihypertensive therapy. A third goal of treatment is the prevention of upward progression of blood pressure. Data from the Veterans' Administration Cooperative Study indicate that this is a reasonable expectation. A final goal, in more advanced cases, is the reversal of complications. Certainly, there is ample evidence that complications such as retinopathy, acute encephalopathy, and hypertensive heart disease are modified or completely reversed by adequate treatment.

ROLE OF DIET

SODIUM

There is no doubt that the sodium ion is an important element in the pathophysiology of high blood pressure. Whether it plays a primary role in the causation of essential hypertension in man, however, is uncertain. Rats which develop hypertension on a high salt diet have been bred, but epidemiologists have had difficulty demonstrating a relationship between sodium intake and blood pressure within human populations. Nevertheless, the amount of salt in the diet of a hypertensive patient under treatment may be of considerable importance. The antihypertensive efficacy of diuretic agents may be blunted by excessive sodium intake, particularly when they are used in combination with sodium-retaining drugs such as vasodilators or guanethidine. Blood pressure control in mild hypertensives being treated with diuretics alone is better when patients are also restricting their sodium intake. As a general rule, patients with high blood pressure should eat a "no-added salt" diet (approximately 4.0 grams NaCl per day).

CALORIES

Epidemiologic studies consistently reveal a positive correlation between weight and blood pressure. In most populations the average blood pressure of obese individuals is higher than that of those with normal weight. There are also data which reveal that blood pressure falls as weight falls during reducing programs for obesity. Although there are some conflicts about this latter point, it is prudent to emphasize weight reduction as part of the management plan of all obese hypertensives. This advice may be of particular value to the obese young adult with borderline hypertension.

HYPERLIPIDEMIA PROBLEM

High blood pressure is more dangerous in patients with hypercholesterolemia and hypertriglyceridemia. It is for this reason that blood lipids are measured routinely during the basic evaluation of patients in the hypertension clinic. If abnormalities are found, they should be treated. Recommendations to such patients invariably involve dietary manipulations with emphasis on total caloric intake, the balance between carbohydrate and fat ingestion, and the kinds of fat in the diet.

IMPORTANCE OF REST AND EXERCISE

Before the availability of specific antihypertensive agents, there was little to do for the patient with high blood pressure other than to place him at rest. Blood pressure declines with rest and falls dramatically during sleep in both normal and hypertensive subjects. It is for this reason that sedatives used to be prescribed for hypertensive patients and that hospitalization with enforced bed rest is still of value in the management of severe cases. But there is no justification for the prescription of sedatives for the control of blood pressure in the ambulatory patient today. Potent antihypertensive agents are available and a major challenge of therapy is keeping patients active with a minimum of drug side effects. Sedatives and tranquilizers are not contraindicated in hypertensive patients but should be used appropriately.

Exercise may be deleterious to the uncontrolled hypertensive because it increases blood pressure and may place undue stress on the heart and blood vessels. Isometric exercise is a particularly potent stimulus in that regard. Patients with sustained diastolic hypertension should be advised to avoid exercise until their blood pressure has returned to normal with treatment. Once the blood pressure is under control, however, exercise should not be restricted unless cardiac function is impaired. The situation may be somewhat different in individuals with borderline hypertension. There is evidence to suggest that physical training may return blood pressure to normal in such patients.

MEDICAL THERAPY OF THE AMBULATORY PATIENT

General Principles

VALUE OF TREATMENT

Evidence now exists indicating that drug therapy can improve the prognosis of the patient with high blood pressure. Initially, such evidence was available only in relation to malignant and severe hypertension. Recent studies have shown that patients with diastolic blood pressures between 105 and 120 mm Hg are also helped. Although solid data relating to those with blood pressures from 90 to 105 mm Hg are not yet available, existing information suggests that their prognosis will be improved by treatment also. The treated hypertensive has a decreased risk of stroke, heart failure, and acceleration of hypertension. Patients need to know these facts, as well as do those who direct their therapy.

HYPERTENSION AS A CHRONIC DISEASE

There is no convincing evidence that hypertension can be cured by medical therapy. Blood pressure can be lowered by antihypertensive agents and prognosis improved if such treatment is maintained over a long period of time, but if therapy is discontinued the blood pressure invariably rises and the disease returns to its destructive course. All patients must be made aware of that fact when they enter into therapy, and it must be continually reinforced both by health care professionals and others who have contact with the patient in everyday life.

IMPORTANCE OF DRUG COMBINATIONS

There are different classes of antihypertensive agents based on mode of action. It is not good practice to discard a drug from one class if it has not produced the desired effect and prescribe another from a different class. Drugs with differing modes of action often complement each other in the treatment of hypertension, usually in an additive manner but sometimes synergistically. Combinations of two, or occasionally three, different kinds of drugs may be required in the resistant patient.

AVOIDANCE OF THE "PATIENT DROP-OUT"

Most people with hypertension are asymptomatic, and all too frequently antihypertensive medications produce side-effects. There is a strong tendency for patients to take less medication than prescribed or to discontinue treatment altogether. Good care requires an active effort on the part of the physician and his staff to counter this tendency. The therapeutic regimen must be kept as simple and inexpensive as possible; the number of tablets and the number of doses prescribed per day should be kept at a minimum. Patients who miss appointments for any reason should be contacted and rescheduled. The value of therapy should be reemphasized regularly.

Antihypertensive Agents

DIURETIC AGENTS

Diuretics lower blood pressure in hypertensive patients, but their exact mode of action is uncertain. Most evidence suggests that it is linked to their natriuretic effects. Recent studies in communities indicate that roughly 50 per cent of all hypertensives can be managed with diuretics alone. A current pathophysiologic model of the hypertensive, which relates elevated blood pressure to either excess intravascular volume or excess vasoconstriction, suggests that the diuretic-responsive hypertensives are those with inappropriately high volume. However, even in resistant patients diuretics augment the blood pressure lowering effects of other classes of agents. Diuretics are therefore the backbone of all antihypertensive therapy. Table 18–1 lists the avail-

TABLE 18–1   Oral Diuretics

DIURETICS	DOSE (mg per day)	
	Usual	Maximal
SULFONAMIDE DERIVATIVE TYPES		
Thiazides		
Chlorothiazide	1000	1000
Flumethiazide	500	1000
Hydrogenated Derivatives		
Hydrochlorothiazide	100	100
Hydroflumethiazide	50	100
Substituted Compounds		
Bendroflumethiazide	5	10
Benzthiazide	50	100
Trichlormethiazide	4	4
Methyclothiazide	5	10
Polythiazide	2	4
Cyclothiazide	2	4
Chlorthalidone	50	100
Quinethazone	100	100
POTASSIUM-SPARING TYPES		
Spironolactone	100	400
Triamterene	200	300
LOOP TYPES		
Furosemide	80	320
Ethacrynic acid	50	100

able oral diuretics. Potent, long-acting drugs which can be administered once daily, such as chlorthalidone and polythiazide, are the most practical.

Metabolic side effects that are most troublesome include hypokalemia and hyperuricemia. Serum potassium concentration falls in almost all patients taking sulfonamide diuretics, but it drops substantially (to less than 3.0 mEq per liter) in less than 10 per cent of patients. It is debatable whether this abnormality should be treated unless it is accompanied by symptoms such as muscle weakness or cramps. A reasonable approach is to attempt to correct hypokalemia only when it is symptomatic or when the serum level falls below 2.5 mEq per liter. Hypokalemia should not be allowed to develop at all in patients taking digitalis preparations. A simple way to cope with the hypokalemia problem is to prescribe tablets which are a combination of sulfonamide and potassium-sparing diuretics. Hyperuricemia is predictable in patients taking sulfonamide diuretics and may be quite extreme in those with impaired renal function. Most authorities do not attempt to treat it unless symptoms of gouty arthropathy appear.

CNS DRUGS

These drugs are antihypertensive primarily because of effects they produce within the central nervous system. They all have additional effects on peripheral adrenergic nerves. These drugs tend to produce sedation and may disturb intellectual processes. They are less liable to produce orthostatic hypotension than are drugs which act more peripherally. Table 18–2 provides information about dosage.

AGENTS WHICH IMPAIR PERIPHERAL ADRENERGIC NEURON FUNCTION

These drugs decrease the release of norepinephrine at adrenergic nerve endings, either through blockade of autonomic ganglia, disturbance of the function of postganglionic neurons, or by directly interfering with the synthesis, storage, or release of neuronal norepinephrine. Typically, all drugs of this class produce troublesome orthostatic hypotension. The only agent in this class in common use is guanethidine (Table 18–2). Additional effects reported by those who take it include diarrhea, loss of ejaculation, and exercise hypotension.

ADRENERGIC RECEPTOR BLOCKING AGENTS

Beta-receptor Blockers. These drugs compete with catecholamines to occupy beta-receptors. Some, such as propranolol, block both cardiac and vascular beta-receptors; others are specific to one or the other site. All appear to have antihypertensive properties, and the basis

TABLE 18-2   Antihypertensive Agents

AGENTS	USUAL DOSE (mg per day) Initial	Maximal
CNS DRUGS		
Rauwolfia alkaloids		
Rauwolfia (whole root)	100.0	200.0
Alseroxylon	1.0	2.0
Reserpine	0.125	0.25
Deserpidine	0.25	0.50
Rescinnamine	0.25	2.0
Syrosingopine	1.0	3.0
Methyldopa	500.0	2000.0
Clonidine	0.3	4.8
PERIPHERAL ANTIADRENERGIC AGENTS		
Guanethidine	12.5	100.0
Pargyline	10.0	100.0
ADRENERGIC RECEPTOR BLOCKING AGENTS		
Beta Receptor Blockers		
Propranolol	40.0	320.0
Alpha Receptor Blockers		
Phentolamine	30.0	60.0
Dibenzyline	30.0	80.0
VASCULAR SMOOTH MUSCLE RELAXANTS		
Hydralazine	50.0	300.0

for this action is currently the subject of debate. It has been suggested that they lower blood pressure because they inhibit renal renin release, but cardio-selective blockers, which have no effect on plasma renin activity, also are antihypertensive. The only beta-receptor blocker presently in clinical use in the United States is propranolol, and it has not yet received formal approval from the Food and Drug Administration for prescription as an antihypertensive agent. Propranolol (Table 18-2) slows heart rate but does not produce orthostatic hypotension. It rarely produces troublesome side effects.

Alpha-receptor Blockers.   These drugs (Table 18-2) do not lower recumbent diastolic blood pressure in patients with hypertension, other than that produced by pheochromocytoma.

VASCULAR SMOOTH MUSCLE RELAXANTS

These drugs have no direct action on the autonomic nervous system. They lower blood pressure because of their ability to dilate resistance and capacitance vessels through direct relaxation of vascular musculature. They are not good antihypertensive agents when given alone by the oral route, and they tend to produce troublesome tachycardia, headache, and nausea. Hydralazine (Table 18-2) is the only oral agent in this class currently being used to treat hypertension in the

United States. A similar and more potent agent, minoxidil, is under investigation. Chronic administration of all vasodilators is accompanied by sodium retention, which probably is an important factor in the development of tolerance to their antihypertensive effect. Vasodilators should not be prescribed without concomitant diuretic therapy.

Current Therapy

MILD AND MODERATELY SEVERE HYPERTENSION

Treatment of hypertensive patients with diastolic blood pressures less than 120 mm Hg should be approached in a step-wise manner as illustrated in Figure 18–1. The goal of therapy is "normal" blood pressure for a person of that age. Combination therapy should be considered if normal pressure has not been achieved after administration of a maximal dose of a diuretic for four weeks. Choice of drug in step 2 should be based on a variety of factors including blood pressure level, heart rate, and the patient's willingness to take multiple doses of medication in a day. Hydralazine may be added as a third drug in those instances in which pressure has not been completely normalized by a diuretic plus an antiadrenergic agent.

SEVERE AND MALIGNANT HYPERTENSION

Patients with diastolic pressures fixed at levels greater than 120 mm Hg should be treated with a combination of drugs from the start.

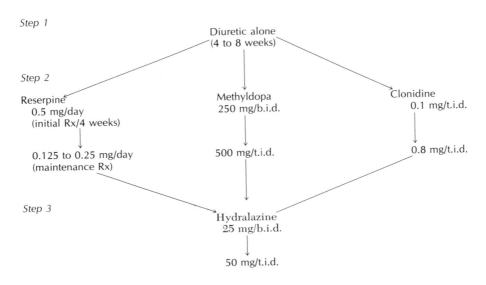

Figure 18–1 Treatment of mild to moderate hypertension.

Patients with very severe cases have usually required the use of guanethidine and a diuretic. Patients with somewhat milder forms may respond to a diuretic plus clonidine or high-dose aldomet. As a general rule, the higher the blood pressure, the higher the dose of antiadrenergic medication required. Blood pressure need not be forced down to normal in a great hurry. Initially it is advisable to aim for a diastolic of from 100 to 110 mm Hg, with the intent to push further after pressure stabilizes in that range.

Ambulatory patients with resistant hypertension, and particularly those with impaired renal function, are often better controlled by the addition of a "loop diuretic" to standard medications. The extra diuresis and natriuresis may prove extremely beneficial. A low-salt diet may also be of value in such cases. Very severe and malignant hypertension demands hospitalization where bed rest, sodium restriction and, if required, parenteral medication can be utilized. Some of these patients may need to be treated with intravenous vasodilating drugs before the blood pressure can be brought under control.

A New Therapeutic Approach

Beta-adrenergic receptor blocking agents are well on their way to revolutionizing the treatment of high blood pressure, both because of their antihypertensive potency and their impressive ability to minimize the side effects of concomitantly administered oral vasodilating agents. Patients with mild and moderately severe hypertension may respond to a beta-blocker administered alone or, if necessary, in combination with either a diuretic agent or a vasodilating drug (Fig. 18–2). Resistant pa-

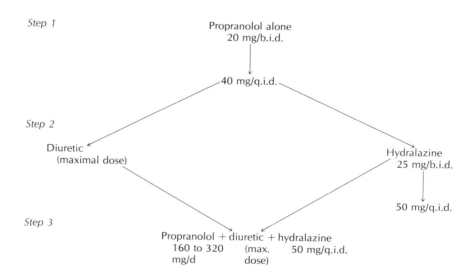

Figure 18–2 Use of propranolol in the treatment of hypertension.

tients and those with severe or malignant hypertension are treated with a combination of all three classes of drug: beta-blocker, vasodilator, and diuretic. Experience to date suggests that this latter therapeutic approach is the best way to lower both lying and standing blood pressure in the most difficult cases, with the added benefit of comparatively few side effects.

TREATMENT OF HYPERTENSIVE EMERGENCY AND URGENCY

Definitions

A *hypertensive emergency* is a situation demanding a decrease in elevated blood pressure within minutes. Conditions which threaten imminent death or permanent disability are properly included in this category. A *hypertensive urgency* exists when the clinical picture is such as to require rapid, but not immediate, lowering of blood pressure. The goal for patients in the latter category is substantial blood pressure reduction within 24 hours. Examples of conditions in the two categories include:

Hypertensive emergencies

1. Hypertensive encephalopathy: severe hypertension with impending or existent convulsions.

2. Pulmonary edema: severe hypertension with acute left ventricular failure.

3. Subarachnoid hemorrhage: hypertension with subarachnoid bleeding of recent onset.

4. Dissecting aneurysm of the aorta.

Hypertensive urgencies

1. Hypertension with hemorrhagic retinopathy or papilledema.

2. Hypertension with heart failure (excluding pulmonary edema).

3. Hypertension with severe headache.

Principles of Therapy

1. The object of treatment is to lower blood pressure without producing any clinically important reduction of blood flow to vital organs (e.g., oliguria, angina, cerebral ischemia). Blood pressure should be dropped to approximately 110 mm Hg diastolic and, when urinary output is stable, ultimately to as near normal as possible.

2. Treatment must be carried out under close supervision. Frequent blood pressure readings are mandatory to guide dosage of medication, and urinary output must be monitored to warn of impending anuria.

3. A rapidly-acting diuretic agent such as furosemide should be administered (orally or intravenously) in addition to the primary antihypertensive agent utilized.

TABLE 18–3 Drugs Used in the Treatment of
Hypertensive Emergency and Urgency

DRUG	MODE *Use in Emergency*	RESPONSE	SIDE EFFECTS
Trimethaphan (Arfonad)	4 to 20 mg/min IV 1 gm/500 ml Begin @ 2 ml/min	Prompt	Ganglion blocker: ileus, bladder atony at 24 hours. Overdose: hypoten- sion.
Sodium Nitroprusside (Nipride)	50 to 400 μg/min 50 mg/liter Begin @ 1.0 ml/min	Prompt	Metabolized to thiocyanate: mental confusion may occur after 24 hours.
Diazoxide (Hyperstat)	300 mg IV injected fast. Follow in 30 min with additional 300 mg if no response.	Prompt	Hyperglycemia, sodium re- tention-precipitation later of heart failure. Furosemide should be given for sodium and water retention.
Hydralazine (Apresoline)	10 to 30 mg IM. Start with 10 mg; if no re- sponse, follow with 20 mg.	Prompt or within ½ hour	Resistance after repeated doses. Tachycardia, head- ache. May cause angina in those predisposed.
	Use in Urgency		
Reserpine (Serpasil)	1.0 to 2.5 mg IM	In 1 to 2 hours	Drowsiness; hypotension. Difficult to follow changes in encephalopathy.
Alpha Methyldopa (Aldomet)	750 mg oral, or 500 mg IV	In 3 to 4 hours	Drowsiness. Often ineffective in severe hypertension.

4. The treatment applied for emergency and urgency is a temporary measure. Chronic treatment must be instituted simultaneously
with acute measures.

Drugs Used in Treatment

Table 18–3 lists the available drugs. Overall, the most practical
agent for the management of emergencies is diazoxide. Large doses of
aldomet are preferred in the treatment of patients in the urgent category.

SELECTED REFERENCES

Kannel, W. B., Costelli, W. P., McNamara, P. M., and Sorlie, P.: The Framingham Study:
Some factors affecting morbidity and mortality in hypertension. Milbank Mem. Fund.
Q., 47:116, 1969.
*The classical longitudinal study of the cardiovascular status of a community. The
risks of both systolic and diastolic blood pressure are quantitated.*
Laragh, J. H.: Vasoconstriction: Volume analysis for understanding and treating hyper-
tension: The use of renin and aldosterone profiles. Am. J. Med., 55:261, 1973.

Exposition of a current hypothesis which attempts to relate pathophysiology to treatment of hypertension. Thought-provoking, but controversial.

Society of Actuaries: Build and Blood Pressure Study, vol. I. Chicago, Illinois, Society of Actuaries, 1959.
Classical documentation of the risks of blood pressure, based on data accumulated by life insurance underwriters.

Veterans Administration Cooperative Study Group on Antihypertensive Agents: Effects of treatment on morbidity in hypertension: Results in patients with diastolic blood pressures averaging 115 through 129 mm Hg. J.A.M.A., *202*:1028, 1967.

Veterans Administration Cooperation Study Group on Antihypertensive Agents: Effects of treatment on morbidity in hypertension: Results in patients with diastolic blood pressures averaging 90 through 114 mm Hg. J.A.M.A., *213*:1143, 1970.
The study which demonstrated that treatment of mild and moderately severe hypertension improves prognosis.

Wilber, J. A., and Barrow, J. G.: Reducing elevated blood pressure: Experience found in a community. Minn. Med., *52*:1303, 1969.
The study which documents the importance of the "drop-out" problem in the therapy of hypertension.

REFERENCES

Chiang, B. N., Perlman, L. V., and Epstein, F. H.: Overweight and hypertension. A review. Circulation, 39:403, 1969.

Dahl, L. K.: Salt and hypertension. Am. J. Clin. Nutr., 25:231, 1972.

Epstein, F. H.: Multiple risk factors and the prediction of coronary heart disease. Bull. N.Y. Acad. Med., 44:916, 1968.

Hamilton, M., Thompson, E. N., and Wisniewsky, T. K. M.: The role of blood pressure control in preventing complications of hypertension. Lancet, 1:235, 1964.

Harrington, M.: Malignant hypertension. Practitioner, 193:35, 1964.

Hypertension Study Group: Guidelines for the detection, diagnosis and management of hypertensive populations. Circulation, 44:A-263, 1971.

Julius, S., and Schork, M. A.: Borderline hypertension: A critical review. J. Chron. Dis., 23:273, 1971.

Kannel, W. B. et al.: Epidemiologic assessment of the role of blood pressure in stroke — The Framingham Study. J.A.M.A., 214:301, 1970.

Koch-Weser, J.: Correlation of pathophysiology and pharmacotherapy in primary hypertension. Am. J. Cardiol., 32:499, 1973.

Oates, J. A., Seligmann, A. W., Clark, M. A., Roussian, P., and Lee, N. E.: The relative efficacy of guanethidine, methyldopa and pargyline as antihypertensive agents. N. Engl. J. Med., 273:729, 1965.

Parijs, J., Joossens, J. V., VanderLinden, L., Verstriken, G., and Amery, A, K.P.C.: Moderate sodium restriction and diuretics in the treatment of hypertension. Am. Heart J., 85:22, 1973.

Veteran's Administration Cooperative Study on Antihypertensive Agents: a double-blind control study of antihypertensive agents. Arch. Int. Med., 106:81, 1960 and Arch. Intern. Med., 110:222, 1962.

Zacest, R., Gilmore, E., and Kock-Weser, J.: Treatment of essential hypertension with combined vasodilation and beta-adrenergic blockade. N. Engl. J. Med., 286:617, 1972.

Chapter Nineteen

RENAL TRANSPLANTATION

John W. Konnak and Jeremiah G. Turcotte

Until the mid-1950s, the course of chronic progressive renal failure was inevitable, whatever the cause. The advent of two new therapeutic procedures, chronic intermittent hemodialysis and renal homotransplantation, has radically changed this prognosis. The technical feasibility of renal transplantation was demonstrated in animals by Alexis Carrel and others in the early 1900s. Following these demonstrations, renal transplants were performed in humans, but graft failure invariably took place owing to immunologic host rejection of the renal homograft. A partial understanding of the rejection phenomenon was attained through the study of skin grafts, and it was shown that skin grafts between identical twins are not rejected. The analogy between skin and renal homografts in identical twins was demonstrated in 1954 when the first successful renal transplant in human identical twins was performed.

The initial attempts at protecting renal homografts in nonidentical individuals were through the use of total body irradiation. While this method suppressed the immune response, the side effects of total body irradiation were usually disastrous. The demonstration of the immunosuppressive effect of 6-mercaptopurine and of its less toxic analogue, azathioprine, together with the discovery of the ability of prednisone to reverse rejection has made human renal homotransplantation a clinically feasible therapeutic procedure. Advances in genetics and immunology with the development of methods of identifying certain "transplantation antigens" plus the use of antilymphocytic globulin have further refined the attack on the immune response.

Although renal transplantation is presently an acceptable therapeutic procedure, serious problems still exist in the realms of immunosuppression, donor organ procurement and preservation, and re-emergence of the original renal disease. The purpose of this chapter is to define the present "state of the art" and the problems involved in renal transplantation.

503

INDICATIONS FOR RENAL TRANSPLANTATION AND SELECTION OF CANDIDATES

The complications of primary irreversible renal failure constitute the major indications for renal transplantation. The initial diseases vary. The histologic diagnoses on 50 consecutive bilateral nephrectomy specimens performed in conjunction with renal transplantation are shown in Table 19–1. The best candidates are relatively young patients whose renal disease is clearly primary and not likely to recur, such as patients with polycystic disease. Intermediate candidates include patients whose initial renal problems may recur, such as those with glomerulonephritis, pyelonephritis, or nephrosclerosis secondary to diabetes or hypertension; most transplant patients fall into this intermediate group. The worst candidates are those with secondary renal disease in which the transplanted kidney is likely to be affected, such as those with congenital oxalosis or uncorrected obstructive uropathy. When the initial disease can be corrected or controlled, the patient becomes a better candidate. Obviously, a complete medical and urologic workup is necessary prior to renal transplantation.

The presence of coexisting diseases and their probable effect on patient longevity and ability to function after transplantation is also taken into account. Patients with active neoplasms, paraplegics, and those with severe debilitating diseases are poor candidates.

There is no definite age limit for receiving a renal transplant. Successful transplants have been performed in infants and young children. Because of coexisting medical problems and limited life expectancy in the aged, few renal transplants are done in patients over 60 years.

Renal transplantation is not done for the presence of impaired renal function alone but for the complications of impaired function. With proper medical management, patients with a fairly marked reduction in renal function can do as well or better than some patients with a renal homograft. Uremia is the most common complication of renal failure corrected by renal transplantation. Other complications which can be effectively treated with a transplant include hypertension, congestive heart failure, pericarditis, peripheral neuropathy, renal osteodys-

TABLE 19–1 Histologic Diagnosis on Kidneys in 50 Cases of End Stage Renal Failure

Diagnosis	Number of Patients
Chronic glomerulonephritis	21
End stage kidney	12
Chronic pyelonephritis	10
Renal dysplasia or hypoplasia with chronic pyelonephritis	3
Polycystic kidney	3
Medullary cystic disease	1
Arteriolar nephrosclerosis	1
Severe nephrocalcinosis	1

trophy, secondary hyperparathyroidism, and failure to grow and thrive in childhood.

It should be remembered that an alternative to renal transplantation exists in the form of chronic hemodialysis. Many patients who are not good transplant candidates can be treated with this method. Some patients do extremely well on dialysis, and in these individuals the risks and complications of transplantation and immunosuppression may not be justified. Long-term survival is possible on chronic hemodialysis although the mortality rate is about 10 per cent per year; this is about the same as the related donor transplant. The long-term cost of a renal transplant and chronic hemodialysis is the same.

RENAL TRANSPLANT DONORS

Of the 12,389 transplanted kidneys reviewed in the Eleventh Report of the Human Renal Transplant Registry, 63.4 per cent were provided by cadavers. Most of the remainder came from related donors, either parent, sibling, or child, a few being donated by more distant relatives or unrelated living donors. In Europe a higher percentage of cadaver kidneys were used (78.8 per cent), while in the United States only 52.6 per cent of the kidneys transplanted came from this source. While the trend is toward the greater use of cadaver kidneys, the overall results of renal transplants from related donor sources are better. The benefits from unrelated living or more distant donors are similar to cadaver sources.

The donor should be of the same ABO blood type as the recipient, and when more than one donor is available, the most compatible tissue match is used. An individual with renal disease, severe infection, hepatitis, or neoplasm (except of the central nervous system or skin) is usually not acceptable as a donor. The transplantation of neoplastic tissue along with the donor kidney has been well-documented.

Related Donors

A related donor should be in excellent health. The usual ages are between 18 and 50, although older individuals can be utilized if they are in good health. Under certain circumstances younger individuals may be used with the consent of the court, as in the case of identical twins. Additional contraindications to donation include the presence of any condition in the donor which constitutes a surgical risk or a future risk to good health with one kidney. It has been estimated that about one of every 1000 kidney donors will die within five years of the operation from early complications or late injury to the remaining kidney. The donor should be well-motivated to give a kidney and have no psychiatric disorders that might be adversely affected by donation. Obligations of the donor to his family are taken into account.

The workup of the donor includes a complete medical evaluation with a history and physical examination, chest film, and electrocardiogram. Routine laboratory testing is done, along with renal function tests, blood typing, and histocompatibility matching. A urine analysis, urine cultures, and 24-hour urine collection for protein are performed. Further x-ray evaluation includes an intravenous pyelogram and finally a renal arteriogram. The donor should be evaluated by the transplant surgeon, nephrologist, urologist, and a social worker. If indicated, a psychiatrist may also see the donor.

Cadaver Donors and Brain Death

The use of cadaver donors is increasing. The advent of organ transplantation has resulted in a redefinition as to the exact moment when death occurs. Again, the basic principle is to protect the donor first. Many cadaver donors are patients with severe irreversible brain damage requiring artificial life support. Because of this damage, brain death has been widely used in the selection of cadaver donors. The definition of brain death varies, but usually the prospective donor must show the usual neurologic criteria of severe cerebral damage, such as fixed dilated pupils, absence of deep pain sensation, areflexia, and the absence of spontaneous respiration and movement. In addition, the absence of electrical activity of the brain by electroencephalography may be used.

The prospective donor must not be on drugs, such as barbiturates, which depress reflexes and electrical activity of the brain, and he must be normothermic. The criteria must be present for a period of time, varying from a few hours to 24 hours. The transplant team usually plays no part in donor therapy and is disassociated from the decision as to the time of death. If cardiac arrest or irreversible shock ensues, the kidneys are usually harvested immediately. Cadavers with primary renal disease, neoplasms excluding central nervous system and skin, or sepsis are usually not employed. Consent for cadaver donation is usually obtained from the next of kin, although a person may donate his own kidneys through the Uniform Anatomical Gift Act.

TISSUE MATCHING

The major histocompatibility antigens on cell walls are determined by the HL-A chromosomal locus in man. The haplotype determined by each parent consists of two gene complexes on subloci located very close together on the chromosome. Each sublocus determines one antigen complex, and around 30 antigen complexes are either known or suspected. Therefore, each individual carries four antigen complexes, two from each parent. The genes on each chromosome are close together and almost never separated, so that they are inherited in pairs,

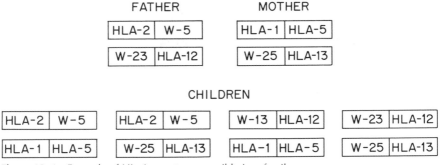

Figure 19–1   Example of HL–A genotypes possible in a family.

one pair from the mother and one pair from the father. Four genotypes are possible in each family as shown in Figure 19–1.

Statistically, one quarter of all siblings will be HL-A identical, one half will share a haplotype in common, and one quarter will have a two haplotype or four antigen mismatch, barring the off chance that the parents shared antigens in common. Offspring will always have one haplotype in common with each parent, but will usually have a haplotype difference with each parent, or a two antigen mismatch. Sometimes one or more antigens cannot be identified and are potentially mismatched. Typing other family members and determining the haplotypes may identify missing antigens. Various classifications have been devised to signify the degree of histocompatibility, taking into account the number of mismatched and potentially mismatched antigens (Table 19–2). The clearest way to state this is to actually state the number of mismatched and potentially mismatched antigens. The system is probably more complex than this, and there may be other histocompatibility loci. The methods of determining these antigens is beyond the scope of this chapter.

The clinical significance of histocompatibility matching is still being defined. Clearly, four antigen identical siblings do better than any degree of mismatch and do as well as identical twins in some series. It may well be that poorly matched siblings (four antigen mismatch) do about the same as cadaver donor recipient pairs. Obviously, good matches are much less common in kidneys from cadaver donors. It is estimated that there may be around 10,000 phenotypes in the population, although some gene complexes are more common than others. HL-A identical cadaver-recipient pairs probably do better than poorer

TABLE 19–2   Match Grades

A = Identical
B = No donor-recipient mismatch, but recipient-donor mismatch
C = 1 donor-recipient group mismatch
D = 2 donor-recipient group mismatch
E = 2 allele difference
F = Positive crossmatch

matches, but not as well as identical siblings. Other as yet unidentified nonHL-A factors are also important in rejection, since HL-A identical grafts are always rejected unless the donor is an identical twin or unless some form of immunosuppression is employed.

Some patients, especially those who have had multiple pregnancies or blood transfusions, have a positive crossmatch, or preformed cytotoxic antibodies against donor cells. The presence of these may, in many cases but not always, lead to hyperacute rejection of the homograft. For this reason, crossmatching between recipient serum and donor cells, usually lymphocytes, is carried out prior to transplantation. Prior sensitization or the presence of preformed antibodies occurs more frequently in cadaveric graft recipients, and this factor helps obscure the correlation of HL-A typing with results in these patients.

Transplantation between ABO incompatible individuals is not done because a form of hyperacute rejection usually occurs. This is thought to take place because of the presence of major blood group antigens on vascular endothelial cells in the kidney. Rh and other minor blood group incompatibilities are probably of no clinical significance.

Mixed Lymphocyte Culture

It has been shown that when lymphocytes of two nonidentical individuals are cultured together a certain percentage are transformed to blast forms. This percentage is inversely proportional to the tissue compatibility of the individuals. This test is of value in predicting histocompatibility and graft survival, but technical problems have limited its use prospectively on a clinical basis. Future advances may expand the role of this test.

HOST RESPONSES TO AN ALLOGRAFT

In higher animals and man, two systems of immunity develop to deal with infections, foreign tissues, and probably tumors. One of these systems is cell-mediated, combats fungi and viruses, and participates in the rejection of foreign tissues and probably tumors. The other is humoral immunity, which combats bacterial infections and viral reinfection. These two systems of immunity derive from two populations of lymphocytes. Both populations originate from hematopoietic stem cells. In adult mammals, there are two "primary" sites of lymphocyte production: the bone marrow and the thymus. The bone marrow is the production site of the so-called *B lymphocytes*, which ultimately produce humoral antibodies. The thymus is the organ of production of the so-called *T lymphocytes*, or thymus-dependent lymphocytes, which are responsible for cell-mediated immunity and organ rejection. There is evidence that these systems interact in a variety of situations.

According to current theory, T lymphocytes originate in or are acted on by the thymus. They multiply rapidly in the thymic cortex and then move to the medulla where they multiply more slowly. They then move out of the thymus and enter a pool of relatively long-lived lymphocytes, which recirculate through the blood, thymus-dependent areas of the spleen and lymph nodes, the lymphatics, and the thoracic duct. They do not recirculate through the thymus. Apparently, only a small number of these cells can respond to a given antigen or class of antigens. When one of these wide-ranging cells encounters an antigen to which its receptors can respond, it returns via the circulation to special regions of the lymph nodes and spleen called thymus-dependent zones. Here it divides repeatedly and develops a clone of cells responsive to the antigen. These T cells then return to the circulation via the lymphatics and thoracic duct. This brief outline of the production of sensitized lymphocytes is speculative, and many of the details are unknown or open to controversy.

When the sensitized lymphocytes return to cells containing the sensitizing antigen, they are capable of destroying these cells. Not only are they cytotoxic to the sensitizing cell, but apparently they are capable of transferring this sensitivity to other lymphocytes and of inhibiting the migration away from, or attracting to the sensitizing cells, mononuclear cells, and other cells that may have a detrimental effect on the sensitizing cells.

B Cells, or bone marrow derived lymphocytes, are capable of responding to sensitizing antigens by producing antibody-producing cells. Circulating cytotoxic antibodies may be produced in the presence of foreign cells. Stimulation may be induced by contact with foreign tissue antigens in the form of an organ transplant, blood transfusion, or pregnancy. Preformed circulating antibodies are often associated with hyperacute allograft rejection. They may also play a part in chronic rejection. In transplantation, certain individuals termed *responders* may have circulating cytotoxic antibodies against a variety of tissue antigens. These individuals tend to reject a transplanted organ more readily than nonresponders.

KIDNEY PRESERVATION

It is necessary to maintain the viability of the donor kidney until the time of transplantation. This period may vary from a few minutes in living related donors to many hours in cadaver donors. Unfortunately, kidneys cannot survive a period of total ischemia at body temperature for more than 60 minutes, and the shorter the warm ischemia the better. If a method of long-term renal preservation were available, it would be possible to build up a bank of living kidneys for elective transplantation. In addition, a large pool of tissue-typed kidneys could be maintained, and the best possible matches used. Bench surgery and testing of the kidney would be possible under excellent conditions, and it might even be feasible to modify the kidney's potential to elicit immune response. Currently, the longest period of preservation that is consistently reliable in humans is approximately 24 hours. Some kidneys have been preserved successfully for as long as 72 hours. All the preservation methods used clinically rely on washing out the formed elements of the blood and cooling to 2 to 4 degrees C. At this temperature the metabolic needs and oxygen requirements of the kidney are markedly decreased. The perfusion solution varies, but the most commonly employed are heparinized Ringer's lactate or a modified intracellular solution such as Collin's solution. Cryoprecipitated plasma is used in continuous perfusion. Various additives such as phenoxybenzamine and steroids are sometimes utilized. After perfusion and cooling, the kidney may be stored at 2 to 4 degrees C until used, or the perfusion may be continued using cooled, pH adjusted perfusate with a pulsatile flow pump and oxygenator. The continuous perfusion systems give somewhat more reliable preservation over 12 hours and a decreased incidence of acute tubular necrosis after transplantation. Another advantage is that the flow rate and pressure of the perfusate through the kidney can be used to predict immediate graft function and even viability. Rising resistance to flow and increasing pressure presage renal failure. The disadvantages of continuous perfusion are the high cost and complexity of the equipment, the loss of potentially usable kidneys using the above criteria, and the possibility of renal damage due to perfusion.

TRANSPLANTATION SURGERY

Recipient Bilateral Nephrectomy

A bilateral nephrectomy may be carried out in the transplant recipient prior to or at the time of transplantation. This is done for the following reasons:

1. To remove the diseased kidneys as a source of infection.

2. To remove polycystic kidneys, which may interfere with the transplant because of their size, future infection, or bleeding.

3. To prevent the urine output from the diseased kidneys from confusing the clinical picture posttransplant.

4. To help control hypertension.

5. To prevent protein or sodium loss by the diseased kidneys.

6. To provide a ureter for transplantation.

This procedure is occasionally done in conjunction with a celiotomy for other reasons and for bleeding following renal biopsy. The procedure may be carried out from the flank or anterior transperitoneal approach (Fig. 19–2). Postoperatively, the anephric patient must be monitored carefully in regard to hydration, blood pressure, and serum potassium. Dialysis is delayed until at least the second postoperative day to minimize the likelihood of bleeding due to heparinization. Currently, most recipient kidneys are left in situ unless a specific indication for nephrectomy exists.

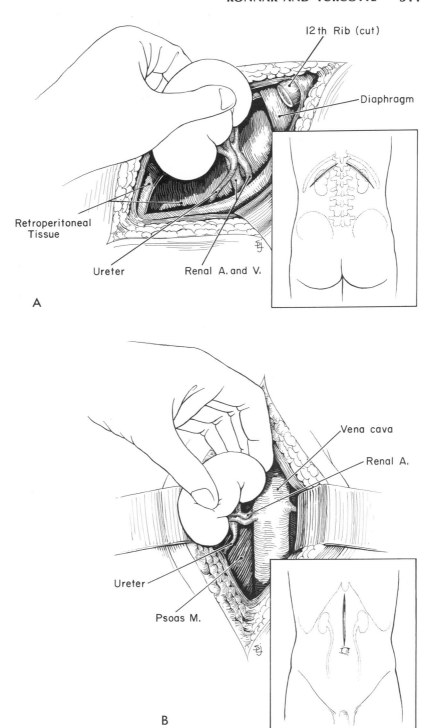

Figure 19–2 *A,* Prone approach for bilateral nephrectomy. *B,* Transabdominal approach for bilateral nephrectomy.

RELATED DONOR NEPHRECTOMY

The related donor is prepared for operation in the manner routine for a major surgical procedure. A general anesthetic is used, and the patient is kept well-hydrated. Mannitol or furosemide may be given during the operation to promote a vigorous diuresis. The kidney is approached either from the flank or from the anterior transperitoneal approach (Fig. 19–3). The kidney is removed quickly and smoothly, with a minimum of manipulation of the kidney, its vessels, and the ureter. The renal vessels are dissected and isolated separately. Then the ureter is mobilized, leaving the blood supply intact with a generous amount of periureteric tissue surrounding it. Finally, the kidney is mobilized and removed. After nephrectomy, the wound is closed in the usual manner. If a diuretic has been used, the donor's bladder should be emptied by a single sterile catherization at the end of the procedure. The rest of the postoperative care is routine.

CADAVER DONOR NEPHRECTOMY

The cadaver donor should be prepared preoperatively if possible. The donor should be well-hydrated so that the central venous pressure, urine output, and blood pressure are normal. The patient is usually

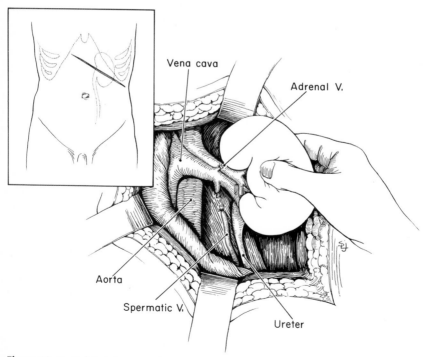

Figure 19–3 Related donor nephrectomy.

given larger quantities of balanced electrolyte solution and albumin and heparinized. Phenoxybenzamine or Regitine and furosemide are often given to produce vasodilatation and promote diuresis, and methylprednisolone is given possibly for its membrane stabilizing effect. If cardiac arrest occurs, resuscitation should be attempted and renal perfusion maintained during the nephrectomy. A midline incision is made from the xyphoid to the pubic symphysis. The kidneys may be removed individually in a manner similar to the living donor, but a more effective method is to reflect the colon and small bowel from the retroperitoneum. The bowel and the peritoneum are reflected off the great vessels; and the kidneys, ureters, aorta, and vena cava are removed en bloc (Fig. 19–4). The celiac, superior mesenteric, spermatic, and lumbar vessels are ligated as encountered. The kidneys are cooled and perfused and further dissection of the kidney, vessels, and ureter is carried out with the kidneys cold.

TECHNIQUE OF RENAL TRANSPLANTATION

In adults, the kidney is placed in either iliac fossa (Fig. 19–5). The iliac vessels are exposed through a low transverse incision, and the in-

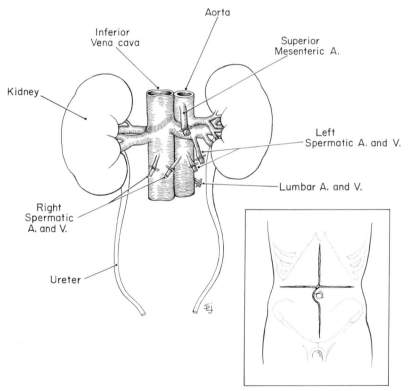

Figure 19–4 En bloc cadaver donor nephrectomy.

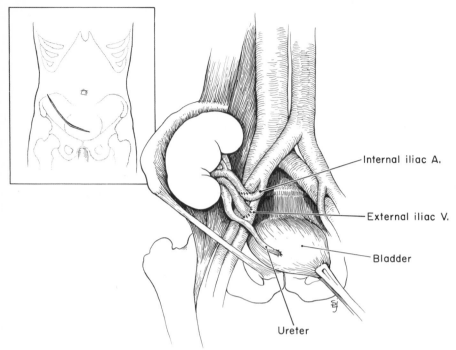

Figure 19–5   Renal transplant into iliac fossa.

ternal iliac artery and common iliac vein are mobilized. The cooled perfused kidney is received, and the renal artery is anastomosed end-to-end to the internal iliac artery, and the renal vein is anastomosed to the side of the common iliac vein. Urine output usually begins in a few minutes. The continuity of the urinary tract is then reestablished. The most common technique used is ureteroneocystostomy. Ureteropyelostomy or ureteroureterostomy are sometimes used, but the complication rate is higher than after ureteroneocystostomy (Fig. 19–6). For the first 24 to 48 hours, a marked diuresis occurs, partly as a result of the patient's increased osmotic load and overhydration. An early defect in sodium reabsorption and an inability of the tubules to respond normally to antidiuretic hormone may also play a part. A good, functioning kidney puts out over 200 ml per hour for the first 24 to 48 hours and decreases serum creatinine to below 2 mg/100 ml, regardless of previous levels, within 48 hours.

IMMUNOSUPPRESSION

Immunosuppression is a general term that refers to various methods of prolonging homograft survival; immunosuppressive as well as some nonimmunosuppressive drugs may accomplish this. These agents act by increasing tolerance to the homograft, or they prevent, modify, or reverse rejection. The exact mechanisms of their actions are not known. The most commonly used drugs are listed as follows.

Azathioprine. This is an analogue of 6-mercaptopurine. This antimetabolite is the one most commonly used agent in prolonging homograft survival. The usual dose is 3 mg/kg, and the major side effect is bone marrow depression. Cyclophosphamide, an alkylating agent, is sometimes substituted when intolerance to azathioprine occurs.

Prednisone. This is a corticosteroid and antiinflammatory agent. This drug is commonly employed to prolong graft survival, and its major use is in reversing acute rejection. It does this very effectively in high doses. It is often given as a "pulse" of 15 to 30 mg/kg intravenously over a short period of time. The main side effect of chronic corticosteroid therapy is the development of Cushing's syndrome.

Antilymphocyte Serum. For human use, this agent is produced by injecting human lymphocytes or thymocytes into a horse. The hyperimmune horse serum is then purified by various absorption and fractionation techniques. Its effectiveness varies with the techniques used in its production, the mode of administration, and the investigator using the product. It has a wide range of toxicity, from pain at injection sites to serum sickness.

COMPLICATIONS OF RENAL TRANSPLANTATION

Complications are frequently more common in renal transplant recipients because of the morbidity of accompanying long-standing renal insufficiency and because of the side effects of presently available immunosuppressants.

Surgical Complications

Those complications that occur include the following.

Thrombosis or Infection at the Vascular Anastomotic Sites. Occasionally, thrombosis of the renal artery or vein occurs. By the time the complication is fully recognized, irreversible renal damage has usually taken place, and nephrectomy is necessary. Infection of the anastomosis has also occurred, especially in cadaver transplants. This has led to mycotic aneurysm formation and blow-out of the anastomosis.

Ureteric Obstruction or Urinary Extravasation. Prompt recognition of these complications is important if repair is to be successful. The diagnosis is usually made with the aid of intravenous pyelography, but cystography and retrograde pyelography may be useful. Treatment consists of exploration of the ureter and revision of the anastomosis if obstruction has occurred. If extravasation is evident, the cause is determined and appropriate surgical correction made. This may involve re-

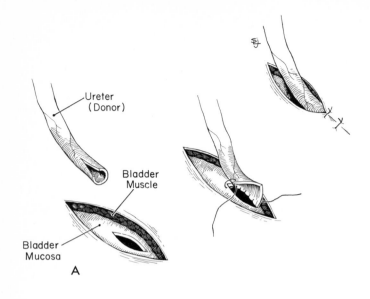

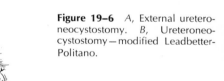

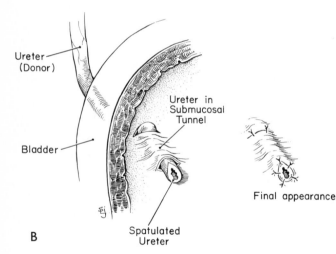

Ureter
(Donor)

Bladder
Muscle

Bladder
Mucosa

A

Ureter
(Donor)

Ureter in
Submucosal
Tunnel

Bladder

Spatulated
Ureter

B

Final appearance

Figure 19–6 *A*, External ureteroneocystostomy. *B*, Ureteroneocystostomy—modified Leadbetter-
Politano.

doing the anastomosis and providing temporary urinary diversion with a
stent or nephrostomy tube, but occasionally simple drainage is sufficient.
A more serious complication is necrosis of the ureter, which is usually
caused by ureteric devascularization at the time of donor nephrectomy
but may also be caused by rejection. The usual treatment is nephrectomy,
but the authors have treated two cases successfully with vesicopyelosto-
my.

   Infection, Sepsis, and Hemorrhage. These present more
frequently in the renal transplant patient owing to the coagulation
defects associated with azotemia and the need for immunosuppression.
Appropriate technical care minimizes these complications.

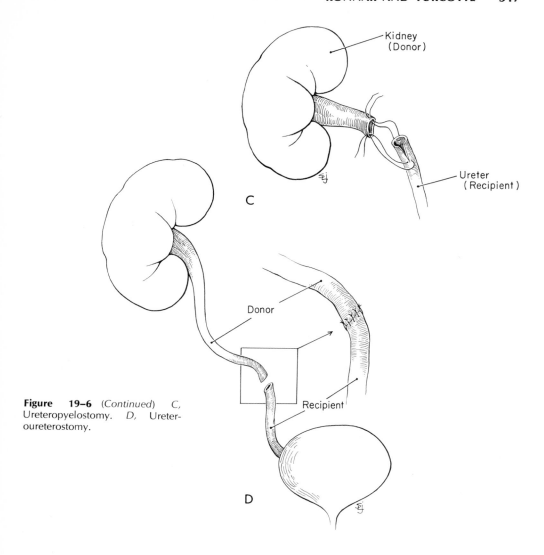

Figure   19–6 (Continued)   C, Ureteropyelostomy.   D,   Ureter-oureterostomy.

Medical Complications

Acute Tubular Necrosis.   This occurs much more frequently in transplantation from cadaver donors due to the circumstances surrounding the donor's death and the longer ischemia and perfusion time. The result is oliguria, which may be prolonged. A useful rule of thumb is that if the kidney does not produce 200 ml of urine per hour in the immediate postoperative period, a variable amount of acute tubular necrosis is present and the kidney will probably shut down. Recovery usually occurs in two to four weeks but can occasionally take longer. During this time the patient requires dialysis. If recovery does not take place, a nonviable kidney may have been transplanted. This kidney should be removed, and the patient prepared for a second transplant. The patient with acute tubular necrosis usually does not have total anuria. If this occurs, vascular or ureteric obstruction or a nonviable kidney should be considered as the cause. Hyperacute or acute rejection is also in the differential diagnosis of oliguria.

Rejection. This is a general term referring to the response of the graft to immunologic attack by the host. In hyperacute rejection, circulating antibody reacts with the transplant endothelium and triggers the coagulation cascade. The allograft becomes cyanotic and mottled, and the vessel soon undergoes thrombosis. Platelets, polymorphonuclear leukocytes, fibrin, and probably complement accumulate on the vascular endothelium. Preformed circulating antibodies are usually found, although the presence of these antibodies does not invariably result in hyperacute rejection.

Acute rejection is far more common clinically and is characterized by oliguria, decreasing renal function, and increasing size and tenderness of the kidney. Fever, leukocytosis, and hypertension may also be present. Histologically, there is a perivascular accumulation of mononuclear cells, usually with varying degrees of vascular endothelial injury, platelet accumulation, and tubular necrosis. Acute rejection occurs most frequently in the immediate posttransplant period, after the seventh postoperative day. After three or four weeks, the likelihood of this occurring becomes less, but it may happen anytime. It is usually completely reversible if promptly treated. The steroid "pulse" has been a valuable tool in treating this process.

Chronic rejection probably takes place to a varying degree in all renal homografts. It is characterized by a slowly progressive deterioration in renal function. Histologically, it is characterized by interstitial fibrosis, glomerular basement membrane thickening, and intimal proliferation in small arterioles. The cause is unknown, but it may be due to a humoral response. Eventually, perhaps over a period of years, it will lead to graft failure.

Complications of Immunosuppressive Therapy. These include an increased susceptibility to infection and sepsis, with opportunistic organisms as well as with common pathogens. Some of the more exotic infections seen include pneumonitis associated with toxoplasmosis, cytomegalic inclusion virus, or pneumocystis carinii; cryptococcal meningitis; candidiasis with fungus balls in the urine; and others. Infection is the most common cause of patient death after transplantation. Wound healing is impaired in the immunosuppressed patient. High doses of steroids result in the development of Cushing's syndrome, and azathioprine may cause bone marrow depression.

Recurrence of the Original Renal Disease. This occurs especially as glomerulonephritis.

Other Complications. Peptic ulcers and pancreatitis occur in transplant patients probably as a result of steroid therapy. Osteoporosis, aseptic necrosis of the hips, and lenticular opacities may also result. Lymphomas and other malignant tumors occur more frequently in transplant patients, possibly as a result of immunosuppression.

RESULTS IN RENAL TRANSPLANTATION

There is a problem in interpreting the results in renal transplantation. The usual data, which speak in terms of graft or patient survival over a number of years, may fail to reflect recent improvements in technique and patient management. Recent statistics have insufficient follow-up. Overall figures fail to show the really superior results in certain groups such as HL-A identical siblings, while inclusion of these patients may make some series look deceptively good. Survival figures do not reflect the quality of the patient's life. A detailed analysis of all aspects of the result of renal transplantation is beyond the scope of this chapter. The one and two-year graft survival figures given by donor type on transplants done in 1971 as reported in the Eleventh Report of the Human Renal Transplant Registry are shown in Figure 19–7.

FUTURE ADVANCES

Future advances in transplantation will come in the fields of immunology and organ preservation. Ideally, the host's immune response might be modified so that only the transplanted organ is tolerated, with no compromise of the immune response against infection and neoplasms, no impairment in wound healing, and no disabling side effects. Possibly, the transplanted organ could be modified immunologically so that it would be tolerated more easily.

Organ preservation time should be extended so that organ banks

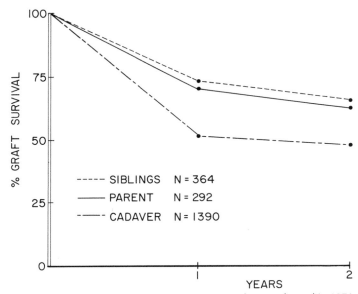

Figure 19–7 Two year renal graft survival by donor type in 2046 transplants performed in 1971 and reported in the Eleventh Report of the Human Renal Transplant Registry.

could be developed and organ supplies expanded. Preservation time needs to be in months rather than in days.

When these problems are overcome, a variety of organs in addition to kidneys will lend themselves to transplantation, including heart, lung, pancreas, blood vessels, bone marrow, liver, and bowel. Considering the present state of the art, these advances will probably occur over decades rather than years.

SELECTED REFERENCES

Calne, R. V.: Clinical Organ Transplantation. Oxford and Edinburgh, Blackwell Scientific Publications, 1971.
    This is a short basic text on organ transplantation. It contains many practical points in technique and management. In most chapters the references are limited to the standard ones.
Hamburger, J., Crosnier, J., Dormont, J., and Bach, J. F.: Renal Transplantation: Theory and Practice, Baltimore, Williams & Wilkins Co., 1972.
    This brief text covers all aspects of renal transplantation; it has brief and exceptionally clear chapters on transplant immunology, graft antigens, and their practical application.
Hume, D. M., and Rapaport, F. T.: Clinical Transplantation. New York, Grune and Stratton, 1972, 1973.
    This text is a collection of papers by a variety of noted authors on all aspects of clinical transplantation.
Najarian, J. S., and Simmons, R. L.: Transplantation. Philadelphia, Lea and Febiger, 1972.
    This reference text has 25 chapters by 54 contributers on all aspects of transplantation of kidneys and other organs. It is divided into two parts; entitled "Immunobiology of Transplantation" (7 chapters) and "Clinical Transplantation" (18 chapters). The chapters contain extensive references.
The Eleventh Report of the Human Renal Transplant Registry. J.A.M.A., 226:1197, 1973.
    This report is published annually. Two hundred forty-six institutions report to the registry, and it presents an average of the results of these institutions. A variety of data is presented, from graft and patient survival rates to data on tumors and pregnancy in transplant patients.

REFERENCES

Bach, J. F., Debray-Sacks, M., Crosmier, J. et al.: Correlation between mixed lymphocyte culture performed before renal transplantation and kidney function. Clin. Exp. Immunol., 6:821, 1970.
Belzer, F. O., and Kountz, S. L.: Preservation and transplantation of human kidneys. Ann. Surg., 172:394, 1970.
Fine, R. N., Korsch, B. M., Brennan, L. P. et al.: Renal transplants in young children. Am. J. Surg., 125:559, 1973.
Lowve, E. G., Lazarus, J. M., Mocelin, A. J. et al.: Survival of patients undergoing chronic hemodialysis and renal transplantation. N. Engl. J. Med., 288:863, 1973.
Murray, J. E., Wilson, R. E., Tilney, N. L. et al.: Five years experience in renal transplantation with immunosuppressive drugs: Survival, functions, complications, and the role of lymphocyte depletion by thoracic duct fistula. Ann. Surg., 168:416, 1968.
Opelz, G., and Terasaki, P. I.: HL-A and kidney transplants: Reexamination. Transplantation, 17:371, 1974.
Penn, I., Halgrimson, C. G., Ogden, D., and Starzl, T. E.: Use of living donors in kidney transplants in man. Arch. Surg., 101:226, 1970.
Santiago-Delphin, E. A., Moberg, A. W., Mozes, M. F. et al.: Comparative analysis of perfusion and nonperfusion methods for renal preservation. Surgery, 72:793, 1972.
Starzl, T. E., Porter, K. A., Andres, G. et al.: Long term survival after renal transplantation in humans: (With special reference to histocompatibility matching, thymectomy, homograft glomerulonephritis, heterologous ALG and recipient malignancy). Ann. Surg., 172:437, 1970.
Turcotte, J. G.: Infections and renal transplantation. Surg. Clin. North Am., 52:6, 1972.
Weil, R., Simmons, R. L., Tallent, M. B. et al.: Prevention of urologic complications after kidney transplantation. Ann. Surg., 174:154, 1971.

Chapter Twenty

MALE INFERTILITY

Robert Anderson

The fertile male produces a number of normal, motile spermatozoa that are capable of transport through patent pathways to be stored in specialized portions of the vasa deferentia and to be discharged from the urethra on ejaculation. The spermatozoa must be deposited in the female, together with secretions of the prostate and seminal vesicles, in such a way that they reach and penetrate the cervical secretions, ascending the uterus to the fallopian tube at a time in the cycle appropriate for fertilization of the ovum. The spermatozoa must also be capable of penetrating the zona pellucida of the ovum if fertilization is to result. Complex biochemical and enzymatic processes must take place to allow the sperm to achieve this end. The production of sperm and the process by which they reach the ovum depend on hormonal stimulation by an intact hypothalamic-pituitary-gonadal axis and a closely integrated, well-functioning neurologic reflex mechanism mediated through peripheral and central stimuli.

When any of the production, maturation, transport, or fertilizing capacities are absent, defective, or deficient, the result may be an infertile or subfertile male.

The investigation of fertility usually involves a couple who have been unsuccessful in achieving pregnancy after 12 to 18 months of unprotected intercourse at a frequency of two to three times per week.

INCIDENCE OF INFERTILITY

Approximately 15 per cent of all marriages are infertile. The male is responsible in 30 per cent of these instances and contributes to the problem in an additional 20 per cent.

EVALUATION OF FERTILITY IN THE MALE

The male patient who appears for evaluation of fertility should receive the same diagnostic consideration as a patient who presents any other complicated medical problem. A general history and physical examination, with special reference to sexual and reproductive health, should be obtained. Appropriate laboratory investigation, including a semen analysis, should also be done. Assuming no abnormalities are found, attention may be further directed to the female and to the couple.

In some instances, the physician may feel that a semen examination alone is adequate to assess the fertility of the male, and if this assessment is normal, he should focus his attention on the female. When abnormalities are detected in the physical examination or examination of the semen, appropriate laboratory studies must be done. It must be remembered that spermatozoa examined in the ejaculate began their formative process 74 days before when the maturation from spermatogonia to mature sperm began. Consequently, a history of illness two to three months before evaluation may suggest temporarily depressed semen quality. A discussion of investigative procedures in the male suspected to be infertile follows later in this chapter.

Factors Affecting Fertility

AGE

Age plays a minor role in patients presenting with fertility problems. Hypospermatogenesis does occur in aged males, but late in the aging process. Reliable reports of fertility in men from the ages of 70 to 90 are documented.

NUTRITION

Nutritional deficiencies are known to affect testicular function. Malabsorption syndrome may result in deficiency of vitamins, amino acids, or other vital nutrients. Vitamin A deficiency produces germinal hypoplasia. Vitamin B is necessary for normal pituitary function, and vitamin C is necessary as a reducing agent in the semen to prevent sperm agglutination.

Trace metals such as zinc and magnesium may be important but are difficult to evaluate. Studies on men confined to concentration camps in World War II revealed marked testicular atrophy associated with starvation, followed by a return to normal functioning after adequate nutrition was restored.

HEAT

The temperature of the scrotum is about 2.2° C cooler than that of the abdominal cavity. Frequent hot baths may impair spermatogenesis, and, therefore, avoidance of heat may improve semen quality. Excessive, prolonged exposure to sauna baths may result in a similar depression of spermatogenesis. Tight underwear, athletic supports, or similar garments have long been suspected of altering spermatogenesis.

Febrile illnesses may suppress spermatogenesis beginning 25 to 55 days after illness. Sperm counts are maintained at low levels from 12 to 50 days and are then followed by a recovery period of from 25 to 30 days.

A serious, deleterious effect of heat occurs in the undescended testis. If it remains outside of the scrotum beyond the age of five years, irreversible damage occurs in the form of fibrosis. If the testis is not brought into the scrotum before puberty, the testis is incapable of spermatogenesis. Early correction of the undescended testis is, therefore, imperative if fertility is to be possible. Even if the testis is promptly corrected, dysgenetic testes and subfertility may occur. The effect of a varicocele on spermatogenesis is very significant in some subfertile men but is mediated by mechanisms other than heat effects. Similarly, large hydroceles do not affect intrascrotal temperature.

SYSTEMIC DISEASE

Systemic disease may affect spermatogenesis by specific involvement of the testes or suppression that results from generalized toxic effects on body tissue.

Diabetes may impair fertility by accelerating aging changes in testicular basement membrane, by impotence, or by retrograde ejaculation secondary to diabetic neuropathy.

Temporary suppression of spermatogenesis may occur in tuberculosis, collagen disorders, and viral illnesses such as viral hepatitis or infectious mononucleosis.

Direct invasion of testicular tissue by a neoplasm such as lymphoma may result in destruction of normal germinal epithelium.

Mumps orchitis, when bilateral, may lead to infertility. In studies of adult mumps, about 70 per cent of orchitis is unilateral, with about 50 per cent resulting in atrophy. With one normal, uninvolved testis, fertility is usually preserved. If atrophy of an involved testis does not occur, fertility may return to normal within several months. In view of the 30 per cent incidence of bilateral orchitis and its possible production of sterility, young men who have not had mumps should be encouraged to receive mumps vaccine.

Systemic allergic reactions have been shown to temporarily suppress spermatogenesis. Documented allergic reactions to merthiolate and penicillin have been reported.

Liver disease may impair spermatogenesis by failure to detoxify estrogens, thereby resulting in suppression of normal spermatogenesis.

Renal disease impairs both fertility and sexual function, and males with impending renal failure frequently are impotent and infertile. Immunosuppressive agents used in association with renal transplantation may affect spermatogenesis. Males maintained on renal dialysis frequently experience impotence caused by psychologic factors. Neuropathy and suppression of gonadotropins occur in uremic patients and are factors in fertility. However, several posttransplantation patients have fathered normal children.

Testicular atrophy associated with paraplegia and quadriplegia is slow and progressive due, probably, to denervation of the lumbar spinal nerves, which control vascular tone and testicular temperature.

STRESS

Under situations of stress, alterations in sperm production may occur, probably mediated by hypothalamic factors. Such situations may involve fear of parenthood, job stress, marital discord, or psychosexual disturbance. Many pregnancies in previously subfertile couples occur during times of vacation or periods of reduced stress. Stressful situations occurring three to four months, or longer, prior to evaluation may contribute to decreased sperm production.

DRUGS

The following drugs have been shown to affect fertility.

DRUG	SITE OF ACTION
Busulfan (Myleran)	Early sperm maturation
T E M (Triethylenemelanine)	Early and late stages of spermatogenesis
Arsenic	Replaces phosphorus in synthesis of DNA
Colchicine	Arrests cell division at metaphase
Methotrexate	Interferes with folic acid in nucleic acid metabolism
Testosterone	Inhibits gonadotropins
Depo Provera	Direct effect on testes
Nitrofurantoin	Interferes with carbohydrate metabolism in the germinal epithelium, producing arrest at primary spermatocyte stage
Monoamine oxidase inhibitors	Azoospermia (mechanism unknown)
Immunosuppressive azathioprine	Spermatogenic arrest
Antihypertensives	May affect potency and ejaculatory competence

ALCOHOL, TOBACCO AND ILLICIT DRUGS

Excessive use of alcohol may affect fertility through impaired liver function or by altering normal sexual function.

The use of large amounts of tobacco has long been suspected as a toxic factor in spermatogenesis, but this has not been scientifically documented.

Evidence has recently been published to suggest impaired testicular function in users of marijuana and narcotics. Both spermatogenesis and sexual function are impaired by heavy usage of these agents.

IRRADIATION

While Leydig cells and Sertoli cells are relatively radiation resistant, the germinal cells are extremely sensitive to radiation, resulting in the complete breakdown of spermatogenesis.

Hypospermatogenesis related to radiation exposure is reversible in most cases, and the damage is proportionate to the dosage received. In general, initial recovery time after radiation exposure appears to be about two years, although a return to levels capable of fertility may take a total of four to five years.

Frequent, high-dosage exposure to x-rays without genital shielding may impair spermatogenesis. Exposure to high voltage electrical shocks or microwaves may also decrease sperm production.

SEXUAL PROBLEMS

Specific sexual problems are found in about 5 per cent of infertile males. These men have normal semen, which make specific questions regarding potency and sexual frequency important. Has the individual been impotent, and how often and under what circumstances? Infrequent coitus may miss the fertile period, while too frequent intercourse in a male with poor quality semen may result in ineffective sperm density at times of ovulation.

Either excessive premature ejaculation or ejaculatory incompetence may result in the inability to deposit semen in the vaginal vault. Anatomic defects such as epispadias or severe penoscrotal hypospadias may also preclude normal fertilization.

Retrograde ejaculation implies retrograde flow of semen into the bladder. It may be diagnosed readily by "the empty condom" sign and by observing postcoital urine loaded with sperm. The causes for retrograde ejaculation involve disturbances of the urethrovesical junction. They include diabetic neuropathy, surgery of the bladder neck, surgical dissections deep in the pelvis, and retroperitoneal node dissections with injury to sympathetic ganglia. Spinal cord injuries and the use of ganglionic blocking agents may also result in retrograde ejaculation.

ENDOCRINE DISEASE

Endocrine causes of subfertility account for approximately 10 per cent of cases. These include pituitary, adrenal, thyroid, and testicular abnormalities. The normal hypothalamic-pituitary-gonadal axis has been described elsewhere. Alterations in this normal pattern can result in abnormalities in spermatogenesis or sexual competence.

Many specific endocrine syndromes are recognized. Examples include the Sertoli cell only syndrome or syndrome of Del Castillo, in which no germinal elements are present. In Klinefelter's syndrome, hyalinization of the testicular tubules occurs, resulting in impaired spermatogenesis. Germinal aplasia in association with hypospadias occurs in Reifenstein's syndrome.

An overproduction of adrenal androgens in adult adrenogenital syndrome results in impaired testicular function by suppression of gonadotropins. Kallman's syndrome is a specific deficiency of gonadotropins in association with an impairment of the sense of smell.

VARICOCELE

Presence of a varicocele may be a very important factor in male subfertility. Approximately 18 to 20 per cent of all males beyond the age of 18 have been found to have a left varicocele. In 1952 the first case of restored spermatogenesis in an azoospermic man by ligation of a varicocele was reported. Since then, numerous similar reports have occurred in the literature. However, it was not until 1965 that the specific seminal pattern seen in subfertile men with varicoceles was reported. A varying degree of oligospermia was described, but more importantly the suppression of motility and a marked increase in immature and tapering forms in the ejaculate was found. This evidence has become known as the *stress pattern* but may also be seen in the presence of elevated levels of 17-ketosteroids, as in adrenogenital syndrome.

The specific cause of subfertility in men with varicocele has not been elucidated. A countercurrent heat effect that results from stasis and increased heat has been described. Subsequent studies using thermocouples have convincingly disputed this allegation, showing no increased heat effect.

Present knowledge clearly shows that there is a retrograde flow of blood from the left renal vein down the left internal spermatic vein. The man with a varicocele has a collateral circulation from the left to right testis that causes an admixture of blood in that direction. A toxic metabolite is probably carried retrograde from the left renal vein to the testis. A high concentration of potential spermatogenic inhibitors from the left adrenal and left renal veins may thus be carried to both testes where they act to suppress spermatogenesis or sperm maturation. The exact nature of the substances is not known.

Right angle insertion of the left internal spermatic vein into the renal vein or squeezing of the superior mesenteric artery and aorta on the renal vein, which causes increased pressure on the valves at the junction of the internal spermatic and left renal veins, are anatomical factors which may contribute to production of the varicocele effect. The size of the varicocele is of no consequence in subfertility. A small varicocele is just as significant as a large one.

The results of varicocele ligation have been very rewarding and are discussed under the section on therapy.

Ligation of an internal spermatic vein in the absence of a varicocele has not been helpful.

INFECTION

Venereal disease, especially gonorrhea, may produce occlusion of the transport system. Urinary tract infections, prostatitis, and seminal vesiculitis may impair normal spermatogenesis. Escherichia coli has been shown to be particularly deleterious to normal spermatozoa.

DISORDERS OF SEMEN

Volume Disturbance. Approximately 12 per cent of male infertility cases are due to semen volumes which are too small or too large for effective fertility. Very small volumes are mechanically ineffective in covering the cervical os, despite vaginal accommodations which occur in the sexual cycle of the female.

In men with large semen volume (over 5 ml), a dilutional effect may effectively decrease fertility. It may be corrected by the use of the first fraction of the ejaculate, to be described under therapeutic considerations.

Liquefaction Disturbance. Failure of semen to liquefy may result in a highly viscous semen which may be observed as a thick, rubbery glob. The sperm count in a highly viscous semen is often incorrect due to varying concentrations of sperm in the specimen. It is not necessarily an infertile semen unless the spermatozoa remain trapped and sluggish in motility.

Motility Disturbance. Normal semen contains not only an adequate density of sperm, but sperm of which at least 70 per cent exhibit progressive, forward motility. Spermatozoa gain their motility in the epididymis. Factors such as infection, scarring, neurologic dysfunction, or biochemical changes may prevent development of normal motility. Decreased levels of intraepididymal androgens or an absence of 5 α-reductase necessary for the conversion of testosterone to dihydrotestosterone may influence motility. Allergies, drug therapy, or adrenogenital syndrome should be further considered as possible causes.

Sperm Density—Normal Values. Progressively less significance has been attached to the sperm count. The standard accepted for minimal fertility for many years has been 20 million sperm per milliliter and 60 million per ejaculate. However, current studies indicate that many men successfully impregnate their wives with counts in the range between 10 and 20 million per milliliter. *Indeed, a male with any motile spermatozoa should not be considered sterile.*

Morphology. The morphology of the sperm cells should be given as much consideration as count and motility. Unusual numbers of immature or abnormal cells may indicate impaired fertility.

Transport Problems

Obstruction of the transport system at any site from the seminiferous tubule to the urethral meatus may result in infertility. The most common cause of this type of obstruction is congenital or inflammatory scarring of the epididymis from gonorrhea or tuberculosis. A congenital absence of the vas deferens and seminal vesicle may occur. Since the vas and seminal vesicle arise from different embryonic tissue than do the testis and epididymis, a normal testis and epididymis may be present despite an absent or undeveloped vas and seminal vesicle. In congenital absence of the kidney or ureter, the vas is frequently absent as well. It has recently been shown that patients with cystic fibrosis also frequently have congenital absence of the vas deferens.

Immunologic Considerations

Antibodies to sperm cells may be found in the serum of many men with previously unexplained infertility. They are present in a majority of vasectomized men. Specific antibodies are now recognized: one which agglutinates spermatozoa, one which immobilizes spermatozoa, and one which is cytotoxic to spermatozoa. Evidence to date suggests that titers of agglutinating antibodies tend to decrease with time following vasectomy or injury. However, immobilizing antibody, once formed, tends to remain and offers a serious prognosis to restoring fertility.

Specific laboratory methods are available to detect antibodies. Manifestations of the immune response are currently under investigation, and a multitude of antigenic substances has been identified within the seminal plasma and specific portions of the sperm cell.

Current research into immunoreproductive control of fertility in the male offers promise of future contraceptive control in man. Possibilities include utilizing one of the many sperm-specific antibodies or manipulating normal spermatogenesis by utilizing antibodies against hypothalamic and pituitary hormones.

EVALUATION OF THE INFERTILE MALE

The couple beginning an infertility workup should be informed of the likelihood that extensive, time-consuming, and often expensive tests might be required. They should also understand that since therapy is based on the long maturation process of spermatogonia, any one form may require three months or more to be effective.

History

A careful medical history will frequently yield important clues to the cause of infertility in the male patient. A general health history,

past medical history, social history, and detailed sexual history are vital
to proper evaluation.

Factors of particular significance are

1. A history of known or suspected fertility or infertility in self or
spouse in the present or previous sexual relationships.

2. A history of abnormal sexual development, delayed puberty, or
use of hormonal agents during childhood or adolescence.

3. A history of mumps orchitis, especially if bilateral, or other
acquired diseases of the genitalia such as venereal disease or tuberculosis.

4. A history of prolonged fever or prolonged use of pharmaceu-
ticals.

5. A history of trauma to the genitalia.

6. A history of accidental or occupational exposures to chemicals,
x-ray or other radiation, or extreme thermal changes. Evaluation of the
work environment may reveal factors such as excessive heat in foundry
work.

7. A history of impaired nutritional status, such as severe malnu-
trition, vitamin deficiency, or alcohol excess.

8. A history of surgery in infancy or childhood for cryptorchidism, inguinal hernia, or other surgical corrections that might impair
the blood supply to the testes. Specific information regarding age of
surgery, procedures done, and surgical sequelae may help evaluate
causative factors.

9. A history of behavioral patterns such as habitual exposure to
thermal factors in prolonged hot baths or saunas. A history of use of
lubricants, douches, or feminine hygiene products that may be spermi-
cidal.

10. A detailed sexual history may disclose decreased libido or impaired erectile or ejaculatory competence. A history of severe premature ejaculation or unusual sexual practices may suggest infertility.

Physical Examination

A general physical examination should be done with special emphasis on endocrine and genital abnormalities. The body habitus may
lead to a suspicion of hypogonadism, Klinefelter's syndrome, or other
endocrinopathies associated with subfertility. Gynecomastia may be
seen with Klinefelter's syndrome, and pale pink nipples may indicate
pituitary insufficiency. The ratio of arm span to height may be a clue to
hypogonadism.

The amount and distribution pattern of hair may indicate adequacy
or deficiency of androgen production. Hair patterns may vary with eth-
nic groups such as the American Indian or Oriental. However, reces-
sion of temporal hairline, midline extension of pubic hair, and presence
of axillary, chest, and facial hair are frequently indicators of hormonal
activity. Severe hypothyroidism, manifested clinically by dry skin and

hair, may contribute to subfertility, but minor depression of thyroid function rarely causes infertility.

The genitalia should be carefully examined for congenital defects, such as absence of the vas deferens, hypospadia, epispadia, and cryptorchidism.

Size and consistency of the testes may be important if there is a history of previous trauma, mumps orchitis, or other testicular disease. While some patients with Klinefelter's syndrome may have testes which are small, firm, and rubbery and other patients with hypogonadism may have small and soft testes, it is unwise to correlate fertility potential with gonadal size.

The presence of a varicocele is usually not significant, but in the subfertile male it may be of extreme importance. The patient should be examined in a standing position, with Valsalva's maneuver performed to detect the presence of reflux into the varicocele, especially in the left hemiscrotum.

An enlarged, indurated, and tender epididymis may indicate acute infection or chronic inflammatory changes associated with obstruction of the vas. Palpation of the vas deferens may reveal an absence of the vasa, a small immature vas, or thickened, indurated vasa resulting from vasitis or chronic inflammatory disease.

Examination of the prostate may reveal evidence of low grade prostatitis known to be deleterious to the metabolism of spermatozoa.

Evaluation of Semen

A complete semen analysis is essential for the male.

COLLECTION OF SPECIMEN

The period of continence prior to obtaining the semen specimen should be related to frequency of intercourse. If such is twice weekly, the period of continence should be approximately three days. Abstinence beyond three days may reveal abnormal volume and motility. At least two, and preferably three, specimens should be studied.

The entire specimen should be collected by masturbation in a dry, clean, wide-mouthed jar. If this is not possible, coitus interruptus may be used, and the specimen brought promptly to the office. Routine condom collection should be avoided. Where religious restrictions prevent direct collection, a perforated, polyethylene, seminal pouch is available, known as a Milex sheath.

MOTILITY

A small drop of thoroughly mixed semen is placed on a glass slide under a cover slip. Estimation of motility with 500 times magnification (high, dry field) may be made. If desired, this preparation may be sealed with petroleum jelly and motility observed for six to eight hours or longer. The normal ejaculate should have at least 60 per cent of the cells actively motile two to three hours after ejaculation. The type of motility should be observed. Healthy spermatozoa have a distinct forward progression. The estimate of sperm motility may range from "zero" for absent motility to "four plus" for active, healthy spermatozoa with forward progression.

Motility may be more quantitatively assessed as a part of the sperm count.

CELL COUNT

Technique. Freshly ejaculated semen is observed as a tapiocalike coagulum which liquefies in 15 to 20 minutes, leaving a fluid of variable viscosity.

After the semen has liquefied and has been mixed thoroughly, use a white blood cell diluting pipette and proceed as follows:

1. Draw the semen up to the 0.5 mark, giving a final dilution of 1:20. If the count is low, draw up to the 1.0 mark, giving a dilution of 1:10. Carefully wipe off the end of the pipette with tissue, and recheck the accuracy of the amount drawn.

2. Dilute with normal saline if differential motile and nonmotile count is desired. If counting is desired with all cells immobilized, dilution is accomplished with sodium bicarbonate solution containing 1 per cent phenol or 1 per cent formalin.

In the latter method, it is necessary to depend upon an estimate of motility from the direct drop observation.

3. After careful mixing in the pipette, gently flood the Neubauer hemacytometer chamber.

4. Under high, dry magnification, the center ("red blood cell") field (Fig. 20–1) and the technique for red blood cell counts are used, counting the four corners and center block of the red cell chamber. Since there are five blocks and 16 squares per block, a total of the 80 smallest squares is counted.

If a 1:10 dilution is used, the total count for the five blocks is equal to the count in millions per milliliter.

A differential count of motile and nonmotile cells can be made simultaneously, as the example below indicates:

Square	Motile	Nonmotile
A	4	2
B	5	1
C	4	2
D	3	1
E	5	2
	21	8
	$\times 10^6$	$\times 10^6$
	21,000,000 per ml	8,000,000 per ml

(9 square millimeters)

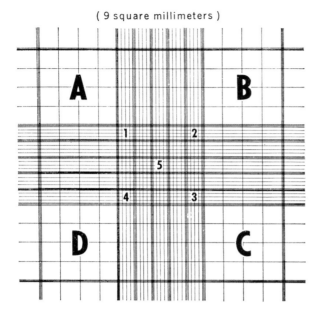

Figure 20–1 Hemacytometer showing areas 1 to 5 used in doing sperm counts. When the counting chamber has been filled with the semen diluted in the white cell pipette, areas 1, 2, 3, 4, and 5 are counted for motile and nonmotile sperm.

By multiplying the per milliliter count by ejaculate volume, the total motile and nonmotile count may be obtained.

MORPHOLOGY

While the Papanicolaou staining technique is admirable for the research laboratory, it is too cumbersome for the average office laboratory. A simple staining technique involves making a smear and allowing it to air dry. The slide is fixed for one minute in 10 per cent formalin and then rinsed with water. The slide is stained for one to two minutes with hematoxylin, Mayer's, hematoxylin-eosin, or Wright's stain. The stained slide is now examined under oil immersion.

The spermatozoa are classified as shown in Figures 20–2 and 20–3:
1. Oval
2. Large (macrocytic)
3. Amorphous
4. Small (microcytic)
5. Tapering forms
6. Duplex (bicephalic)
7. Double tail

Immature forms of the spermatozoa may be seen and must be differentiated from white blood cells. This can usually be done by identification of nuclear material, but in difficult cases special stains may be used to demonstrate the acrosome of the sperm cell.

Eighty per cent of spermatozoa evaluated should be of normal, oval form.

Structure of a Sperm

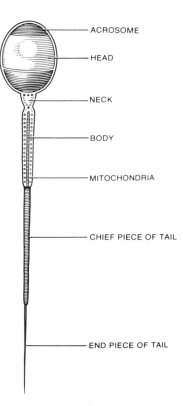

- ACROSOME
- HEAD
- NECK
- BODY
- MITOCHONDRIA
- CHIEF PIECE OF TAIL
- END PIECE OF TAIL

Figure 20–2   Structure of normal sperm.

Abnormal Sperm

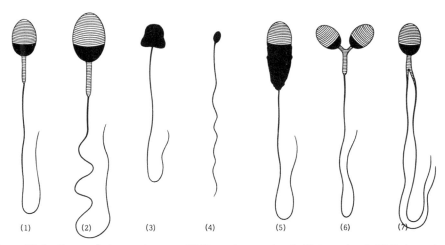

(1)   (2)   (3)   (4)   (5)   (6)   (7)

Figure 20–3   Forms of abnormal sperm: (*1*) Normal sperm (oval), (*2*) Large head, (*3*) Deformed head (amorphous), (*4*) Pinhead (microhead), (*5*) "Cigar-shaped" head (tapering form), (*6*) Double head (duplex), and (*7*) Double tail.

OTHER LABORATORY PROCEDURES

In patients with azoospermia, a test for fructose is essential. Seminal fructose is a product of the seminal vesicles, which are, embryologically, an out-pouching of the vasa deferentia. Consequently, if there is a congenital absence of the vasa, there is no fructose in the semen, and the ejaculate does not coagulate. This finding is also seen with occlusion of the ejaculatory ducts, in which case the ejaculate consists largely of prostatic secretions and fructose, and coagulation is likewise absent.

A simple test for fructose may be performed as follows: The testing reagent is made by mixing 50 mg of powdered resorcinol with 33 ml of concentrated hydrochloric acid and diluting to 100 ml with distilled water. Five milliliters of this reagent are added to 0.5 ml of semen and brought to a boil.

In the presence of fructose, an orange-red color will appear within 60 seconds after boiling. In the absence of fructose, the mixture remains colorless.

GONADOTROPINS

Since spermatogenesis and androgen production by the testes are controlled by hormonal stimulation from pituitary and hypothalamic hormones, assays of gonadotropic hormones are helpful in determining normal functioning of the pituitary-gonadal axis. Measurements of follicle-stimulating hormone (FSH) and luteinizing hormone (LH) within the normal range of 4 to 19 m I.U. for FSH and of 5 to 20 m I.U. for LH indicate a normal pituitary-gonadal axis.

Measurement of serum testosterone in a normal range of 5.96 ± 2.02 nanograms per milliliter indicates a normal, end-organ response to LH. Significance should not be attached to one abnormal determination, since diurnal variations do occur, as well as surges of hormonal release.

Measurements of 17-ketosteroids may be important in the detection of mild forms of adrenogenital syndrome. In this instance, the large amount of adrenal androgen produced by excessive stimulation of the adrenal cortex results in feedback suppression of pituitary gonadotropins and subsequent suppression of spermatogenesis.

Spermatogenesis may be suppressed by systemic disease, and consequently, appropriate laboratory tests should be done to exclude such possibilities. In some cases, blood count, urinalysis, glucose, and renal function tests may be specifically indicated.

Testicular Biopsy

INDICATIONS

1. Unexplained oligospermia.
2. Azoospermia when it is necessary to distinguish between ob-

structive azoospermia and the absence of spermatozoa due to impaired production.

3. May define those patients who do not respond to treatment so that time, expense, and hope are not wasted.

COMMON HISTOLOGIC CLASSIFICATIONS OF TESTICULAR BIOPSY

Normal.   This pattern is found in many oligospermic males and in some azoospermic males when ductal obstruction occurs.

Spermatogenic Arrest.   In many cases of oligospermia, there is an arrest of normal maturation of spermatozoa.

In general, spermatogonia are found to be normal, but the maturation process breaks down at the primary spermatocyte level. Consequently, an increased number of primary spermatocytes are present, but marked decrease is seen in further maturation. The exact nature of this arrest is unknown. Factors suspected to be active are enzymatic, biochemical, and chromosomal defects.

Peritubular Fibrosis.   In this process, seminiferous tubules are surrounded by fibrous tissue with subsequent atrophy of spermatogenic elements. The process is usually permanent and progressive and may be associated with testicular trauma, severe infection such as mumps orchitis, and impaired blood supply to the testes.

An unusual peritubular fibrosis associated with administration of testosterone propionate disappears after cessation of treatment.

Germinal Aplasia or Hypoplasia.   The testes of these men may be normal in size and consistency but they are azoospermic and show an absence of germinal cells with only Sertoli cells present in the tubule. The Leydig cells may be slightly increased.

In germinal cell hypoplasia, there is some spermatogenesis, but the number of germinal cells is markedly reduced, and the germinal epithelium presents a loosely bound network of cells.

Sloughing of Immature Cells.   Sloughing of immature cells for unknown reasons may occur and result in immature cells being prematurely extruded into the tubular lumen. There is usually prominent disorganization in the maturation process.

Radiologic Procedures

In azoospermic men with histologically normal testes, an x-ray procedure known as vasography may be done by instilling contrast material into the vasa and observing their patency.

GENERAL APPROACH TO MANAGEMENT OF THE SUBFERTILE MALE

PROPHYLACTIC MEASURES

1. Adequate nutrition in childhood and youth.
2. Early correction of congenital defects such as cryptorchidism.

3. Mumps immunization for children who have not had the disease by puberty.

4. Adequate scrotal protection for boys and men participating in contact sports.

5. Avoidance of habits which interfere with normal spermatogenesis, e.g., prolonged, hot baths.

6. Adequate examination of children and youths to detect genital abnormalities, e.g., cryptorchidism and the congenital absence of vasa.

7. Early and specific care for injuries to the gonads.

SPECIFIC MEASURES BASED ON HISTORY OF SUBFERTILE MALE

1. Careful review and counseling regarding sexual function, i.e., sexual techniques, coital frequency, avoidance of lubricants and douche solutions.

2. Proper nutrition, well-rounded diet, and vitamin supplements, if indicated.

3. Cessation of hot baths, sauna baths, or steam cabinets.

4. Change to boxer shorts. Significance of tight underwear has received wide lay publicity. To date, this factor has not been adequately evaluated.

SPECIFIC MEASURES RELATED TO FINDINGS ON PHYSICAL EXAMINATION

1. Reduce weight to optimal level.

2. Correct infectious states such as epididymitis, urethritis, or prostatitis. The role of infections caused by Escherichia coli or Mycoplasma is mentioned below under Specific Measures Based on Laboratory Findings.

3. Detection and correction of varicocele.

SPECIFIC MEASURES RELATED TO SEMEN ABNORMALITIES

1. Volume disturbance. Low volume (less than 1 ml) may respond to chorionic gonadotropin, 2000 to 4000 units twice each week for 10 weeks. High volume (over 6 ml) may respond to split ejaculate techniques or homologous artificial insemination. When asked to produce a split ejaculate, the majority of males with a large volume of semen will show a much higher sperm density in the first portion (2 to 3 ml) of ejaculate. This method may be helpful in accomplishing pregnancy. The couple are instructed to have intercourse, deposit the first portion of ejaculate and then withdraw the penis. This first fraction may also be used for homologous artificial insemination.

2. Viscosity. Highly viscid semen which fails to liquefy may trap

sperm. Attempts to liquefy semen by the use of liquefying agents, such as mucolytics, have resulted in minimal success. A few patients have reported some benefit from clomiphene. The mechanism of this latter approach is not understood.

3. Autoagglutination due to decreased activity of the reducing substance, which prevents sperm agglutination, may respond to vitamin C therapy. Care should be taken to use a well-cleaned slide and to observe the semen long enough to observe agglutination.

4. Sperm count. Oligospermia and azoospermia require a complete workup. Specific measures are discussed under endocrine replacement therapy and nonspecific therapy for oligospermia.

5. Motility. Decreased motility is frequently seen in patients with varicocele and adrenogenital syndrome. Marked improvement may be noted by high ligation of the left internal spermatic vein or by steroid suppression of elevated 17-ketosteroids. Chorionic gonadotropin in a dosage of 4000 units twice weekly for 10 weeks may improve motility. Therapy with arginine has been effective in some men with motility problems, and recent experimental work with caffeine has not yet been fully evaluated.

6. Abnormal forms. These frequently are immature sperm cells and are reduced following varicocele ligation or steroid suppression.

SPECIFIC MEASURES BASED ON LABORATORY FINDINGS

1. Decreased FSH. Human menopausal gonadotropin is difficult to obtain and expensive, but it has been shown to effectively maintain spermatogenesis following hypophysectomy. Clomid may be effective in some cases. The specific nature of this effect is not known. Adequate vitamin B in the diet is essential to gonadotropin production. Hypothalamic releasing factors are only currently being elucidated but offer promise of benefit to selected patients.

2. LH can be effectively replaced by chorionic gonadotropin, which is much more readily available and less expensive than the menopausal form.

3. Testosterone decrease in the presence of a low LH level usually responds to stimulation by chorionic gonadotropin. In the presence of normal or elevated LH, it may be necessary to give replacement testosterone. It is extremely important to use a low dosage of testosterone, since this drug in dosages above a critical level is suppressive to gonadotropin and, consequently, also to spermatogenesis.

4. Decreased 17-ketosteroids may imply an androgen deficiency if concomitant 17-hydroxysteroids are normal. Elevated 17-ketosteroids may represent an adult adrenogenital syndrome. Pregnanetriol determination may be helpful to confirm this. Decreasing the ketosteroids by suppression with steroids may increase spermatogenesis by increasing gonadotropin.

5. Presence of infection in the genital system should be documented and specific treatment implemented. Controversial data have emerged regarding the significance of infectious agents such as Mycoplasma. Acting on this data, some investigators have reported success in prolonged treatment with broad spectrum antibiotics in men who have otherwise unexplained leukocytes in the semen. Because of the frequent occurrence of this organism in the reproductive tract of humans, the above-mentioned success is difficult to evaluate.

In vitro studies of the effect of Escherichia coli on spermatozoa have revealed a significant, deleterious effect, and justify vigorous attempts to eradicate the infection.

6. In the azoospermic male, a simple test for fructose may be done, which, if absent, supports the diagnosis of congenital absence of the vasa deferentia. Since there is no surgical procedure for correcting this entity, further diagnostic studies are not warranted.

Nonspecific Measures in the Oligospermic Male

Nonspecific measures in the oligospermic male with a normal history and physical examination, normal hormone assays, and no evidence of other organic disease are as follows:

1. Counseling, emotional support, and supportive therapy.

2. Adequate nutrition and proper health habits. Avoidance of hot baths, tight underwear, fatigue, tension, lubricants, douches, and illicit drugs.

3. Multivitamins.

4. Empiric use of therapeutic agents.

It has been shown that the extended use of small doses of cortisone acetate, 2.5 mg, three times a day, results in a pregnancy rate of 19 per cent, and 56 per cent of those using it showed significant improvement.

Empiric trials on chorionic gonadotropin, low-dosage testosterone, clomid, and, more recently, arginine, have all been effective in some instances.

Perhaps the most important factor is the patient's awareness that the physician is interested in improving his fertility. The couple must be aware of the likelihood that the diagnostic and treatment process may be prolonged. They must be aware of the fact that treatment is not always successful. In one study, cumulative conception rates for infertile couples after medical evaluation only were 35 per cent after one year, 55 per cent after three years, and 63 per cent after five years. By comparison, 73 to 90 per cent of normal couples were able to conceive during their first year of unprotected intercourse. Major research in the field of male infertility is continuing, and further knowledge in diagnosis and treatment can be anticipated.

SELECTED REFERENCES

Amelar, R.: Infertility in Men: Diagnosis and Treatment. Philadelphia, F.A. Davis Co., 1966.

Amelar, R., and Dubin, L.: Male infertility. Urology, *1*:1, 1973.
Cochran, J.: Immunobiology of reproductive processes in men. Urology, *4*:367, 1974.
   *A review of historical and current knowledge about the immunology of male
   reproduction.*

REFERENCES

Amelar, R., and Dubin, L.: Etiologic factors in 1,294 consecutive cases of male infertility.
   Fertil. Steril., *22*:469, 1971.
Amelar, R., Dubin, L., and Schoenfeld, C.: Semen analysis: An office technique. Urology,
   2:605, 1973.
Amelar, R., and Hotchkiss, R. S.: The split ejaculate: Its use in management of male in-
   fertility. Fertil. Steril., *16*:46, 1965.
Ansbacher, R., Manarang-Pangan, S., and Srivannaboon, S.: Sperm antibodies in infertile
   couples. Fertil. Steril., *22*:298, 1971.
Jefferies, W. M., Weir, W. C., Wein, D. R., and Prouty, R. C.: The use of cortisone and
   related steroids in infertility. Fertil. Steril., *9*:145, 1958.
MacLeod, J.: Human male infertility. Obstet. Gynecol. Surv., *26*:335, 1971.
MacLeod, J.: Seminal cytology in the presence of varicocele. Fertil. Steril., *16*:735, 1965.
MacLeod, J.: The parameters of male fertility. Hosp. Pract., *8*:43, 1973.
Mann, T.: The Biochemistry of Semen and of the Male Reproductive Tract. New York,
   John Wiley and Sons, Inc., 1974.
Patil, Z.: Clomiphene therapy in defective spermatogenesis. Fertil. Steril., *21*:838, 1970.
Schackler, A., Goldman, J. A., and Zucherman, Z.: Treatment of oligospermia with the
   amino acid arginine. J. Urol., *110*:311, 1973.

INDEX

Note: Page numbers in *italic* indicate illustrations.
Page numbers accompanied by (t) indicate tables.